SURGICAL TECHNIQUES IN OTOLARYNGOLOGY HEAD AND NECK SURGERY

Series Editor: **Robert T Sataloff** MD DMA FACS

SINONASAL SURGERY

SURGICAL TECHNIQUES IN
OTOLARYNGOLOGY
HEAD AND NECK SURGERY

Series Editor: **Robert T Sataloff** MD DMA FACS

SINONASAL SURGERY

Authors

Spencer C Payne MD
Associate Professor of Otolaryngology—Head and Neck Surgery and
Allergy and Clinical Immunology
Department of Otolaryngology—Head and Neck Surgery
University of Virginia Health System
Charlottesville, Virginia, USA

Ameet Singh MD
Associate Professor of Otolaryngology and Neurosurgery
Director, Rhinology and Skull Base Surgery
Co-Director, Endoscopic Pituitary and Skull Base Surgery
The George Washington University Medical Center
Washington, District of Columbia, USA

Bradford A Woodworth MD
James J Hicks Associate Professor of Surgery
Division of Otolaryngology
Director of Otolaryngology Research and Associate Scientist
Gregory Fleming James Cystic Fibrosis Research Center
University of Alabama School of Medicine
Birmingham, Alabama, USA

JAYPEE The Health Sciences Publisher
New Delhi | London | Philadelphia | Panama

Jaypee Brothers Medical Publishers (P) Ltd

Headquarters
Jaypee Brothers Medical Publishers (P) Ltd.
4838/24, Ansari Road, Daryaganj
New Delhi 110 002, India
Phone: +91-11-43574357
Fax: +91-11-43574314
E-mail: jaypee@jaypeebrothers.com

Overseas Offices
J.P. Medical Ltd.
83, Victoria Street, London
SW1H 0HW (UK)
Phone: +44-20 3170 8910
Fax: +44(0)20 3008 6180
E-mail: info@jpmedpub.com

Jaypee-Highlights Medical Publishers Inc.
City of Knowledge, Bld. 237, Clayton
Panama City, Panama
Phone: +1 507-301-0496
Fax: +1 507-301-0499
E-mail: cservice@jphmedical.com

Jaypee Medical Inc.
The Bourse
111, South Independence Mall East
Suite 835, Philadelphia, PA 19106, USA
Phone: +1 267-519-9789
E-mail: jpmed.us@gmail.com

Jaypee Brothers Medical Publishers (P) Ltd.
17/1-B, Babar Road, Block-B, Shaymali
Mohammadpur, Dhaka-1207
Bangladesh
Mobile: +08801912003485
E-mail: jaypeedhaka@gmail.com

Jaypee Brothers Medical Publishers (P) Ltd.
Bhotahity, Kathmandu, Nepal
Phone: +977-9741283608
E-mail: kathmandu@jaypeebrothers.com

Website: www.jaypeebrothers.com
Website: www.jaypeedigital.com

Inquiries for bulk sales may be solicited at: jaypee@jaypeebrothers.com

Surgical Techniques in Otolaryngology—Head and Neck Surgery: Sinonasal Surgery

First Edition: **2015**

ISBN: 978-93-5152-462-5

Printed at: Ajanta Offset & Packagings Ltd., New Delhi

Dedication

To my wife Elizabeth, the B whose guidance, love and support truly helps me be an A.
To Becca and Amanda, my lovely daughters who put a smile on my face and graciously share their Daddy with the hospital and his office.
And to my mentors Drs Benninger, Catalano, and Yaremchuk who have shared their talents and skills in order to hone my own.

— Spencer C Payne

To my lovely wife Sonalee, for her endless love, wisdom and encouragement.
To my adorable boys, Rohan and Aman, who are my infinite source of pride and joy.
To my beloved parents, Mohini and Karam and my brother, Uminder for their love, sacrifice, and teaching me how to think critically.
To my Shah family for their love and understanding, especially my exhaustion during every family vacation!
To my mentors, Drs Vijay Anand and Arthur Hengerer, to whom I will be forever grateful for shaping my career in Otolaryngology.

— Ameet Singh

To my wife Lesley, who is my constant source of inspiration. Without her love and support, my career would not have been possible.
To my sons Austen, Brandon, and Holden, who provide purpose in my life and round with me on weekends.
To my parents Ronald and Sigrid, who gave their support and constant encouragement.
To my mentors Drs Cohen, Chiu, Kennedy, Palmer, and Schlosser, who were gracious to offer their tremendous talents for my surgical and research training.

— Bradford A Woodworth

Contributors

Seth A Akst MD MBA
Assistant Professor
Department of Anesthesiology and Critical Care Medicine
The George Washington University
Washington, District of Columbia, USA

Dane M Barrett MD
Resident
Department of Otolaryngology
University of Virginia
Charlottesville, Virginia, USA

Mohamad R Chaaban MD
Division of Otolaryngology Head and Neck Surgery
University of Alabama at Birmingham
Birmingham, Alabama, USA

Anita Cucchiaro MD
Resident
Department of Anesthesiology and Critical Care Medicine
The George Washington University
Washington, District of Columbia, USA

Brian A Fishero MD
Resident, Department of Otolaryngology—Head and Neck Surgery
University of Virginia
Charlottesville, Virginia, USA

Devon C Flaherty MD
Resident Physician
Department of Anesthesiology
The Mount Sinai Hospital
New York, New York, USA

Anand V Germanwala MD
Assistant Professor
Department of Neurological Surgery
Loyola University School of Medicine
Maywood, Illinois, USA

Joseph Gorodenker MD
Neuroradiology Fellow
Department of Radiology
The George Washington University
Washington, District of Columbia, USA

Tarik Ibrahim MD
Resident
Department of Neurological Surgery
Loyola University School of Medicine
Maywood, Illinois, USA

Elisa A Illing MD
Resident, Division of Otolaryngology—Head and Neck Surgery
University of Alabama—Birmingham
Birmingham, Illinois, USA

John A Jane, Jr MD
Associate Professor of Neurosurgery and Pediatrics
Department of Neurosurgery
University of Virginia
Charlottesville, Virginia, USA

Arjun Joshi MD
Associate Professor of Surgery
The George Washington University
Washington, District of Columbia, USA

Alexandra Kejner MD
University of Alabama
Birmingham, Alabama, USA

Ning-Wei Li MD
Division of Otolaryngology—Head and Neck Surgery
The George Washington University
Washington, District of Columbia, USA

Zachary N Litvack MD MCR
Assistant Professor
Department of Neurosurgery
The George Washington University
Washington, District of Columbia, USA

Robert G Louis MD
Program Director—Minimally Invasive Brain Tumor Skull Base and Pituitary Surgery
Hoag Hospital
Newport Beach, California, USA

Nitin Patel MD MPH
Resident
The George Washington University
Washington, District of Columbia, USA

Spencer C Payne MD
Associate Professor of Otolaryngology—Head & Neck Surgery and Allergy & Clinical Immunology
Department of Otolaryngology—Head & Neck Surgery
University of Virginia Health System
Charlottesville, Virginia, USA

James D Phillips MD
Department of Surgery
Division of Otolaryngology
University of Alabama, Birmingham
Birmingham, Alabama, USA

Madeleine R Schaberg MD MPH
Assistant Professor Icahn School of Medicine at Mount Sinai
Department of Otolaryngology—Head and Neck Surgery
The New York Eye and Ear Infirmary of Mount Sinai
New York, New York, USA

Ameet Singh MD
Associate Professor of Otolaryngology and Neurosurgery
Director, Rhinology and Skull Base Surgery
Co-Director, Endoscopic Pituitary and Skull-Base Surgery
The George Washington University
Washington, District of Columbia, USA

Sinonasal Surgery

Alan Siu MD
Resident
Department of Neurosurgery
The George Washington University
Washington, District of Columbia, USA

Abtin Tabaee MD FACS FARS
Director of Rhinology and
Endoscopic Sinus Surgery
Department of Otolaryngology—
Beth Israel Medical Center
Associate Professor of Otolaryngology—
Head and Neck Surgery
Icahn School of Medicine at
Mount Sinai
New York, New York, USA

M Reza Taheri MD PhD
Assistant Professor
Department of Radiology
The George Washington University
Washington, District of Columbia, USA

Nilesh A Vyas MD FAANS
Director
Cerebrovascular and Skull Based
Neurosurgery
Department of Neurosurgery
Inova Fairfax Hospital
Falls Church, Virginia, USA

Erika McCarty Walsh MD
Resident Physician
Division of Otolaryngology—
Head and Neck Surgery
University of Alabama, Birmingham
Birmingham, Alabama, USA

Joseph C Watson MD
Associate Professor
Department of Neurosurgery
Virginia Commonwealth University
Inova Campus
Vienna, Virginia, USA

Aaron P Wessell MD
Neurosurgery Resident
Department of Neurosurgery
University of Maryland
Baltimore, Maryland, USA

Bradford A Woodworth MD
James J Hicks Associate Professor of
Surgery, Division of Otolaryngology
Director of Otolaryngology Research
and Associate Scientist
Gregory Fleming James Cystic Fibrosis
Research Center
University of Alabama School of Medicine
Birmingham, Alabama, USA

Philip E Zapanta MD FACS
Associate Professor of Surgery
Otolaryngology Residency Program
Director
Division of Otolaryngology—
Head and Neck Surgery
The George Washington University
Washington, District of Columbia, USA

Foreword

Surgical Techniques in Otolaryngology—Head and Neck Surgery is a six-volume compendium. In addition to being an integral component of the compendium, each volume was written to stand alone, as well. The volumes in this work include Atlases of Otologic and Neurotologic Surgery, Rhinologic and Sinus Surgery, Laryngeal Surgery, Facial Plastic and Reconstructive Surgery, Pediatric Otolaryngologic Surgery, and Head and Neck Surgery. The authors of each volume have included not only background information and step-by-step details of surgical technique, but also "pearls" gleaned through vast experience. Each volume contains extensive illustrations and intraoperative photographs that illustrate and simplify the techniques described.

Surgical Techniques in Otolaryngology—Head and Neck Surgery is intended to provide clinicians with thorough, accessible and clinically useful details of surgery for nearly all disorders cared for by otolaryngologists. The work also serves as a companion to Sataloff's six-volume *Comprehensive Textbook of Otolaryngology—Head and Neck Surgery*, which was written simultaneously with the compendium on surgical techniques. Hopefully, Surgical Techniques will prove useful for otolaryngologists by making it easier to provide (and teach) state-of-the-art otolaryngologic surgery.

Robert T Sataloff MD DMA FACS
Series Editor
Professor and Chairman
Department of Otolaryngology—Head and Neck Surgery
Senior Associate Dean for Clinical Academic Specialties
Drexel University College of Medicine
Philadelphia, Pennsylvania, USA

Preface

The introduction and broad adoption of endoscopic technology has revolutionized the field of rhinology. Over the last 40 years, our appreciation of sinonasal anatomy afforded by magnified endoscopic views has allowed us to continually modify and adapt our techniques to old and new challenges. Despite continued advancements in surgical methods and research, our understanding of the pathophysiology behind chronic rhinosinusitis (and many other rhinologic diseases) remains in its infancy and the road ahead is unpredictable. However, we are assured that the evolving technologies and tinkering spirits that attracted most of us to this subspecialty will fuel continued refinement of the surgical procedures described in this Atlas.

Although this Atlas is not intended to be completely comprehensive, the content contains a broad array of procedures that reflect the accumulated expertise over the course of our training and careers. An exhaustive tome that comprises the infinite modifications described by those who have preceded us would be impossible. Instead, we have provided the pearls and subtleties that we have found most useful. It is our hope that this foundation will serve the readers as a guide for their own rhinology training, and also stimulate them to pursue further modifications of surgical technique as they accumulate expertise in this rapidly advancing field.

Spencer C Payne MD
Ameet Singh MD
Bradford A Woodworth MD

Contents

Section 1: Basic Principles

Section 5: Endoscopic Skull Base Surgery

Section 1

Basic Principles

Chapters

CHAPTER

1 The History and Evolution of Sinus Surgery

Spencer C Payne

FROM THE BEGINNING

Although this textbook will describe the latest techniques and innovations in endoscopic sinus surgery, the history of sinus surgery is one that dates back to ancient civilization. The Egyptians are known to have practiced transnasal surgery to remove cranial contents on the recently deceased in order to help prepare for the process of mummification. The initial description of the use of endoscopes for sinus visualization comes much later, however. It was 1903 when Hirschmann first described the use of a primitive endoscope, originally designed for cystoscopy, to examine the maxillary sinus through an oroantral fistula.[1] Many years passed without much advance and so it was not until 1959, with the patenting of a rigid optic rod lens system, which came to be known as the "Hopkins Rod", that surgical endoscopy truly became a real possibility. The rigid system represented a departure from previous flexible fiberoptic technologies and allowed for significant improvement in light and image transmission. Seeing the promise in this technology, the Karl Storz company purchased the patent and began a long process, which continues to this day, of refining the rigid endoscope. Introduction of angled lenses and the view they afforded allowed the technology to be applied to the field of rhinology and sinus surgery and is what in essence enabled a major paradigm shift in this realm.

Through a series of magnificent experiments, Prof. Walter Messerklinger of Graz, Austria was able to examine the nasal cavity and sinuses of fresh cadavers. Using a variety of powders applied to the nasal lining, the natural patterns of mucous transport were able to be determined. Although many of his early experiments were performed with microscopes, Prof. Messerklinger began using endoscopes to study the mucous flow endonasally on patients during surgery. It was through this technique that he was able to postulate that disease of the frontal and maxillary sinuses was secondary to disease of the anterior ethmoid and, as a result of this, believed that surgery directed to this latter structure without alteration of the other, larger sinuses was preferable to prevailing techniques.[2] Prior to this, surgery on the paranasal sinuses, while via microscope or bare eye, via internal or external approaches, was based on radical alteration of the sinuses, creation of large openings, and frequent injudicious removal of sinonasal mucosa. The addition of the endoscope to these surgeries not only enabled superior visualization of the anatomy under manipulation, but facilitated a greater understanding of the goals of the operation as a whole. It was not long before others, such as Wigand,[3] further espoused the importance of the endoscopic approach and tissue preservation.

The Messerklinger technique quickly caught on and through the work of David Kennedy,[4] who brought the concept to the United States in 1985, Functional Endoscopic Sinus Surgery or FESS was born. It became clear, however, that as this new approach represented a significant departure from a prior lack of concern for the sinus mucosa and the supposition of its condemnation, that newer instrumentation would be necessary. It is this overriding precept, the minimalization of sinonasal trauma, that has likely fomented the technological evolution that continues today in sinus surgery. Initially, it came in the form of smaller and thru-cutting instruments. Originally developed for orthopedic cartilage removal, these devices greatly facilitated the targeted removal of bone and overlying mucosa compared with the prior tearing and stripping seen with earlier grasping forceps. These cutting instruments also greatly facilitated the safer and more effective dissection of the sphenoid ostium and frontal recess.

POWERED INSTRUMENTS

Powered instrumentation, yet another technology borrowed from orthopedic joint surgery, furthered this cause.

Separately described by Setliff[5] and Parsons[6] in 1996, the tissue microdebriders introduced real time suction to the dissection process. Additionally, with their use of disposable blades, which provided a consistently sharp interface, the microdebrider optimized tissue removal. Early reports, however, quickly revealed that the power of this instrumentation could also have dire consequences with orbital and intracranial injuries.[7] As the technology in this arena advanced, curved blades and eventually drills were also introduced. Although slower than conventional drill systems, the suction irrigation drills now available with most microdebrider systems enable removal of boney tumors or osteitic septations not amenable to standard forceps. Further, these drills have greatly facilitated the removal of the bone underlying soft tissue tumors such as inverted papilloma as well as normal bone in the purposeful transgression of the skull base through endonasal routes.

NAVIGATION

With these increasingly powerful instruments, the paranasal sinuses became an ideal "theater" for the use of stereotactic navigation. Originally developed for neurosurgical procedures in the late 1980s, it was not until 1994 when its use in endoscopic sinus surgery was first published by Anon et al.[8] Using a combination of reference frames and specialized instrumentation, the technology allowed for real time confirmation of sinus anatomy to aid in surgical planning and progression. Significant anecdotal evidence indicates the benefit of image guidance systems with regard to establishing orientation and landmarks in either the previously operated individual or patient with extensive disease. Although it is generally thought of as a means to reduce complications and operative time, studies showing its definitive benefit in this regard are lacking and likely not feasible given the already low rate of orbital and intracranial complications that the technology would be expected to reduce.[9] Where we might truly be able to "prove" benefit, however, is with the integration of intraoperative imaging. The ongoing minimization of CT and/or magnetic resonance imaging has resulted in their increasing use. With the ability to immediately supplement any navigational system with real time data, its likely, as one study indicated, to increase the completeness of the sinus dissection by up to 30%.[10] Additionally, the development of low-dose, volumetric scanners has allowed for a decrease in data acquisition time while minimizing radiation risk.

BALLOON DILATION

Over time our understanding of the pathophysiology of sinus disease, like our surgical approaches, has continued to evolve. Although Messerklinger's work focused on key anatomical areas that necessitated addressing during surgery, we have also come to appreciate that chronic sinusitis is more of a spectrum of disorders than an individual disease and that while anatomical issues may play a role, the underlying inflammatory process must also be addressed. It is in this setting that balloon dilation of the sinuses was introduced, somewhat controversially, in the last decade. Stammberger wrote that addressing of the sinus "prechambers" was necessary and that mucosal preservation was of utmost importance. As such, the use of a balloon to dilate these "prechambers" seems logical. Using concepts from dilational procedures in the gastrointestinal tract and cardiac specialties along with a specialized catheter system containing a nondeformable balloon, the Balloon Sinuplasty system was introduced by Acclarent in the early 2000s. Initial reports of its use from 2006 to 2008[11-13] confirmed its safety and efficacy at dilating the ostia of the sphenoid, frontal, and maxillary sinuses. These studies, along with multiple others, further indicate a significant improvement in quality of life for the patients undergoing these procedures, but given the physiological issue noted above, it remains difficult to fully extrapolate the applicability of the technology across the spectrum of chronic sinusitis.

SKULL BASE

As endoscopic sinus surgical technology has advanced, so has the concept of natural orifice and minimally invasive skull base surgery. With improvement in visualization and tissue removal, the identification and repair of skull base defects endoscopically[14] quickly became superior to prior intracranial routes. Jankowski later described the endoscopic approach to the pituitary in 1994. The technology was further applied to removal of intranasal tumors. In the case of inverted papilloma, the endoscope allows a much more specific identification of the site of origin[15] aiding in full removal. Application of the endoscopic technique has been further utilized with malignant tumors, and the advent of arterially based flaps such as the Hadad-Bassagasteguy nasoseptal flap[16] has greatly facilitated skull base reconstruction. Although multiple initial reports indicate good local control for endoscopic resection of nasal and skull base tumors, the data do remain somewhat heterogenous. Although very promising, further long-term results will also be needed before the endoscopic route might be considered standard of care.[17]

NEW FRONTIERS

New technologies for endoscopic sinus surgery are added daily. As our understanding of the interplay between anatomical and physiological predispositions to sinonasal disorders continues to change, we will undoubtedly find new techniques and technologies to optimize patient healing and outcomes. At present, the burgeoning technologies appear to be in the area of local drug delivery with topical therapies and dissolvable drug infused stents revolutionizing medical therapies.[18] Only time will tell which of the latest technologies will become tomorrow's antiquities, but the effect of these innovations on our understanding and management of our patients will always make rhinology an exciting field of study.

REFERENCES

1. Hirschmann A. über Endoskopic dcr Nase und deren Nebenhöhlen: Eine neue Untersuchungsmethode. Arch Laryngol Rhinol (Berl). 1903;14:195-7.
2. Messerklinger W. Nasenendoskopie: DER mittlere Nasengang und seine unspezifischen Entzündungen. HNO. 1972; 20:212 5.
3. Wigand ME, Steiner W, Jaumann MP. Endonasal sinus surgery with endoscopical control: from radical operation to rehabilitation of the mucosa. Endoscopy. 1978;10:255-60.
4. Kennedy DW. Functional endoscopic sinus surgery: technique. Arch Otolaryngol. 1985;111:643-9.
5. Setliff RC 3rd. The hummer: a remedy for apprehension in functional endoscopic sinus surgery. Otolaryngol Clin North Am. 1996;29:95-104.
6. Parsons DS. Rhinologic uses of powered instrumentation in children beyond sinus surgery. Otolaryngol Clin North Am. 1996;29:105-14.
7. Hackman TG, Ferguson BJ. Powered instrumentation and tissue effects in the nose and paranasal sinuses. Curr Opin Otolaryngol Head Neck Surg. 2005;13:22-6.
8. Anon JB, Lipman SP, Oppenheim D, et al. Computer assisted endoscopic sinus surgery. Laryngoscope. 1994;104:901-5.
9. Ramakrishnan VR, Orlandi RR, Citardi MJ, et al. The use of image-guided surgery in endoscopic sinus surgery: an evidence-based review with recommendations. Int Forum Allergy Rhinol. 2013;3(3):236-41.
10. Jackman AH, Palmer JN, Chiu AG, et al. Use of intraoperative CT scanning in endoscopic sinus surgery: a preliminary report. Am J Rhinol. 2008;22:170-4.
11. Brown CL, Bolger WE. Safety as feasibility of balloon catheter dilation of paranasal sinus ostia: a preliminary investigation. Ann Otol Rhinol Laryngol. 2006;115:293-9.
12. Bolger WE, Brown CL, Church CA, et al. Safety and outcomes of balloon catheter sinusotomy: a multicenter 24-week analysis in 115 patients. Otolaryngol Head Neck Surg. 2007; 137:10-20.
13. Weiss RL, Church CA, Kuhn FA, et al. Long-term outcome analysis of balloon catheter sinusotomy: Two-year follow-up. Otolaryngol Head Neck Surg. 2008;139:S38-46.
14. Wigand WE. Transnasal ethmoidectomy under endoscopic control. Rhinology. 1981;19:7 15.
15. Schneyer MS, Milam BM, Payne SC. Sites of attachment of Schneiderian papilloma: a retrospective analysis. Int Forum Allergy Rhinol. 2011;1:324-8.
16. Hadad G, Bassagasteguy L, Carrau RL, et al. A novel reconstructive technique after endoscopic expanded endonasal approaches: vascular pedicle nasoseptal flap. Laryngoscope. 2006;116:1882-6.
17. Lund VJ, Stammberger H, Nicolai P, et al. European position paper on endoscopic management of tumours of the nose, paranasal sinuses and skull base. Rhinol Suppl. 2010;22: 1-143.
18. Harvey RJ, Schlosser RJ. Local drug delivery. Otolaryngol Clin North Am. 2009;4:829-45.

CHAPTER

2 Physiology of the Nose and Paranasal Sinuses

Erika McCarty Walsh, Bradford A Woodworth

INTRODUCTION

The nose is a dynamic unit that works to purify and condition air while functioning as a sensory organ. The sinonasal unit conditions inhaled air, and nasal conditioning is a direct consequence of the unique anatomy and physiology of the upper airway. The sinonasal cavity is an efficient barrier against constant bombardment by pathogens. However, transient or chronic aberrations in the structure and function of the sinonasal cavity may result in rhinosinusitis and other sinus and nasal disorders. This chapter details sinonasal physiology as it relates to air flow dynamics, host defense, and olfaction.

AIR FLOW DYNAMICS

Advances in technology, particularly computational fluid dynamics, have improved our understanding about the structure and function of the nose. Airflow into the nasal vestibule is laminar, or smooth and linear, in nature. However, once air encounters the resistance of the nasal valve and turbinates, the flow pattern becomes transitional. Transitional air flow has mixed laminar and turbulent properties, increasing the exposure of respiratory debris, including antigens and olfactants, to respiratory mucosa. Notably, turbulence is nearly absent during expiration, underlining its importance in filtration of inhaled air.[1] The nasal valve is the flow limiting structure for inhaled air, providing at least half of the total resistance of inspired air to the lungs.[2] The nasal valve is small, with a cross-sectional area of approximately 40 mm^2, and has external and internal components. The external nasal valve exists between the lateral and medial crura of the lower lateral cartilage, and the internal nasal valve resides between the upper lateral cartilage and the septum. At high inspiratory velocities, the nasal valve may completely collapse secondary to the Bernoulli effect. An additional example of the dynamic properties of the sinonasal unit is the nasal cycle. The nasal cycle refers to an alternating pattern of congestion whereby the total nasal resistance remains unchanged but the resistance of each nasal cavity reciprocally increases and decreases (Fig. 2.1). Although the functional significance of the nasal cycle is uncertain, it is controlled by inputs from the hypothalamus, suggesting a homeostatic or autoregulatory role.[3] The turbinates are three shelves of bone and soft tissue attached to the lateral nasal wall. The turbinates add surface area to the nasal epithelium, providing greater territory for conditioning. The nasal mucosa and inferior and middle turbinates especially serve to warm and humidify the air, preparing it for gas exchange in the alveoli.[4] Even at high air flow rates and

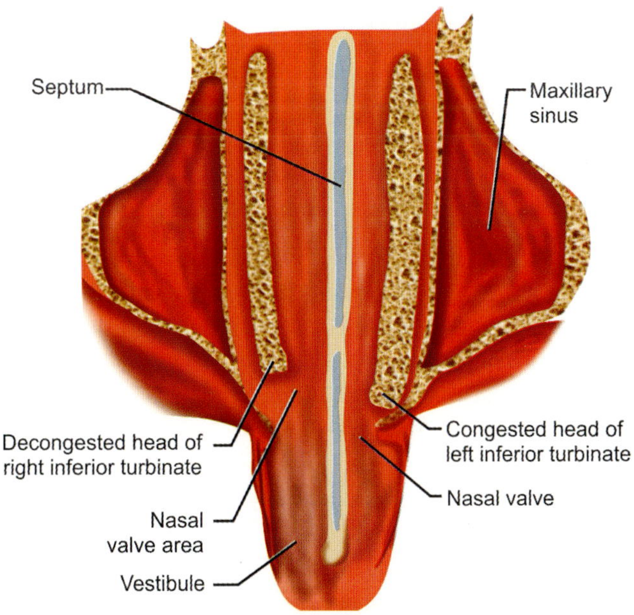

Fig. 2.1: Axial cross-sectional anatomy of the nasal cavity and maxillary sinuses. The nasal cycle results in alternate swelling and decongestion of the inferior turbinate as demonstrated. The head of the inferior turbinate is a component of the internal nasal valve that can significantly affect nasal air flow.

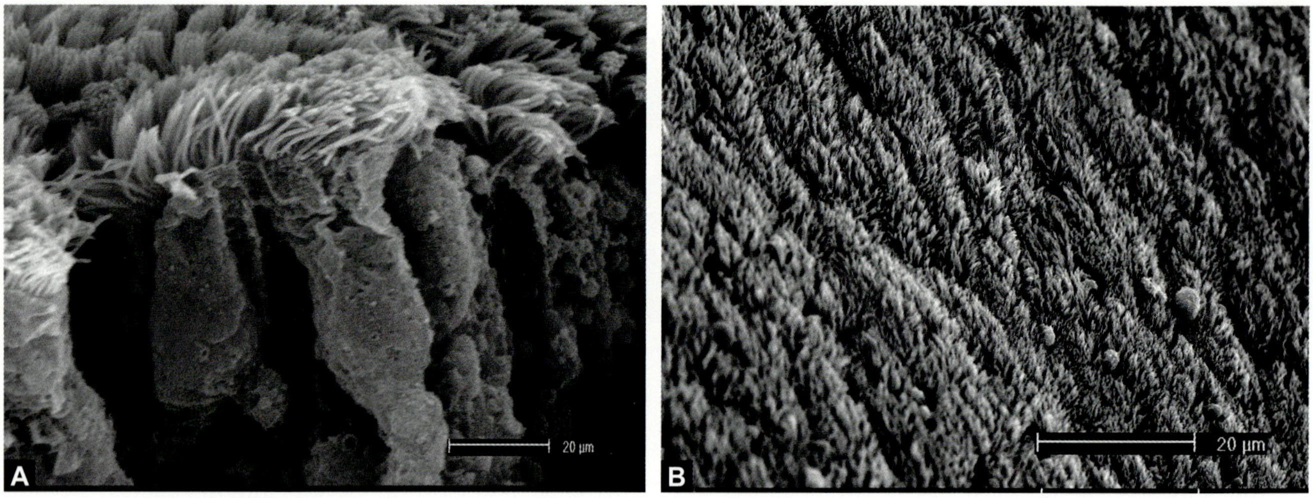

Figs. 2.2A and B: Scanning electron micrographs of sinonasal ciliated respiratory epithelium from lateral (A) and superior (B) views.

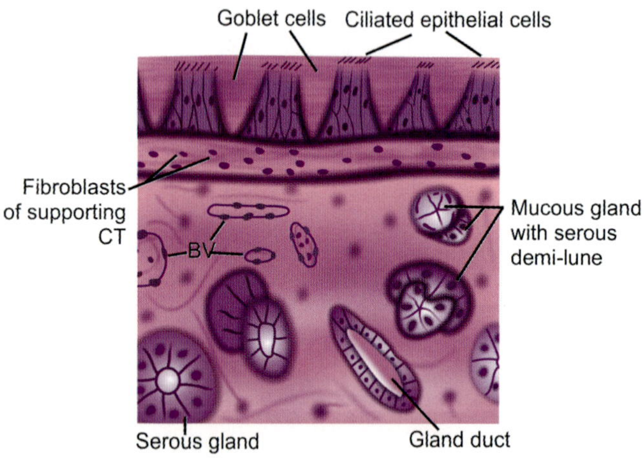

Fig. 2.3: Histology and compositional layers of the nasal mucosa. BV: Blood vessel; CT: Connective tissue.

low ambient temperatures, air can be warmed to an optimal 38°C.[5] After passing through the sinonasal unit, inhaled air is prepped for gas exchange, and deviations from normal anatomy, such as those seen in chronic rhinosinusitis or septal deviation, have deleterious effects on nasal conditioning.[6]

SINONASAL HOST DEFENSE

Given that humans are preferentially nose breathers, air purification is an essential function of the sinonasal unit. Nasal air filtration is a stepwise process—vibrissae, the coarse hair lining the nasal meatus anterior to the nasal valves, trap large particles while progressively smaller particles are trapped more proximally in the mucus layer of the sinonasal epithelium. Particles on the order of 1–10 μm in diameter are effectively trapped by this method.[7] Sweat and sebaceous glands located in the nasal vestibule further help sequester debris caught by vibrissae. Proximal to the nasal valves, the nonciliated stratified squamous epithelium of the anterior nose gives way to ciliated, pseudostratified columnar epithelium (Figs. 2.2A and B). The cilia work synergistically with the mucus layer of the nose to herd trapped debris toward the nasopharynx to be swallowed. Cilia are composed of axonemes, which exist in a 9 plus 2 configuration with two single central microtubules wreathed with 9 pairs of microtubules. Outer doublets interact via motile dynein arms, which produce the characteristic beating motion central to ciliary function.[8] Evidence suggests that decreased mucociliary clearance is seen in a number of disease states, including diabetes and hypertension,[9] suggesting a causative role in the increased frequency and severity of respiratory tract infections seen in certain patient populations and emphasizing the protective role of mucociliary clearance. Similarly, patients with chronic rhinosinusitis have decreased mucociliary clearance.[10]

Intimately related to ciliary function, sinonasal secretions are of considerable functional significance in health and disease. The nasal mucosa consists of, from deepest to most superficial: periosteum, lamina propria, and its associated glands, acellular basement membrane, and pseudostratified columnar ciliated epithelium with interspersed goblet cells (Fig. 2.3). Paranasal sinus epithelium, in contrast, is simple, ciliated, and columnar. Inhaled particles, after passing through the nasal valve, are subject to nasal secretions produced by the nasal mucosa.

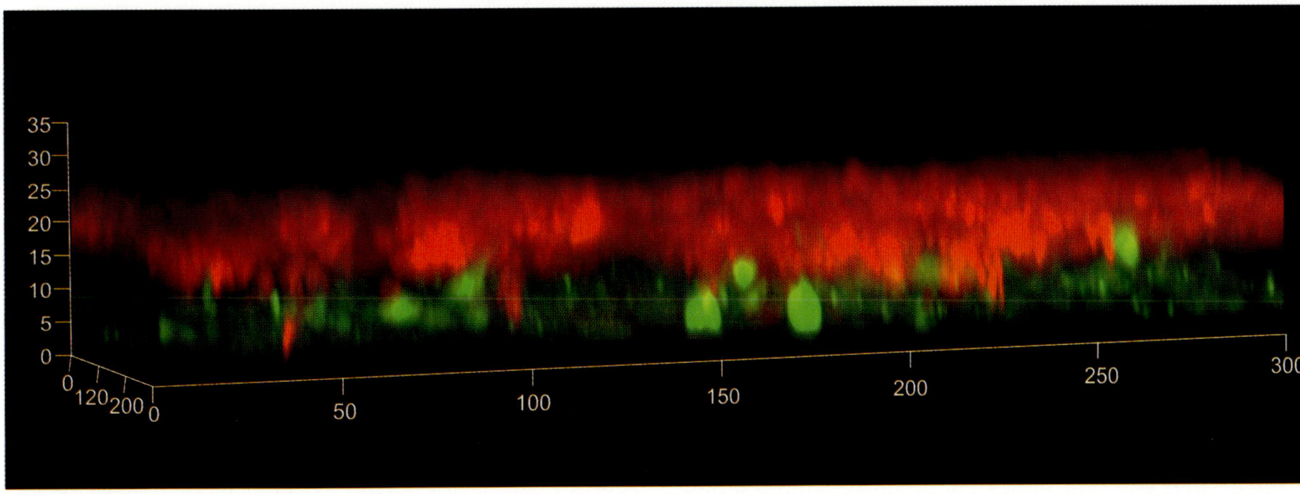

Fig. 2.4: Confocal scanning laser microscopy of a sinonasal respiratory epithelial cell culture on a semipermeable membrane. The cells are stained green, while the airway surface liquid is stained red.

These secretions act as an additional line of defense against antigens and their protective qualities have long been recognized; Alexander Fleming first described the antimicrobial properties of nasal secretions in 1922.[11] Nasal secretions are made up of varying quantities of water, ions, and proteins, including immunoglobins. Immunoglobins A and G, secreted by plasma cells found in the submucosa, are found in nasal secretions and are responsible for antigen specific, or adapative, immune function in the sinonasal unit.[12,13] Lysozyme, lactoferrin, uric acid, and peroxidase are just a few of the proteins thought to mediate innate, or nonspecific, immunity in the nose.[12,14,15] Individual differences in the complement of proteins found in nasal secretions exist, and there is growing evidence that chronic carriers of antigens, for example, patients colonized with *Staphylococcus aureus* in the nasopharynx, may have a deficiency in one or several protein mediators of innate immunity.[12] The exact ionic milieu of nasal secretions is an area of active research, but studies suggest sodium and potassium concentrations between 102 and 150 mEq/L, and 41 and 46 mEq/L, respectively.[16] Active chloride secretion and sodium absorption across the apical membrane of airway epithelial and glandular cells drives water into and out of the nasal passages, respectively.[17-19] Free water also enters the sinonasal unit via the nasolacrimal duct, and mechanical obstruction of fluid transport to the nose, as seen in patients with nasolacrimal duct obstruction, results in expected hypertonic nasal secretions.[20] Nasal fluid over the respiratory epithelia is called airway surface liquid and is composed of two layers: a gel, or mucus-containing, layer, and a less viscous sol layer adjacent to the cilia.[21-25] The composition and depth, usually 5–20 μm in healthy subjects, of nasal secretions are of considerable physiologic significance (Fig. 2.4).[18] Cilia beat through the thin sol layer, effectively propelling the mucus to the oropharynx; the exception is the most anterior portion of the sinonasal unit, where mucus is relatively stationary and nasal secretions rely on innate antimicrobial properties to fight infection.[12,14] Mucus aids in the trapping and transport of inhaled pathogens, and the essential role mucus plays in the upper respiratory tract is highlighted by disorders of mucus production, like cystic fibrosis (CF).[26-31] Caused by mutations in the cystic fibrosis transmembrane conductance regulator (CFTR) gene, patients with CF have impaired transmembrane chloride transport, and CF appears to decrease the depth and volume of nasal secretions secondary to perturbations in ion secretion.[32-36] One theory suggests the decreased secretion of chloride lowers the diffusion gradient, decreasing the amount of free water in nasal secretions.[37] Similarly, it is postulated that lower salt concentrations in nasal secretions may predispose patients to infection by interfering with neutrophil-mediated destruction of bacteria.[37,38] Mucins, which are secreted by goblet cells, are proteins bonded to oligosaccharides; these carbohydrates make up the overwhelming majority of the molecular weight of mucus.[39] The properties of mucins and, therefore, mucus depend on the unique glycosylation pattern. Variations in the composition of these glycoproteins determine the viscosity of mucus. Inflammatory conditions, like chronic rhinosinusitis, result in alterations in glycoproteins that are responsible for the thicker, more tenacious secretions seen in these diseases.[40]

OLFACTION

Olfaction, too, is a function of air dynamics within the nose. Sniffed air travels preferentially to the olfactory groove in the superior portion of the nasal cavity.[41] Located in the roof of the sinonasal unit and shielded by the ethmoid bone, the ciliated, pseudostratified, columnar bipolar cells of the olfactory groove transform stimulation from olfactants into electrical potentials that are processed by the olfactory cortex.[42] These cells provide a nonstop conduit from environment to brain without synapsing—resulting in efficient transmission for both olfactory stimuli and neuropathogens.[43] Olfactory mucus has a complex and distinct composition, with proteins that perform anti-inflammatory, antimicrobial, and signaling functions.[44] In order for odorants to be exposed to their receptors in the olfactory mucosa, these typically hydrophobic particles must move from air into the mucus overlying the olfactory mucosa, and soluble proteins in olfactory secretions may be responsible for mediating the phase change.[45,46] Olfactory receptors are phylogenetically conserved seven transmembrane domain receptors that come in a wide variety of flavors.[47] Each receptor cell expresses only one olfactory receptor, which in turn may respond to a wide range of olfactants.[42,45] When an odorant binds to its receptor, the resultant increase in cyclic AMP leads to opening of ion channels and receptor cell depolarization.[48] The electrical signal is then transmitted to the central nervous system for processing by the olfactory cortex.

CONCLUSIONS

The sinus and nasal cavities have developed effective physiologic processes to control air flow; purify the air of aerosolized pathogens, environmental toxins, and miscellaneous debris; and eliminate filtered waste via mucociliary clearance. These highly evolved physiologic mechanisms arm the respiratory system with the capability to adapt despite constant alteration of environmental conditions and continuous bombardment with respiratory pathogens.

REFERENCES

1. Ishikawa S, Nakayama T, Watanabe M, et al. Visualization of flow resistance in physiological nasal respiration: analysis of velocity and vorticities using numerical simulation. Arch Otolaryngol Head Neck Surg. 2006;132:1203-9.
2. Proctor DF, Adams GK, 3rd. Physiology and pharmacology of nasal function and mucus secretion. Pharmacol Ther B. 1976;2:493-509.
3. Mirza N, Kroger H, Doty RL. Influence of age on the 'nasal cycle'. Laryngoscope. 1997;107:62-6.
4. Bailie N, Hanna B, Watterson J, et al. A model of airflow in the nasal cavities: Implications for nasal air conditioning and epistaxis. Am J Rhinol Allergy. 2009;23:244-9.
5. Mirza N, Lanza DC. The nasal airway and obstructed breathing during sleep. Otolaryngol Clin North Am. 1999; 32:243-62.
6. Liu T, Han D, Wang J, et al. Effects of septal deviation on the airflow characteristics: using computational fluid dynamics models. Acta Otolaryngol. 2012;132:290-8.
7. Heyder J. Deposition of inhaled particles in the human respiratory tract and consequences for regional targeting in respiratory drug delivery. Proc Am Thorac Soc. 2004;1: 315-20.
8. Hard R, Blaustein K, Scarcello L. Reactivation of outer-arm-depleted lung axonemes: evidence for functional differences between inner and outer dynein arms in situ. Cell Motil Cytoskeleton. 1992;21:199-209.
9. de Oliveira-Maul JP, de Carvalho HB, Miyuki Goto D, et al. Aging, diabetes, and hypertension are associated with decreased nasal mucociliary clearance. Chest. 2013; 143:1091-7.
10. Passali D, Ferri R, Becchini G, et al. Alterations of nasal mucociliary transport in patients with hypertrophy of the inferior turbinates, deviations of the nasal septum and chronic sinusitis. Eur Arch Otorhinolaryngol. 1999;256: 335-7.
11. Fleming A. On a remarkable bacteriolytic element found in tissues and secretions. Proc R Soc Lond (Biol). 1922; 93:306-17.
12. Cole AM, Dewan P, Ganz T. Innate antimicrobial activity of nasal secretions. Infect Immun. 1999;67:3267-75.
13. Meredith SD, Raphael GD, Baraniuk JN, et al. The pathophysiology of rhinitis. III. The control of IgG secretion. J Allergy Clin Immunol. 1989;84:920-30.
14. Kaliner MA. Human nasal respiratory secretions and host defense. Am Rev Respir Dis. 1991;144:S52-56.
15. Kaliner MA. Human nasal host defense and sinusitis. J Allergy Clin Immunol. 1992;90:424-30.
16. Boucher RC. Human airway ion transport. Part one. Am J Respir Crit Care Med. 1994;150:271-81.
17. Diamond JM. Osmotic water flow in leaky epithelia. J Membr Biol. 1979;51:195-216.
18. Widdicombe JH, Bastacky SJ, Wu DX, et al. Regulation of depth and composition of airway surface liquid. Eur Respir J. 1997;10:2892-7.
19. Zhang S, Fortenberry JA, Cohen NA, et al. Comparison of vectorial ion transport in primary murine airway and human sinonasal air-liquid interface cultures, models for studies of cystic fibrosis, and other airway diseases. Am J Rhinol Allergy. 2009;23:149-52.

20. Naiboglu B, Deveci I, Kalaycik C, et al. Effect of nasolacrimal duct obstruction on nasal mucociliary transport. J Laryngol Otol. 2010;124:166-70.
21. Lucas A, Douglas L. Principles underlying ciliary activity in the respiratory tract. II. A comparin of nasal clearance in man, monkey, and other mammals. Arch Otolaryngol. 1934;20:518-41.
22. Sanderson MJ, Sleigh MA. Ciliary activity of cultured rabbit tracheal epithelium: beat pattern and metachrony. J Cell Sci. 1981;47:331-47.
23. Reissig M, Bang BG, Bang FB. Ultrastructure of the mucociliary interface in the nasal mucosa of the chicken. Am Rev Respir Dis. 1978;117:327-41.
24. Yoneda K. Mucous blanket of rat bronchus: an ultrastructural study. Am Rev Respir Dis. 1976; 114:837-42.
25. Puchelle E, Beorchia A, Menager M, et al. Three-dimensional imaging of the mucus secretory process in the cryofixed frog respiratory epithelium. Biol Cell. 1991;72:159-66.
26. Alexander NS, Blount A, Zhang S, et al. Cystic fibrosis transmembrane conductance regulator modulation by the tobacco smoke toxin acrolein. Laryngoscope 2012;122: 1193-7.
27. Alexander NS, Hatch N, Zhang S, et al. Resveratrol has salutary effects on mucociliary transport and inflammation in sinonasal epithelium. Laryngoscope. 2011;121:1313-9.
28. Azbell C, Zhang S, Skinner D, et al. Hesperidin stimulates cystic fibrosis transmembrane conductance regulator-mediated chloride secretion and ciliary beat frequency in sinonasal epithelium. Otolaryngol Head Neck Surg. 2010; 143:397-404.
29. Blount A, Zhang S, Chestnut M, et al. Transepithelial ion transport is suppressed in hypoxic sinonasal epithelium. Laryngoscope. 2011;121:1929-34.
30. Chaaban MR, Kejner A, Rowe SM, et al. Cystic fibrosis chronic rhinosinusitis: a comprehensive review. Am J Rhinol Allergy. 2013;27:387-95.
31. Virgin F, Rowe SM, Wade MB, et al. Extensive surgical and comprehensive postoperative medical management for severe, recalcitrant cystic fibrosis chronic rhinosinusitis. Am J Rhinol Allergy. 2012;26.
32. Boucher RC. Molecular insights into the physiology of the 'thin film' of airway surface liquid. J Physiol. 1999;516 (Pt 3):631-8.
33. Matsui H, Grubb BR, Tarran R, et al. Evidence for periciliary liquid layer depletion, not abnormal ion composition, in the pathogenesis of cystic fibrosis airways disease. Cell. 1998;95:1005-15.
34. Smith JJ, Travis SM, Greenberg EP, et al. Cystic fibrosis airway epithelia fail to kill bacteria because of abnormal airway surface fluid. Cell. 1996;85:229-36.
35. Vanthanouvong V, Kozlova I, Johannesson M, et al. Composition of nasal airway surface liquid in cystic fibrosis and other airway diseases determined by X-ray microanalysis. Microsc Res Tech. 2006;69:271-6.
36. Zabner J, Smith JJ, Karp PH, et al. Loss of CFTR chloride channels alters salt absorption by cystic fibrosis airway epithelia in vitro. Mol Cell. 1998;2:397-403.
37. Hull J, Skinner W, Robertson C, et al. Elemental content of airway surface liquid from infants with cystic fibrosis. Am J Respir Crit Care Med. 1998;157:10-4.
38. Stutts MJ, Canessa CM, Olsen JC, et al. CFTR as a cAMP-dependent regulator of sodium channels. Science. 1995; 269:847-50.
39. Ali MS, Pearson JP. Upper airway mucin gene expression: a review. Laryngoscope 2007;117:932-8.
40. Berger G, Kogan T, Ophir D, et al. Glycoconjugate expression of sinus mucosa in chronic rhinosinusitis: a lectin histochemical study. Am J Rhinol. 2008;22:349-55.
41. Ishikawa S, Nakayama T, Watanabe M, et al. Flow mechanisms in the human olfactory groove: numerical simulation of nasal physiological respiration during inspiration, expiration, and sniffing. Arch Otolaryngol Head Neck Surg. 2009;135:156 62.
42. Doty RL. The olfactory system and its disorders. Semin Neurol. 2009;29:74-81.
43. Doty RL. The olfactory vector hypothesis of neurodegenerative disease: is it viable? Ann Neurol. 2008;63:7-15.
44. Debat H, Eloit C, Blon F, et al. Identification of human olfactory cleft mucus proteins using proteomic analysis. J Proteome Res. 2007;6:1985-96.
45. Johnson BA, Leon M. Chemotopic odorant coding in a mammalian olfactory system. J Comp Neurol. 2007;503:1-34.
46. Pevsner J, Hou V, Snowman AM, et al. Odorant-binding protein. Characterization of ligand binding. J Biol Chem. 1990;265:6118-25.
47. Hoover KC. Smell with inspiration: the evolutionary significance of olfaction. Am J Phys Anthropol. 2012;143 (Suppl 51):63-74.
48. Jenkins PM, McEwen DP, Martens JR. Olfactory cilia: linking sensory cilia function and human disease. Chem Senses. 2009;34:451-64.

CHAPTER

3 Anatomy and Interpretation of Nasal and Sinus Radiology

Joseph Gorodenker, Ameet Singh, M Reza Taheri

NASAL FOSSA, SEPTUM, AND TURBINATES

The nasal fossae are air-filled cavities separated by the vertically oriented midline nasal septum. The nasal septum is principally composed of the vomer, the perpendicular plate of the ethmoid, the quadrangular cartilage, and the membranous septum, with contribution from the palatine processes of the maxillae and the horizontal plates of the palatine bones. The columella, a strip of skin that separates the nostrils, also contributes to the anterior nasal septum.[1]

The hard palate forms the floor of the nasal cavity, of which the maxillary palatine process contributes the anterior two thirds, whereas the horizontal portions of the palatine bones form the posterior third. The bilateral cribriform plates and the fovea ethmoidalis (ethmoid roof) of the ethmoid bone form the roof of the nasal cavity. The cross-shaped ethmoid bone projects above the horizontal cribriform plate as the crista galli ("cock's comb") and extends below as the perpendicular plate of the ethmoid. The perpendicular plate articulates with the quadrangular cartilage anteroinferiorly and with the grooved vomer posteroinferiorly to form the nasal septum. The free posterior edge of the vomer divides the posterior choanae. Of note, the vomer may be bilaminar, and both it and the perpendicular plate of ethmoid may be pneumatized. The crista galli may also be aerated or may contain fat. Anterior to the crista galli lies the foramen cecum, a normally regressed developmental canal containing fibrotic tissue. Nasal dermoid cysts, nasal gliomas, and meningoencephaloceles may be associated with patency of the foramen cecum and/or a bifid crista galli. Patency may also allow venous communication from the nasal mucosa to the superior sagittal sinus, furnishing a potential route for infection.[2]

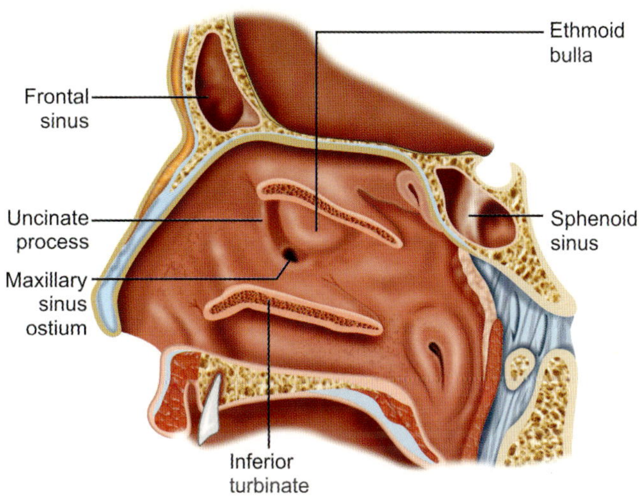

Fig. 3.1: Major landmarks of the lateral nasal wall.

The turbinates or nasal conchae (inferior, middle, superior, and the variable supreme) are paired scrolled bony projections from the lateral nasal wall, which are covered by sinus mucosa, and serve to warm and humidify inspired air (Fig. 3.1). The space below and lateral to a turbinate is the meatus named after it. The inferior turbinate has a different embryological origin (maxilloturbinal) and attaches to the medial maxillary and palatine bones. The middle turbinate and its attachments, the anterior and posterior buttresses and projecting lamellae, are important anatomic landmarks.

The anterior buttress of the middle turbinate attaches to the lateral nasal wall in the agger nasi region. The middle turbinate attaches to the ethmoid roof and cribriform plate by the vertical lamella, which extends cephalad from the anterior aspect of the middle turbinate to the lateral cribriform plate lamella (LCPL), that is, the lateral wall of the olfactory groove. The LCPL is a very thin (0.05–0.2 mm), fragile, usually vertically oriented bone

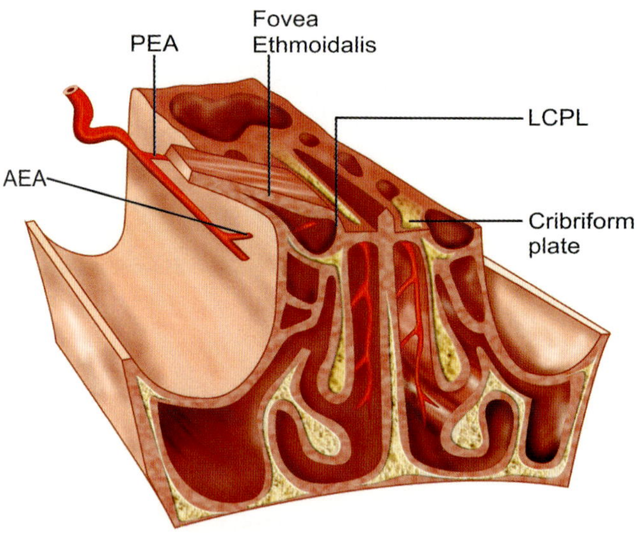

Fig. 3.2: Fovea ethmoidalis (ethmoid roof) and LCPL (lateral cribriform plate lamella). PEA: Posterior ethmoid artery; AEA: Anterior ethmoid artery.

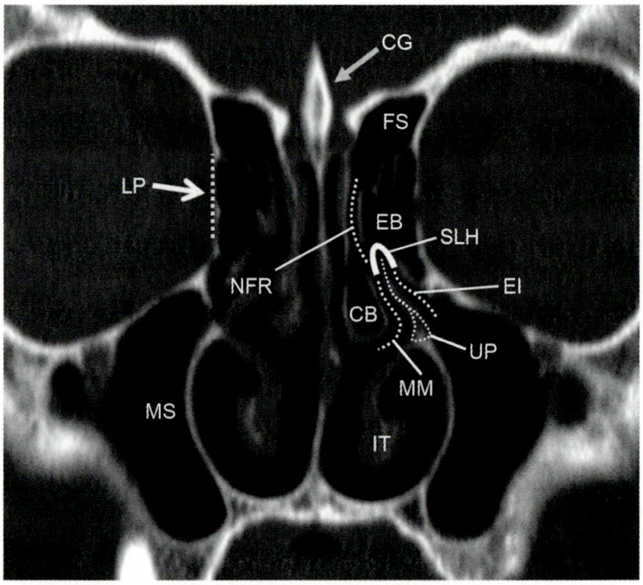

Fig. 3.3: Anterior ostiomeatal complex (OMC): uncinate process (UP), semilunar hiatus (SLH), nasofrontal recess (NFR), ethmoid bulla (EB), ethmoid infundibulum (EI), middle meatus (MM), concha bullosa (CB) = pneumatized middle turbinate, frontal sinus (FS). Also note right maxillary sinus (MS), left inferior turbinate (IT), crista galli (CG), and right lamina papyracea (LP).

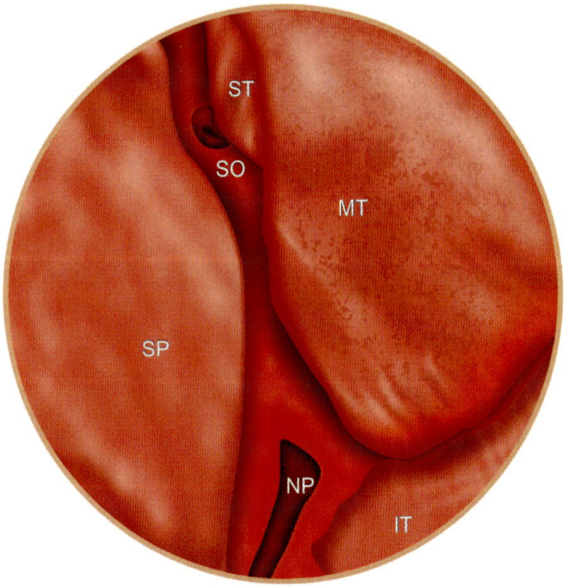

Fig. 3.4: Sphenoethmoidal recess. Superior turbinate (ST), middle turbinate (MT), inferior turbinate (IT), nasal septum (SP), sphenoid ostium (SO), and nasopharynx (NP).

that forms the medial ethmoid roof. It joins the cribriform plate medially and inferiorly, and the fovea ethmoidalis laterally and superiorly (Fig. 3.2). The horizontal lamella and posterior buttress of the middle turbinate attach to the lateral nasal wall in the sphenopalatine region.

The horizontal lamella (also called the basal lamella or ground lamella) marks the division between the anterior and posterior ethmoidal cells.[3] Preserving the anterior buttress, posterior buttresses and vertical lamella of the turbinate during surgery is important to prevent lateralization of the turbinate and consequent obstruction of outflow. Preservation of the inferior portion of the horizontal lamella further decreases the risk of turbinate lateralization. Pneumatization of a turbinate is called a concha bullosa (typically pneumatization of a middle turbinate by a posterior ethmoid air cell), which may cause nasal obstruction or chronic sinusitis (Fig. 3.3).

The superior and the inconstant supreme turbinate lie above and posterior to the middle turbinate, anterior to the face of the sphenoid sinus. The perpendicular attachment of the superior turbinate divides the anterior wall or face of the sphenoid sinuses into unequal medial third and lateral two thirds. The open medial third, referred to as the free intranasal surface, is bounded by the nasal septum medially, the cribriform plate superiorly, and the upper surface of the posterior choanae inferiorly. The sphenoethmoidal recess refers to the space limited by the free intranasal surface of the sphenoid and the superior turbinate (Fig. 3.4). The lateral two thirds of the anterior sphenoid sinus wall are contiguous with the posterior walls of the ipsilateral ethmoid air-cells.[4,5]

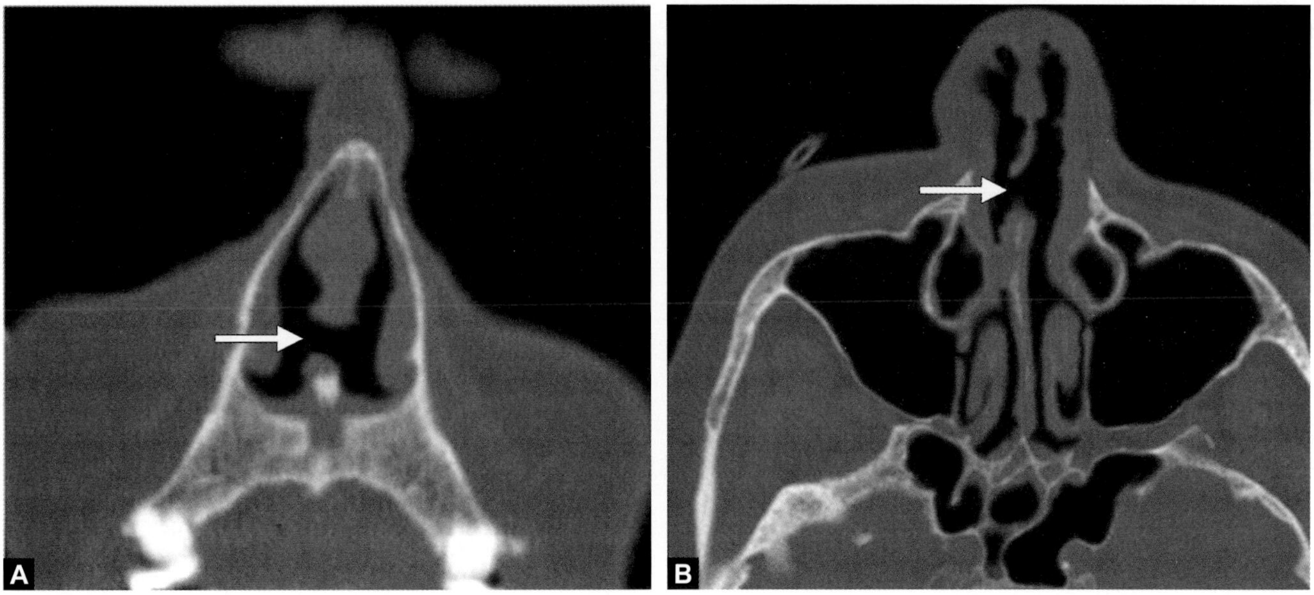

Figs. 3.5A and B: Nasal septal perforation (A) coronal and (B) axial CT images demonstrate nasal septal perforation (arrows) caused by invasive fungal disease. Absence of apparent mass suggests a non-neoplastic etiology, such as infection or granulomatous disease.

Some of the anatomic variants of the nasal fossa, which may cause sinonasal obstruction, include clinically significant nasal septum deviations, paradoxic middle turbinates, and concha bullosa of the middle or superior turbinates.

The presence of a nasal septal defect is concerning. The differential for cartilaginous nasal septal perforation is wide, ranging from trauma (including surgical resection), neoplasm (especially lymphoma, previously termed *polymorphic reticulosis* and *lethal midline granulomatosis*), typical granulomatous disease (sarcoidosis, Wegener's preferentially affect the septum), inhaled toxins (including cocaine, beryllium, chromates, etc.), and infection. Of infectious agents, TB, syphilis, and leprosy are most common, although accompanying bony sclerosis may reflect yaws. Of note, earlier in granulomatous disease, especially Wegener's but also in sarcoidosis and lymphoma, the cartilaginous septum may be swollen rather than eroded. Despite this, it is critical to recognize that any mass lesion in the nasal septal region should be presumed aggressive until proven otherwise. If a mass lesion is identified, it is important to consider its likely origin and to carefully evaluate extent. On the other hand, if no mass lesion is seen, granulomatous disease or infection should be suspected (Figs. 3.5A and B).

Diagnosis is often made by clinical history or direct visualization and histopathology; however, certain imaging features may be helpful. For example, the presence of a central diffusion-weighted imaging (DWI)-hyperintense mass on magnetic resonance imaging (MRI) is typical of T-cell lymphoma, an uncommon sinonasal tumor, whereas a hyperdense lesion on computed tomography (CT) with signal dropout on T2 weighted MRI sequences suggests fungal disease.

Nasal septal abscess is usually associated with suppressed immune status, history of trauma or postsurgical septoplasty and is rarely related to extension of dental infection or sinusitis. Early recognition of this entity is critical, as delayed management complicated by septal cartilage ischemia may lead to cosmetic deformity as well as sepsis.[6]

PARANASAL SINUS ANATOMY AND DRAINAGE

The ostiomeatal complex (OMC) is key to understanding paranasal sinus anatomy and drainage. The complex is composed of anterior and posterior ostiomeatal units.

The anterior ostiomeatal unit is composed of the frontal sinus ostium, the frontal recess, the maxillary sinus ostium, the infundibulum, and middle meatus. Together, these link the drainage systems of the frontal, anterior ethmoid, and maxillary sinuses. Mucociliary clearance in each sinus is naturally directed toward the respective sinus ostium. In the maxillary sinus, mucus from the floor of the antrum is directed toward the maxillary sinus ostium, which is typically located anteromedially. The mucus is then directed through the ethmoid infundibulum to the

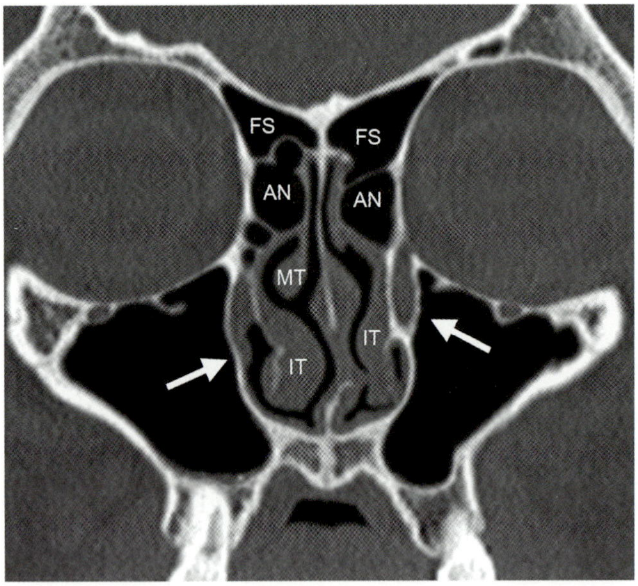

Fig. 3.6: Anterior coronal CT through the frontal sinuses (FS) demonstrates paired Agger nasi (AN) cells. Agger nasi cells are very common (90% prevalence), and represent the most anterior variable ethmoidal air cells. They are located within the lacrimal bone, and above the attachment of the middle turbinate (MT). Note arrows denoting nasolacrimal ducts draining into the inferior meati, lateral to the inferior turinates (IT).

hiatus semilunaris, and then on to the middle meatus and ultimately to the nasopharynx. The primary ostium of the frontal sinus lies medial and inferior, at the floor of the sinus. Drainage proceeds down the nasofrontal recess into the middle meatus, where it joins flow from the ipsilateral maxillary sinus. The anterior ethmoid cell ostia converge unto the middle meatus. Their drainage joins mucus from the frontal sinus (via the nasofrontal recess) and the maxillary sinus (from the maxillary ostium via ethmoidal infundibulum).[7]

Of note, some sources list the uncinate process (and/or the ethmoid bulla) as part of the anterior OMU; however, although very important to the function of the complex, this inclusion may confuse uninitiated readers as the uncinate process is a bony structure while the remainder of the listed components are air-filled spaces. Naturally, the bony walls of these listed spaces effectively contribute to the complex by outlining the air-filled cavities.

The posterior ostiomeatal unit consists of the sphenoid sinus ostium, the sphenoethmoidal recess, and the superior meatus. The posterior ethmoid air cells and the sphenoid sinus drain via the sphenoethmoidal recess into the superior meatus.

The nasolacrimal duct drains separately to the inferior meatus (Fig. 3.6). The superior, middle, and inferior meati collectively drain to the nasopharynx. The remainder of this section reviews the relationships of these and related structures in further detail.

Frontal Sinus

The frontal sinus is contained in the frontal bone superior to the eyes in the forehead. It is formed by superior movement of anterior ethmoid cells after the age of 2 years. Growth of this sinus increases at the age of 6 years and continues until the late teenage years. The frontal sinuses are funnel-shaped structures with their ostia located in the most dependent aspect of the cavities. The posterior wall of the frontal sinus, which separates the sinus from the anterior cranial fossa, is much thinner than its anterior wall. The posterior wall lies near the superior sagittal sinus, which drains the superior cerebral and frontal *diploic veins of Breschet.* This wall represents a potential route of intracranial spread of infection with complications such as sagittal sinus thrombosis and empyema. The frontal sinus is supplied by the supraorbital and supratrochlear arteries of the ophthalmic artery. It is innervated by the supraorbital and supratrochlear nerves of the first division of the trigeminal nerve (V1).

The frontal sinuses are usually asymmetric, with the larger sinus often extending across the midline, and may contain several septations, usually better developed in larger sinuses. These septations may create partially hidden recesses, which are important to identify preoperatively, as failure to do so may result in the formation of a mucocele. Likewise, it is important to identify bullae, which are deformations of the frontal sinus floor, which may be related to contralateral frontal sinus extension or protrusion by an underlying ethmoid cell. The frontal sinuses are intimately related to adjacent anatomic structures; remodeling of the superomedial orbital margin may be related to expansile frontal sinus pathology, such as mucocele, pneumocele, or tumor.

Persistence of a metopic suture results in small or absent frontal sinuses, whereas a frontal sinus is often greatly enlarged in case of early insult to the ipsilateral frontal lobe (e.g., Dyke-Davidoff-Masson syndrome).[8] The intersinus septum, the residual frontal bone between the frontal sinuses, may be thickened or may contain focal acquired or congenital dehiscence.

Nasofrontal Recess

In broad anatomic terms, the nasofrontal recess is bordered posteriorly by the sloping anterior skull base and anteriorly by the beak of the frontal process. Its anatomy is made complex by the wide variety of anterior ethmoidal cells that inhabit the space. Some of the more common frontal recess cells include the agger nasi cell, supraorbital ethmoid cell, interfrontal sinus septal cell, frontal bulla cell, suprabullar cell, and four types of frontal cells (types I–IV). The most prominent cells include the agger nasi cell, supraorbital cell, and the frontal cells.

Although the exact configuration and pathway of the frontal recess vary, this structure is usually bounded anteriorly by the posterior wall of the agger nasi cell (the most anterior ethmoid air cell), superiorly by the frontal sinus, medially by the LCPL (i.e., the lateral wall of the olfactory groove) and vertical lamella of the middle turbinate, laterally by the lamina papyracea, and posteriorly by the anterior wall of the ethmoidal bulla, or suprabullar recess. The risk of a cerebrospinal fluid leak from the olfactory fossa or damage to the anterior ethmoidal artery, with potential visual loss and orbital injury, make dissection in the frontal recess particularly challenging for the endoscopic sinus surgeon.

Ethmoid Sinus

The ethmoid sinuses arise in the ethmoid bone, forming several distinct air cells between the eyes. They are a collection of fluid-filled cells at birth that grow and pneumatize until the age of 12 years. The ethmoid cells are shaped like pyramids and are divided by thin septa. The basal lamella is a bony strut which extends laterally from the posterior middle turbinate to the lamina papyracea and separates the ethmoid air cells into the more numerous and smaller anterior cells and the larger and fewer posterior cells, which drain into the middle and superior meatus, respectively. Of note, the basal lamella is also attached posteroinferiorly to the crista ethmoidalis, which represents the most consistent landmark for the sphenopalatine foramen.

The ethmoid labyrinth may extend above the orbit, lateral and superior to the sphenoid, above the frontal sinus, and into the roof of the maxillary sinus.

Medially the ethmoid sinus is bound by the vertical lamella (of the middle turbinate). The lateral wall of the ethmoid sinus is formed by the lacrimal bone (anterior third), and by the lamina papyracea (posterior third), which separates the ethmoid from the orbit. The lacrimal bone, which is commonly pneumatized, lies between the ascending process of the maxilla anteriorly, where it covers the nasolacrimal duct, and the lamina papyracea and anterior ethmoid air cells posteriorly, where it covers the lacrimal process of the inferior turbinate. Superiorly, the lacrimal bone articulates with the frontal bone.

The ethmoid sinuses are supplied by the anterior and posterior ethmoidal arteries from the ophthalmic artery (internal carotid system), as well as by the sphenopalatine artery from the terminal branches of the internal maxillary artery (external carotid system).

Uncinate Process and Ethmoid Infundibulum

The uncinate process (of the ethmoid) is a cutlass-shaped superior bony projection. The uncinate lies lateral to the middle turbinate, articulates with the inferior turbinate, and attaches to the posterior wall of the lacrimal bone anteriorly. This is useful in locating the nasolacrimal duct, which drains into the anterior superior aspect of the inferior meatus (Fig. 3.6).

The uncinate process is a critical bony structure of the lateral nasal cavity. With the ethmoid bulla it contributes to the ethmoid infundibulum and the hiatus semilunaris, a common drainage pathway for the anterior ethmoid and maxillary sinuses (and potentially the frontal sinus; see below). Hence, its anatomic configuration may cause anterior ethmoid, frontal recess, and/or infundibular (maxillary) sinus obstruction. A pneumatized uncinate, typically related to extension of an agger nasi cell, is termed an uncinate bulla. This may cause obstruction but is relatively uncommon.

The unfortunately named ethmoid infundibulum is a channel that drains the maxillary sinus. It lies between the uncinate process (caudally and medially) and the inferomedial margin of the orbit (cranial and lateral). The infundibulum drains to the hiatus semilunaris, a space that lies medial and superior to the infundibulum, and above the uncinate process (see below). If the free edge of the uncinate process deviates laterally, it may narrow or obstruct the hiatus semilunaris and/or the infundibulum. The infundibulum may also be narrowed or obstructed by Haller cells (see below).

The uncinate process usually attaches to the medial orbital wall superiorly but may attach to the skull base or the middle turbinate, and these various patterns of attachment are variously categorized[7] (e.g., Landsberg and Friedman); however, essentially the site of superior attachment of the uncinate influences the drainage pattern of the frontal sinus in relation to the ethmoidal infundibulum (Figs. 3.7A to C):

- If the uncinate process bends laterally (most frequent configuration) and inserts superiorly into the lateral nasal wall (a common location of agger nasi cells) or the lamina papyracea, the ethmoidal infundibulum is separated from the frontal recess. In this case, the

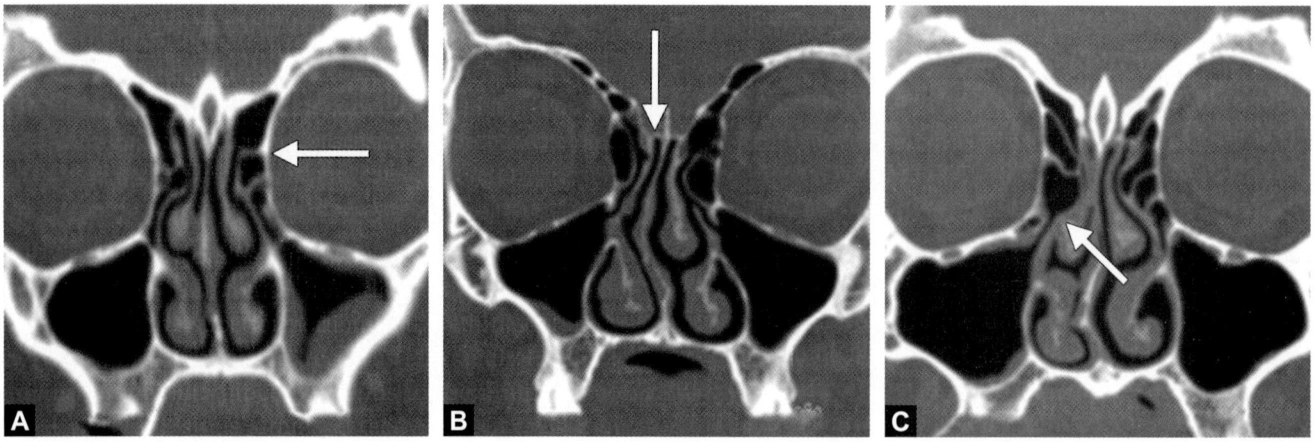

Figs. 3.7A to C: The superior attachment of the uncinate process (white arrows) affects the drainage pattern of the frontal sinus. (A) Attachment to the lamina; (B) Attachment to cribriform plate/skull base; (C) Attachment to middle turbinate.

frontal recess drains separately into the middle meatus, medial to ethmoidal infundibulum. The resultant blind-ending superior portion of the ethmoidal infundibulum is termed the recessus terminalis.

- If the uncinate process extends to the ethmoid roof, the frontal sinus drains directly into the ethmoid infundibulum. Excessive traction during uncinectomy in such configuration may cause injury to the ethmoid roof and result in cerebrospinal fluid (CSF) leak or other complications. If the uncinate process extends to the roof of the anterior ethmoid, the superior infundibulum is closed superiorly, and the infundibulum drains via the posterior middle meatus.
- If the uncinate process turns medially and attaches to the middle turbinate, the frontal sinus drains into the ethmoid infundibulum.

Ethmoid Bone

The medial portion of the ethmoid bone is a cruciate membranous bone that is composed of the crista galli, the cribriform plate and the superior portion of the nasal septum. The crista galli is a thick portion of bone, shaped like a cock's comb, that projects superiorly into the cranial cavity and serves as an attachment of the falx cerebri. If pneumatized, the crista galli air cell drains into either the left or right frontal sinus. The cribriform plate contains several perforations that transmit olfactory fibers to the middle turbinate, superior turbinate, and the superior nasal septum. The perpendicular plate of the ethmoid articulates with the quadrangular cartilage anteroinferiorly and with the vomer posteroinferiorly to form the nasal septum.

Ethmoid Roof

The vertical lamella (of the middle turbinate) divides the anterior skull base into the cribriform plate medially and the roof of the ethmoid, or fovea ethmoidalis, laterally.

The fovea ethmoidalis slopes inferiorly when traveling in an anterior-to-posterior or lateral-to-medial direction along the skull base. Understanding this orientation is important for preventing inadvertent entry into the skull base during endoscopic sinonasal procedures. The roof of the ethmoid is primarily composed of a thicker horizontal portion, called the orbital plate of the frontal bone, and a thinner vertical portion, called the LCPL (also known as the lateral wall of the olfactory groove). The height of the LCPL defines the depth of the olfactory cleft where dura is closely adherent to the bone. The bony thickness of the LCPL ranges from 0.05 to 0.2 mm and provides little resistance to injury (*see* Fig. 3.2).[3]

The depth of the olfactory cleft may be graded by the Keros system as Type I (1–3 mm), Type II (3–7 mm), or Type III (8–16 mm). Deeper olfactory clefts are at greater risk during surgery, including CSF leak, pneumocephalus, or intracranial injury.[9] The most common location of iatrogenic CSF leak is the thinnest portion of the LCPL in the region of the anterior ethmoid artery (AEA), which courses along the anterior ethmoid roof, from the orbit to the olfactory groove.

Of note, an anatomic variant exists in which the orbital plate is relatively thin and the LCPL runs in a more horizontal direction. A great risk of inadvertent injury exists if the surgeon perceives the thinner orbital plate to be part of a superior ethmoid cell, rather than the skull base.

Ethmoid Bulla and Semilunar Hiatus

The ethmoid bulla is the largest of the anterior ethmoidal cells and is a constant landmark during endoscopic surgery. It lies posteromedial to the uncinate process, superior to the ethmoidal infundibulum, and anterior to the basal lamella (of the middle turbinate), which separates the anterior from the posterior ethmoidal cells.

The ethmoid bulla often extends cephalad all the way to the skull base, however, it may be separated from the skull base by a suprabullar cell or a cleft named the suprabullar recess. Alternatively, it is sometimes attached to the skull base via the bulla lamella. The anterior ethmoidal artery usually courses superomedially in the region of the bulla lamella.

The air space between the inferolateral surface of the ethmoidal bulla and the superior surface of the uncinate process is called the hiatus semilunaris (or semilunar hiatus). This common space joins the infundibulum (and potentially the nasofrontal recess, depending on the configuration of the uncinate process) with the middle meatus, allowing maxillary sinus (and possibly frontal sinus) mucus to drain with the anterior ethmoid cells into the middle meatus, and then to the nasopharynx (*see* Fig. 3.3).

If the ethmoidal bulla has a posterior surface separate from the basal lamella, the space between them is called the retrobullar recess or sinus lateralis. The retrobullar recess may communicate with the suprabullar recess, a space that may exist between the superior surface of the ethmoidal bulla and the fovea ethmoidalis (skull base).

Haller Cell (Infraorbital Ethmoid Cell)

The Haller cell, or infraorbital ethmoid cell, is an anterior ethmoidal cell that pneumatizes into the maxillary sinus ostium just below the medial floor of the orbit (Fig. 3.8). A Haller cell may contribute to recalcitrant maxillary sinus disease in some cases of chronic sinusitis. This is usually secondary to mucosal inflammation of the common wall between the Haller cell and the maxillary sinus ostium.

Patterns of Sinus Disease

Sinus disease often takes the form of a recognizable pattern that reflects the location of obstruction. Obstruction at the middle meatus results in the OMC pattern (per Sonkens' classification[10]) and involves the maxillary sinus, the anterior ethmoid group and variably the frontal sinus, depending on the insertion of the anterior uncinate process, as discussed above. Obstruction at the middle meatus may be related to mucosal edema, structural lesions such as concha bullosa or septal deviation, or mass effect from a benign or malignant process.

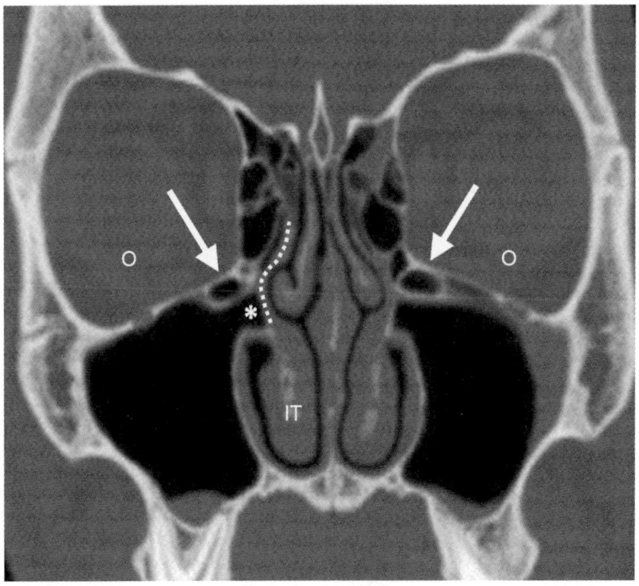

Fig. 3.8: Haller cells (arrows) are anterior ethmoid air cells which pneumatize and potentially narrow the maxillary sinus ostium (*) just below the medial floor of the orbit (O). Note the relationship of the Haller cell on the right to the uncinate process (dashed line).

The frontal recess inflammatory pattern, a variant of the OMC pattern above, refers to the isolated involvement of the frontal sinus in case of isolated involvement of a frontal recess or direct drainage of the frontal recess into the middle meatus.

The infundibular pattern of sinus disease refers to the isolated obstruction of the ethmoid infundibulum and/or the maxillary sinus. In this pattern, the frontal and/or ethmoid sinuses are not involved. The underlying etiology may likewise include mucosal edema, polypoid lesions or structural lesions such as Haller cells.

Not uncommonly, diffuse obstruction develops, sparing the inferior meatus, with extensive polyps throughout the nasal cavity and the paranasal sinuses (Figs. 3.9A and B). This sinonasal polyposis pattern should be distinguished from the sporadic pattern, which refers to no apparent pattern of paranasal sinus pathology.

Agger Nasi Cell

The agger nasi cell, when present, is the most anterior of the ethmoidal cells (*see* Fig. 3.6). Located within the lacrimal bone, it is found in over 90% of CT scans. Agger nasi cells are found medial to the nasolacrimal duct,

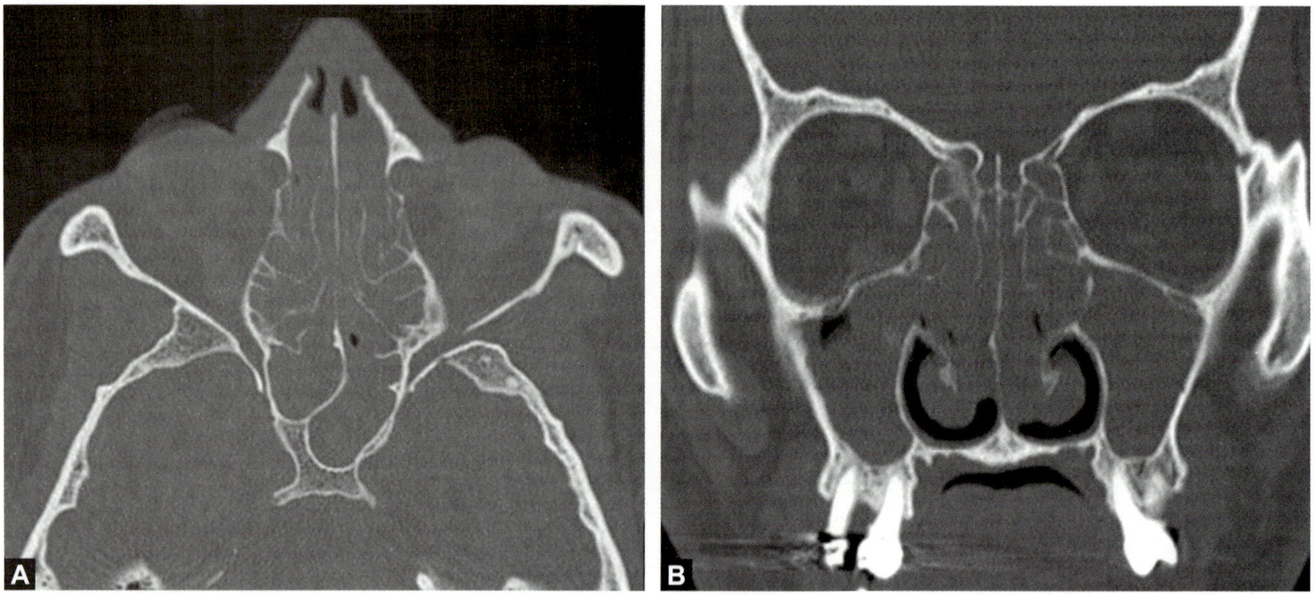

Figs. 3.9A and B: Diffuse polyposis. (A) Axial and (B) coronal CT demonstrate generalized homogeneous opacification of the sinuses with no evidence of bony involvement (no erosion, bulging, or dehiscence). The appearance of convex, outward margins to the fluid density in the opacified structures suggests polyposis rather than mere sinusitis.

and anterior and superior to the anterior buttress of the middle turbinate. The medial wall and roof of the agger nasi cell often lie in close association with the vertical lamella of the middle turbinate and the anterior skull base, respectively, whereas the posterior wall often represents the anterior face of the nasofrontal recess. The superior surface (or cap) of the agger nasi cell, if left in place during frontal recess surgery, may contribute to iatrogenic frontal sinus obstruction.

Frontal Sinus Cells

Four types of frontal sinus cells may pneumatize above the agger nasi cell, and potentially contribute to the complexity of frontal recess anatomy. A type I frontal sinus cell lies above the agger nasi cell. A type II frontal sinus cell is a configuration of two cells stacked above the agger nasi cell. A type III cell is a large frontal sinus cell that pneumatizes into the frontal sinus and occupies nearly 50% of the sinus. Finally, a type IV frontal sinus cell is a single isolated cell that exists completely within the frontal sinus and has no connection to the frontal recess.[7]

Supraorbital Ethmoid Cell

The supraorbital ethmoid cell is an anterior ethmoidal cell that pneumatizes into the orbital plate of the frontal bone, occasionally involving the lateral wall of the orbit. When extensively pneumatized, this cell may be mistaken for the frontal sinus or a septate frontal sinus.

Maxillary Sinus

The maxillary sinus is the largest of the paranasal sinuses. It is situated within the body of the maxillary bone below the orbits. The shape of the sinus is a pyramid with the base along the nasal wall and the apex pointing laterally toward the zygoma. Embryologically, it is the first sinus to form and usually grows symmetrically. Its growth is biphasic, where the first phase occurs during the first 3 years and the second during years 6–12. Pneumatization is initially directed horizontally and posteriorly during the first phase and inferiorly toward the maxillary teeth during the second phase.

Maxillary hypoplasia is uncommon, and may be related to prior trauma, infection, surgical intervention, irradiation, or underdevelopment related to branchial arch anomalies (e.g., Treacher-Collins s., mandibulofacial dysostosis) or erythropoetic demand, such as thalassemia major.[8]

The medial wall of the maxillary sinus is the inferolateral wall of the nasal cavity, whereas the posterolateral wall separates the sinus from the pterygopalatine fossa and infratemporal fossa. The roof of the maxillary sinus is also the floor of the orbit.

The natural maxillary sinus ostium varies in precise location, but usually lies at the superior aspect of the medial wall, and measures up to 4 mm in diameter. It drains indirectly into the nasal cavity via the infundibulum (see *Ostiomeatal Complex* above). Multiple structures contribute to the maxillary hiatus (ostium): portions of the ethmoid bone (forming the uncinate process), the perpendicular plate of the palatine bone (posteriorly), the lacrimal bone (anterior and superior), and inferior turbinate (inferior).

The lateral nasal wall has two areas deficient in bone that lie anterior and posterior to the uncinate process. These areas are called fontanelles, or accessory ostia that may be confused with the natural maxillary sinus ostium. Although sometimes functional, these ostia rarely function as the true ostium because the mucociliary clearance pattern of the maxillary sinus preferentially flows to the natural ostium. A posterior ethmoid cell can invade the posterior maxilla and divide the maxillary antrum into anterior and posterior compartments, which may drain separately into the nasal fossa via accessory ostia. Rarely, the antrum is divided by a horizontal or vertical septum.

The maxillary nerve (canal) lies within the maxillary sinus roof, diving anteriorly to exit 1 cm below the inferior orbital rim on the anterior face of the maxilla via the infraorbital foramen. The thinnest portion of the anterior maxillary wall is above the canine tooth, called the canine fossa. This area is an ideal entry site for addressing various disease processes of the maxillary sinus if endoscopic surgery is not sufficient. The maxillary sinus is supplied by branches of the internal maxillary artery, which include the infraorbital, alveolar, greater palatine and sphenopalatine arteries. It is innervated by branches of the mandibular nerve (second branch of the trigeminal), the infraorbital nerve and the greater palatine nerves.

The maxillary sinuses contain several named recesses. The lateral or zygomatic recess extends into the malar eminence of the zygoma. The tuberosity recess extends inferiorly and posterior to the third maxillary molar. The alveolar recess extends to the alveolar process of the maxilla. The variable palatine recess extends into the hard palate. Notably, the inferior pneumatization of the sinus is intimately related to tooth eruption; bone overlying the tooth roots may be dehiscent with only mucosal covering.

Sphenoid Sinus

The sphenoid sinuses are a large pair of paranasal sinuses located in the sphenoid bone posterior to the ethmoid sinuses. These paired sinuses develop separately from the nasal capsule of the embryonic nose, often divided by a single vertical intersinus septation. However, multiple complete and incomplete bony septations, with vertical, horizontal, or oblique orientations, may further subdivide the sinus. In one radiologic study, 80% of sphenoid sinuses were found to have a single sphenoid septation, and 20% were found to have a double septation. These septations often localize to the carotid artery, underscoring the importance of atraumatic dissection to avoid a catastrophic vascular injury.

Sphenoid Pneumatization Patterns

Pneumatization of the sphenoid sinus is highly variable and can extend as far as the clivus inferiorly, the sphenoid wings laterally and the foramen magnum inferiorly. Pneumatization of the sphenoid sinuses is rarely absent, with lack of pneumatization suggesting underlying abnormal erythropoetic demand (e.g., thalassemia).[9] Pneumatization of the vast majority of sinuses reaches the sella turcica by the age of 7 years. The major pneumatization patterns for sphenoid sinus include sellar (55%), presellar (20%), conchal (3%), and postsellar (22%) (Fig. 3.10).[11]

A sellar sphenoid sinus has pneumatization anterior and inferior to the sellar prominence. A presellar sphenoid sinus has pneumatization only anterior to the sella. A conchal sphenoid sinus has minimal to no pneumatization, and poses the greatest anatomic challenge to the endoscopic management of sphenoid, pituitary, or anterior skull base pathology. A postsellar configuration consists of presellar pneumatization followed by a smaller pneumatization behind the sella. This pattern is important to recognize during endoscopic skull base surgery.

The degree of sphenoid sinus pneumatization determines the relative location of the foramen rotundum and vidian canal, which may lie outside the sinus or protrude into the lower lateral sinus wall. Likewise, the cartotid artery may lie outside the sinus, lie within a sinus septum or may be covered by a partially dehisced wall, predisposing it to injury. It is thus critical to identify the carotid artery on preoperative imaging.[12] The sphenoid sinus commonly (50%) extends laterally to involve the greater sphenoid wing (lateral recess), underlying the middle cranial fossa and the posterior orbital wall. The pterygoid process is less commonly pneumatized (25%). These represent common sites of spontaneous CSF leak into the sphenoid sinus.[13]

Onodi Cell

The Onodi, or sphenoethmoid cell, is a posterior ethmoidal cell that pneumatizes the sphenoid bone, posterior, lateral, and superior to the sphenoid face. It is present

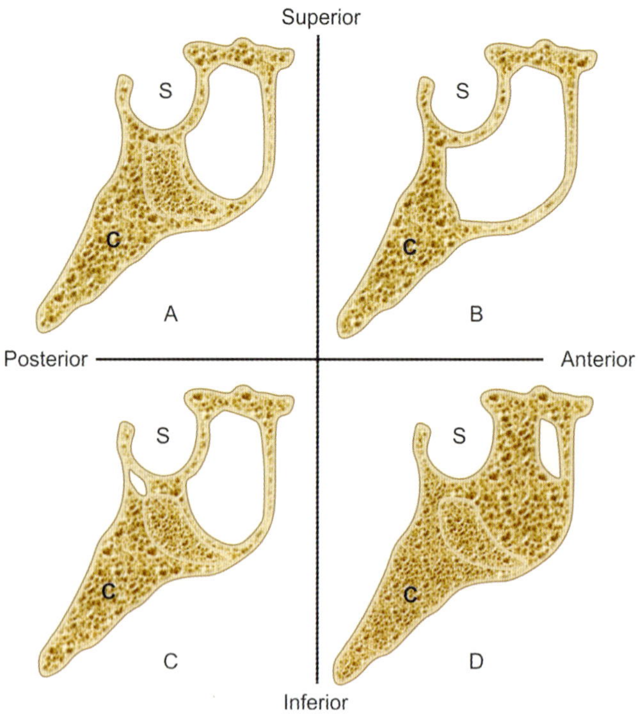

Fig. 3.10: Sphenoid pneumatization patterns: (A) sellar, (B) presellar, (C) conchal, and (D) postsellar. Note the clivus (C) and sella (S).

in 7–25%, with higher prevalence in patients from the Far East and the Indian subcontinent. Recognizing the presence of this cell before and during endoscopic sinus or skull base surgery is important. An Onodi cell may encompass the optic nerve laterally in the posterior ethmoid sinus, making it potentially vulnerable to injury. The presence of an Onodi cell places the sphenoid sinus in a more medial and inferior position, thereby increasing the risk of intracranial penetration if the surgeon expects the sinus to be behind the last posterior ethmoid cell.

Endoscopic Sphenoid Sinus Anatomy

The endoscopic anatomy of the sphenoid sinus has several anatomic landmarks that are important for the endonasal endoscopic surgeon. The midline posterior wall of the sphenoid sinus reveals the sellar protuberance, inferior to which lies the clivus, separated by the sellar-clival junction. Superior and anterior to the sella lies the planum sphenoidale, separated by a thick ridge of bone called the tuberculum sellae, which corresponds to the chiasmatic sulcus intracranially.

The lateral wall of the sphenoid sinus reveals four prominences and three depressions. The prominences, from superior to inferior, are the (1) optic nerve, the (2) parasellar internal carotid artery, the (3) maxillary division, V2 and the (4) mandibular division, V3 of the trigeminal nerve. The three bony depressions of the lateral sphenoid sinus wall are the lateral opticocarotid recess, the depression between the cavernous sinus apex and the maxillary nerve, and the depression between the maxillary and mandibular divisions of the trigeminal nerve (Fig. 3.11).

In addition, the space medial to the junction between the optic nerve and the carotid arteries, called the medial opticocarotid recess, has been labeled the "anatomic keyhole" in endonasal skull base surgery.[14] Nearly 25% of patients may have a bony dehiscence over critical structures such as the optic nerve and the carotid artery. Caution must be exercised in the removal of these septations in order to prevent visual or vascular injury.

Sphenoid Ostium and Sphenoethmoid Recess

The natural sphenoid sinus ostium is located 1.5 cm superior to the posterior choanae on the anterior sphenoid sinus wall. The natural ostium is elliptical in shape and is found in close association with the superior turbinate in the sphenoethmoid recess. In 83% of cases, the ostium is located medial to the superior turbinate and may be visualized with gentle lateralization of the superior turbinate. To further aid craniocaudal localization, if the superior turbinate is divided into horizontal thirds, the natural ostium lies at the junction of the inferior and middle thirds of the superior turbinate.

The sphenoethmoid recess is the narrow vertical corridor enclosed by the septum medially and the superior turbinate laterally. It is defined superiorly by the cribriform plate and inferiorly by the floor of the nasal cavity. The natural sphenoid ostium drains into this corridor, as do the posterior ethmoid cells. Thereafter, mucus continues to the superior meatus, and on to the nasopharynx.

RADIOLOGIC APPROACH

Computer-aided tomography is a volumetric modality that is based on the differential attenuation of X-rays by tissues. Although plain film offers higher spatial resolution, CT benefits from its superb and 3D-capable anatomic definition and density discrimination. CT is additionally valuable as a screening modality for its sensitivity to early osseous involvement, a critical feature in the characterization of sinusitis and sinonasal lesions.[15]

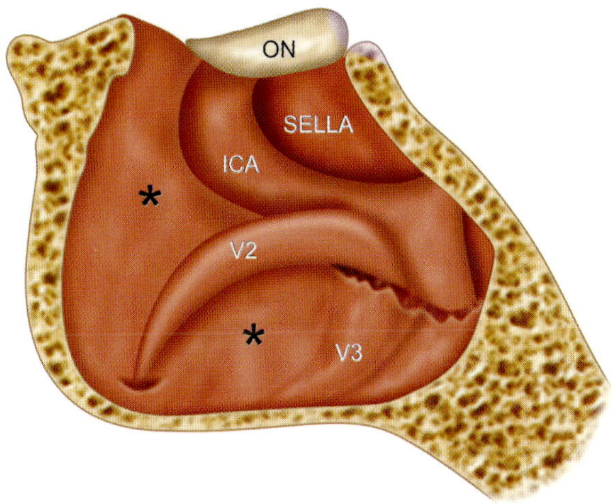

Fig. 3.11: Bony depressions* of the lateral sphenoid sinus wall. Optic nerve (ON), internal carotid artery (ICA), V2 = maxillary nerve, V3 = mandibular nerve.

CT Bone

Effective evaluation of abnormal bone relies on acquiring images with an appropriate bone kernel, a scanner-specific bone-optimized algorithm, and using suitable viewing windows. Bones on a sequence acquired with a "soft-tissue" kernel will appear diffusely sclerotic and thickened, and fine osseous changes may not be apparent. Likewise, fine osseous changes are also difficult to appreciate on contrast-enhanced CT images, which are usually acquired with a soft-tissue kernel.

Bone Thickening and Sclerosis

Bone thickening, as related to the paranasal sinuses, generally reflects a benign process, most frequently chronic sinus disease, whether allergic, odontogenic or polypoid, and may be focal or diffuse. Sclerosis typically accompanies bone thickening, and is recognized by the hyperintensity, or brightness, of dense bone on CT. The presence of sclerosis also suggests an indolent, benign process, whether a reaction to chronic inflammation or a pathologic imbalance between osteoblastic and osteoclastic activity. The recognition of bone thickening and sclerosis often benefits from asymmetry.

Chronic sinus obstruction commonly results in both periosteal thickening and sclerosis of the involved sinus walls. This may affect a single sinus due to ostial obstruction or may present in a pattern involving several sinuses (see *Patterns of Sinus Disease*). Occasionally, a mass may cause obstruction of only a portion of a sinus with focal underlying mural thickening and sclerosis. Such an obstructing mass would most likely be benign, given the necessarily indolent, chronic nature of the associated findings, and may represent a polyp or a fungus ball. Aside from a suggestive rounded contour or subtly higher internal density such a lesion may be difficult to distinguish from adjacent trapped mucus secretions on non-contrast CT imaging.

Occasionally, chronic obstruction results in a pattern of "silent sinus," an incompletely understood sclerotic collapse or atelectasis of the maxillary sinus, associated with cosmetic deformity and enopthalmos (Fig. 3.12).[16] In contrast, the apparent absence of a sinus likely reflects a congenital abnormality, and may be associated with other significant clinical findings (e.g. thalassemia, Kartagener syndrome, Trisomy 21).

Benign Bony Expansion

Reactive bony thickening should be distinguished from bony expansion, a characteristic appearance of several uncommon but benign entities. Fibrous dysplasia is a rare process that represents abnormal fibrous bone tissue filling and expanding the medullary cavity of bone (Figs. 3.13A and B). When present, fibrous dysplasia commonly affects bones of the skull and has a typical hazy "ground-glass" appearance on CT. It is usually limited to one bone (80%), although polyostotic forms occur and may be associated with McCune-Albright syndrome.

Paget's disease (of the bone, i.e. *osteodystrophia deformans*) may also simulate thickening or sclerosis related to sinusitis. This is a benign multistage process of imbalanced bone formation and resorption, resulting in expanded characteristically heterogeneous "woven-bone" appearance, although imaging findings vary with disease stage.

Other lesions that have more focal appearance of bony expansion include osteoma, one of the most common benign tumors of the nose and paranasal sinuses. An osteoma represents a densely sclerotic protruding bone growth which may cause obstruction or deformity (commonly proptosis) if large or unfortunately located.

Odontogenic fibromyxomas are exceedingly rare benign tumors, usually affecting the posterior mandible but occasionally the maxilla, from where they may extend cephalad into the maxillary sinus. They do not have a characteristic appearance on CT and have been described as having a "lacelike," "honeycomb," and "soap bubble" appearance, but also simply "lucent," a generic term for low density on CT.[17] Hemangiomas are much more common, and may have a similar appearance.

Thinning and Remodeling

Thinning and remodeling of the osseous sinonasal structures, whether diffuse or focal, is associated with benign processes, such as mucoceles, allergic fungal sinusitis (AFS) and polyposis.[17] The diffuse expansion of a fluid-filled air cell is a common appearance of a mucocele, which represents a mucus-filled sac that slowly fills up with mucus. Mucoceles should be distinguished from the much more common mucus retention cysts, fluid-filled sacs that do not typically cause mass effect and usually do not remodel adjacent bone. Most mucus retention cysts remain unchanged or shrink over time but rarely may become displaced and cause obstruction. Focal remodeling may also reflect a benign polyp (Figs. 3.14A and B). An "antrochoanal" polyp, referring to its maxillary sinus origin, often causes isolated medial bulging of the medial maxillary sinus wall.

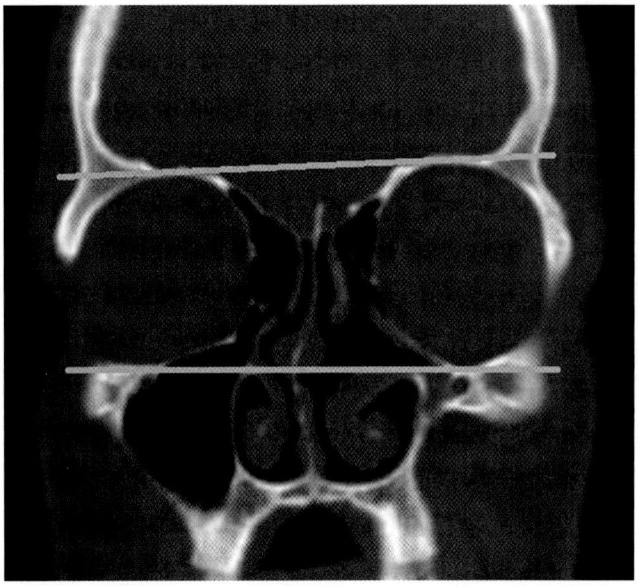

Fig. 3.12: "Silent Sinus" syndrome. Coronal CT demonstrates a shrunken left maxillary sinus with increased craniocaudal diameter of the left orbit as compared with the right (note guide-lines diverging to the left). These are the findings of "silent sinus," maxillary sinus atelectasis that is often accompanied by deformity of the orbital floor, or enopthalmos. This should be distinguished from maxillary sinus hypoplasia, which has normal-appearing orbits.

Notably, certain osseous structures are less able to remodel in response to chronic pressure. These include the floor of the anterior cranial fossa and the skull base. In these locations, mucoceles and AFS instead cause pressure demineralization, which appears as lucent or absent bone (Figs. 3.15A and B).[18] Pressure demineralization is expected to have smooth, mildly bulging margins and may result in appearance of dehiscence or "a hole," which may reverse on removal of the offending process. Pressure demineralization must be carefully distinguished from erosion, which suggests an aggressive or malignant process.

Erosion

Osseous erosion is pathognomonic for an aggressive process, which may reflect neoplasm or infection, and

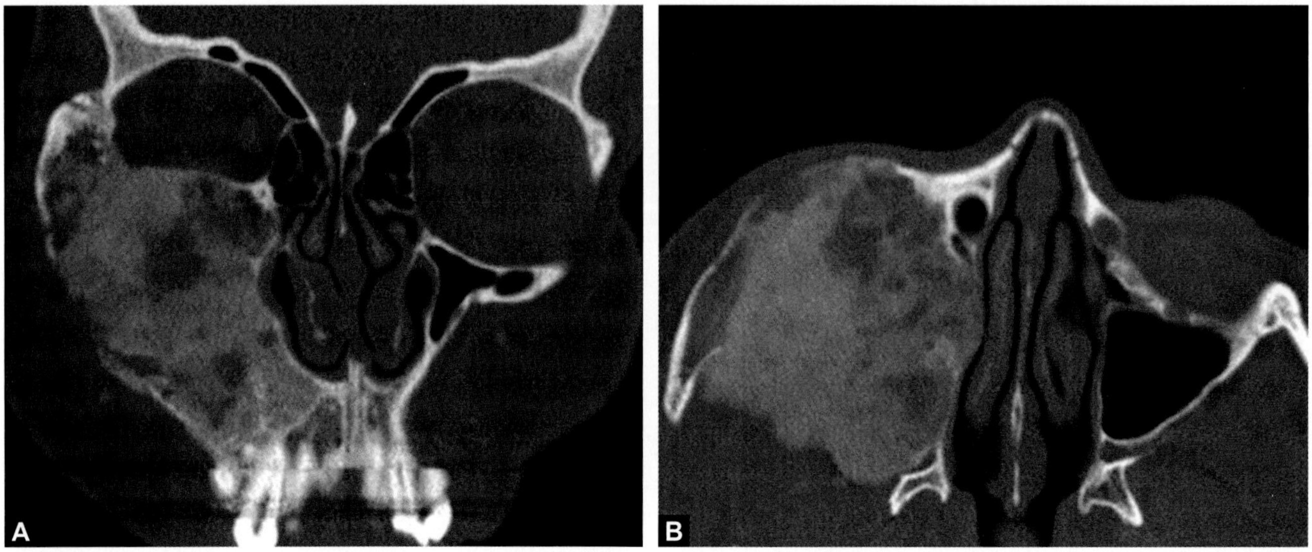

Figs. 3.13A and B: Fibrous dysplasia. (A) Coronal and (B) axial CT demonstrate heterogeneous sclerotic bone expansion of right maxillary marrow space, extending beyond the sinus, with characteristic "ground-glass" appearance that is pathognomonic for fibrous dysplasia, a benign process.

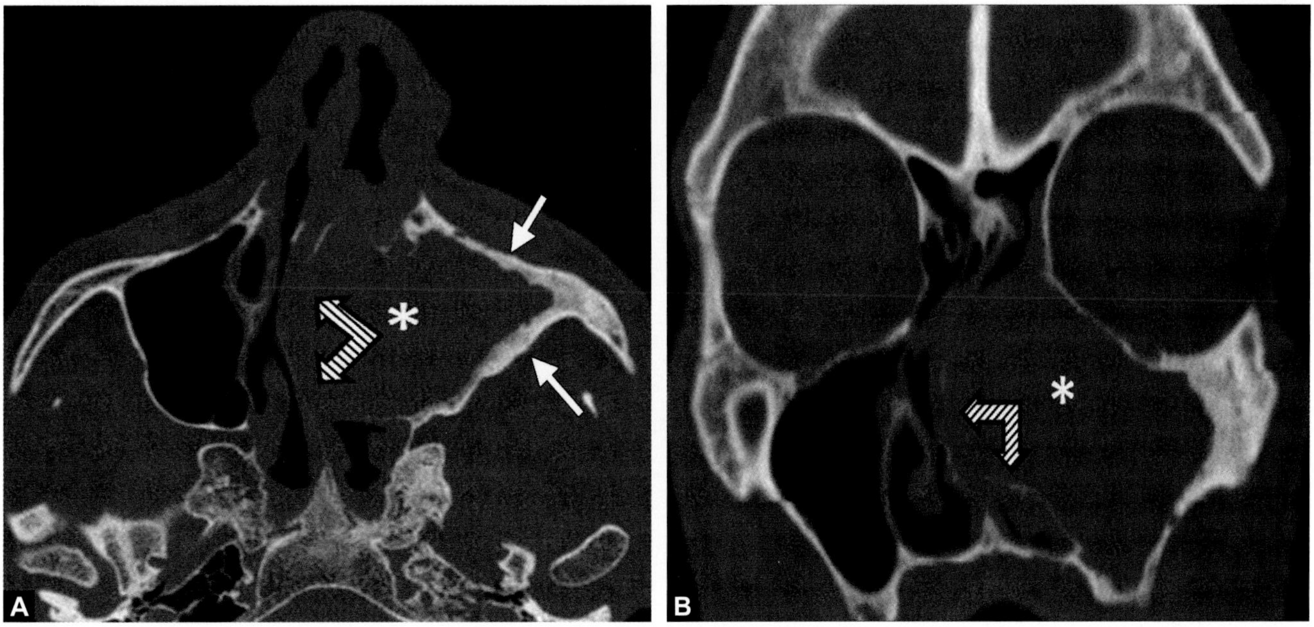

Figs. 3.14A and B: (A) Axial and (B) coronal CT demonstrate periosteal thickening (white arrows), implying a chronic obstructive process. There is focal remodeling (double arrows) of the nasal septum, the medial wall of the left maxillary sinus, and the left middle and inferior turbinates. This represents indolent mass effect, related to chronic obstruction by an antrochoanal polyp (*).

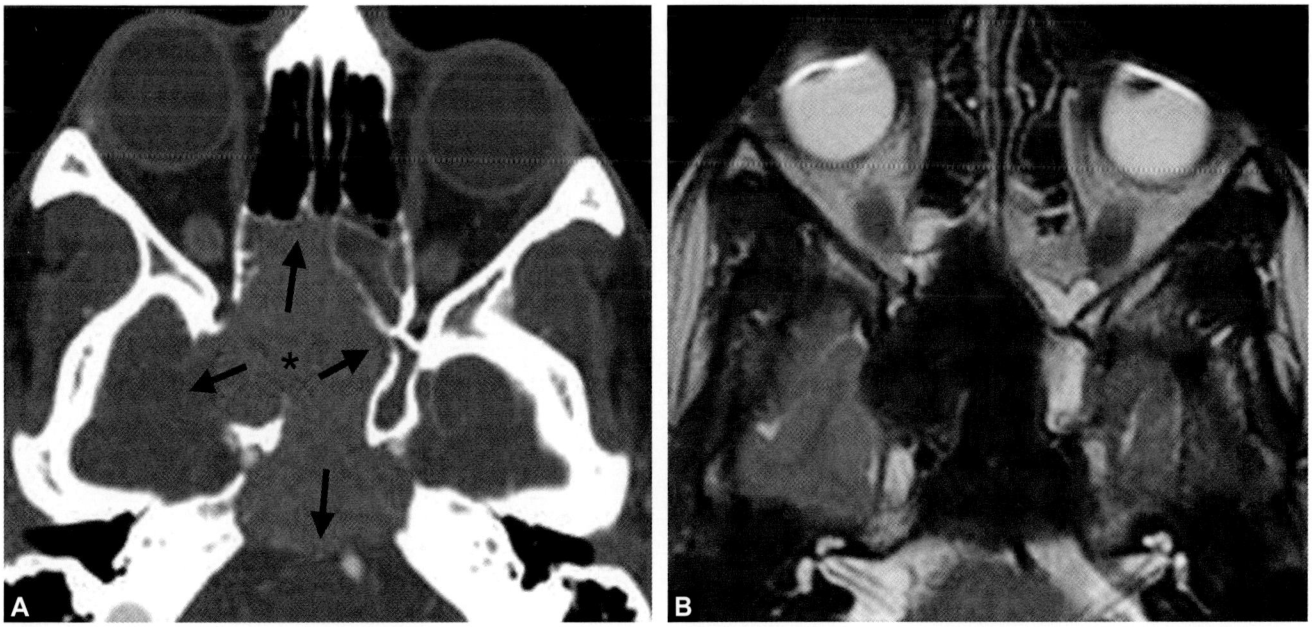

Figs. 3.15A and B: Pressure demineralization. (A) Axial CT demonstrates marked expansion of the right sphenoid sinus (black arrows), a finding fairly specific for mucocele. High density on CT (*) suggests fungal colonization, further supported by (B) T2 signal loss or "drop-out." Postoperative CT better demonstrates the smooth demineralization consistent with a non-aggressive process (not shown).

is best identified as absent bone with sharp or shaggy, irregular margins (Fig. 3.16). Fine irregular calcifications may be seen in place of eroded bone, which may represent residual fragments or tumoral calcification. Erosion must be carefully distinguished from pressure demineralization or remodeling, which are characterized by smooth contours and bulging, implying chronicity and hence benignity. Appearance of bone destruction without

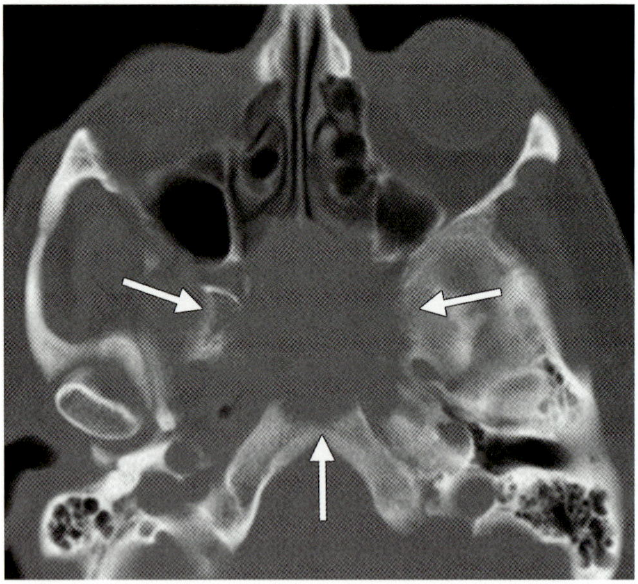

Fig. 3.16: Osseous erosion. Axial CT demonstrates a sphenoid sinus lesion eroding the clivus. Note the margin is irregular and infiltrative (arrows), highly suggestive of an aggressive tumor.

accompanying mass may reflect chronic granulomatous disease or prior surgery. While specific for aggression, absence of bone erosion should not dissuade further work-up; approximately 20% of squamous cell carcinomas (SCC), the most common malignant sinonasal tumors, do not demonstrate osseous destruction on presentation.[19]

CT Soft Tissues

Density

Much as the celsius temperature scale is defined by the freezing and boiling points of water at 0° and 100°, respectively, density on CT is measured in Hounsfield units (HU), a linear scale of electron density where 0 corresponds to water and the much lower density of air is defined as -1,000. Bone is typically 200–400 HU, whereas fat usually measures -100 to -20 HU, varying with contents, such as water from edema, and soft tissue elements.

Fat Density

The differential for a fat density lesion is relatively short and includes: herniated fat related to a bony defect, such as dehiscence of the lamina papyracea with medial protrusion of orbital fat into the ethmoid sinus, fat-packing from prior surgery, or a fat-containing mass, such as dermoid, teratoma, lipoma, or rarely liposarcoma. Certain midline structures may normally but unexpectedly contain fat.

Fluid Density

Normal sinus secretions are predominantly water, with scant protein, and hence normally measure approximately water in density (typically 0 to 20 HU). With accretion and dehydration, sinus secretions may become heterogeneous and significantly denser, although inspissated mucus may be surrounded by relatively hypoattenuating new secretions.

The appearance of a rounded, homogeneous fluid density on CT (typically 0 to 20 HU) is most compatible with a mucus retention cyst or mucocele. Mucoceles, while benign, are typically associated with bulging and thinning (or demineralization) of adjacent bone, and may expand intracranially or intraorbitally, generating symptoms through mass effect (Fig. 3.15). Mucus retention cysts, which are much more common, usually do not remodel adjacent bone, but rarely may become displaced and cause obstruction.

A fluid density mass with smooth, lobulated, or polypoid contours may also represent a polyp (Figs. 3.17A and B). Specifically, extension of a polypoid fluid density mass through the maxillary ostium with nonerosive bony remodeling (possibly inclusive of the septum and turbinates) is strongly suggestive of an "antrochoanal polyp."

Diffuse opacification of the sinuses may reflect sinusitis or polyposis, which may or may not be distinguished by contours, pattern of enhancement or presence of osseous involvement.

Fluid density within the paranasal sinuses does not always represent mucoid secretions, and may instead reflect a CSF leak or meningocele. It is especially important to evaluate for underlying bone dehiscence at the anterior cranial fossa and pterygoid process of the sphenoid sinus, where CSF leaks are relatively common.[13] CT cisternography may be useful in identifying the site of a CSF leak if a diagnosis remains elusive. In this procedure, intrathecal contrast is administered through a lumbar puncture and is expected to pool at the site of a putative CSF leak, extending through the defect and into the sinus (Figs. 3.18A and B). Certain MRI protocols (specifically heavily-T2 weighted sequences such as 3D FIESTA) may also be helpful in better defining local anatomy, and assist in distinguishing a CSF leak from other lesions, such as a mucocele or simple sinus disease (Fig. 3.19).[20,21]

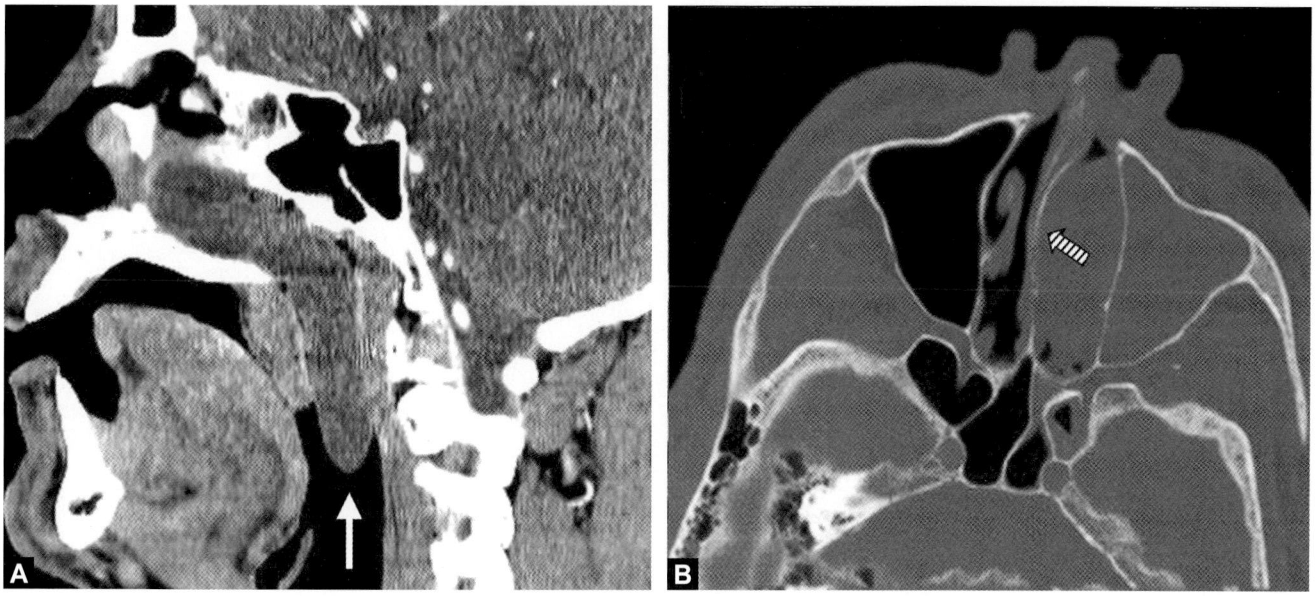

Figs. 3.17A and B: Polyp. (A) Sagittal CT (reconstruction) demonstrates a homogenous fluid density (HU 0-20), with smooth, ovoid contours drooping into the oropharynx (white arrow). (B) Bone kernel axial CT demonstrates benign-appearing bony remodeling (striped arrow) without evidence of erosion compatible with a polyp.

Soft Tissue Density

The appearance of soft tissue density (HU greater than what would be expected for water but less than 80) is most suggestive of cellular or proteinaceous contents, such as a tumor, although history of recent trauma, evidence of traumatic injury or layering density should suggest the possibility of blood products.

The most common sinonasal tumors in adults include: SCC, inverted papilloma (IP), adenocarcinoma, adenoid cystic carcinoma (ACS), sinonasal undifferentiated carcinoma (SNUC), esthesioneuroblastoma, melanoma, sarcoma, lymphoma, and metastases. In children, the most common sinonasal tumors include: juvenile nasopharyngeal angiofibroma (JNA), neurogenic tumors, papilloma, Langerhan's cell hystiocytosis, sarcoma, carcinoma, lymphoma, esthesioneuroblastoma, and metastases (especially neuroblastoma).

Tumors are typically soft tissue in density, although they may contain cystic (fluid-density) components, which may or may not be related to necrosis. It may be difficult to distinguish the borders of a soft tissue density mass from trapped mucus secretions on CT, a role better suited for MRI. Tumors may also contain calcifications, which may reflect the residua of eroded bony walls or nonspecific tumoral calcification.

The apparent center of a lesion, with consideration of mass effect and anatomic impedance to growth, may suggest underlying histology, as certain tumors have strong predispositions to origin or common patterns of disease extension.

Inverted papillomas for example are most commonly centered at the lateral wall of the nasal cavity, often near the middle turbinate and maxillary ostium (Figs. 3.20A to D).

Juvenile nasopharyngeal angiofibromas are hypervascular masses thought to arise from the sphenopalatine foramen. They typically expand the pterygopalatine fossa and subsequently may extend to the masticator space (Chandler's, Fisch's, and Radkowski's stage II). In advanced, stage III disease, intraorbital or intracranial extension may also be seen. Of note, involvement of the skull base is associated with early recurrence.[22,23]

A destructive, heterogeneous lesion centered at the cribriform plate is a common appearance of an esthesioneuroblastoma (olfactory neuroblastoma). These masses may extend to the orbit, which may underly exophthalmos, ophthalmoplegia, and visual loss. Inferior extension may also be seen, with erosion of the nasal septum. Cysts may be seen along the superior tumor margin, especially within the anterior cranial fossa.[24]

Hyperdensity

Very dense sinus contents (>80 HU) should strongly suggest the presence of fungus, with its elevated mineral content. This may reflect simple AFS, which may be accompanied by wall thickening or chronic deformation/expansion (Figs. 3.21A and B), or aggressive fungal

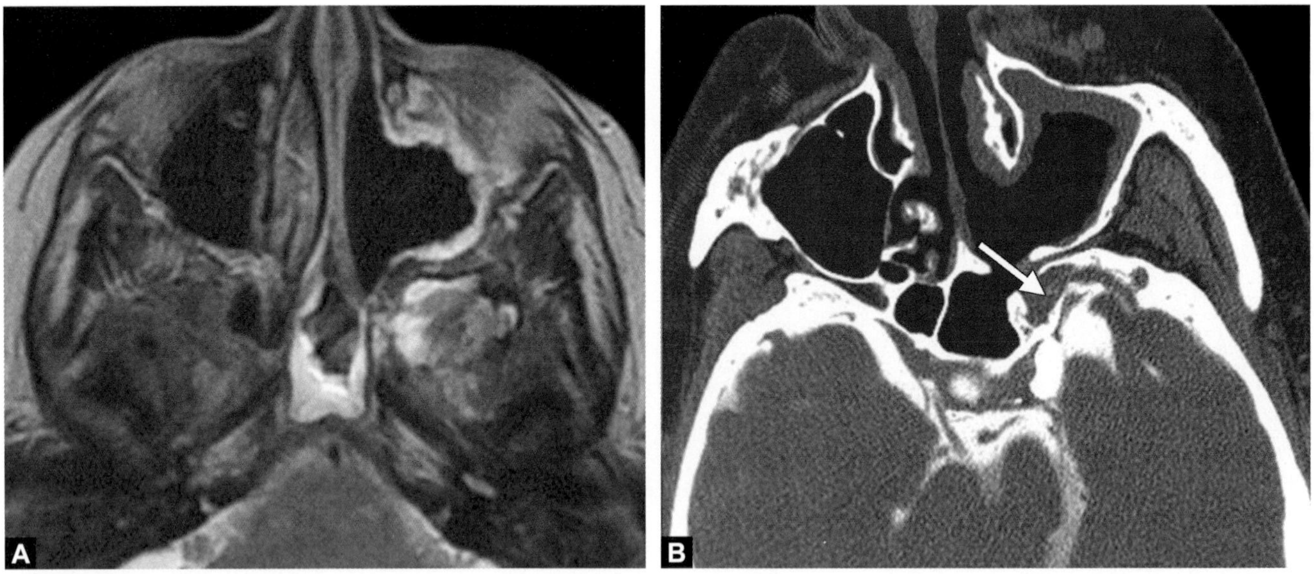

Figs. 3.18A and B: Four years following repair of a CSF leak patient returns with rhinorrhea and concern for recurrent CSF leak. Postoperative changes make the interpretation of this area difficult on (A) axial T2 MRI. (B) Axial CT cisternogram demonstrates hyperattenuating contrast (arrow) extending from the left middle cranial fossa into the lateral recess of the left sphenoid sinus, consistent with CSF leak.

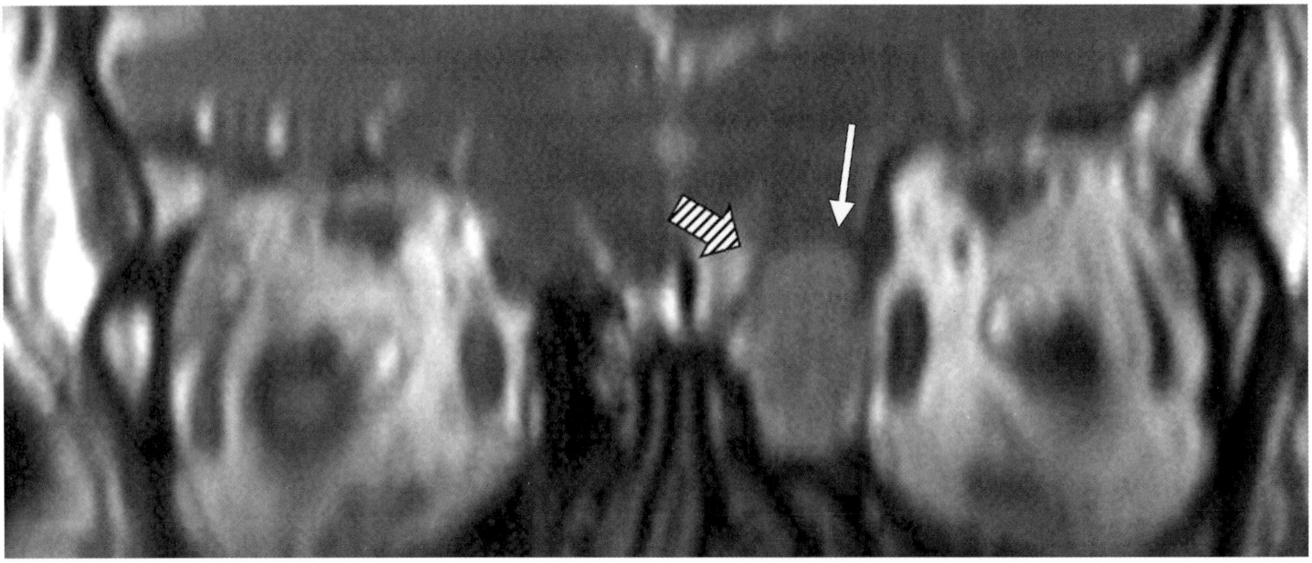

Fig. 3.19: High resolution coronal 3D FIESTA, a fluid-sensitive sequence, can be helpful to better visualize adjacent structures. In this patient with ethmoid mucocele (white arrow), the integrity of the olfactory groove (striped arrow) and the olfactory bulb can be demonstrated to better advantage.

disease, which is expected to demonstrate accompanying bony erosion. Desiccated mucus secretions may also be relatively hyperdense.

Enhancement

Enhancement on CT is related to a structure gaining density through perfusion by intravenously administered hyperdense contrast. Hence, the degree of enhancement is intimately related to contrast dose and vascularity, which equates with the propensity of a mass to bleed after biopsy. Any linear or branching avidly enhancing structure should be suspected of being vascular, and should not be biopsied or otherwise violated without due precaution.

Typically, tumors demonstrate internal "mass-like" and often heterogeneous enhancement, whereas mucosa

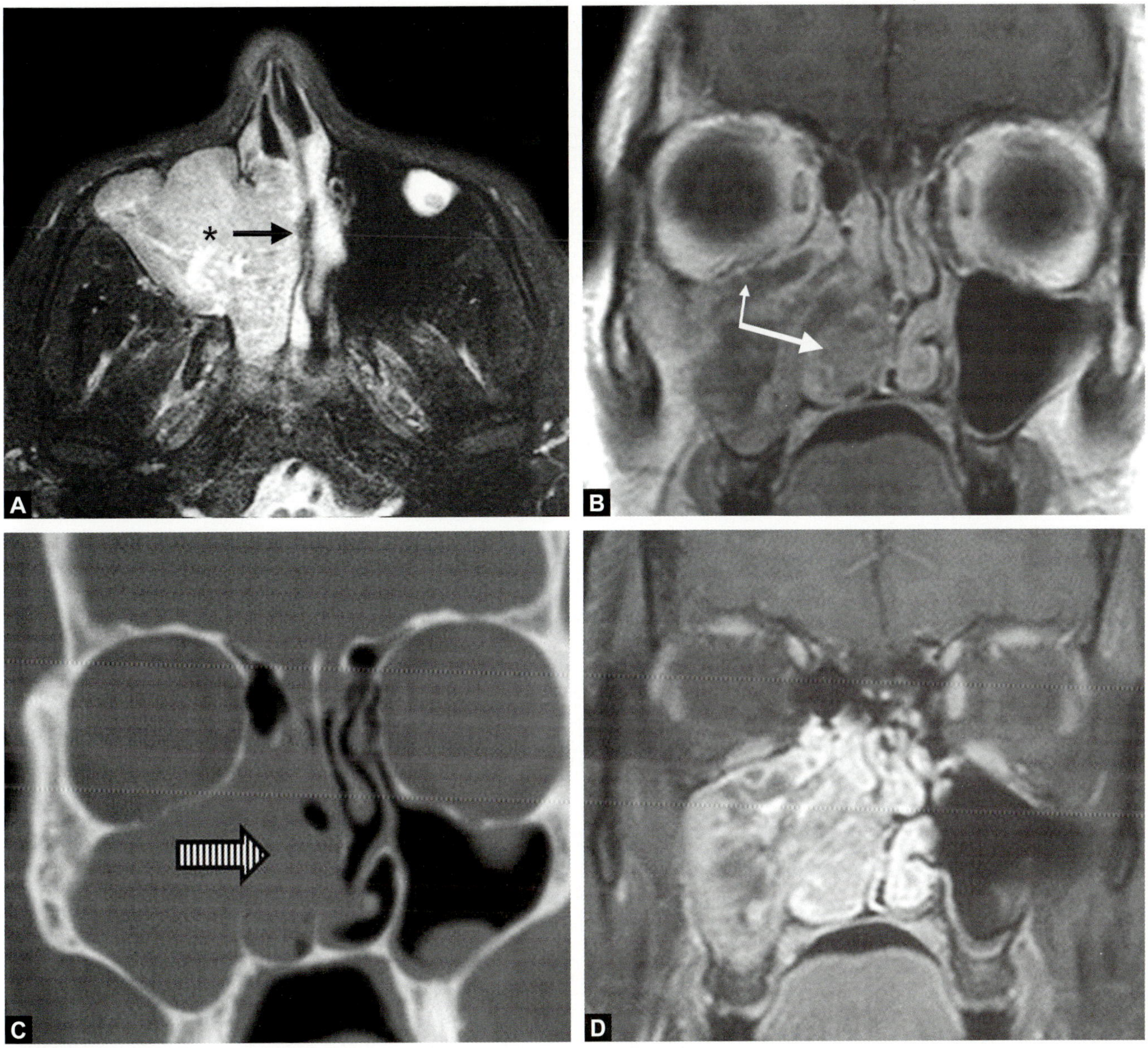

Figs. 3.20A to D: Inverted papilloma (IP) with focal transformation into squamous cell carcinoma (SCC). (A) Axial T2 demonstrates a hyperintense mass lesion expanding the right maxillary sinus (*), with bowing of the nasal septum (black arrow). (B) Coronal T1 precontrast shows remodeling of the orbital floor, with suggestion of destruction of the right inferior and middle turbinates and as well as the medial wall of the right maxillary sinus (double white arrows). Erosive changes are confirmed on (C) Coronal CT (striped arrow), suggesting an aggressive process concurrent with more indolent mass effect. (D) T1 postcontrast shows mass-like enhancement centered in the nasal cavity, as well as nonenhancing trapped sinus secretions in the maxillary sinus.

and abscesses demonstrate relatively homogeneous peripheral enhancement.

Hypervascular tumors, such as JNAs, demonstrate intense homogeneous enhancement, whereas nonhypervascular tumors may heterogeneously or minimally enhance. Differences in pattern of enhancement may be related to heterogeneity in feeding vessel vascularity, necrosis, or presence of cystic components, which do not enhance. Angiography is a useful adjunct modality that can more directly demonstrate the vascularity of a lesion, and may assist in preoperative planning, including embolization.

Magnetic Resonance Imaging

Magnetic resonance imaging relies on the differences in magnetic properties of hydrogen in various molecular

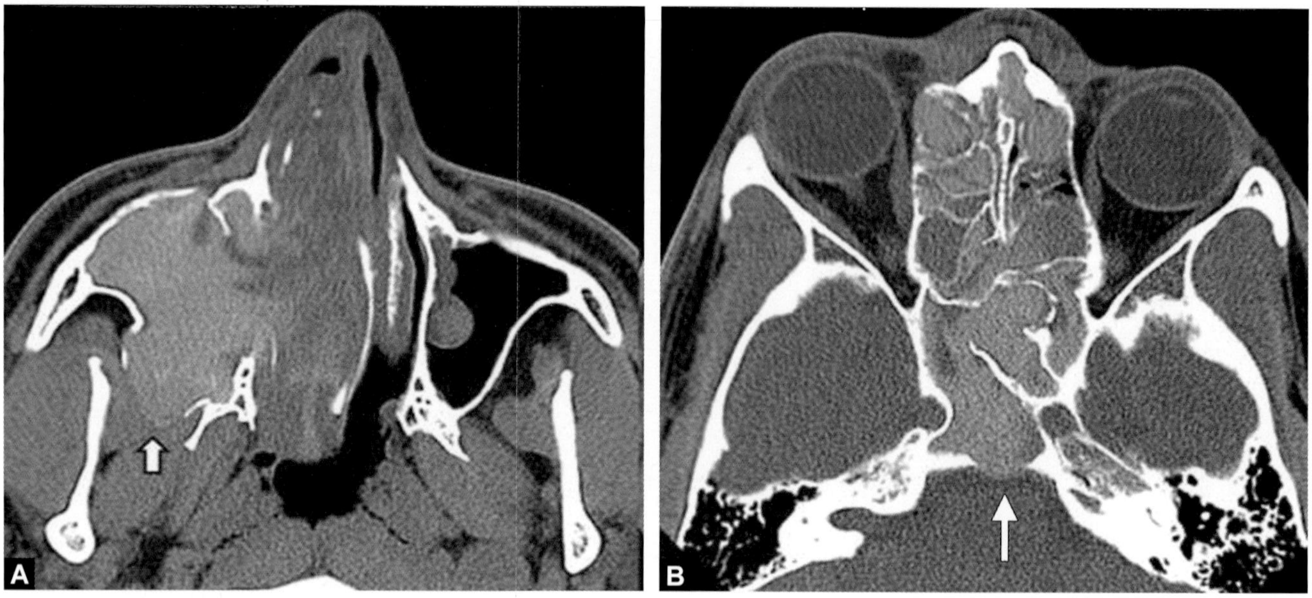

Figs. 3.21A and B: Axial CT images demonstrate diffuse sinus disease with focal expansion and pressure demineralization of the posterior walls of the (A) right maxillary and (B) right sphenoid sinuses (arrows) compatible with chronic, and specifically allergic fungal sinusitis (AFS). Hyperdensity of sinus contents, appreciated on these soft-tissue windows, further supports the presence of fungus.

environments to generate contrast between tissues. While lacking the spatial resolution of CT, and suffering from local field distortion related to paramagnetic effects (iron, air, calcium), MRI has excellent soft tissue contrast as well as the ability to typify molecular environment (e.g., DWI and spectroscopy).

Magnetic resonance imaging particularly excels in characterizing soft tissue masses, such as in discriminating between postobstructive secretions, tumor tissue and scarring, and is able to precisely define tumor extent, including early bone marrow involvement and perineural spread.[25,26] MRI may demonstrate intraosseous extension of a tumor or aggressive infection even before osseous changes in the form of cortical erosion are apparent on CT, especially at the skull base.[25]

It should be emphasized that MRI is not a screening tool, but rather a problem-solving tool. This is because osseous cortical erosion, a hallmark of aggressive sinonasal pathology, is often exceedingly subtle or invisible on MRI, while usually adequately visualized on CT. Nevertheless, lesion appearance and extent on both CT and contrast-enhanced MRI is useful in refining a differential diagnosis if a lesion is identified, and may critically impact the therapeutic approach.

Different MRI sequences or protocols rely on various molecular properties of tissues, and have distinct strengths and weaknesses. In concert, they are very useful in solving a variety of diagnostic problems.

T2

This primary diagnostic sequence is especially sensitive to fluid content. Fluid-containing structures are hyperintense (bright) on T2-weighted sequences, hence inflammatory lesions are often homogeneous and T2-hyperintense.[27] As fluid is replaced by protenaceous content or hemorrhage, whether inspissated mucus or tumor, T2 signal decreases.

Although the majority (80%) of malignant sinonasal cavity tumors are SCC, which have intermediate T2 signal, 10% are hypercellular tumors (lymphomas, olfactory neuroblastomas/PNET, etc.), which have little water content, and appear low to intermediate signal intensity on T2-weighted imaging. Conversely, salivary gland tumors usually have intermediate to high T2-signal, whereas schwannomas are often T2-hyperintense, occasionally with a "*target sign*" appearance typical of an epineurial capsule: low central T2 signal surrounded by high T2 signal intensity. In contrast, neurofibromas are usually not encapsulated, and hence do not demonstrate peripheral T2 hyperintensity.[28] These examples illustrate that both signal intensity and overall appearance may be helpful in refining a differential diagnosis. They furthermore stress that T2-hyperintensity is not equivalent to fluid collection, as some tumors may be T2-hyperintense, but are distinguished by contrast enhancement.[29]

Tissues lacking water, including bone, air and cartilage, appear dark on T2-weighted sequences, as do structures

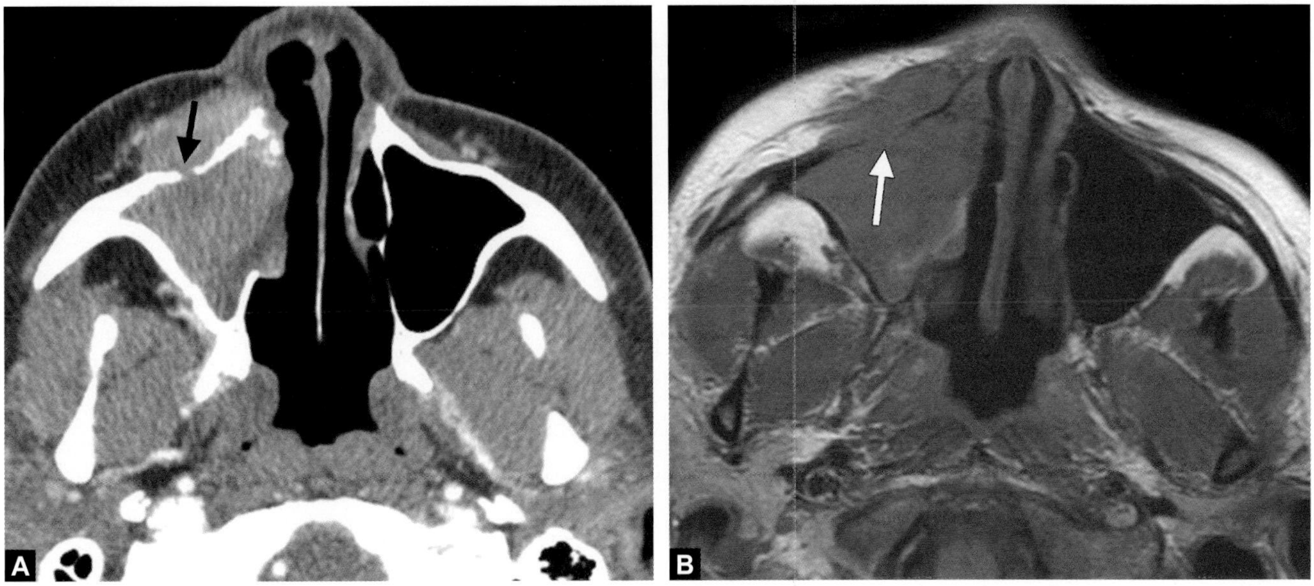

Figs. 3.22A and B: (A) Axial postcontrast CT demonstrates a soft tissue mass in the right maxillary sinus, eroding through the anterior wall (black arrow), which highlights the aggressive nature of this lesion. Although noncontrast axial T1-weighted imaging (B) also demonstrates the osseous erosion (white arrow), the replacement of the expected T1 hyperintense preantral fat by tumor is more apparent.

where signal is lacking for reasons related to high-velocity flow ("flow voids") or magnetic distortion. Magnetic distortion or signal loss may be caused by macroscopic metal (from hardware, foreign bodies), or microscopic minerals within cells, whether related to iron-avid fungus or macrophages associated with hemorrhage or abscess.

T1

This sequence primarily benefits from the native T1-hyperintensity of fat-containing tissues, including the regions surrounding the maxillary sinuses, the orbital contents, and bone-marrow. Replacement of the normally T1-bright premaxillary fat may be the first sign of an aggressive process within the maxillary sinus (Figs. 3.22A and B). Similarly, loss of expected T1-hyperintensity in the orbital apex can be an early indication of aggressive fungal sinusitis. Abnormal marrow signal can be more difficult to interpret, as aggressive and reactive changes may appear similar, and subtle bony erosion may be difficult to appreciate on MRI. In such cases, correlation with CT can be of great value.

In addition to fat, highly protenaceous collections, recent blood products, and various biological cations associated with necrosis (including copper, iron, and manganese) may appear bright on T1-weighted sequences, as can melanin and slow vascular flow. These can usually be distinguished by findings from other MRI sequences, as well as by additional information obtained from CT.

It should be noted that the MRI appearance of calcification varies by the specific molecular form of calcium, which is often not visible for technical reasons. If calcification is seen it usually appears (1) T2-hypointense due to associated paramagnetic ions, (2) dark on all sequences due to lack of mobile water, or (3) hyperintense on T1-weighted imaging.

Contrast-Enhanced MRI

Contrast-enhanced sequences usually refer to T1-weighted sequences obtained following IV administration of gadolinium-containing contrast and employing fat-saturation techniques. Hence, it is important to compare postcontrast sequences to fat-saturated precontrast T1-weighted sequences to evaluate enhancement and to avoid diagnostic blunders.

Contrast-enhanced T1-sequences are superb in delineating lesion extent and margins, which may critically impact therapeutic approach. Postcontrast sequences are helpful in differentiating a T2-hyperintense mass from a cyst, and are likewise useful in distinguishing mass from adjacent retained secretions and scar tissue. Diagnostically it is especially important to distinguish the smooth contours of mucosal enhancement, and thick rim enhancement of abscesses, from mass-like enhancement

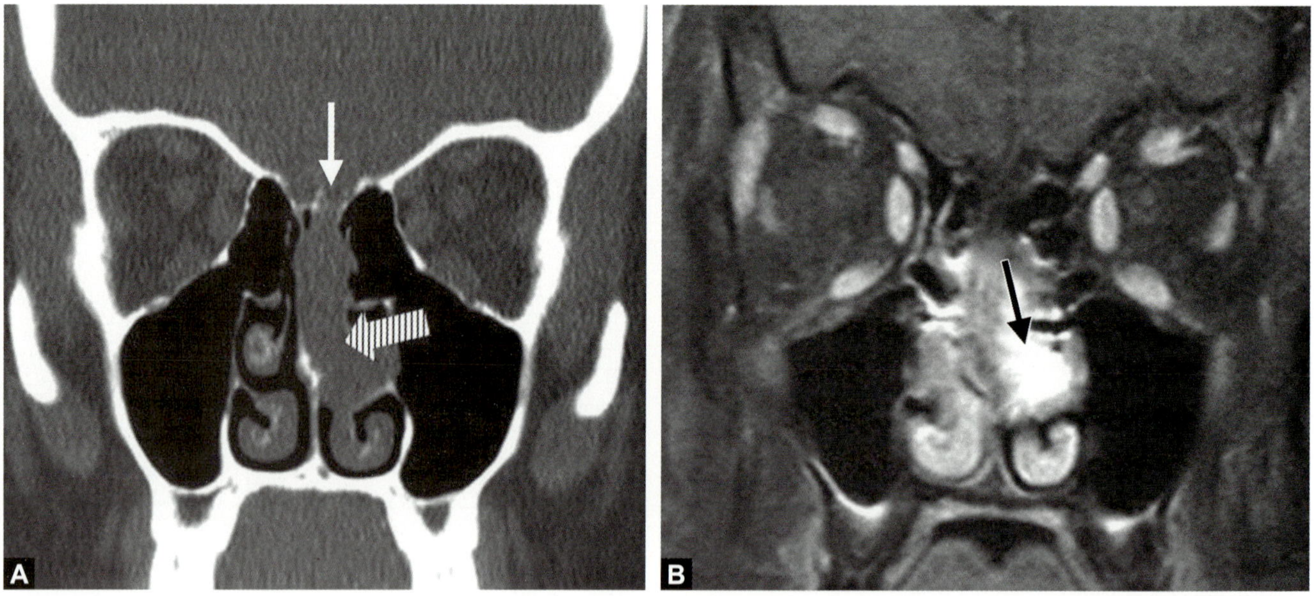

Figs. 3.23A and B: (A) Coronal CT demonstrates nonspecific opacity below the left cribriform plate (white arrow), which can be easily mistaken for sinus secretions. Note the absence of left middle turbinate (striped arrow) which is worrisome for erosion from an aggressive process. Postcontrast coronal T1 (B) demonstrates an enhancing mass (black arrow). The differential for mass enhancement in this region includes squamous cell carcinoma (SCC), hemangipericytoma, esthesioneuroblastoma, sinonasal undifferentiated carcinoma (SNUC), and lymphoma.

of tumors (Figs. 3.23A and B). Contrast-enhanced MR imaging may also help to grade mass vascularity, which may be useful for preoperative planning.

Postcontrast images can also improve detection of perineural spread of a tumor. In patients with tumors such SCC and sinonasal ACC, which have a high predilection for perineural spread, close attention should be paid to trigeminal nerve branches within the pterygopalatine fossa, as enhancement within foramen rotundum, infraorbital fissure (V2), and foramen ovale (V3) are strongly suggestive of perineural spread.

Diffusion-Sensitive Sequences

Diffusion-weighted imaging is a T2-weighted sequence that is sensitive to the microscopic flow of water molecules. In regions where this flow is limited or "restricted" the DWI signal will be bright. The same region will appear dark on a mathematically calculated complementary sequence called apparent diffusion coefficient (ADC).

Restricted diffusion typically reflects hypercellularity (decreased extracellular water, and high nuclear to cytoplasmic ratio in a mass) or (highly protenaceous) viscous fluid.

A diffusion-restricting, enhancing mass centered within the sinonasal cavity most likely represents lymphoma, a prototypical hypercellular mass, which often has a bulky appearance, demonstrates hypointense signal on T2-weighted imaging, and moderate enhancement (Figs. 3.24A to C). Lymphomas, especially high grade lymphomas, may remodel or destroy bone (e.g., nasal septal perforation is often associated with nasal T-cell lymphomas), hence it is important to look for signs of osseous involvement on CT bone windows and MRI T1 sequences. Other typically hypercellular tumors include neuroblastoma, fibrous histiocytoma, and sarcoma.

Viscous fluid collections, such as highly proteinaceous mucous retention cysts and abscesses, will also restrict diffusion. Postcontrast sequences can help distinguish these from hypercellular masses, which should demonstrate solid, "mass-like" enhancement, as opposed to rim enhancement of fluid collections (Figs. 3.25A to D).[30]

The appearance of DWI signal hyperintensity without corresponding low signal on ADC sequences likely reflects "T2 shine-through," an artifact related to underlying T2 signal hyperintensity rather than restricted diffusion.

Complementary Modalities

Positron emission tomography (PET) is a physiologic test, which measures relative glucose metabolism in tissues, and relies on the notion that standard uptake values are elevated in tumors and inflammatory processes

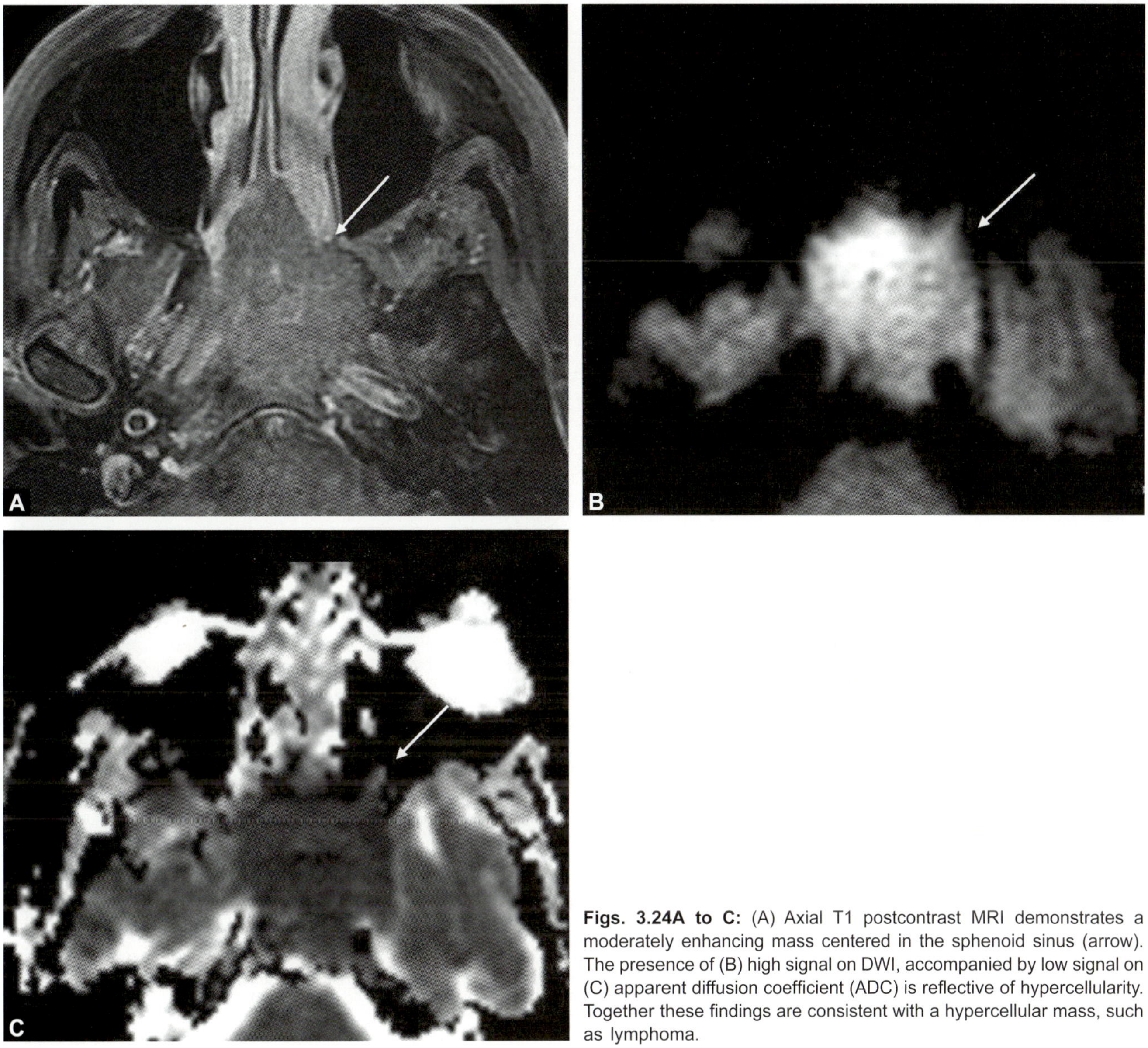

Figs. 3.24A to C: (A) Axial T1 postcontrast MRI demonstrates a moderately enhancing mass centered in the sphenoid sinus (arrow). The presence of (B) high signal on DWI, accompanied by low signal on (C) apparent diffusion coefficient (ADC) is reflective of hypercellularity. Together these findings are consistent with a hypercellular mass, such as lymphoma.

(Fig. 3.26). PET may be useful for discriminating between postirradiative changes and tumor recurrence; however, its low spatial resolution limits its sensitivity for local disease and small masses. Although PET may confirm presence of a tumor in the sinonasal cavity, its primary role is the detection of distal metastases or systemic involvement in granulomatous disease.[31]

Angiography is an adjunct modality that may lead to a more accurate diagnosis if a vascular mass is suspected, and which may facilitate preoperative embolization to reduce risk of hemorrhage (Figs. 3.27A to C).

CONCLUSIONS

The essence of an effective radiologic approach to the sinonasal region rests on a thorough knowledge of the anatomy and a basic understanding of the relevant imaging modalities combined with a reasoned, systematic reading pattern. While knowledge of typical features of common entities may be helpful in narrowing the differential diagnosis, the goal of imaging should be to solve essential problems of screening: distinguishing normal from abnormal, chronic versus acute, focal from diffuse, and indolent from aggressive.

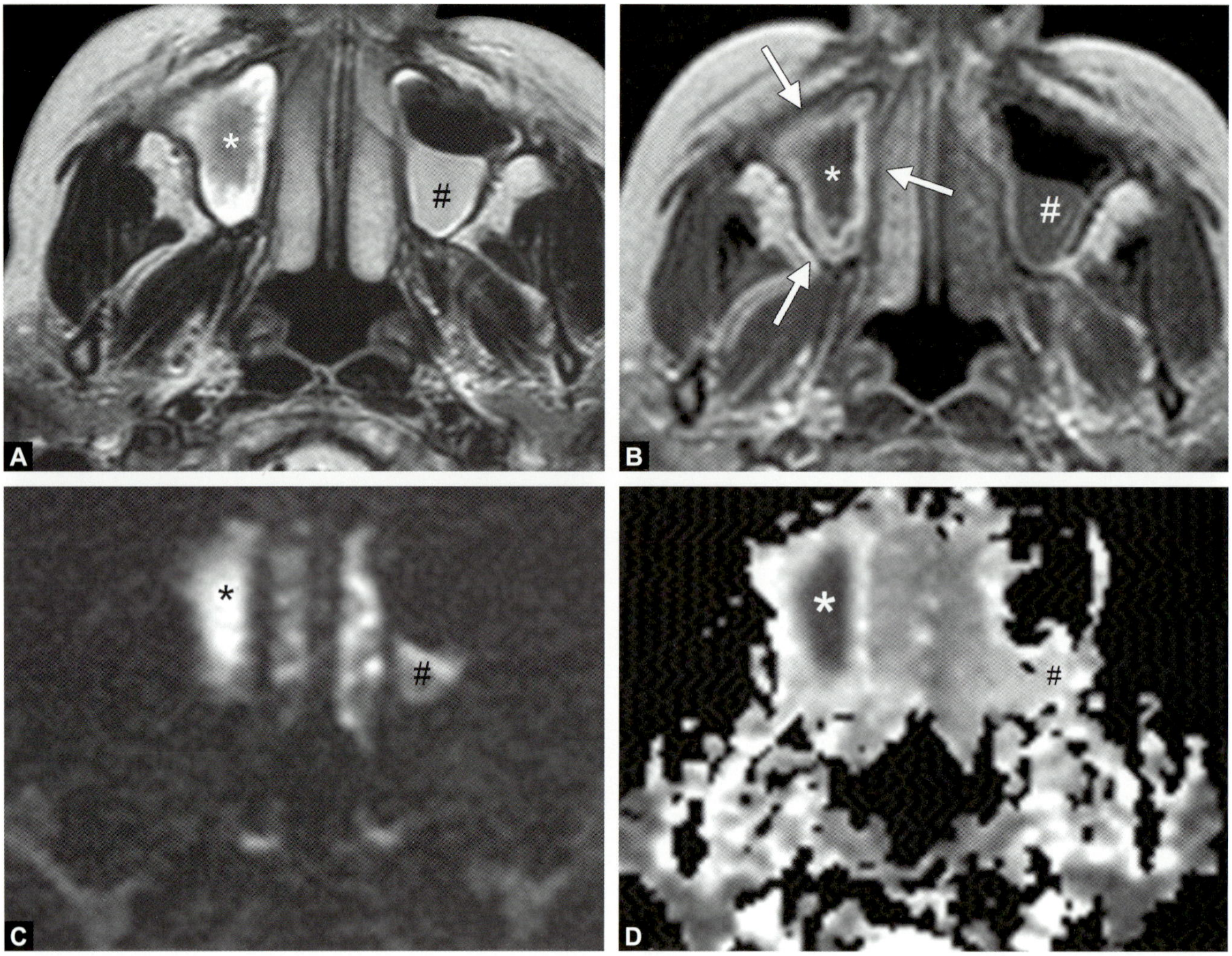

Figs. 3.25A to D: (A) Axial T2-weighted, (B) T1 postcontrast, (C) DWI, and (D) ADC images demonstrate that restricted diffusion does not always relate to hypercellularity. In this case, flow is restricted due to a viscous effusion reflecting acute on chronic sinusitis. This is supported by the rim enhancement (arrows) of the sinus mucosa and absence of enhancement of the area that demonstrates restricted diffusion (*). An abscess would also demonstrate restricted diffusion and rim enhancement but would be centrally T2 hyperintense reflecting its fluid content, rather than T2 hypointense reflecting inspissated fluid. Note the relatively simple fluid in the left maxillary sinus (#).

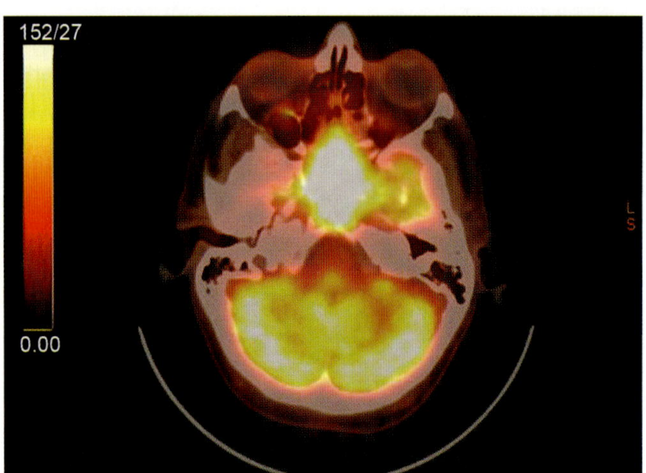

Fig. 3.26: Fusion of axial CT and PET demonstrates marked FDG uptake in the sphenoid sinus representing a hypermetabolic mass, in this case a biopsy-proven lymphoma.

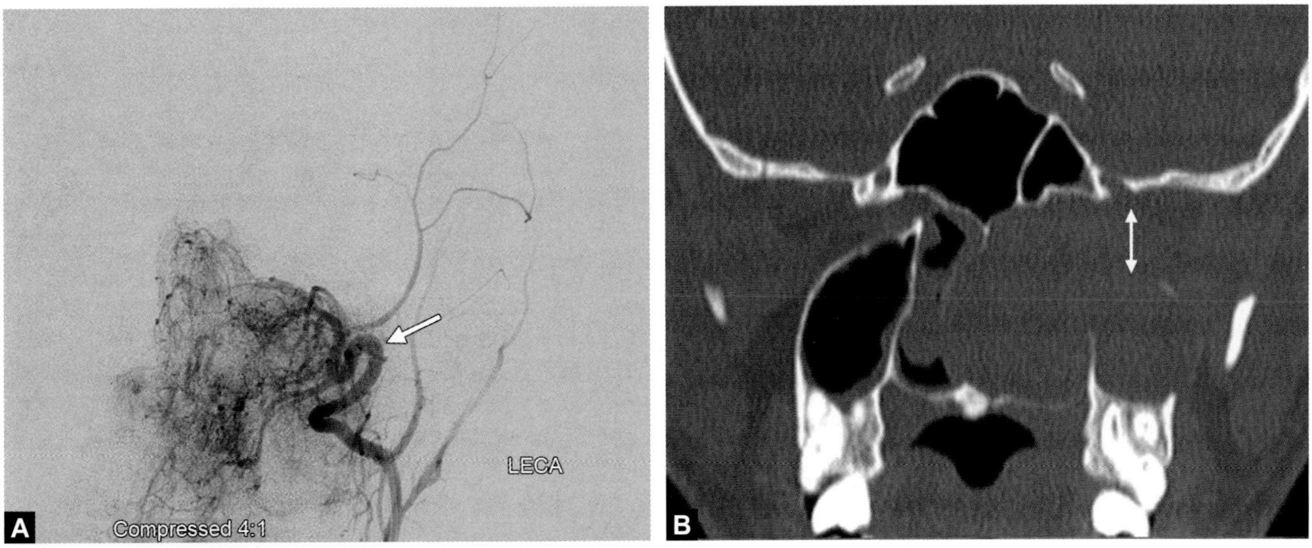

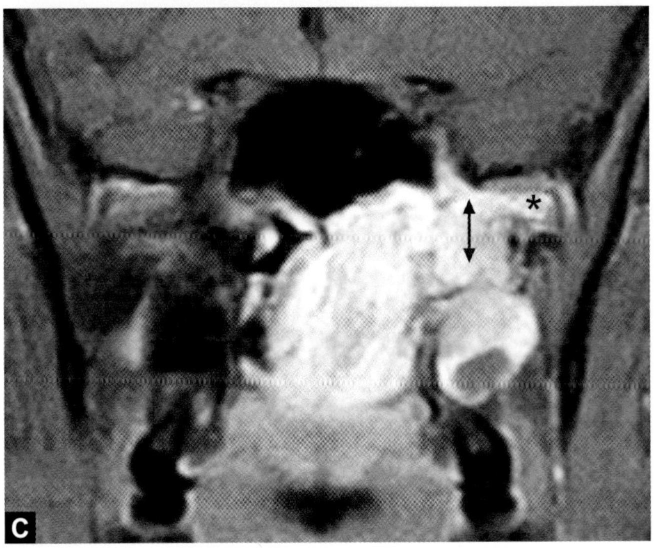

Figs. 3.27A to C: Juvenile angiofibroma. (A) AP angiography view following injection of the left ECA (arrow) demonstrates the characteristic hypervascular appearance of a juvenile angiofibroma (JNA). Preoperative embolization reduces intraoperative blood loss, minimizes the need of blood transfusion, and makes resection easier.[32] (B) Coronal CT and (C) postcontrast MRI demonstrate expansion of the left pterygopalatine fossa (double arrows) without destruction, with enhancing soft tissue seen extending to the infratemporal fossa (*), a classic appearance of JNA.

REFERENCES

1. Som PS, Curtin HD (Eds). Head and Neck Imaging, Vol. 1. St. Louis: CV Mosby; 2003. pp. 87-147.
2. Ruíz DSM, Gailloud P, Rüfenachta DA, et al. Anomalous intracranial drainage of the nasal mucosa: a vein of the foramen caecum? AJNR Am J Neuroradial. 2006;27:129-31.
3. Singh A, Wessell AP, Anand VK, et al. Surgical anatomy and physiology for the skull base surgeon. Operative Techn Otolaryngol. 2011;22:184-93.
4. Beale TJ, Madani G, Morley SJ. Imaging of the paranasal sinuses and nasal cavity: normal anatomy and clinically relevant anatomical variants. Semin Ultrasound CT MR. 2009;30(1):2-16.
5. Reddy UD, Dev B. Pictorial essay: Anatomical variations of paranasal sinuses on multidetector computed tomography-How does it help FESS surgeons? Indian J Radiol Imaging. 2012;22(4):317-24.
6. Santiago R, Villalonga P, Maggioni A. Nasal septal abscess: A case report. Int Pediatr. 1999;14:229-31
7. Maroldi R, Nicolai P (Eds). Imaging in Treatment Planning for Sinonasal Diseases. Berlin: Springer-Verlag; 2005.
8. Reeder MR, Bradley, WG Jr., Merritt CR. Reeder and Felson's Gamuts in Radiology and 4.0 Web Version: Comprehensive Lists of Imaging Differential Diagnoses; 2003.
9. Keros P. On the practical value of differences in the level of the lamina cribrosa of the ethmoid. Z Laryngol Rhinol Otol. 1962;41:809-13.
10. Sonkens JW, Harnsberger HR, Blanch GM, et al. The impact of screening sinus CT on the planning of functional endoscopic sinus surgery. Otolaryngol Head Neck Surg. 1991; 105:802-13.
11. Sirikci A, Bayazit YA, Bayram M, et al. Variations of sphenoid and related structures. Eur Radiol. 2000;10(5):844-8.
12. Fernandez-Miranda JC, Prevedello DM, Madhok R, et al. Sphenoid septations and their relationship with internal

carotid arteries: anatomical and radiological study. Laryngoscope. 2009;119(10):1893-6.
13. Shetty PG, Shroff MM, Fatterpekar GM, et al. A retrospective analysis of spontaneous sphenoid sinus fistula: MR and CT findings. AJNR Am J Neuroradiol. 2000;21:337-42.
14. Sindou M (Ed). Practical Handbook of Neurosurgery: From Leading Neurosurgeons, Vol. 1. New York: Springer-Verlag; 2009. p. 203.
15. Rao VM, El-Noueam KI. Sinonasal imaging. Radiol Clin North Am. 1998;36(5):921-39.
16. Illner A, Davidson HC, Harnsberger HR, et al. The silent sinus syndrome: clinical and radiographic findings. AJR 2002;178:503-6.
17. Reddy GSP, Kumar BS, Muppa R, et al. Odontogenic fibromyxoma of maxilla: a rare case report. Case Rep Dent. 2013; 2013:345479.
18. Jackson AR. Bone thinning in frontal mucocele. Br J Radiol. 1977;50(591):181-4.
19. Kennedy DW, Bolger WE, Zinreich SJ (Eds). Diseases of the Sinuses: Diagnosis and Management. Ontario: BC Decker; 2001. p. 145.
20. Stone JA, Castillo M, Neelon B, et al. Evaluation of CSF leaks: high-resolution CT compared with contrast-enhanced CT and radionuclide cisternography. AJNR 1999;20:706-12.
21. Tyagi I, Syal R, Goyal A. Cerebrospinal fluid otorhinorrhoea due to inner-ear malformations: clinical presentation and new perspectives in management. J Laryngol Otol. 2005;119(9):714-8.
22. Radkowski D, McGill T, Healy GB, et al. Angiofibroma. Changes in staging and treatment. Arch. Otolaryngol. Head Neck Surg. 1996;122 (2):122-9.
23. Kania RE, Sauvaget E, Guichard JP, et al. Early Postoperative CT scanning for juvenile nasopharyngeal angiofibroma: detection of residual disease. AJNR 2005;26:82-8.
24. Broich G, Pagliari A, Ottaviani F. Esthesioneuroblastoma: a general review of the cases published since the discovery of the tumour in 1924. Anticancer Res. 1997;17(4A):2683-706.
25. Nemzek WR, Hecht S, Gandour-Edwards R, et al. Perineural spread of head and neck tumors: how accurate is MR imaging? AJNR Am J Neuroradiol. 1998;19:7016.
26. Shy CG, Chen CC, Chen WH, et al. Comparison of CT with MRI for the evaluation of the juxta-oral tumor. Chin J Radiol. 2003;28:1-8.
27. Hurt CJ, Yousem DM, Beauchamp NJ (Eds). Head and Neck. Holland-Frei Cancer Medicine, 6th edition. Hamilton, Ontario: BC Decker; 2003.
28. Koga H, Matsumoto S, Manabe J, et al. Definition of the target sign and its use for the diagnosis of schwannomas. Clin Orthop Relat Res. 2007;464:224-9.
29. Genden EM, Varvares MA (Eds). Head and Neck Cancer: An Evidence-Based Team Approach. Thieme, 2008. Carcinoma of the Nasal Cavity and Paranasal Sinus.
30. Chawla S, Kim S, Wang S, et al. Diffusion-weighted imaging in head and neck cancers. Future Oncol. 2009;5(7): 959-9.
31. Ramakrishnan VR, Lee JY, O'Malley BW Jr. et al. 18-FDG-PET in the initial staging of sinonasal malignancy. Laryngoscope. 2013;123(12):2962-6.
32. Giavroglou C, Constantinidis J, Triaridis S, et al. Angiographic evaluation and embolization of juvenile nasopharyngeal angiofibroma. HNO. 2007;55(1):36-41.

CHAPTER 4

Patient Selection and Evaluation

Abtin Tabaee

INTRODUCTION

Integral to any surgical procedure is a comprehensive understanding of its indications. Although the role of a given surgery may be generally defined by disease- and patient-related factors, the decision-making process is often complex. Indeed, often the most difficult question is not how to perform a given procedure but whether to perform the procedure in the first place. Algorithms and treatment guidelines are available and are based on clinical outcome studies and position statements by thought leaders in the field. However, the application of these principles to a specific patient requires individualized analysis and appropriate diagnostic testing. Compounding the complexity of this process is the constantly evolving nature of medicine as scientific research and developing technologies continue to advance surgical procedures. This chapter aims to review the available methods in evaluating a patient with sinonasal symptoms and discuss the indications for surgery in different clinical scenarios.

PATIENT EVALUATION

History and Examination

A systematic method of evaluating a patient with sinonasal symptoms is critical for successful treatment. Although there is variability among clinicians, common principles apply and an understanding of the various diagnostic tests is necessary. The initial and most important step is performing a thorough clinical history. This entails obtaining a description of the presenting symptoms, associated symptoms, temporal trends in the symptoms, past medical and surgical history, medication usage, recreational and social habits, and occupational exposures. The patient's use of prior therapies for the current condition and clinical response should be assessed. A prior history of sinonasal disorders, therapies, and surgeries should be discussed. Although each patient presentation is unique, common sinonasal symptoms suggestive of inflammatory sinusitis should be queried including nasal congestion/obstruction, facial pain/pressure, mucopurulent rhinorrhea, postnasal drip, fatigue, malaise, and hyposmia. Pulmonary symptoms concerning for reactive airway disease should be discussed including cough, shortness of breath, wheeze, and chest tightness. Otologic symptoms including hearing loss, ear popping, imbalance, and ear pain may represent Eustachian tube dysfunction, referred otalgia, or possible otitis media. Symptoms typical of allergic rhinitis should be reviewed including sneezing, itchiness (eyes, throat, nose, ear, skin), watery rhinorrhea, watery epiphora, and nasal congestion. Finally, atypical symptoms including epistaxis, facial swelling, cranial nerve symptoms, severe headache, fever, and orbital symptoms may raise the suspicion for a more serious condition including neoplasm or impending infectious complication from sinusitis (orbital, intracranial).

Evaluation of a patient with sinonasal pathology includes a complete otolaryngologic examination. Specific findings that are common in patients with sinonasal disorders are outlined in Table 4.1. Nasal endoscopy is a routine and critical tool in the evaluation of a patient with sinonasal pathology. This is reviewed elsewhere in this text and will only be briefly discussed here. The primary goal of nasal endoscopy is to assess anatomic- and pathologic-related findings of the nasal cavity, middle meatus, sphenoethmoid recess, nasopharynx, and, in patients with a prior history of sinus surgery, the paranasal sinus cavities. The procedure is generally well tolerated and is technically easy to perform. Simultaneous instrumentation including suctioning, palpation, culture, and biopsy increase the diagnostic utility of the procedure. The incorporation of both flexible and rigid endoscopes allows for a more versatile examination. Diagnostic findings can be identified including those related to anatomic, inflammatory, and neoplastic disorders.

Table 4.1: Examination findings in patients with sinonasal disorders

Organ System	*Findings*
General appearance	Toxicity level, nutritional status, communication, overall well being, nasality
Face	Swelling, erythema, focal tenderness over the forehead and malar areas
Ears	Tympanic membrane and middle ear inflammatory changes, hearing loss
Oropharynx	Posterior pharyngeal wall inflammation, cobblestoning, postnasal drip-related secretions, possible concomitant pharyngitis
Neck	Cervical lymphadenopathy
Eyes	Orbital swelling, proptosis, extraocular muscle function, visual acuity, gross visual fields, pupil function
Nasal cavity	Nasal septum deviation, anterior mucosal inflammatory changes (erythema, edema, purulence), inferior turbinate hypertrophy
Neurologic	Cranial nerve dysfunction, mental status evaluation including olfactory evaluation
Respiratory	Inflammatory findings on auscultation of the chest, respiratory status

Radiography

Radiographic testing of sinonasal disorders is an essential adjunct to history and examination. Several imaging modalities are available depending on the clinical needs. Plain film studies have largely been replaced by computed tomography (CT) and magnetic resonance imaging (MRI) given the improved anatomic detail, sensitivity, and specificity. Additional studies including angiography, positron emission testing, cisternography, and radionuclide studies have a role in specific clinical situations and are used selectively. For patients with suspected inflammatory sinusitis, CT ideally details the relationship between mucosal changes and the surrounding bony sinonasal framework. Diagnostic assessment focuses largely on the location, severity, and radiographic qualities of the inflammatory changes. Various patterns of disease can be noted including polypoid, fungal, anatomic variants, and odontogenic etiologies. Detailed inspection of the images additionally provides a triplanar road map for surgical planning. This includes identification of the extent of disease and associated extent of surgery. Critical neurovascular structures, anatomic variants, and specific bony landmarks are detailed in preparation for surgery. Image acquisition protocols with 1 mm thin slices provide data sets that can be used for intraoperative image guidance. The inclusion of intravenous contrast with the CT scan is useful in patients with possible infectious intraorbital or intracranial complications.

In patients with complex sinonasal and skull base disorders including neoplasm, a combination of CT and MRI is considered for complete pretreatment evaluation of disease extent and location. CT is superior in delineating expansion of neurovascular foramina and the bony integrity of the orbit and skull base, but has a limited ability to differentiate soft tissue lesions from inflammatory changes including postobstructive sinusitis. Conversely, MRI provides superior detail in evaluation of the soft tissue extension of the lesion and surrounding neurovascular structures, but is limited in bony detail (Figs. 4.1A and B). Inclusion of MRI should be considered in patients with sinonasal and skull base neoplasms and infectious complications of sinusitis involving the orbit or intracranial cavities (Fig. 4.2).

Tissue and Mucous Analysis

In addition to clinical and radiographic evaluation of sinonasal disorders, diagnostic information in the form of tissue and mucous analysis is critical in determining appropriate treatment. In patients with inflammatory sinusitis, endoscopic guided, transnasal culture of the middle meatus, or paranasal sinus cavities is associated with similar diagnostic yield when compared with specimens obtained through maxillary sinus aspirate.[1] The identification of specific microbiologic organisms and their antimicrobial sensitivity pattern has critical clinical utility in the medical management of patients with chronic rhinosinusitis (CRS), especially refractory disease. Cultures may be repeated throughout the course of therapy and are especially useful in patients with resistant organisms.

Tissue histopathology in patients with CRS is useful in phenotypic subcategorization including distinction among polypoid, eosinophillic, and fungal variants. The tissue is most commonly obtained at the time of surgery and diagnostic clarity is aided by close communication with the pathology team. Specialized histopathologic testing in the form ciliary beat frequency is necessary in patients with suspected ciliary dyskinesia.

The other primary role of tissue histopathology is in patients with suspected sinonasal neoplasm. Pretreatment biopsy of sinonasal lesions is necessary to differentiate among the greater than 25 types of neoplasms, as described by the World Health Organization.[2] Given the

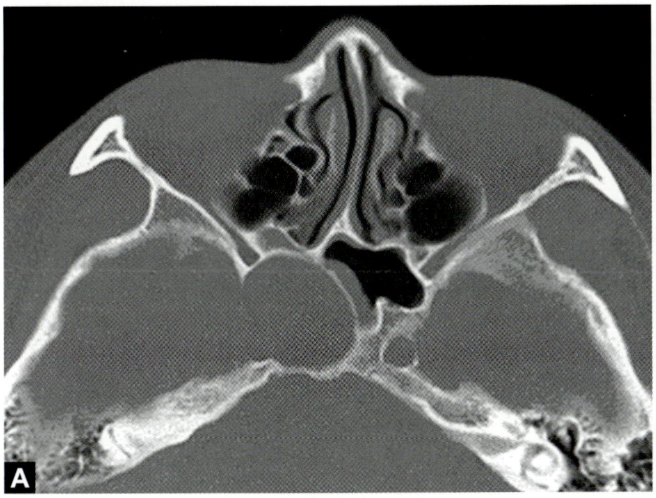

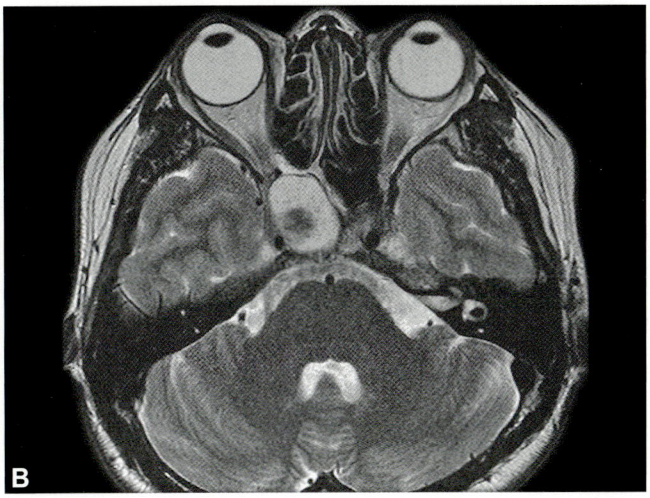

Figs. 4.1A and B: (A) Noncontrast axial CT scan and (B) noncontrast axial T2 weighted MRI of a patient with a mucopyocele of the right sphenoid sinus with extensive bony skull base erosion. The two imaging studies are complementary in this patient with improved detail of the bony skull base dehiscence and relationship of the lesion to the paranasal sinus architecture conferred by the CT scan. Conversely, MRI conveys the nature of the lesion (inflammatory versus neoplastic process) and its relationship to the soft tissues of the intracranial and orbital cavities.

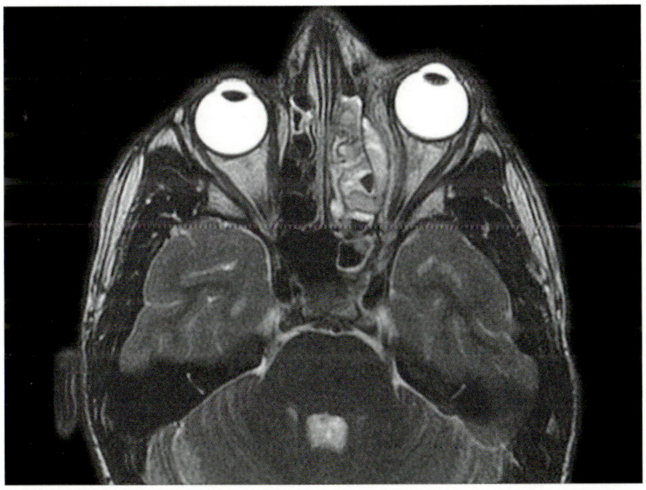

Fig. 4.2: Noncontrast, axial T2 weighted MRI of a patient with acute left-sided sinusitis (primarily ethmoid, frontal) with associated subperiostial orbital abscess. CT in this case would detail the paranasal sinusitis and would adequately identify the abscess changes in the medial orbit. However, the location and extent of the abscess and its relationship to the other orbital structures is more ideally shown with MRI.

differences in treatment protocols and clinical outcomes associated with the different types of tumors, pretreatment histopathologic diagnosis is critical. The procedure can be performed routinely in the office setting with appropriate set-up measures. Prebiopsy imaging studies should be performed to identify the lesion, its relationship to the intracranial cavity and its vascularity. Contraindications to office based biopsy include highly vascular appearing lesions (juvenile nasopharyngeal angiofibroma) and possible meningoencephalocele. The procedure should be performed with adequate local anesthesia and with cutting instrumentation to minimize tissue pulling. Significant biopsy-related bleeding, though rare, should be anticipated with proper set-up and equipment. Finally, although the sensitivity and specificity of office-based biopsy is high, potential false positives, and false negatives may occur. If the biopsy results are not consistent with the clinical and radiographic findings, repeat biopsy in the operating room setting is appropriate prior to treatment planning.[3]

Other Diagnostic Testing

Additional diagnostic testing in patients with inflammatory CRS is indicated in a number of clinical settings. Patients who present with pulmonary symptoms benefit from dedicated evaluation by a pulmonologist. In addition to ascertaining the nature of the pulmonary symptoms through clinical evaluation, pulmonary function testing and selective chest imaging, a team-based approach to pulmonary care is invaluable in the management of the respiratory symptoms throughout the course of the disease. Further, patients with CRS often benefit from comprehensive evaluation by specialists in allergy and clinical immunology. In patients with suspected allergic rhinitis as a comorbid factor, allergy testing and management is integral to the overall treatment plan. Evaluation in the form of various skin and serologic tests can identify possible environmental allergies. This information can be translated into consideration of the various therapeutic options including environmental measures, medical therapy, and desensitization. The integration of allergy care is especially useful in patients with complex polypoid CRS. An additional role for allergist evaluation involves performing immunologic evaluation in patients with refractory CRS and recurrent acute rhinosinusitis. Occult immune deficiency, while uncommon, accounts for a subset of difficult to manage sinusitis and requires appropriate identification through serologic testing. Finally, sweat test or genetic testing for cystic fibrosis should be considered if clinically appropriate.

INDICATIONS FOR SURGERY

Primary Surgery for CRS

Chronic rhinosinusitis remains the most common indication for endoscopic sinus surgery (ESS) and balloon sinuplasty. Understanding how sinus surgery integrates with the other treatment options for CRS is critical in defining its indications. The natural history of a patient with CRS commonly progresses through a series of steps. The patient initially presents with symptoms and examination findings consistent with sinusitis. A course of medical therapy is initiated which, if unsuccessful, is repeated until "maximal medical therapy" has failed. Diagnostic testing is initiated for persistent symptoms, primarily in the form of paranasal sinus CT. If inflammatory CRS findings are identified, a surgical procedure is contemplated. Although this has historically represented ESS, an increasing number of patients are offered balloon sinuplasty at this point. Following the surgical procedure, continued medical therapy is provided based on specific disease and patient factors. Persistent symptoms and inflammatory changes at this point are treated with additional medical therapy options, and possibly with a consideration of revision surgery. Of note, clinical response to therapy is assessed at each of these steps. If patient improvement is noted, maintenance therapy and surveillance are instituted.

The primary indication for primary ESS for CRS is a failure of "maximal medical therapy". Although this principle is conceptually straightforward, the exact definition of "maximal" remains unclear. In a survey of American Rhinologic Society members, Dubin et al.[1] reported variability in the medical therapy used by respondents prior to recommending surgery. The most frequently used interventions were oral antibiotics, nasal steroid sprays, oral steroids, saline irrigation, and allergy testing. The median antibiotic length was reported to be between 3.1 and 4 weeks.[4]

Heterogeneity in CRS variants and patient presentations likely necessitates individualized care and precludes a strict algorithmic approach. Following diagnosis of CRS by a combination of symptoms and objective findings (e.g. nasal endoscopy or CT scan),[5] the majority of patients with CRS should be treated with a minimum 3–4 week course of broad spectrum antibiotics (ideally culture directed), nasal steroids sprays, and saline irrigation. Consideration of systemic steroids is indicated, especially in patients with significant inflammatory changes. Additional consideration should be given to evaluation and management of various CRS comorbid factors including allergic rhinitis. Surgery may be considered if there has been a failure of medical therapy.

The overall goal of ESS for CRS is to mediate improvement in patient symptoms and sinonasal inflammatory changes as a part of multimodality therapy. In contrast to resection type surgeries such as tonsillectomy or appendectomy that aim to remove the diseased organ as a means of "curing" the disorder, ESS primarily aims to assist in the return to normal physiology. There are multiple identified benefits of ESS for CRS, both diagnostic and therapeutic. Endoscopic examination of the sinonasal cavities during the course of surgery allows for assessment of the severity and nature of the disease. Tissue and mucous analysis in the form of histopathology and microbiologic culture studies allow for improved subclassification and for more targeted postsurgical medical therapy. The primary therapeutic benefit of ESS is to create widely patent outflow tracts that facilitate both a return to normal sinonasal physiology and delivery of postoperative medical therapy, including topical therapy.

Revision Surgery for CRS

The role of revision surgery in patients with refractory CRS is highly individualized. A number of different clinical situations may result in the consideration of revision surgery. The overall unifying indication, however, is the persistence of clinical symptoms and inflammatory changes despite prior therapies. In the setting of revision surgery, the prior therapies most commonly include, in order, presurgical medical therapy, surgical therapy, and additional postsurgical medical therapy. The amount and nature of the medical therapy that should be used following the initial surgery and prior to consideration

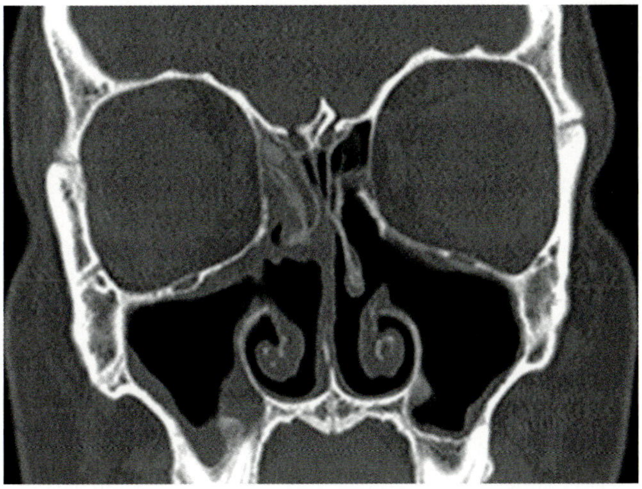

Fig. 4.3: Noncontrast coronal CT scan of a patient with a prior history of endoscopic sinus surgery (ESS) being considered for revision surgery. Note the ethmoid cavity obstruction by osteitic bone on the right side.

of revision surgery is poorly defined and varies based on the clinical situation. This commonly encompasses a prolonged course of culture directed systemic antibiotics and anti-inflammatory therapy. A heavier reliance on topical therapy is often appropriate in the postsurgical setting given the improved access to the sinonasal cavities.

In patients who have initially undergone dilation-based therapy (balloon sinuplasty) as their only form of surgical therapy, ESS may be considered as a next step for persistent disease. Performing ESS in this situation is similar to primary ESS since the anatomic structures that define the sinonasal outflow tracts have been minimally shifted with the prior balloon therapy.

Revision surgery in patients with nonpolypoid CRS who have undergone prior ESS has the same goals as primary surgery, namely, the creation of widely patent outflow tracts. However, the anatomic targets differ in primary versus revision surgery. In the former, the outflow tracts are obstructed by normal structures including the uncinate process, ethmoid cell partitions, and bony ostial boundaries. In revision surgery, these structures have been previously manipulated to a varying degree. The targets in revision surgery may include the partially retained structures that are ideally cleared in primary ESS (ethmoid cavity partitions, uncinate process, agger nasi cell) in addition to synechia, osteitis, stenosis, lateralization of the middle turbinate[6] (Fig. 4.3). Determining whether a patient with persistent CRS symptoms would benefit from revision ESS in this setting is clinically challenging but can be greatly facilitated by objective information including evidence of both inflammatory changes and areas of outflow tract obstruction on nasal endoscopy and CT sinus. The initial surgical records should also be reviewed for the initial extent of surgery and technical issues encountered.

Revision ESS is also common in the natural course of patients with polypoid CRS. The indication for revision surgery in this cohort encompasses the same concepts as described above for patients with nonpolypoid CRS. Additionally, unique to patients with polypoid CRS is the need for clearance of obstructive polypoid soft tissue even in the presence of widely patent bony outflow tracts. The timing of revision surgery in this cohort is individualized and may be indicated by poorly controlled symptoms despite medical therapy including systemic steroids.

Complications of Rhinosinusitis

Patients presenting with infectious complications of sinusitis involving the orbital and intracranial structures require aggressive medial and surgical therapy given the potential for permanent sequelae. Multidisciplinary care in an in-patient setting is typically required. Although the management of orbital and intracranial infections secondary to sinusitis is beyond the scope of this chapter, consideration of early performance of ESS should be given in these patients. The extent of surgery is dictated by the inflammatory changes on CT scan and the goals of surgery in this setting include endoscopic guided culture and histopathologic tissue analysis, creation of widely patent outflow tracts to promote drainage of the mucopurulent secretions and, if appropriate, drainage of the abscess collection. Although increased vascularity and inflammatory changes is expected in this setting, the potential morbidity of the disease process warrants aggressive intervention. In terms of timing, the majority of patients presenting with advanced disease states including abscess formation warrant early surgical intervention. In patients with mild infectious findings without sequelae (e.g. early staged orbital cellulitis), aggressive medical therapy and close observation may be indicated initially with consideration of surgery if rapid improvement does not occur.

Recurrent Acute Rhinosinusitis

Recurrent acute rhinosinusitis (RARS) represents a subset of patients with chronic inflammatory sinusitis. Although the definition of RARS continues to evolve, the current clinical criteria include a frequency of greater than four acute bacterial rhinosinusitis episodes in a 12 month period with complete resolution of symptoms and inflammatory changes between acute episodes. Implicit in this definition is that the acute episodes are distinguished from viral upper respiratory tract infections.[5] The exact incidence of RARS is incompletely defined, but has been estimated to occur in approximately 77,000 adults per year in the United States.[7] Although this is clearly a smaller population than CRS, it may be an underestimation given the previously limited attention RARS has received in the medical literature. The condition is also likely under reported by primary care physicians who are typically the first level of care. Regardless, the societal burden associated with the care of these patients appears to be significant given the similar negative impact on quality of life when compared with CRS and estimated direct medical cost of $1000 per patient per year.[7,8]

The two goals of therapy for RARS are to treat each individual acute episode and to decrease the frequency and severity of future RARS episodes. Treatment of individual acute rhinosinusitis episodes is largely similar to treatment models that apply to the general population. However, improved surveillance and follow up strategies are appropriate to track the recurrent nature of the condition. Strategies for decreasing the frequency of acute episodes include evaluation of medical, social, and occupational risk factors, evaluation of allergic rhinitis and immune deficiencies, and consideration of ESS.

In patients that have otherwise well-controlled ARS risk factors, ESS does have a beneficial role in reducing the severity and frequency of recurrent episodes. Poetker et al.[8] reported overall significant improvement in a cohort of 22 patients with RARS who underwent ESS including overall quality of life scores, symptom scores, and medication usage. Similar improvement in symptom scores, rhinosinusitis quality of life measures, and number of infections were noted in a separate study of 19 patients with 1-year follow up.[9] Finally, a 61% decrease in antibiotic usage was noted in 21 patients undergoing ESS for RARS in a multi-institutional study.[10] The role of ESS in patients with RARS requires additional investigation, but the limited studies to date to support this indication.

Sinonasal and Intracranial Neoplasms

One of the major advances in rhinology over the past two decades has been the application of endoscopic surgery to different sinonasal and skull base pathologies. This has represented a major paradigm shift in the way these conditions are managed and is associated with several theoretical benefits. Endoscopic surgery for these lesions through a transnasal approach precludes transfacial and transcranial incisions with a resultant decreased in the invasiveness of the approach. Additionally, the robust visualization afforded by modern endoscopic systems is an improvement over the cavitary and limited angulation issues associated with external microscopic approaches. Finally, the development of instrumentation with adequate functionality has allowed for the management of the technical challenges associated with these lesions including the vascularity, skull base defects, and proximity to critical neurovascular structures that may be associated with these lesions.

Although it is beyond the scope of this chapter, endoscopic skull base surgery has become a well-defined treatment consideration for a number of different pathologies. In deciding whether a given skull base lesion will be addressed through an endoscopic approach, a number of anatomic-, disease-, and surgeon-related factors are considered. The anatomic limits of endoscopic approaches have been continuously expanded throughout its history. Sub-sites that are routinely amenable to endoscopic surgery include the nasal cavity, paranasal sinuses, infratemporal and pterygopalatine fossae, medial and inferior orbit, sellar and suprasellar cavities, subfrontal region, medial cavernous sinus, and petrous apex. Certain anatomic locations are more easily addressed through open approaches given limitations in angulation of a transnasal approach including far-lateral aspects of the maxillary sinus, frontal sinus, infratemporal fossae. Additionally, the anterior wall of the maxillary sinus is more easily addressed through a Caldwell-Luc type approach. Involvement of certain anatomic locations is a contraindication to endoscopic surgery including facial soft tissues and extensive involvement of the orbit and brain parenchyma.

The evolution of endoscopic surgery has reflected the complexity of the disease pathologies that have been successfully managed. Endoscopic surgery is currently used to manage fibro-osseous sinonasal lesions, cerebrospinal fluid rhinorrhea and meningoencephalocele, orbital pathology (Graves' disease, orbital fracture) benign sinonasal neoplasms (inverted papilloma, juvenile nasopharyngeal angiofibroma), benign intracranial neoplasms (pituitary adenoma, meningioma). Little controversy exists at this point in time in the application of endoscopic surgery to these pathologies given the favorable outcome studies and the theoretical benefits of endoscopic surgery for benign pathology. The past decade has also witnessed the successful application of endoscopic surgery to management of appropriately selected, often early staged sinonasal and skull base malignancies. Although this remains an active area of debate and investigation, the collective literature exploring early cancer-related outcomes have been positive. The controversy associated with endoscopic surgery for malignancy has centered largely on the concern for a detrimental impact on oncologic outcomes by performing piece meal resection. Although the favorable early experience has allayed some of these concerns, management of skull base malignancy still requires strict adherence to oncologic principles including clearance of adequate tumor margins. Appropriate case selection based on preoperative imaging studies, tissue diagnosis, and multidisciplinary discussion remain paramount.

The final consideration in deciding whether to manage advanced lesions endoscopically has to do with the experience and skills of the surgical team. Endoscopic skull base procedures represent advanced techniques significantly different from surgery for inflammatory sinusitis. Although ESS for CRS represents an important foundation for endoscopic skull base surgery, additional components are required. The primary determinant for a given surgeon has to do with technical skills and experience. A step-wise approach is appropriate with performance of endoscopic surgery for benign sinonasal lesions, meningoencephalocele, posterior epistaxis, benign intracranial neoplasms (pituitary adenoma) prior to advancing to surgery for malignancy, or surgery in complex anatomic skull base corridors. A team approach is also necessary given the complexity of the perioperative and surgical care of these patients.

CONCLUSION

Paramount to any successful surgery is a thorough approach to pretreatment evaluation including medical history, examination, and diagnostic testing. Within rhinology, this includes an understanding of the various clinical presentations, expertise in the interpretation of examination and endoscopy findings, appropriate use of imaging studies including CT and MRI. Consideration of the potential differential diagnosis and the role of various treatment options is critical for both accurate diagnosis and optimization of therapy. Following appropriate evaluation, the indications for surgery are considered. The surgical management of sinonasal disorders has largely evolved toward endoscopic approaches, including its application to complex pathologies and anatomic sites. Chronic inflammatory rhinosinusitis remains the most common indication for ESS, but the surgical principles have continued to evolve. Endoscopic surgery for sinonasal and skull-base neoplasms represents the most recent frontier and has been associated with favorable early outcomes. As the field has grown from proof of concept, to refinement of technique, to widespread adoption, the next step will be defined by the long-term outcomes and ultimately a robust understanding of the indications and limitations of the procedure.

REFERENCES

1. Dubin MG, Ebert CS, Coffey CS, et al. Concordance of middle meatal swab and maxillary sinus aspirate in acute and chronic sinusitis: a meta-analysis. Am J Rhinol. 2005;19:462-70.
2. Barnes L, Eveson J, Reichart P, et al. WHO Classification of Tumors. Pathology & Genetics. Head and Neck Tumors. Lyon, France: IARC Press; 2005.
3. Tabaee A, Hsu A, Kacker A. Indications, technique, safety and accuracy of office-based nasal endoscopy with biopsy for sinonasal neoplasm. Int Forum Allergy Rhinol. 2011;1: 225-8.
4. Dubin MG, Liu C, Lin SY, et al. American Rhinologic Society member survey on "maximal medical therapy" for chronic rhinosinusitis. Am J Rhinol. 2007;21:483-8.
5. Rosenfeld RM, Andes D, Bhattacharyya N, et al. Clinical practice guideline: adult sinusitis. Otolaryngol-Head Neck Surgery. 2007;137:S1-31.
6. Musy PY, Kountakis SE. Anatomic findings in patients undergoing revision endoscopic sinus surgery. Am J Otolaryngol. 2004;25:418-22.
7. Bhattacharyya N, Grebner J, Martinson NG. Recurrent acute rhinosinusitis: epidemiology and health care cost burden. Otolaryngol Head Neck Surg. 2012;146:307-12.
8. Poetker DM, Litvack JR, Mace JC, et al. Recurrent acute rhinosinusitis: presentation and outcomes of sinus surgery. Am J Rhinol. 2008;22:329-33.
9. Bhattacharyya N. Surgical treatment of chronic recurrent rhinosinusitis: a preliminary report. Laryngoscope. 2006; 116:1805-8.
10. Bhandarkar ND, Mace JC, Smith TL. Endoscopic sinus surgery reduces antibiotic utilization in rhinosinusitis. Int Forum Allergy Rhinol. 2011;1:18-22.

CHAPTER 5

Nasal Endoscopy

Spencer C Payne

INTRODUCTION

Nasal endoscopy is a crucial component in the evaluation of the patient with sinonasal symptoms and is essentially a requirement for true diagnosis of chronic rhinosinusitis.[1-3] Information regarding the extent of inflammation, edema, mucous discharge, presence, and extent of polyps can be acquired and used to stage patients (Table 5.1).[4] Additional information can also be obtained through sinus cultures when applicable in the acute or exacerbated chronic sinusitis scenario. In addition to diagnostic opportunities, in-office endoscopy can also be utilized to perform a variety of procedures that escalate with physician experience and skill. These can include steroid injection, control of minor epistaxis, endoscopic biopsy and debridement, and eventually even limited revision sinus surgery depending on patient comfort and willingness.

The variety of endoscopes now available enables a wide selection from which the surgeon can choose to examine the nose. This selection includes any combination of diameter (2.7, 3, or 4 mm), angulation (0°, 30°, 45°, and 70°), and light post placement (standard and reversed). Each combination carries its own inherent advantages and disadvantages. Although the smaller 2.7 ("pediatric") diameter scopes are ideal for children or adults with narrow or sensitive passageways, they tend to be more flimsy and provide a narrower field of view. In contrast, the larger, standard 4 mm endoscopes often used in the operating room provide a much nicer field of view and magnification, but can be difficult to use in some noses even with adequate topical preparation. As such, the authors prefer the recently available 3 mm scopes, which seem to optimally blend the tradeoffs between strength, size, and optimal view and use them frequently without the need for topical analgesics. Although 30° endoscopes are essential for evaluation of the postoperative and often preoperative nose and sinuses, they can be more difficult with which to co-instrument, and we recommend the surgeon have access to a zero degree endoscope as well. Standard endoscopes place the post for the light cable attachment on the opposite side of the angled view. Reverse-post scopes simply move the light post to the opposite side of the standard scope such that the angled view and the light-post are on the same side. This reverse functionality is extremely useful in the operative setting as it permits free passage of the operative hand below the scope when utilizing the angled view to engage the frontal sinus or anterior ethmoid roof. In the clinic setting, however, this benefit is likely not realized.

Table 5.1: Lund-Kennedy endoscopic staging system

Characteristic	*Left*	*Right*
Polyp		
Edema		
Discharge		
Scarring		
Crusting		
Total Score		

Scoring: For polyps: 0, absence of polyps; 1, polyps in middle meatus only, 2, polyps beyond middle meatus. For edema, scarring, and crusting: 0, absent; 1, mild; 2, severe. For discharge: 0, no discharge; I, clear, thin discharge; 2, thick, purulent discharge. Reprinted with permission from Lund and Kennedy.[4]

SURGICAL TECHNIQUE

The patient is generally seated in a comfortable position, often with the chair back at 60°–75°. Depending on surgeon preference, the patient may also be fully reclined but the authors find that this is often unnecessary, limited by space in the office, and adds additional time to the procedure. If used in conjunction with a video system with television display, the chair is left at its default position

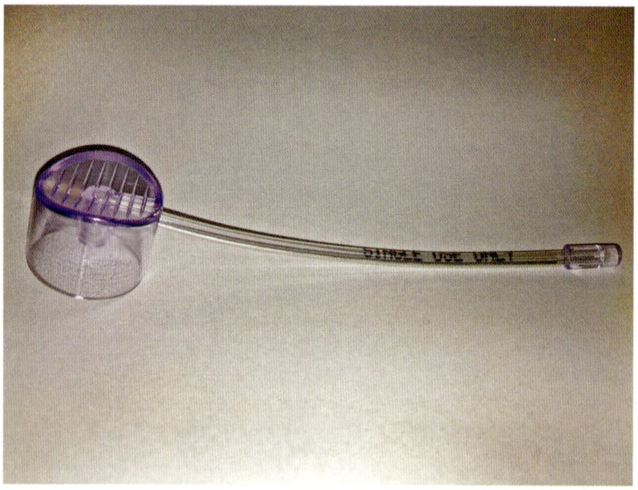

Fig. 5.1: Disposable nasal atomization device. Use of the atomization device may help prevent cross-contamination and is often better tolerated than the higher pressure venturi devices.

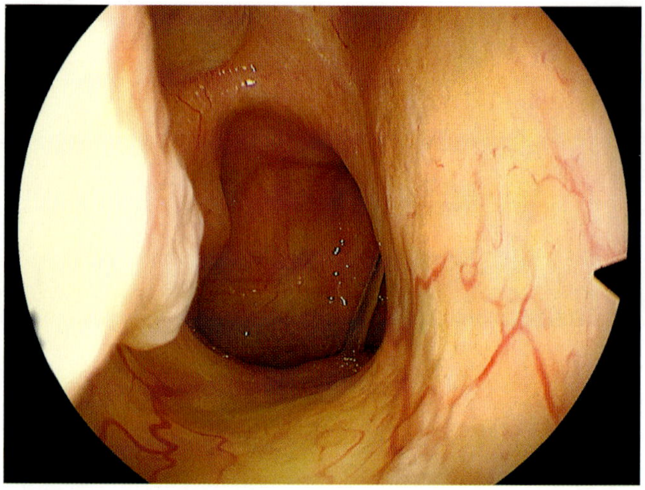

Fig. 5.2: First pass along nasal floor to nasopharynx. Note any issues with septum, turbinate, torus tubarius, and fossa of Rosenmuller.

as this is the most comfortable and puts less strain on the surgeon's shoulder. For "bare-eye" visualization, the chair is raised until the nostril is about eye level. For the initial visit, it is essential to gauge the state of the patient's nose before any topically administered medications are applied. This can be achieved through standard rhinoscopy or with a quick "shallow" inspection with the endoscope. Following this, two to three sprays each of a decongestant and topical analgesic are applied. The authors prefer a disposable atomization device (Fig. 5.1) in order to minimize patient discomfort and potential for device contamination as can be seen with the traditional Venturi sprayers.[5] In terms of drugs, a variety of studies indicate that oxymetazoline may be safer than phenylephrine[6] and that 4% tetracaine (or pontocaine) may be more effective than topical lidocaine.[7] Tetracaine, however, is more difficult to obtain and may require supplying through compounding pharmacies. The author has often found that in the postoperative patient, the application of these medications may not be required for most diagnostic (culture) and limited therapeutic (mucous suctioning) purposes.

Once positioning and preparation are complete, the surgeon should stand or sit on the same side of the patient as their handedness. For a diagnostic procedure, either hand can be used but in the event that culturing or suctioning may occur, the scope is better utilized in the nondominant hand. The author prefers to use his dominant hand for diagnostic endoscopy, freeing up his nondominant hand to make the first contact with the patient's shoulder. Not only is this less jarring for the patient, but also provides proprioceptive feedback to facilitate stabilization while acting in the two-dimensional world inherent to current endoscopic technologies.

The examination begins with introduction of the endoscope into either nostril. Generally, three passes are taken through the nose in order to fully examine all areas of potential concern. A first pass is made from anterior to posterior along the nasal floor. One should note the position and shape of the septum including the presence of any spur, deviation, or slippage of the quadrangular cartilage off the maxillary crest. Additionally, the size and color of the inferior turbinate and whether it remains engorged even after decongestant. In the patient with facial pain, noting the presence of a contact point between any spur and turbinate or evidence of such (often after decongestant no further contact may be seen, but an indentation can be noted in the inferior turbinate). As one makes their way back to the nasopharynx, the presence of any secretions can be noted and their location (e.g., sphenoethmoidal recess, middle meatus, superior meatus) may indicate the likely set of sinuses from which they may be originating. Finally, the nasopharynx is examined, the appearance of the torus tubarius and fossa of Rosenmuller are noted (Fig. 5.2). At this time, the patient can be asked to swallow and patency of the Eustachian tube can be evaluated. A 30° scope is particularly useful in this setting.

At this point, the scope can be fully withdrawn and reintroduced in a more superior, but continued medial course to evaluate the superior meatus and sphenoethmoidal recess. We prefer to instead start posteriorly and angle the scope superiorly so that the rounded aspect of the shaft can more delicately slip into this medial

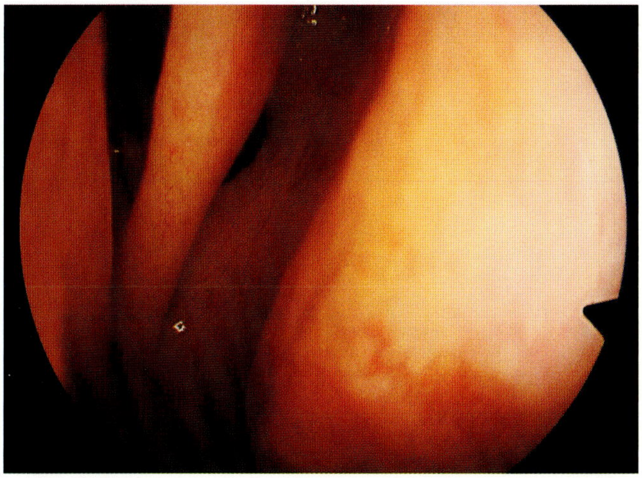

Fig. 5.3: Second pass and visualization of sphenoid ostium. The slit like opening of the sphenoid is seen superiorly with an opening to a posterior ethmoid cell through superior meatus seen to the left.

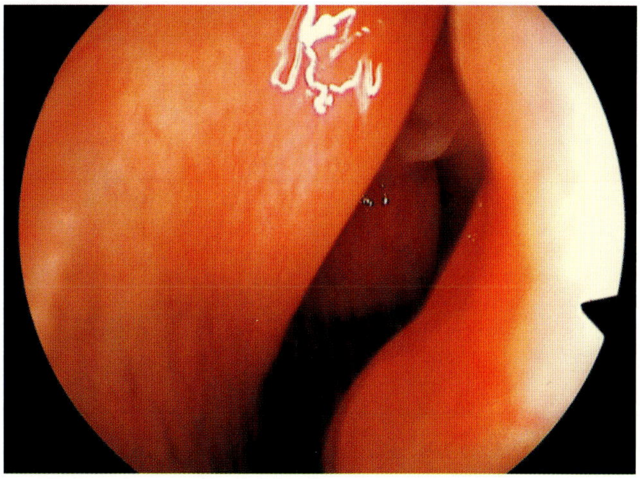

Fig. 5.4: Third pass and visualization of middle meatus. Note any edema of uncinate process and ethmoid bulla. Here, we see a polyp superiorly between the uncinate and bulla.

corridor. The sphenoethmoidal recess and hopefully the sphenoid os can be examined, often requiring a 30° scope (Fig. 5.3). As the scope is then withdrawn, the presence of any polyps, inflammation, drainage or masses in the superior meatus or along the septum can be noted.

A final third pass is made to evaluate the middle turbinate and meatus (Fig. 5.4). We start with a superior approach and attempts are made to visualize the axilla of the middle turbinate. Difficulty in doing so can indicate a higher, more dorsal deflection of the septum even if it appears more midline inferiorly. Additionally, the nasal fault and anterior aspect of the cribriform can be evaluated at this point. With adequate anesthesia, and utilizing a small diameter scope, the middle meatus can be evaluated. A paradoxical or lateralized middle turbinate, or one with a concha bullosa may render this portion of the exam impossible however. Instead of a direct "entry" into the meatus, which will typically result in excoriation of the middle turbinate with subsequent bleeding and view limitation, two other alternatives exist. The first is the inferior "roll-in" technique where the tip of the scope is introduced below the middle turbinate and rolled laterally and superiorly into the middle meatus from below, thus "bluntly" displaces the middle turbinate medially. The second, which is also quite useful in the postoperative patient with a lateralized middle turbinate, is what we have dubbed the "nose-up" or "landing-the-plane" technique. With a 30° endoscope and while obtaining a view of the area above the axilla of the middle turbinate, hence the "nose-up" moniker, the scope is advanced posteriorly through the meatus with the "under-belly" of the scope breaking the vertical plane between the middle turbinate head and the lateral nasal wall, thus "landing-the-plane" into the middle meatus. Note can then be made of any drainage, edema, polyps, or erythema of the ethmoid bulla and uncinate process. Similarly in the postoperative scenario, attempts should be made to evaluate for the adequacy of prior ethmoidectomy, frontal exploration, uncinectomy, and/or maxillary antrostomy as these may be common areas responsible for surgical failure.

The scope is then withdrawn and the contralateral side examined in a similar fashion. Any bleeding that may have resulted from the procedure can either be observed or controlled with temporary placement of decongestant soaked cotton packs with or without the use of gentle silver nitrate cautery if necessary.

REFERENCES

1. Rosenfeld RM, Andes D, Bhattacharyya N, et al. Clinical practice guideline: Adult sinusitis. Otolaryngol Head Neck Surg. 2007;137:S1-S31.
2. Meltzer EO, Hamilos DL, Hadley JA, et al. Rhinosinusitis: Developing guidance for clinical trials. Otolaryngol Head Neck Surg. 2006;135:S31-S80.
3. Fokkens WJ, Lund VJ, Mullol J, et al. European position paper on rhinosinusitis and nasal polyps 2012. Rhinology. 2012;50(Suppl 23):1-298.
4. Lund VJ, Kennedy DW. Staging for rhinosinusitis. Otolaryngol Head Neck Surg. 1997;117:S35-S40.
5. Bossart PJ, Wolfe T. Venturi atomizers as potential sources of patient cross-infection. Am J Infect Control. 2003;31:441-4.
6. Higgins TS, Hwang PH, Kingdom TT, et al. Systematic review of topical vasoconstrictors in endoscopic sinus surgery. Laryngoscope. 2011;32:55-63.
7. Noorily AD, Noorily SH, Otto RA. Cocaine, lidocaine, tetracaine: which is best for topical nasal anesthesia? Anesth Analg. 1995;81:724-7.

CHAPTER 6

Anesthesia for Endoscopic Surgery

Anita Cucchiaro, Ameet Singh, Seth A Akst

INTRODUCTION

Anesthetic techniques utilized during endoscopic sinus and skull base surgery can significantly influence the surgical field and affect patient outcome. Inadequate visualization and excessive bleeding during endoscopic sinus and skull base surgery can not only lead to suboptimal results (incomplete surgery, residual opacified cells), but also result in catastrophic complications (e.g., orbital and/or intracranial injury). The type of airway, anesthetic agents used, and the degree of hypercapnia can heavily impact the amount of bleeding in the surgical field and consequently the surgical result. Coughing and bucking during emergence from anesthesia can lead to bleeding, possible aspiration, or laryngospasm. Meaningful partnership between the anesthesiologist and the surgeon can enhance patient outcomes.

PREOPERATIVE RISK ASSESSMENT

Endoscopic, endonasal surgery requires a surgical field with minimal bleeding to achieve good results. Toward this end, patient medical histories are investigated, controlled hypotension is cautiously enforced with respect to end organ perfusion, and local (topical and injectable) vasoconstriction is administered.

Every patient presents to surgery with individual risk factors for perioperative events, so the intraoperative control of bleeding starts with being aware of a patient's coagulopathy, medications, and/or other conditions that would increase this risk. If the patient is on anticoagulation or antiplatelet therapy, a determination must be made on whether the patient should continue this therapy perioperatively, and if not, when in the preoperative period they should stop. This decision should be made between the anesthesiologist, the surgeon, and the patient's physician who has placed them on anticoagulation. Detailed discussion of the perioperative timing of antiplatelet agents in patients with coronary stents is outside the scope of this chapter, but the reader is referred to an article by Jaffer[1] and a Practice Alert published by the American Society of Anesthesiologists.[2]

Patients on herbal medications or other over-the-counter substances known to impact bleeding through platelet aggregation inhibition are usually asked to stop these medications 3 weeks prior to surgery, although this is an arbitrarily chosen time course as no definitive studies have shown benefit or complication with herbal medications.[3] Patients with coagulopathies such as von Willebrand's disease or Hemophilia A should be treated preoperatively with appropriate therapies such as DDAVP and Factor VIII, or Factor IX for Hemophilia B. For patients with complicated coagulopathies, discussion with the patient's hematologist is recommended.

GENERAL ANESTHESIA TECHNIQUES

Type of Airway

The type of airway used during endoscopic surgery has been studied in the otolaryngologic and anesthetic literature. The use of a laryngeal mask airway (LMA) has been shown to be superior to endotracheal intubation (ETT) in numerous studies with regard to airway, hemodynamics, and control of bleeding.[4] This has been thought to be secondary to decreased stimulation and less sympathetic activation with LMA placement versus placement of an ETT via direct laryngoscopy. Lower blood pressure and heart rate are usually achievable following LMA placement compared with intubation; therefore, patients can have a more rapid onset of controlled hypotension and decreased surgical bleeding. In addition, patients were observed to cough less on extubation when using an LMA—an important point of consideration in endoscopic sinus and skull base procedures.[5,5a]

The LMA sits in a supraglottic position, and the absence of an inflated cuff within the trachea does lead to risks of laryngospasm or aspiration. However, because of less traumatic placement methods, there may be less hypopharyngeal blood following LMA placement than following intubation. One study demonstrated a decreased instance of blood in the upper airway with LMA as compared with ETT (20% vs. 85%).[6] Although lower airway blood/debris was found to occur at a rate of 2% with LMA in a prospective observational study of 200 patients undergoing nasal surgery, no airway contamination symptoms were noted.[7] This study excluded patients with gastroesophageal reflux or hiatal hernia due to increased aspiration risk, reinforcing the importance of appropriate patient selection when choosing any aspect of anesthetic management.

As noted earlier, because of its supraglottic position, a LMA is less likely to produce coughing during emergence from general anesthesia. Whether the anesthetic is conducted with a LMA or an ETT, a smooth emergence can minimize risk for surgical rebleeding and reduce its attendant complications such as delayed epistaxis, acute sinusitis, persistent blood/crusting, and/or cerebrospinal fluid (CSF) leak. One method to reduce coughing during emergence is to remove the airway while the patient is still deeply anesthetized, when the cough reflex is blunted. Although often preferred by the surgeon, a "deep extubation" does pose concerns for the anesthesiologist. Upper airway obstruction, laryngopasm, or central apnea can occur with resultant hypoxemia and poor outcome. Supportive continuous positive airway pressure (CPAP) or assisted positive-pressure mask ventilation may be required after a "deep extubation." While contraindicated after middle-ear surgery, application of positive pressure to the pharynx is less of a concern following endoscopic endonasal surgery. It should be remembered that postoperative nasal packing reduces the available routes for air exchange.

Loss of the airway is not the only risk of extubating while the patient is still anesthetized. While the cough reflex is blunted, so is the gag reflex. Reflux or emesis can lead to aspiration and severe lung injury. The Difficult Airway Society Guidelines for the management of tracheal extubation states that "deep extubation" is contraindicated in patients with a full stomach, unstable cardiovascular physiology, acid–base derangements, temperature derangements, head/neck surgery that required an awake fiberoptic intubation, obstructive sleep apnea (OSA), and mechanical or other airway obstruction arising during surgery. Any benefits of maintaining a bloodless environment would be lost with emergent reintubation or the inability to mask ventilate.[8]

If awakening from anesthesia will precede removal of the airway, there are pharmacologic methods to reduce coughing and bucking. Remifentanil titration during emergence may eliminate coughing. Researchers at the Yonsei University College of Medicine in South Korea found an effect site concentration of Remifentanil 2.14 ng/mL to be effective at preventing cough during emergence after thyroid surgery.[9] Transition from volatile to intravenous (IV) anesthetic may also reduce the hyper-reflexic "stage 2" of emergence. Use of lidocaine as a local anesthetic in the trachea has been shown to reduce the cough reflex; it has successfully been administered topically, via instillation into the ETT cuff, or intravenously during emergence. The authors prefer IV lidocaine, administered during emergence and prior to extubation, to smooth awakening and reduce coughing. It has mild general anesthetic effects that blunt the hyper-reflexia of emergence, and is more easily dosed than topical or cuff-instilled anesthetics.

Ventilation

Hypercapnia acts to cause smooth muscle relaxation and vasodilation, with resultant increases in cerebral blood flow as well as nasal mucosa blood flow. Therefore, controlled ventilation toward low or normal CO_2 levels can theoretically avoid mucosal hyperemia and improve surgical conditions. Control of ventilation is made more difficult with a LMA, when positive pressure ventilation is limited because of the lack of differentiation between air flow into the esophagus rather than the trachea. Reduction in use of opioids will better preserve the patient's spontaneous respiratory drive and allow for normal levels of carbon dioxide. The theoretical advantage of hypocapnia in terms of reducing surgical blood loss was not shown in one study published about this technique.[10] Ventilation with lower mean airway pressures may enhance venous return, with reduced nasal mucosal engorgement and improvement in surgical conditions. A small study by Gilbey et al.[11] showed a statistically significant reduction in blood loss during endoscopic sinus surgery, along with surgeons' report of improved operating conditions, when high-frequency jet ventilation was used in order to lower mean airway pressures. Following this logic, it would seem that the use of positive end-expiratory pressure could worsen surgical conditions.

Any ventilation procedures to optimize surgical conditions must also take into account the patient's respiratory status and oxygenation requirements. Patients with OSA cause special concern. Those that require a CPAP device postoperatively will require more vigilance with regard to possible disruption to the surgical site with use of the device. As well, such patients may not be suitable for LMA placement due to their habitus/size or other confounding ventilatory disturbances.

Hemodynamic Modulation

Controlled hypotension can reduce mucosal blood flow and surgical bleeding, but the benefits of this technique must be weighed against the risk of organ hypoperfusion. The success of the technique may partially depend upon which antihypertensive agent is used to achieve the target blood pressure. When using sodium nitroprusside, a potent vasodilator, Boezaart et al.[12] found that the mean arterial pressure (MAP) must be reduced to a target less than 50 mm Hg in order to reduce surgical bleeding. Not every patient is a candidate for MAP this low; in fact, the risk of cerebral ischemia, coronary ischemia, renal injury, and other end-organ damage with a MAP < 50 mm Hg is significant, particularly for patients with comorbid conditions or chronic hypertension. However, the same authors found that hypotension induced with esmolol, a selective β1-blocker, can achieve reduction in bleeding and improvement in surgical conditions at MAP goals higher than 65 mm Hg. The authors speculate that esmolol attenuates sympathetic tone, whereas a reflexive increase in sympathetic tone occurs with hypotension induced by a vasodilator such as nitroprusside.[12]

The importance of relative bradycardia and diminished sympathetic tone rather than absolute blood pressure control is also demonstrated in several other studies. Hypotension accomplished with vasodilators (prostaglandin E1 or nitroprusside) results in reflex tachycardia and no improvement in bleeding, respectively, when compared with normotensive anesthesia.[13,14] In contrast, Nair et al.[15,16] show a relationship between decreased heart rate and decreased bleeding in the surgical field. Centrally acting α2-agonists such as clonidine and dexmedetomidine work at presynaptic receptors to diminish sympathetic tone; premedication with clonidine[13] and infusion of dexmedetomidine[17] improve the surgical field during endoscopic sinus surgery.

While discussing hemodynamics during sinus surgery, an additional point bears mention. Systemic absorption of topical phenylephrine can lead to significant hypertension. Because of the focused effect of phenylephrine on α1 receptors, this hypertension is due solely to increases in afterload, with no change or even decrease in cardiac output. Use of a beta blocker to treat phenylephrine-induced hypertension will further worsen cardiac output by limiting β1-mediated cardiac contractility and also potentially blocking β2-mediated compensatory vasodilation. Significant pulmonary edema and even cardiac arrest may result.[18] Hypertension induced by systemic absorption of nasal phenylephrine is better countered with β1-blockers or other direct vasodilators. It is suggested by the Commissioner of Health in New York State that the initial dose of phenylephrine should not exceed 0.5 mg in adults, and should not exceed 20 mcg/kg in children.[18]

Finally, just as with patient-specific ventilatory concerns, hemodynamic altering procedures must keep in mind individual patients. Hypertensive patients whose MAP is consistently above 100 through poor blood pressure control, and or obesity and a higher concomitant cardiac output, are not good candidates for controlled profound hypotension. Patients with prior end-organ perfusion deficiencies, for example, renal insufficiency or prior stroke as a limited example, are also not appropriate candidates for variations in blood pressure exceeding 20% from their baseline.

Inhalational versus IV Anesthetics

As discussed above, dexmedetomidine has been shown to improve surgical conditions, possibly through its reduction in sympathetic tone. Another potential advantage of dexmedetomodine relates to its sedative effects. While not potent enough to function as a sole IV anesthetic, the addition of dexmedetomidine can reduce the necessary dose of volatile anesthetic. The veno- and vasodilatory properties of volatile anesthetics such as isoflurane, sevoflurane, and desflurane may encourage increased mucosal blood flow and engorgement. Therefore, substitution of IV anesthetics in place of volatile anesthetics may theoretically enhance operating conditions for the endoscopic surgeon.

There has been no definitive study showing an advantage of IV rather than volatile anesthetic. A small prospective, double-blinded study showed decreased blood flow in endoscopic sinus surgery when a Propofol–Remifentanil regimen was administered versus a Sevofluorane–Remifentanil regimen. However, this did not correlate with decreased blood loss or improved surgeon-rated visualization scores (VAS).[19] A more positive result was seen with dexmedetomidine; a study of forty patients in Turkey showed decreased intraoperative bleeding, increased hemodynamic stability and lower nausea complaints by patients who were given dexmedetomodine infusions as opposed to patients given identical amounts of saline solution.[20] Another small study of 62 patients in Turkey also showed similar results along with significantly decreased postoperative nausea and vomiting (PONV).[21] More studies are continuing to evaluate the utility of dexmedetomidine in FESS. A randomized controlled clinical trial performed by Yonsei University at Severance Hospital in Seoul, South Korea to compare the effect of dexmedetomidine to remifentanil on intraoperative bleeding, propofol requirement and postoperative profiles just entered Phase 4 with published results pending.

Although the clinical significance of these findings is unknown, it should be noted that different anesthetic agents have differing effects upon platelet function. Some of the inhalational anesthetics (isoflurane and desflurane) do not affect platelet function, whereas sevoflurane and nitrous oxide both appear to prevent platelet aggregation.[22] Intravenous anesthetics such as propofol are thought to inhibit platelet aggregation, whereas the narcotics do not appear to have the same effect.[22] A direct comparison of the effects of propofol, isoflurane, and sevoflurane found propofol to have a larger platelet aggregation inhibitory effect than sevoflurane or isoflurane.[23] These findings have been demonstrated in vitro, but not linked to changes in clinical outcome.

LOCAL ANESTHESIA TECHNIQUES

Local Anesthesia for Endoscopic Surgery

Certain select endoscopic sinus procedures may be performed under local anesthesia alone, without systemic sedatives or anesthesia. Advantages of pure local anesthesia include increasing patient safety during dissection at the periorbita and dura, operating in a drier surgical field, and increasing endoscopic surgery to patients deemed unfit for general anesthesia. As local anesthesia is ineffective at the periorbita and dura, patients may warn the surgeon by complaining of pain. The vasodilatory effects of general anesthesia and consequent increased bleeding in the surgical field are eliminated when operating under local anesthesia. In addition, local anesthesia may provide vasoconstriction (dependent upon choice of local anesthetic), with resultant decrease in surgical bleeding. Finally, patients who are high-risk candidates for general anesthesia may still benefit from limited endoscopic sinus surgery.

A primary disadvantage of performing sinus surgery under local anesthesia is a surgeon's divided attention between the surgical procedure and patient comfort. In addition, certain anatomic areas (frontal, sphenoid) are difficult to anesthetize with local anesthesia alone. Finally, even minor amounts of bleeding may trigger the gag reflex, especially if the swallowing reflex has been suppressed. Patient discomfort and movement may result.

Sedation may be used as an adjunct during endoscopic sinus surgery performed under local anesthesia. Oral, intramuscular, or IV administration of benzodiazepines, such as midazolam, or narcotics, such as morphine, may be used.[24] Depending on the substance and dosage, the depth of the sedation will vary and may require monitoring. Both benzodiazepines and opioids suppress respiratory drive, and diminished consciousness may also reduce airway patency and protection. Great caution must be exercised with sedative techniques used in patients undergoing endoscopic surgery with local anesthesia.

Topical Anesthesia

Regardless of whether endoscopic surgery is performed under local or general anesthesia, numbing, decongestion, and vasoconstriction of the surgical field are essential for reducing blood loss, lowering the general anesthetic requirement, and providing immediate postoperative pain relief. A number of topical anesthetic agents are utilized either alone or in combination for endoscopic sinus and skull base surgery. Epinephrine produces a dose-dependent response at both $\alpha 1$ and $\alpha 2$ adrenergic receptors leading to vasoconstriction of both arterial and venous vasculature.[25] The authors use topical epinephrine in concentrations as high as 1:1,000 without causing any significant hemodynamic response.

Cocaine is the only local anesthetic agent that has intrinsic vasoconstrictive properties, mediated via blockade of norepinephrine reuptake at synaptic junctions. Its use has been limited by some surgeons given its risk of cardiotoxicity and death in patients.[26] Oxymetazoline and phenylephrine are partial α agonists, with largely $\alpha 1$ effects, and therefore are less likely to provide hemostasis for venous vasculature during endoscopic sinus surgery.[25] If used with epinephrine, partial α agonists like oxymetazoline may compete with epinephrine for the same receptors, thereby limiting its efficacy. The authors frequently use cocaine in conjunction with a solution of

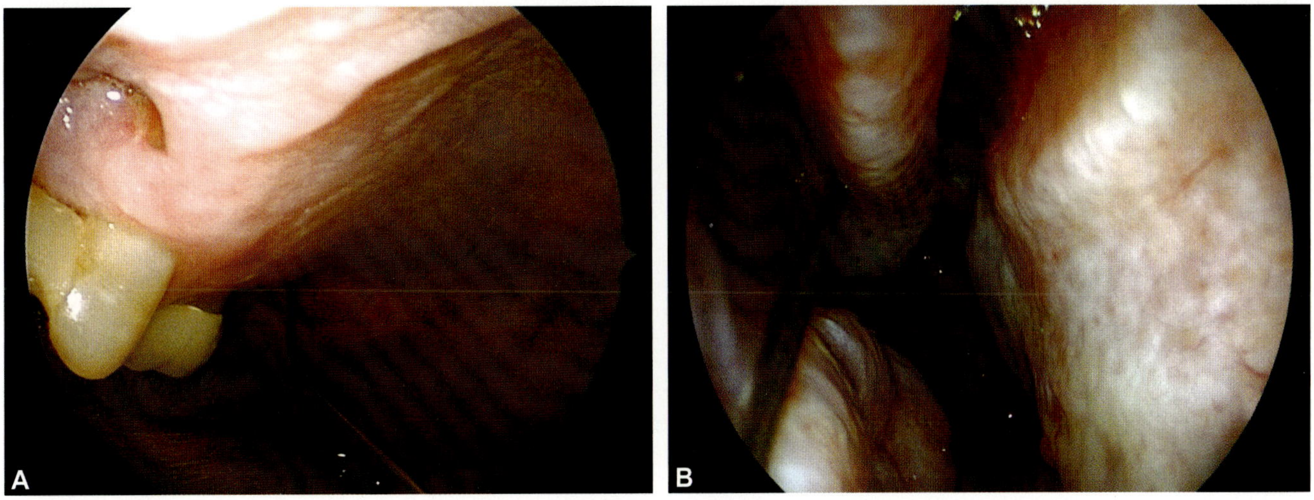

Figs. 6.1A and B: (A) Local anesthesia delivered to the pterygopalatine fossa via the greater palatal canal through a transoral approach. (B) Local anesthesia injected to the pterygopalatine fossa via the sphenopalatine foramen near the horizontal lamella of the middle turbinate.

thrombin with 1:1,000 epinephrine during endoscopic endonasal procedures. Epinephrine use is avoided during the intracranial portion of endoscopic skull base procedures. In a recent randomized blinded control study, no difference in decongestion and quality of the surgical field was found between cocaine and epinephrine.[27]

Injection of Local Anesthesia

Infiltration of the nasal and paranasal sinus mucosa with combination of epinephrine with local anesthetics has complex vascular effects. The relative individual effects of epinephrine and local anesthetic are difficult to ascertain during endoscopic surgery. Epinephrine in low doses causes vasodilation and hypotension likely due to activation of β2 receptors in skeletal muscle. At higher doses, increasing vasoconstrictive effects in the vasculature, skin, and mucosa, as well as activation of cardiac β1 receptors, result in hypertension.[28] Direct intravascular injection can result in a rapid increase in blood pressure. In a study examining the role of local anesthetic, infiltration with a lidocaine/epinephrine mixture resulted in an improved surgical field with less bleeding compared with saline.[29] Local anesthetics are critical to maintaining a bloodless surgical field during endoscopic sinus surgery. Their beneficial effects have to be carefully balanced with potential deleterious hemodynamic side effects.

Decreased bleeding in the surgical field has been shown when local anesthesia is delivered to the pterygopalatine fossa (PPF) via the greater palatine canal (Fig. 6.1A).[30] Local anesthesia delivered to the PPF via the root of the horizontal lamella of the middle turbinate has a similar effect (Fig. 6.1B). With either mechanism, vasoconstriction of the terminal branches of the internal maxillary artery results in decreased blood flow and improvement of the surgical field. Multiple clinical studies have described good control of posterior epistaxis with injection of xylocaine or gylcerine into the PPF,[31] cementing the utility of delivering local anesthesia to PPF during endoscopic surgery.

ENDONASAL APPROACH TO SKULL BASE SURGERY

Hemostasis is as important during an endonasal approach to facilitate neurologic surgery at the skull base as it is during endoscopic sinus surgery. Therefore, the above discussion of anesthetic techniques and use of local anesthetics and vasoconstrictors is applicable to endonasal approaches to the skull base as well. Hypercapnia will increase cerebral blood flow and intracranial pressure, so ETT is preferred in order to control ventilation. Endotracheal intubation rather than placement of an LMA also allows for use of neuromuscular blockade to reduce the incidence of patient movement, given the importance of structures near the surgical field. It is the authors' preference to maintain complete neuromuscular blockade throughout skull base neurosurgery, as it is with other intracranial surgery. At times, the endonasal approach is used for patch repair of CSF leak, and a lumbar drain may be placed in order to drain CSF and thereby reduce internal pressure against the repair.

In these cases, the lumbar drain is generally placed by the neurosurgeon, but managed intraoperatively by the anesthesiologist. Working knowledge of the stopcock and drainage system of the particular CSF collection system being used is vital in order to prevent accidental overdrainage of CSF and also to be able to drain controlled amounts of CSF at the request of the surgical team.

PONV AND PAIN CONTROL

All postsurgical patients require adequate pain and nausea avoidance, and this is especially true for endoscopic sinus surgery patients. Pain is experienced via multiple pathways—somatically as well as viscerally through surgical incisions and nerve disruption. All of these pathways must be considered, with a plan to avoid sedation and protect airway reflexes as much as possible. As soon as surgically appropriate, cyclo-oxygenase (COX) inhibitors should be used in order to control pain as well as inflammation. Acetaminophen and judicious use opioids should be employed in appropriate patients. Any new bleeding should be investigated, and nausea secondary to opioids should be quickly controlled.

Antiemetic control can be started preoperatively and/or intraoperatively depending on the patient and plan of anesthetic. Consistent with multiple pathways for pain, nausea is experienced due to multiple sites in the brain. These sites are triggered by various neurotransmitters.[32] Using the 2003 Consensus Guidelines for Managing Postoperative Nausea and Vomiting, four independent predictors help triage patients for risk of PONV: (1) female, (2) a history of PONV, (3) nonsmokers, and (4) postoperative opioid use.[33] In addition to these risk factors, patients undergoing ear, nose, and throat procedures were also at an increased risk of postoperative nausea and emesis (double control group).[33] As mentioned earlier, intraoperative medications can increase or decrease this risk, and a plan must be made accordingly. Antimuscarinics such as a scopolamine patch, steroids for both anti-inflammatory and antiemetic effect, and 5-HT3 receptor antagonists can be used together or individually in this endeavor.

CONCLUSIONS

Endoscopic sinus surgery is a routine case for an anesthesiologist, and good anesthetic care of the patient for ESS rests upon the foundation of good anesthetic care for any patient. Careful attention to bleeding and the optimization of the surgical field does set ESS slightly apart from other general anesthetics. Thorough communication between the surgeon and the anesthesiologist can best achieve a balance between potentially competing goals, facilitate optimal care of even complex patients with an eye toward patient safety, and maximize surgical outcomes. Preoperative discussion of anticoagulants or antiplatelet agents, attention to the airway and extubation procedures, careful titration of blood pressure and cardiac output, knowledge of vasoconstrictors and local anesthetics, and avoidance of postoperative nausea can all contribute to good surgical outcomes. Teamwork, communication, and respect between the sinus surgeon and the anesthesiologist are vital to working toward these optimal results.

REFERENCES

1. Jaffer AK. Perioperative management of warfarin and antiplatelet therapy. Cleve Clin J Med. 2009;76(4):S37-44.
2. Practice alert for the perioperative management of patients with coronary stents. Anesthesiology. 2009;110(1):1-2.
3. Ang-Lee MK, et al. Herbal medicines and perioperative care. JAMA. 2001;286(2):208-16.
4. Atef A, et al. Comparison of laryngeal mask with endotracheal tube for anesthesia in endoscopic sinus surgery. Am J Rhinol. 2088;22:653-7.
5. Barak M, et al. Hemodynamic and catecholamine response to tracheal intubation: direct laryngoscopy compared with fiberoptic intubation. J Clin Anesth. 2003;15:132-6.

5a. Oczenski W, et al. Hemodynamic and catecholamine stress responses to insertion of the combitube, laryngeal mask airway or tracheal intubation. Anesth Analg. 1999;88:1389-94.

6. Kaplan A, Crosby GJ, Bhattacharyya N. Airway protection and the laryngeal mask airway in sinus and nasal surgery. Laryngoscope. 2004;114(4):652-5.
7. Ahmed MZ, et al. The reinforced laryngeal mask airway (RLMA) protects the airway in patients undergoing nasal surgery—an observational study of 200 patients. Can J Anaesth. 2002;49:863-6.
8. Popat M, et al. Difficult airway society guidelines for the management of tracheal extubation. Anaesthesia. 2012;67(3):318-40.
9. Lee B, et al., Target smooth emergence: the effect site concentration of remifentanil for preventing cough during propofol-remifentanil anaesthesia for thyroid surgery. Br J Anaesth. 2009;102:775-8.
10. Nekhendzy V, Lemmens HJM, Vaughan WC, et al. The effect of deliberate hypercapnia and hypocapnia on intraoperative blood loss and quality of surgical field during functional endoscopic sinus surgery. Anesth Analg. 2007;105:1404-9.
11. Gilbey P, et al. The quality of the surgical field during functional endoscopic sinus surgery—the effect of the

mode of ventilation—a randomized, prospective, double-blind study. Laryngoscope. 2009;119(12):2449-53.

12. Boezaart AP. Comparison of sodium nitroprusside- and esmolol-induced controlled hypotension for functional endoscopic sinus surgery. Can J Anaesth. 1995;42:373-6.
13. Okuyama K, Inomata S, Toyooka H. The effects of prostaglandin E1 or oral clonidine premedication on blood loss during paranasal sinus surgery. Can J Anaesth. 2005;52(5):546-7;
14. Jacobi KE, Bohm BE, Rickauer AJ, et al. Moderate controlled hypotension with sodium nitroprusside does not improve surgical conditions or decrease blood loss in endoscopic sinus surgery. J Clin Anesth. 2000;12:202-7.
15. Nair S, Collins M, Hung P, et al. The effect of beta-blocker premedication on the surgical field during endoscopic sinus surgery. Laryngoscope. 2004;114(6):1042-6;
16. Wormald PJ, Renen Gv, Perks J, et al. The effect of the total intravenous anesthesia compared with inhalational anesthesia on the surgical field during endoscopic sinus surgery. Am J Rhinol. 2005;19(5):514-20.
17. Durmus M, But AK, Dogan Z, et al. Effect of dexmedetomidine on bleeding during tympanoplasty or septorhinoplasty. Eur J Anaesthesiol. 2007;24(5):447-53.
18. Groudine S, et al. New York state guidelines on the topical use of phenylephrine in the operating room. Anesthesiology 2000;92:859-64.
19. Gomez-Rivera F, et al., Pilot study comparing total intravenous anesthesia to inhalational anesthesia in endoscopic sinus surgery: novel approach of blood flow quantification. Ann Otol Rhinol Laryngol. 2012;121(11):725-32.
20. Guven DG, et al. Evaluation of outcomes in patients given dexmedetomidine in functional endocscopic sinus surgery. Ann Otol Rhinol Laryngol. 2011;120(9):586-92.
21. Goksu S, et al. Effects of dexmedetomidine infusion in patients undergoing functional endoscopic sinus surgery under local anesthesia. Eur J Anaesthesiol. 2008;25(1):22-8.
22. Kozek-Langenecker SA, Kozek-Langenecker SA. The effects of drugs used in anaesthesia on platelet membrane receptors and on platelet function. Current Drug Targets [Review]. 2002;3(3):247-58.
23. Dogan IV, Ovalı E, Eti Z, et al. The in vitro effects of isoflurane, sevoflurane, and propofol on platelet aggregation. Anesth Analg. 1999;88:432-6.
24. Singh A, Sjorgen E, Becker S, Brenkman. "Anesthesia, Pre- and Post-Operative Care For Nasal Surgery." Integrative Rhinology: From the Lab to the Operating Room. New York, Thieme Publishers; 2013.
25. Corboz MR, Rivelli MA, Varty L, et al. Pharmacological characterization of postjunctional alpha-adrenoceptors in human nasal mucosa. Am J Rhinol. 2005;19(5):495-502.
26. Liao BS, Hilsinger RL Jr. Rasgon BM, et al. A preliminary study of cocaine absorption from the nasal mucosa. Laryngoscope 1999;109(1):98-102.
27. Valdes CJ, Bogado M, Rammal A, et al. Topical cocaine vs adrenaline in endoscopic sinus surgery: a blinded randomized control study. Int Forum Allergy Rhinol. 2014 March 26. doi:10.1002/alr.21325. [Epub ahead of print].
28. Timperley D, Sacks R, Parkinson RJ, et al. Perioperative and intraoperative maneuvers to optimize surgical outcomes in skull base surgery. Otolaryngol Clin North Am. 2010;43(4):699-730.
29. Cohen-Kerem R, Brown S, Villasenor LV, et al. Epinephrine/lidocaine injection vs. saline during endoscopic sinus surgery. Laryngoscope. 2008;118:1275-81.
30. Wormald PJ, Athanasiadis T, Rees G, et al. An evaluation of effect of pterygopalatine fossa injection with local anesthetic and adrenalin in the control of nasal bleeding during endoscopic sinus surgery. Am J Rhinol. 2005;19(3):288-92.
31. Weingarten CZ. Injection of the pterygopalatine fossa with glycerin for posterior epistaxis. Trans Am Acad Ophthalmol Otolaryngol. 1972;76(4):932-7.
32. Williams K. Postoperative nausea and vomiting. Surg Clin N Am. 2005;85(6):1229-41.
33. Gan TJ, et al. Consensus guidelines for managing postoperative nausea and vomiting. Anesth Analg. 2003;97(1):62-71.

CHAPTER

7 Endoscopic Instrumentation and Image Guidance

James D Phillips, Bradford A Woodworth

INTRODUCTION

The application of rigid endoscopes to surgery of the sinuses was the crucial step leading to the conceptual development of functional endoscopic sinus surgery (FESS) in the 1980s.[1-4] Endoscopes were noted to provide excellent visualization at the site of surgical intervention while permitting simultaneous manipulation of tissue with an instrument in the opposite hand.[5] Over the last 30 years, the development of a wide armamentarium of specialized equipment has been central to improving the technical aspects of FESS and endoscopic skull base surgery.

VISUALIZATION

Surgeons who utilize traditional endoscopic technique look directly down the eyepiece of the endoscope because it provides an extra degree of orientation and depth perception.[6] However, the vast majority of sinus surgeons prefer the attachment of a camera to the endoscope eyepiece in order to operate from a video monitor. This provides a few practical advantages.[6] First, the surgeon is allowed increased ergonomic comfort, because he/she is not required to bend at the neck or back to move the scope through the angles of the sinus cavities. In addition, the monitor provides the ability for magnification of pertinent anatomy and delineation of small, delicate structures. A senior surgeon can monitor and teach a trainee, assistants can more readily follow the procedure and anticipate the upcoming need for certain instruments, and the anesthesia team can better correlate their care to the real time needs of the procedure. Finally, utilization of a monitor allows for the participation of the other members of the operative team.

Modifications of current equipment or introduction of novel systems continue to focus on improving visualization for a wide range of sinus and skull base disorders. Modifications of the rigid endoscope include angulation of the tip (30°, 45°, and 70°) for markedly improved visualization around corners (Figs. 7.1A to C), smaller diameters (2.7 or 3 mm), and even three-dimensional endoscopic systems for skull base surgery. Endoscopic visualization is also noticeably enhanced with the development of high definition systems that provide superior image quality. Various lens cleaning systems allow superior visualization by immediately counteracting visual obstruction of the endoscope from blood, mucous, or fogging without having to remove the endoscope from the nose. Finally, robotic surgery is an exciting area of ongoing research and development that could enhance visualization in endoscopic sinus and skull base surgery.

BASIC SINUS INSTRUMENTATION

A basic sinus set of nonpowered instruments includes thumb-controlled suction tips, ball-tipped probes of varying size and angulation, back-biting forceps—either rotating or sided, sickle knife, Freer elevator with and without suction attachment, straight and 45° upturned Blakesley forceps, straight and 45° upturned through-cut forceps, Kerrison punches, and curettes of varying size and angulation. If the frontal sinus is to be addressed, the addition of 45° and 90° giraffe cup forceps, a Hosemann frontal sinus punch, and Kuhn Bolger through-cut forceps of several angulations are critical for complex frontal recess dissections (Fig. 7.2). For a complete list of a comprehensive sinus set, *see* Table 7.1.[6]

As experience grows, surgeons develop greater efficiency with instruments guided by a few select principles: minimization of the number of endoscope changes while still maintaining a broad adequate view of the surgical field, safe removal of tissue while preserving the maximum amount of residual mucosa, and choosing the correct angulation and length of instrument to accomplish the

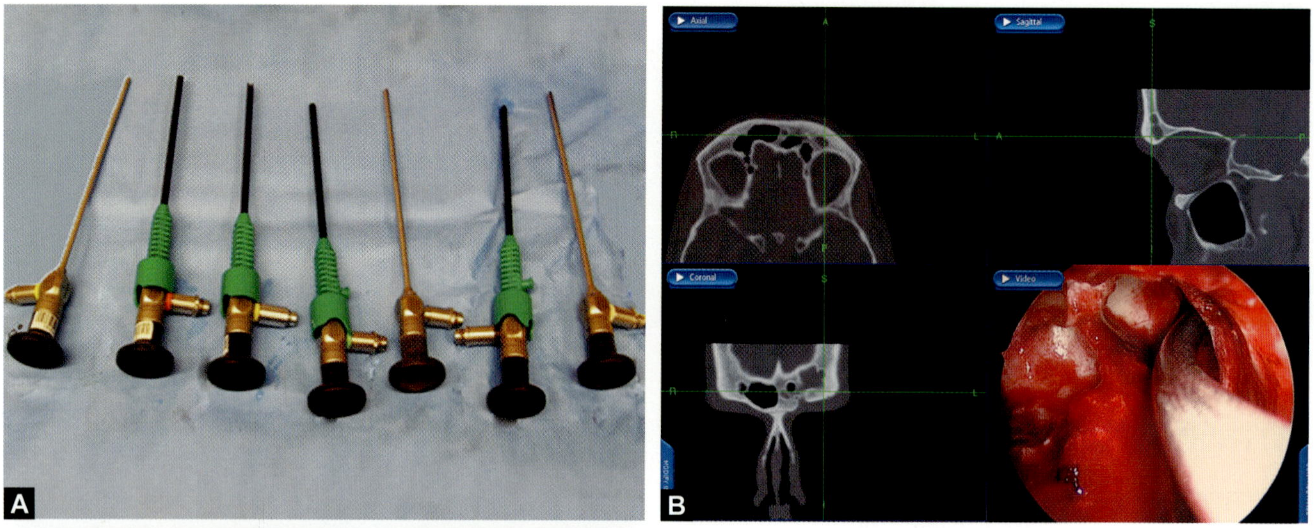

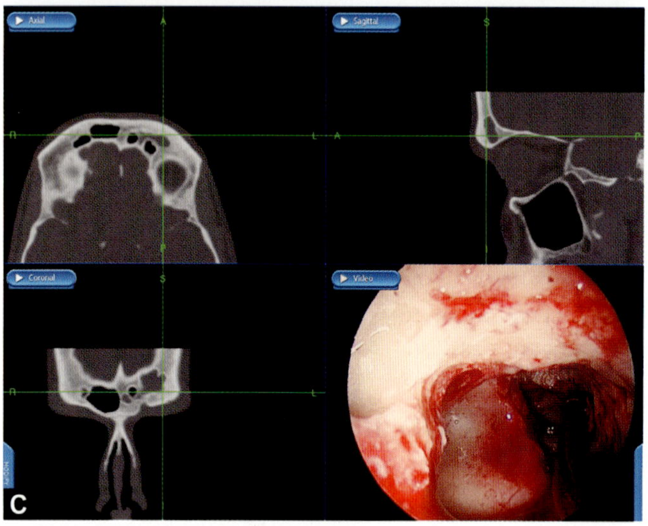

Figs. 7.1A to C: Rigid endoscopes with varying degrees of angulation (A). Angled scopes may have "offset" or "reverse" posts for the light source to accommodate various directions of view without inhibiting the opposite hand. The green attachment on several scopes is a lens cleaning system (Endoscrub II, Medtronic®, Jacksonville, FL). Image-guidance triplanar CT and endoscopic views with a 30° (B) and 70° (C) endoscope of a lateral frontal sinus recess mucocele. Increasing the angulation with a 70° endoscope provided the view necessary for complete visualization.

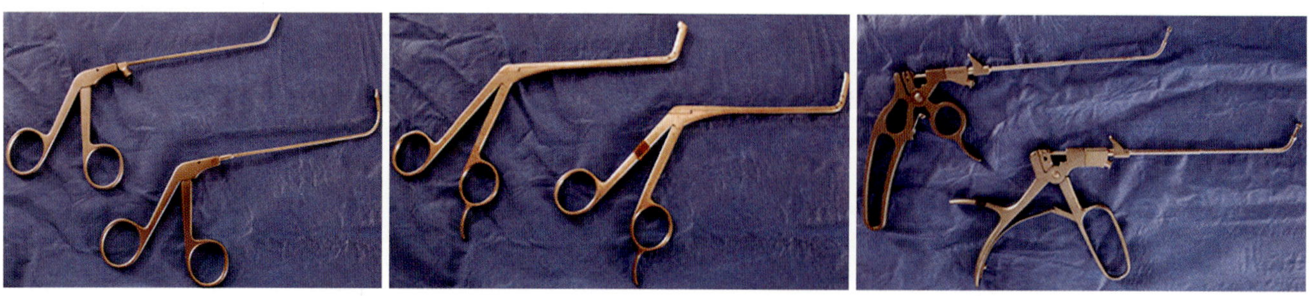

Fig. 7.2: Various sharply angled forceps for use in frontal sinus surgery. Through-cutting instruments allow for the safe removal of bony partitions while maximizing the preservation of normal mucosa to prevent postoperative scarring and restenosis.

desired maneuver. When operating in the frontal sinus, this learning curve can be particularly steep as the degree of angulation can be disorienting to the novice sinus surgeon.

POWERED INSTRUMENTATION

The powered microdebrider was a significant advancement in FESS instrumentation. With parallel circuits

Table 7.1: Endoscopic sinus surgery hand instrument set

Hosemann frontal punch 70°	Freer suction elevator	Adson forceps
Hosemann frontal punch 70° upturn	Frazier suction tip, 10 French	Hemostats
Frontal sinus chain punch 70° upturn backward cutting 3.5 mm	Rhino sinus back-biting forceps	Needle driver
Frontal sinus chain punch 70° upturn backward cutting 5 mm	Rotatable Stammberger antrum punch	Beaver blade scalpel
Frontal sinus thru-cut forceps 60° up backward left opening	Cottle elevator	Nasal speculum
Frontal sinus thru-cut forceps 60° up backward opening, flat jaw 12 cm	Freer elevator	Kerrison 3 mm down biting punch
Kuhn frontal sinus thru-cut forceps 60° up backward opening	Bayonet forceps	Kerrison 2 mm 40° punch
Rhinoforce sinus forcep thru-cut 90° up flat jaw	Mayo scissors	Kerrison 4 mm 40° up-biting punch
Rhoton Sella 1 mm 90° down-biting punch	Straight frontal sinus curette	45° Frontal sinus curette
90° frontal sinus curette	Strumpel Voss forceps 2 mm straight	Right-angled nasal sinus scissors
Straight nasal sinus scissors	Left angled nasal sinus scissors	Straight Blakesley thru cutting forceps
Ferris Smith alligator forceps	Weil-Blakesley 90° up sinus forceps	Frontal sinus recess giraffe forceps 45°
Kerrison 40° 1 mm up-biting punch	Blakesley 45° thru-cut forceps	Weil-Blakesley 45° upturned forceps
Curved sinus suction	Frontal ostium seeker 90°	Sickle knife
Maxillary seeker, doubled ended ball tip probe		

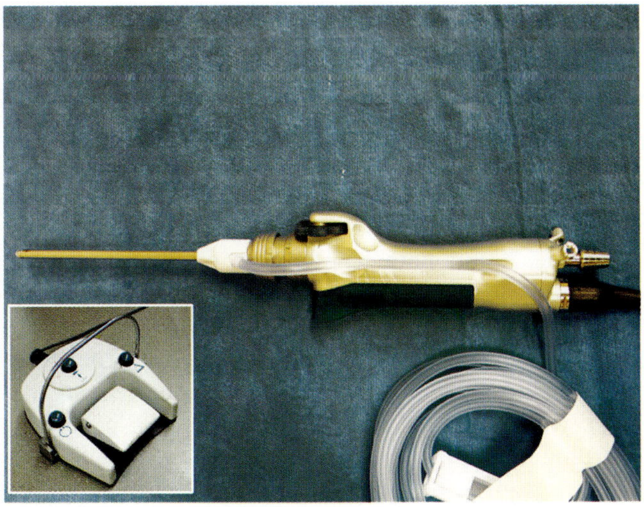

Fig. 7.3: An example of a powered microdebrider with separate ports for suction and saline irrigation. Angled tips may be exchanged for the straight tip to expand access. The wheel on the side may be used to rotate the tip 360°. The pedal (inset) allows for hands-free control of speed as well as various operation modes.

of suction and irrigation, tissue can be drawn into the inner rotating blade of the microdebrider and resected quickly and accurately while preserving the maximum amount of normal mucosa without stripping. The back edge can shield normal anatomy, such as the middle turbinate, while the open blade resects. Because of its efficacy in the rapid removal of tissue and the shortening of operative times, the powered microdebrider is a popular instrument among modern rhinologists (Fig. 7.3). However, the microdebrider must be utilized with great caution. If the debrider is unintentionally administered to an extrasinus location such as the orbit, injury to tissue can occur rapidly. The potential for medial rectus injury and unnecessary visual morbidity with the powered microdebrider is well documented.[7,8]

Endoscopic angled power drills also represent a significant leap forward for expanded endonasal surgery. Utilization of diamond burs with parallel suction and irrigation circuits allow for the precise, safe removal of thick bone that was previously quite tedious. Thicker sections of bone such as the clivus or the ptyergoid plates may be removed rapidly in order to address pathology beyond the sinuses. As with the powered microdebrider, endoscopic drills should be utilized with significant restraint and care in areas where injury may occur. If the depth of dissection is not constantly monitored, nearby structures may be rapidly damaged.

HEMOSTASIS

Hemostasis during and after FESS and expanded endonasal surgery is essential for safe and effective treatment.[9] When visualization is reliant on the integrity of the endoscopic image and the space for additional instrumentation is limited, the importance of maintaining hemostatic control of the surgical field cannot be overemphasized. This is accomplished through multiple ways such as positioning of the patient with the head slightly elevated, maintaining tight control of patient blood pressure by the anesthesia team, and utilizing preoperative and intraoperative topical vasoconstrictive agents such as oxymetazoline or epinephrine.

Hemostatic instruments are indispensable when addressing highly vascular tumors (e.g., juvenile nasopharyngeal angiofibromas) or removing fulminate polyposis. Monopolar cautery (an electrical circuit passed through the patient and converted to heat energy at the tip of the instrument) is typically delivered through a suction cautery device in the nose. It may be used for the prophylactic control of specific vascular structures, such as the septal branch of the sphenopalatine artery when performing sphenoidotomy. Bipolar cautery (the passing of an electrical circuit between the tips of the instrument) is considered more precise, particularly when the tissue or vessel are straddled by the instrument tips, and avoids jump currents to nearby neural structures. Tip guards are necessary for safe utilization of this instrument in the nose. Radiofrequency coblation (ArthroCare ENT, Austin, TX) is another hemostatic instrument for sinus and skull base surgery that utilizes bipolar radiofrequency plasma for the generation of hemostasis (Fig. 7.4). The radiofrequency energy excites electrons through a medium such as saline to create a focused area of plasma energy.[9] This allows for the ablation of tissue while maintaining control of bleeding. Significantly lower thermal energy is delivered when compared with cautery devices so tissue is removed with minimal damage to surrounding structures. This is quite beneficial in the debulking and resection of sinonasal tumors which may have a high degree of vascularity. Additionally, it can be used in the reduction and excision of encephaloceles.[10]

IMAGE GUIDANCE SYSTEMS

Image guidance (IG), the utilization of preoperative imaging triangulated to the real-time location of calibrated instruments within the sinus cavities, has become a popular adjunct in endoscopic sinus surgery. Because

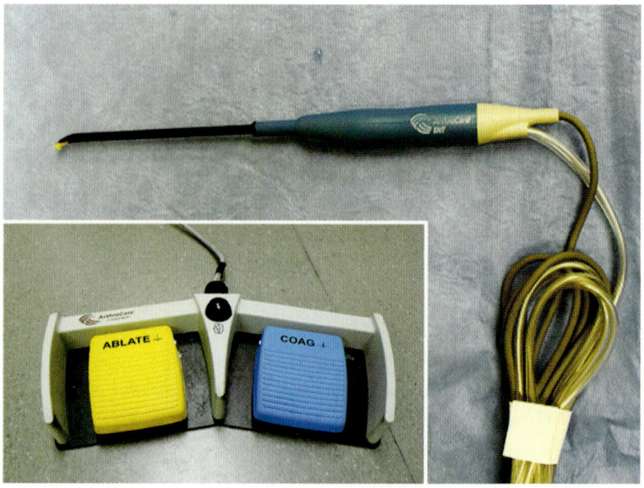

Fig. 7.4: The Coblator (ArthroCare ENT®, Austin, TX) wand. The pedal control (inset) allows for hands-free administration of plasma energy focused for the purpose of ablation with coagulation.

the sinus cavities are surrounded by a number of crucial anatomic structures, IG serves to confirm the position of the instrument as well as the location of nearby areas of danger beyond what is directly visible through the endoscope. When functioning properly, surgeons may expect accuracy up to 2 mm. It has been applied to all complex aspects of rhinologic surgery.[11-15] Fears that the system might be used as a substitute for detailed understanding of anatomy (resulting in increased complications) were premature as a recent meta-analysis indicated that IG systems have decreased the risk of both major and the total number of complication events when compared with non-IG sinus surgery.[16]

Currently, there are two different localization systems commercially available—infrared and electromagnetic (Fig. 7.5).[17] Both types match the position of an instrument within the perioperative spatial field to the three-dimensional repository "map" made from preoperative imaging. In the electromagnetic system, an electromagnetic field is generated about the patient's head, which responds to the movements of calibrated instruments with magnetic landmarks. In the infrared optical systems, the spatial repository is created by two to three infrared cameras that must maintain direct line of sight to the surgical field. Localizing instruments are then outfitted with infrared emitters or sensors which the systems use to calculate the position.[17] Although a useful adjunct for position confirmation, no IG system should be considered a replacement for mastery of the pertinent paranasal sinus anatomy.

Image guidance systems are based on preoperative imaging and thus do not provide real-time information

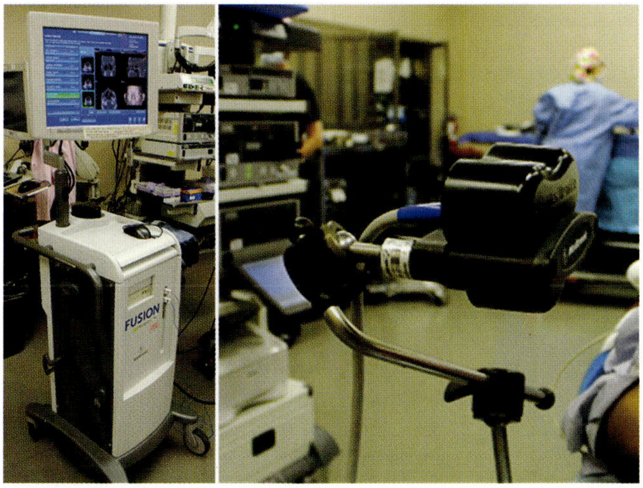

Fig. 7.5: An example of an electromagnetic image guidance system (Medtronic® Fusion, Jacksonville, FL) is displayed (left). The tower includes the input for a tracker that may be attached interchangeably to calibrated instruments. This is also where patient imaging is loaded. The monitor provides real-time correlation of instrument position to the imaging construct. The electromagnetic emitter (right) is attached to the bed near the patient's head.

regarding the progress of a resection. In order to bypass this shortcoming, interest has arisen in intraoperative CT acquisition with real time update of IG systems. The xCAT (Xoran Technologies, Ann Arbor, MI, USA) is a compact, portable CT scanner that can provide 0.4 mm thick images to the sinuses in less than 3 min.[9] The cone beam technology significantly reduces the amount of radiation exposure to the patient.

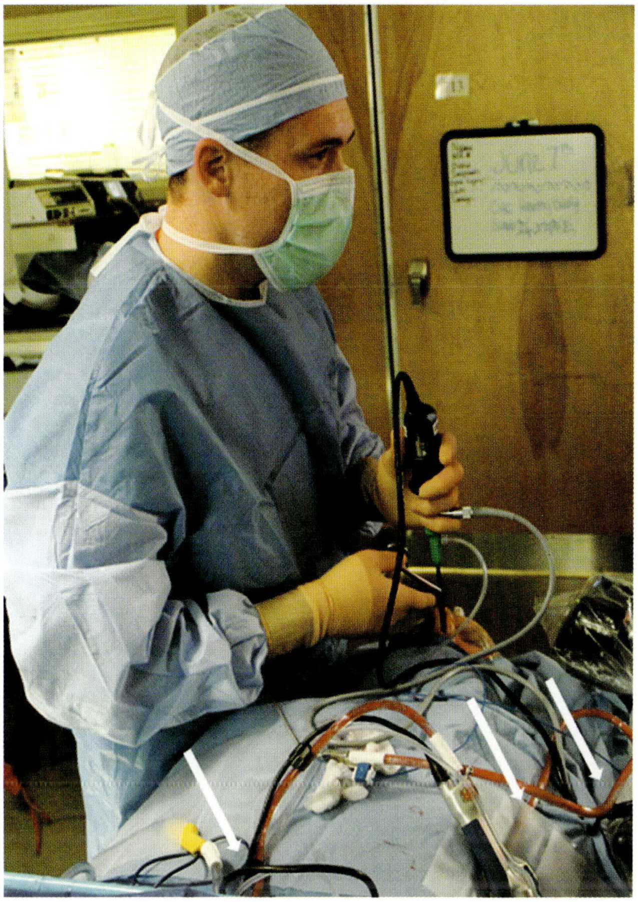

Fig. 7.6: The importance of a consistent, logical system for the organization of the various cables and tubes associated with FESS is paramount. The surgical staff can maintain "lanes" for each element to diminish opportunities for tangling (arrows).

EQUIPMENT ORGANIZATION

An experienced ancillary staff in the operating room, familiar with the instruments and their uses, is critical for streamlined surgical procedures. Multiple suctions, cautery, video cables, a lens cleaning system, and powered instruments (often with multiple ports and cords) can reduce the field to a scrambled nest that hinders the efficiency of the operation. Creating "lanes" for each instrument will minimize tangling (Fig. 7.6). Placement of control pedals should be consistent so that various devices may be deployed without distracting the surgeon's eyes from the surgical field.

CONCLUSION

Innovations such as powered instrumentation, advanced hemostatic devices, and IG have markedly improved endoscopic techniques and made an enormous impact on the management of sinus and skull base pathology. Although thorough knowledge of equipment and instrumentation is imperative for expert endoscopic management, there is no substitute for experience and proficient understanding of the relevant anatomy.

REFERENCES

1. Kennedy DW. Functional endoscopic sinus surgery. Technique. Arch Otolaryngol. 1985;111:643-9.
2. Kennedy DW, Zinreich SJ, Rosenbaum AE, et al. Functional endoscopic sinus surgery. Theory and diagnostic evaluation. Arch Otolaryngol. 1985;111:576-82.
3. Stammberger H. Endoscopic endonasal surgery—concepts in treatment of recurring rhinosinusitis. Part I. Anatomic and pathophysiologic considerations. Otolaryngol Head Neck Surg. 1986;94:143-7.

4. Stammberger H. Endoscopic endonasal surgery—concepts in treatment of recurring rhinosinusitis. Part II. Surgical technique. Otolaryngol Head Neck Surg. 1986;94:147-56.
5. Zada G, Liu C, Apuzzo ML. Through the looking glass: optical physics, issues, and the evolution of neuroendoscopy. World Neurosurg. 2012;77:92-102.
6. Wormald PJ. Endoscopic sinus surgery: anatomy, three-dimensional reconstruction, and surgical technique. New York: Thieme; 2012.
7. Graham SM, Nerad JA. Orbital complications in endoscopic sinus surgery using powered instrumentation. Laryngoscope. 2003;113:874-8.
8. Bhatti MT, Giannoni CM, Raynor E, et al. Ocular motility complications after endoscopic sinus surgery with powered cutting instruments. Otolaryngol Head Neck Surg. 2001; 125:501-9.
9. Virgin FW, Bleier BS, Woodworth BA. Evolving materials and techniques for endoscopic sinus surgery. Otolaryngol Clin North Am. 2010;43:653-72, xi.
10. Smith N, Riley KO, Woodworth BA. Endoscopic Coblator-assisted management of encephaloceles. Laryngoscope. 2010 Dec;120(12):2535-9.
11. Metson R. Image-guided sinus surgery: lessons learned from the first 1000 cases. Otolaryngol Head Neck Surg. 2003;128:8-13.
12. Lam SM, Huang C, Newman J, et al. Computer-aided image-guided endoscopic sinus surgery in unusual cases of sphenoid disease. Rhinology. 2002;40:179-84.
13. Anand VK, Hiltzik DH, Kacker A, et al. Osteoplastic flap for frontal sinus obliteration in the era of image-guided endoscopic sinus surgery. Am J Rhinol. 2005;19:406-10.
14. Gharabaghi A, Krischek B, Feigl GC, et al. Image-guided craniotomy for frontal sinus preservation during meningioma surgery. Eur J Surg Oncol. 2008;34:928-31.
15. Wong WK, Matsuwaki Y, Omura K, et al. Role of intra-operative CT-updates during image-guided endoscopic sinus surgery for sinonasal fibro-osseous lesions. Auris Nasus Larynx. 2011;38:628-31.
16. Dalgorf DM, Sacks R, Wormald PJ, et al. Image-guided surgery influences perioperative morbidity from endoscopic sinus surgery: a systematic review and meta-analysis. Otolaryngol Head Neck Surg. 2013;149:17-29.
17. Pruliere-Escabasse V, Coste A. Image-guided sinus surgery. Eur Ann Otorhinolaryngol Head Neck Dis. 2010;127:33-9.

CHAPTER 8

Optimizing Postoperative Care

Elisa A Illing, Bradford A Woodworth

INTRODUCTION

Functional endoscopic sinus surgery (ESS) has evolved as the gold standard treatment for medically refractory chronic rhinosinusitis (CRS). The goals of the procedure are to restore paranasal sinus drainage tracts and ventilation with mucosal-sparing techniques. Although ESS has well-documented success as a treatment modality, patients may have disease recurrence or complications upon long-term follow-up and surgical intervention should be viewed as a complement to the medical treatment of this chronic inflammatory disease.[1] Complications may include synechiae formation, mucosal overgrowth with stenosis of sinus ostia, and lateralization of the middle turbinates. Preoperative counseling, proper patient selection, and postoperative management strategies are critical to prevent complications and increase likelihood of successful surgical intervention. This chapter will discuss postoperative strategies designed to optimize surgical outcomes in patients after ESS.

NASAL PACKING

Traditionally, nasal packing has been utilized after ESS for hemostasis, with the additional benefits of middle turbinate medialization, prevention of adhesions, and decreasing stenosis. Initially anterior packing with nonabsorbable devices was used, although patients reported presence and removal of this packing to be the most uncomfortable portion of postoperative ESS recovery.[2] For the purpose of hemostasis, some have shown that packing is not necessary without any increase in the risk of postoperative bleeding.[3] Advances in absorbable packing have provided surgeons with options to avoid discomfort issues while also achieving the desirable effects of packing. However, there are concerns regarding increased inflammation at the surgical bed and inferior hemostasis when absorbable packing is used.[4-7] Characteristics both absorbable and nonabsorbable packing strive to achieve include painless removal, adequate hemostasis, nonabrasive qualities, wound healing promotion, and low cost.[8]

Nonabsorbable Packing

Nonabsorbable packing in the middle meatus is used postoperatively in ESS patients to provide middle turbinate medialization, hemostasis, and prevent adhesion formation. Adhesions are one of the most common complications of ESS. They are reported to occur in up to 36% of patients with 2/3 of those with adhesions requiring surgical revision.[9] Patients with nonabsorbable packing in place have been shown to have less synechiae formation compared with control groups where no packing was used at all.[10] Historically, examples of nonabsorbable packing include balloon catheter devices, polyvinyl acetate sponge (Merocel, Metronic Xomed, Jacksonville, FL, USA), Telfa gauze, gloved Merocel nasal packs or petroleum-impregnated gauze. Varied lengths of duration for the packing have been described including removal in the immediate postoperative setting and anywhere up to 13 days after surgery.[11,12]

Complications beyond pain at removal are not uncommon with nonabsorbable packing. Use of petroleum-impregnated gauze is not recommended because of reports of paraffin granulomas and spherulocytosis.[11] Concerns for mucosal lesions including septal perforation and turbinate necrosis have been shown most readily with balloon catheters, and with uncovered Merocel packs, which induce a loss of 50–70% of ciliated mucosal surface area.[13] Using a nonlatex glove finger covering over the Merocel (Figs. 8.1A and B) decreases pain on removal, has less bleeding after removal, and reduces the incidence of synechiae formation compared with Merocel middle meatal spacers without covering.[8] Nonlatex glove use is imperative to avoid latex sensitivity. To prevent

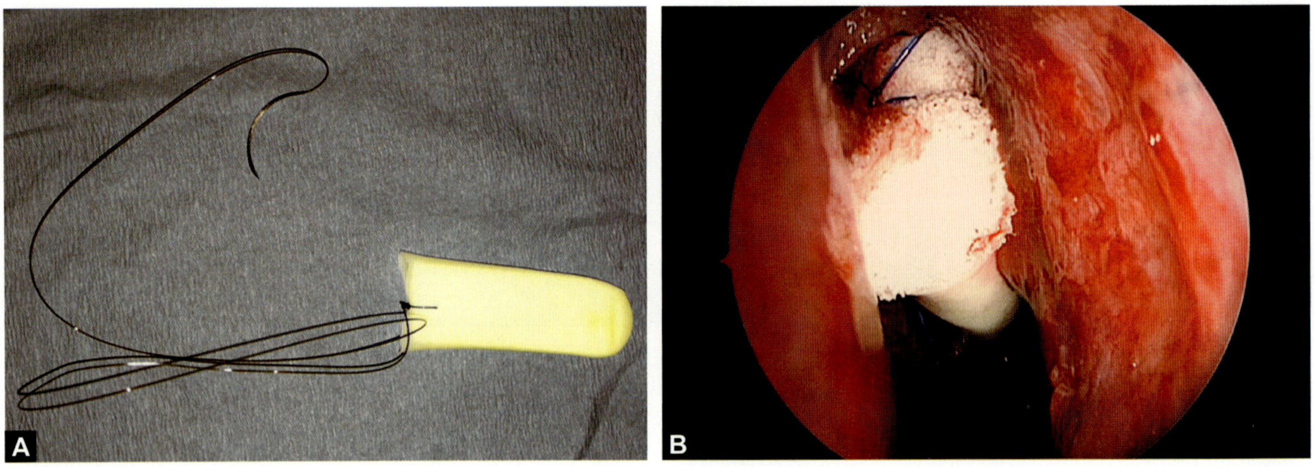

Figs. 8.1A and B: Gloved-Merocel middle meatal spacer. A sterile, nonlatex glove is used to cover the Merocel pack with a prolene suture securing the glove to the Merocel prior to placement in the middle meatus (A). The Merocel is inserted into the ethmoid cavity effectively "spacing" the cavity to prevent accumulation of blood and medializing the middle turbinate (B).

mobilization and aspiration of the pack, a tethering, nonabsorbable stitch placed through the pack and the nasal septum is recommended.[11] Additionally, concern for toxic shock syndrome (TSS) is increased with nonabsorbable packs. Although studies have shown topical and prophylactic antibiotic, administration did not demonstrate decreased incidence of TSS, the authors do recommend empiric antibiotic coverage when nonabsorbable packing is in place.[14,15]

Absorbable Packing

Because of the complications and complaints with nonabsorbable packs, research into absorbable packing options was pursued, using primarily biologic agents such as those derived from blood products, animal, plant, or synthetic materials. Hemostatic efficacy and impairment of wound healing vary amongst products and are summarized in Table 8.1.

Drug-Eluting Packing and Stents

To combat issues with topical medication delivery in the setting of nasal crusting, retained secretions and mucosal edema, as well as patient compliance, recent studies have evaluated the benefit of drug-eluting packing and stents in postoperative ESS patients. Most commonly, surgeons create off-label drug-eluting middle meatal spacers to provide continuous topical therapy, although the pharmacokinetics and systemic absorbance of these medications are not well known. NasoPore soaked with triamcinolone placed within the ethmoid cavity for 7 days after ESS was shown to improve the appearance of nasal mucosa at both early and late postoperative periods, as well as decrease polyp formation.[16] More recently, the use of Sinu-Foam (carboxymethylcellulose) (Figs. 8.2A and B) mixed with dexamethasone placed in the ethmoid sinus at the completion of ESS for patients with CRS without nasal polyposis did not demonstrate advantages over placebo (Sinu-Foam only) with regards to Lund-Kennedy sinus grading system on nasal endoscopy.[17] However, use with triamcinolone acetonide postoperatively in nasal polyposis patients was shown beneficial in improving outcomes and may reduce overall prednisone use for recurrent polyposis.[18,19]

Drug-eluting stents, such as the Propel Sinus Implant (Intersect ENT; Palo Alto, CA, USA) recently approved by the Food and Drug Administration for use in post-ESS patients with CRS with nasal polyposis, are evolving options for postoperative ESS topical drug delivery. The Propel Implant is an absorbable stent impregnated with mometasone furoate placed in the ethmoid cavity at the conclusion of ESS, releasing 370 μg of mometasone over 30 days, with the stent dissolving within 30–45 days. Several studies have demonstrated decreased adhesions, polyp recurrence, and mucosal inflammation, including a meta-analysis that showed reduction in the need of postoperative interventions decreased by 35%, lysis of adhesions by 51%, and use of oral steroids by 40%.[20]

MIDDLE TURBINATE STABILIZATION

In addition to middle meatal spacers, stabilization of the middle turbinate has been described via various

Table 8.1: Absorbable packing

	Components	Advantages	Disadvantages
Blood-derived products			
Fibrin glue	Human-thrombin and fibrinogen combined with amino acids and salts	Reportedly as effective as conventional packing at hemostasis, decreases adhesion formation[53]	
FloSeal	Bovine-derived gelatin matrix with human-derived thrombin	Achieves hemostasis[54]	Increased granulation tissue and adhesion formation noted[54]
Animal-derived products			
MeroGel	Hyaluronic acid ester		No improvement in hemostasis, no significant decrease in adhesions compared with no packing[55-57]
GelFilm	Denatured porcine collagen		
Surgiflo	Absorbable porcine gelatin	As effective as thrombin at hemostasis, no adverse adhesions, infections noted[58]	
Hyaluronan hydrogel products			
PureRegen Gel Sinus	Cross-linked sodium hyaluronate, sodium chloride, phosphate, and water	Decreased adhesions, edema, crusting, and mucopurulent drainage when compared with no packing[59]	
Plant-based products			
Surgicel	Oxidized regenerated cellulose	Achieves hemostasis as well as nonabsorbable packing[60]	
Sinu-FoamTM	Carboxymethylcellulose		No improvement in hemostasis or wound healing compared with no packing[60,61]

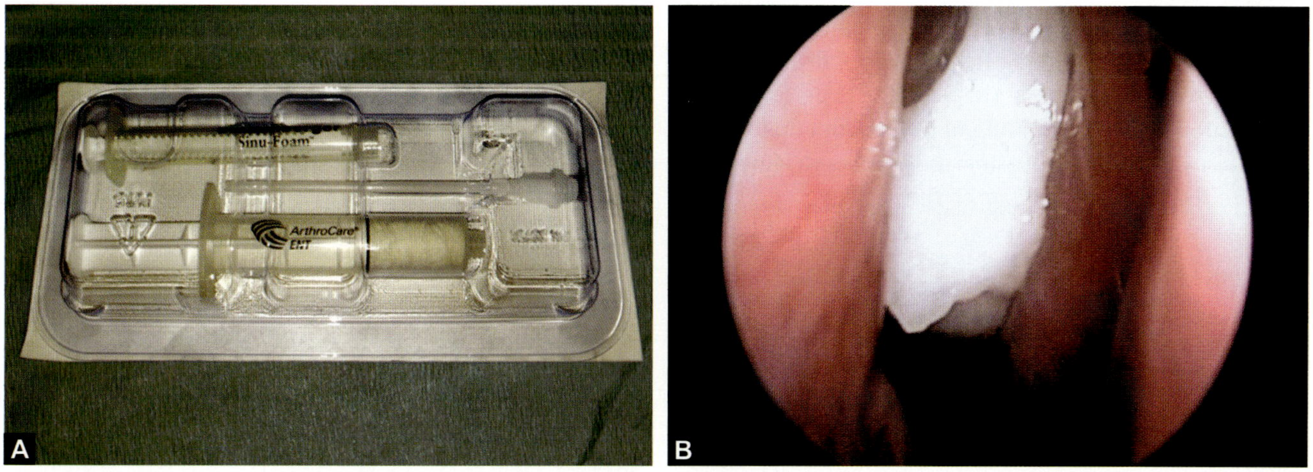

Figs. 8.2A and B: Carboxymethylcellulose foam (Sinu-Foam®, ArthroCare ENT, Austin, Tx) is demonstrated before mixing (A). Transnasal endoscopic view after expulsion of the foam into the ethmoid cavity where it acts as absorbable "spacer" (B).

techniques, including suturing the middle turbinate to the septum (Figs. 8.3A to C), scoring the medial wall of the middle turbinate as well as the adjacent septal mucosa to promote scarring (Bolgerization), use of biological glue to adhere the middle turbinate to the septum, and so on.[21-24] Long-term followup has not been reported regarding outcomes of these methods; however, in the short-term patients have had successful medialization of the middle

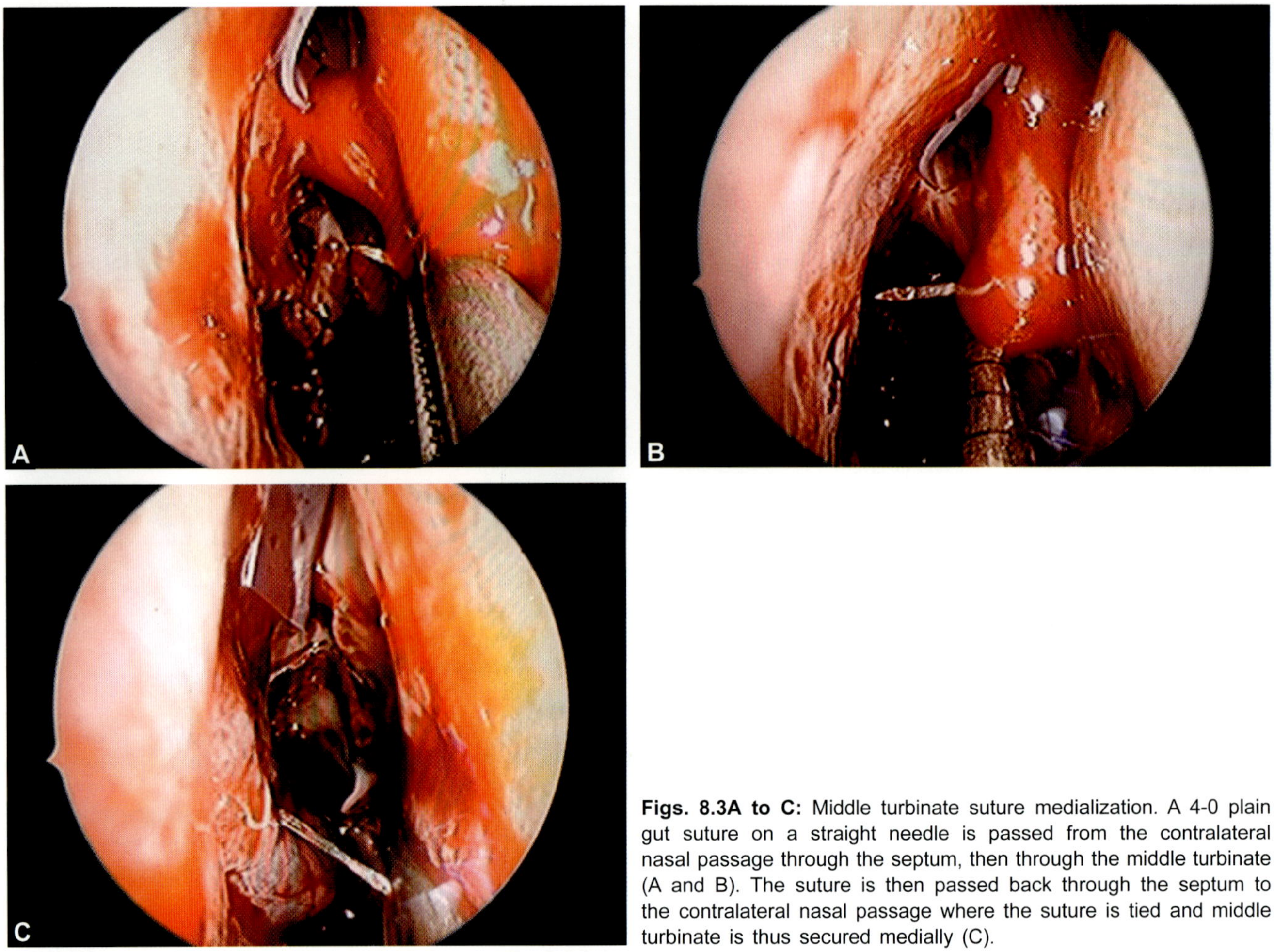

Figs. 8.3A to C: Middle turbinate suture medialization. A 4-0 plain gut suture on a straight needle is passed from the contralateral nasal passage through the septum, then through the middle turbinate (A and B). The suture is then passed back through the septum to the contralateral nasal passage where the suture is tied and middle turbinate is thus secured medially (C).

turbinate without consequences such as disruption of olfaction.[25] In cases where a septoplasty is performed in conjunction with ESS, quilting of the mucoperichondrial flaps may be performed using the same stitch used to stabilize the middle turbinate to the septum.[26]

FRONTAL SINUS STENT

Endoscopic frontal sinus surgery is a challenging procedure, where instrumentation of the frontal recess may cause scarring, synechiae, or osteoneogenesis of the frontal outflow tract. To maintain patency of the frontal recess, the use of frontal sinus stents has been debated in the literature using an assortment of materials for a variable duration of time (Table 8.2). Frontal sinus stenting is not without risks, however, and reports have shown biofilms exist on frontal stents, questioning the propagation of chronic sinus disease in susceptible patients.[27] Additionally, patients may have difficulty with granulation if stents are too short, or nasal crusting, obstruction, and odor if the stent is too long as it protrudes into the nasal cavity. Noting the risks and benefits, we recommend silastic sheeting, formed into a "Liberty Bell" or "T" shape inserted into the frontal recess (Fig. 8.4). The horizontal "T" portion should be introduced first into the frontal outflow tract, and released to allow the flanges to rest within the frontal sinus, effectively securing it in place. The vertical "T" portion should extend into the ethmoid area, but not beyond (Figs. 8.5A to C). The purpose of the stent is to facilitate debridement of the frontal recess in clinic rather than a long-term stenting of the sinus.

PREOPERATIVE AND POSTOPERATIVE SYSTEMIC STEROIDS

Inflammatory changes of the sinonasal mucosa are typical in patients suffering from CRS, with systemic steroids being utilized commonly to try and medically control this

Table 8.2: Frontal sinus stent usage

	Type of frontal stent	*Duration of stent placement*	*Outcome*
Weber et al.	Rains self-retaining, U-shaped silicone tube, H-shaped silicone tube	6 months	70% patency[62]
Blom and Freeman	Freeman frontal sinus stent (biflanged hollow silicone tube)	4 weeks	87% patency[63]
Orlandi	Rains self-retaining	Up to 6 years	78% patency[64]
Neel et al.*	Silicone sheeting		Promotes epithelization, decreases osteoblastic activity, decreases scar formation compared with more rigid plastic tubing[65]
Beule et al.*	Dexamethasone-eluting frontal stents		Decreases granulation[66]

(*Animal models)

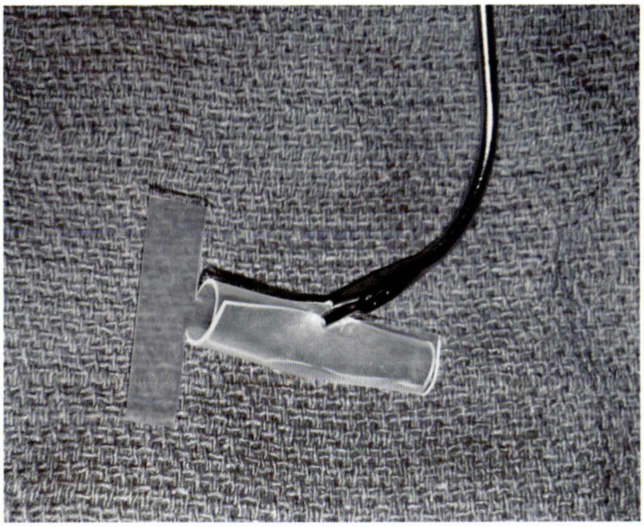

Fig. 8.4: Frontal sinus stenting. Silastic sheeting, formed into a "Liberty Bell" or "T" shape.

disease process. In patients with recalcitrant CRS pursuing ESS, systemic steroids are often suggested to preoperatively optimize patients for surgery, and to maximize postoperative successful outcomes. Systemic steroid usage is not without consequences, with risks of use including hyperglycemia, insomnia, mood changes, gastritis, aseptic necrosis of the hip, increased intraocular pressure, and adrenal insufficiency if used for prolonged periods.[28] To avoid these complications, lower doses of steroids, 30–40 mg, tapered over 7–14 days are typically reported.[29] A randomized, double-blind, placebo-controlled study by Wright and Agarwal using prednisone in patients with history of CRS with polyposis did not show subjective improvement in postoperative symptoms, but did demonstrate postoperative endoscopic appearance improvement most visible at the 2-week postoperative interval.[30] In this study, 30 mg of prednisone was prescribed for 5 days prior to surgery and continued through 9 days following surgery, with no taper. No adverse events were reported with regard to steroid administration. Further studies are needed to conclude the role for steroids systemically in ESS patients; however, for those with CRS with nasal polyposis who are at high risk of polyp formation, edema, and crusting, oral steroids may be indicated.

POSTOPERATIVE SYSTEMIC ANTIBIOTICS AND ANTIFUNGALS

To avoid postoperative delayed wound healing, nasal discharge, mucosal crusting, and other patient symptoms thought to be due to bacterial infection following ESS; 7–21 days of systemic antibiotics have traditionally been prescribed. Although some studies have shown increased amounts of *Pseudomonas aeruginosa* and *Staphylococcus aureus* in patients with history of ESS and chronic sinusitis, others have revealed 97% of asymptomatic post-ESS patients have bacterial colonization with coagulase-negative staphylococci and diphteroids.[31,32] Despite the common use of postoperative systemic antibiotics, little evidence-based research exists to support their use. However, three randomized trials are commonly referenced to direct therapy for perioperative antibiotics (Table 8.3).[28,29]

Antibiotic therapy may have adverse effects, such as gastrointestinal malaise, clostridium difficile, allergic reaction, or bacterial resistance in some patients. Further

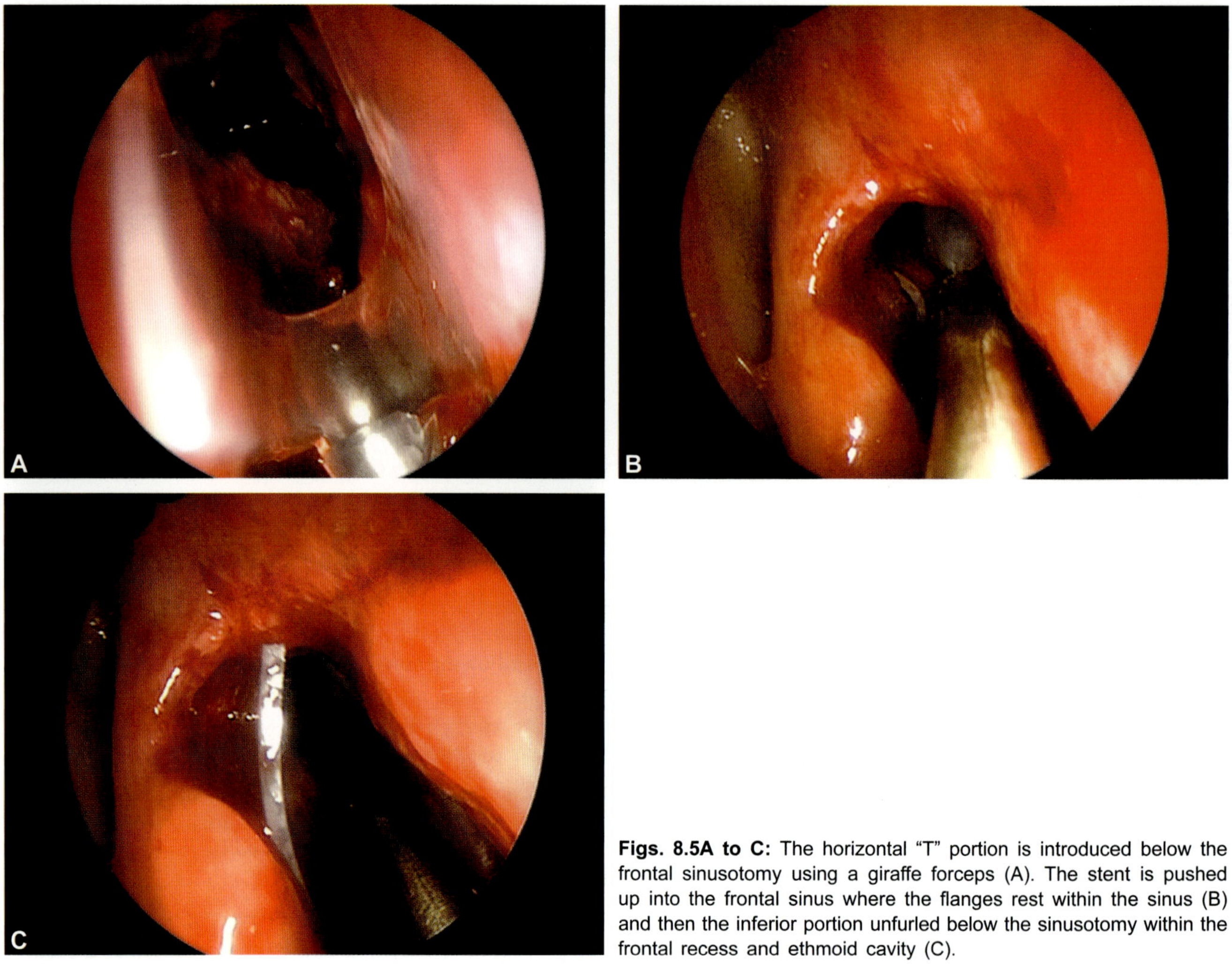

Figs. 8.5A to C: The horizontal "T" portion is introduced below the frontal sinusotomy using a giraffe forceps (A). The stent is pushed up into the frontal sinus where the flanges rest within the sinus (B) and then the inferior portion unfurled below the sinusotomy within the frontal recess and ethmoid cavity (C).

studies are required to establish guidelines on antibiotic therapy, including situations where existing infection is present at the time of ESS.

TOPICAL THERAPIES

Nasal Saline Irrigations

Nasal saline irrigations have a well-established role in postoperative ESS care, although the tonicity, frequency, and delivery of the irrigations vary. Delivery methods range from squeeze bottles, atomizers, and electrical delivery devices, whereas dosing ranges from 2 to 240 mL two to four times per day.[29] Those who promote early nasal saline irrigations state benefits of softening debris and minimizing crusting, allowing for return of mucociliary clearance and improvement in in-office debridement.[29] In general, the saline irrigations are well-tolerated, however, adverse reactions reported include local irritation, epistaxis, nasal burning, headaches, ear fullness, or nasal drainage.[33]

Several studies examined postoperative ESS patients with or without saline irrigations (large and small volume), and found that patient symptoms were improved with irrigations.[28] Liang et al.[34] performed a randomized trial with large volume (240 mL) saline irrigations in the immediate postoperative period and found improvement in patient symptoms for those with mild CRS. However, symptoms of those with severe CRS were unaffected by early irrigations.[34]

To determine ability of nasal irrigations to reach the operative sites following ESS, Wormald and colleagues compared irrigation devices and positioning using Technetium 99 tagged sulfur colloid in saline irrigations.[35]

Table 8.3: Postoperative antibiotic usage

	Study Design	*Antibiotic*	*Duration of Therapy*	*Outcomes*
Annys et al.	Randomized, double-blind placebo	Cefuroxime	2 days	No differences in symptom or endoscopic scores[67]
Jiang et al.	Randomized study	Amoxicillin-clavulanate	21 days	No differences in symptom or endoscopic scores, or of rates of bacterial culture[68]
Albu et al.	Randomized, double-blind placebo	Amoxicillin-clavulanate	14 days	Improvement in patient symptoms at 5 day post-op interval, improvement in endoscopic appearance with decreased crusting at 12 day interval[69]

Devices compared included metered-dose nasal spray, nasal nebulizer, and nasal irrigations (5 mL) in the head down position, or Mygind's position. Nasal irrigations were found to best reach the maxillary and frontal sinuses, though not completely. A subsequent study found that higher volume irrigation (240 mL) better reached the frontal sinus.[36] This study also suggested the head-down position as the most effective for irrigations of the frontal sinus, although no effect of head positioning was seen for irrigation of maxillary, sphenoid, or ethmoid sinuses.

Should irrigations be pursued, careful counseling on how to clean their irrigation delivery devices should be provided, as bacterial colonization is common in these devices.[37] The significance of colonization of the delivery devices is currently controversial, as a recent study demonstrated no increase of post-ESS infections in patients utilizing these devices.[38]

Topical Nasal Steroid Irrigations and Sprays

Integral to the postoperative success of patients with CRS with and without polyps is the control of the inflammatory mechanisms driving disease progression. Topical steroid therapies are utilized commonly in postoperative ESS patients to achieve this goal and offer the advantage of low systemic absorption which enables longer-term usage if necessary. Commonly used topical nasal steroid sprays include fluticasone, budesonide, and mometasone, with off-label use of budesonide and mometasone combined with nasal saline irrigations also common. Other off-label sprays include dexamethasone 0.1% ophthalmic, prednisolone 1% ophthalmic, and ciprofloxacin/dexamethasone (0.3/0.1%) otic drops. Nasal sprays are believed to have adequate coverage of nasal mucosa, with irrigations believed to have better sinus penetration.[29]

Of four randomized, double-blind, placebo-controlled trials evaluating the effect of topical nasal steroid sprays on postoperative ESS outcomes, three showed significant benefit of this therapy in patients with CRS.[39-42] The most noticeable impact was noted in patients with CRS with polyps, with decrease appearance of polyps and increased interval of time until recurrence. The interval of time with which to initiate nasal steroid therapy has not been clearly defined; however, most studies begin therapy within 2–6 weeks postoperatively.[29] Adverse effects of topical steroid use occur in less than 5% of patients and include epistaxis, nasal irritation, headache, and cough.[28]

Off-label usage of topical steroids has been described for use in patients with more severe CRS or concern for ostial stenosis, and has been shown to be very effective in these populations. Lavigne and Kanowitz have both demonstrated that the usage of budesonide irrigations and atomization, respectively, are beneficial in postoperative ESS patient outcomes with improved endoscopic scores, patient symptoms, and use of oral steroids.[43,44] Systemic absorption of budesonide irrigations was studied by Bhalla et al.,[45] who found no significant adrenal suppression with its use. A further study by Welch et al.[46] showed no alteration in serum cortisol levels or 24-h urine cortisol levels in patients using budesonide irrigations.

POSTOPERATIVE DEBRIDEMENTS

Crusting, old blood, retained secretions, and undissolved packing present in the sinonasal cavities of patients after ESS fosters an environment for ostial stenosis, scarring, and lateralization of the middle turbinate. Postoperative debridements are widely utilized to decrease the inflammatory content, lower risk of infection, allow better penetration of topical therapies, and monitor healing progression. Rudmik et al.[28] reviewed the literature on benefits of postoperative debridements and also on timing of these debridements. They noted four randomized controlled studies on the topic, and found that three of these studies demonstrated significant improvements in symptomatology as well as endoscopic appearance with postoperative debridements.[47-50] Bugten et al.[47,51] reported patients had decreased crusting and middle meatal adhesions at 3 months and a subsequent study revealed stable findings at the 56 week interval follow-up. However, some have argued against debridements due to patient discomfort, potential for mucosal stripping, as well as epistaxis and syncope.[52]

CONCLUSION

Postoperative techniques and therapies to optimize patient outcomes have a wide variability amongst clinicians and it is their responsibility to apply them to the appropriate patients. Further clinical research is required to establish high level evidence based guidelines.

REFERENCES

1. Senior BA, Kennedy DW, Tanabodee J, et al. Long-term results of functional endoscopic sinus surgery. Laryngoscope. 1998;108:151-7.
2. Valentine R, Wormald PJ, Sindwani R. Advances in absorbable biomaterials and nasal packing. Otolaryngol Clin North Am. 2009;42:813-28.
3. Orlandi RR, Lanza DC. Is nasal packing necessary following endoscopic sinus surgery? Laryngoscope. 2004;116:83-8.
4. Chandra RK, Conley DB, Kern RC. The effect of FloSeal on mucosal healing after endoscopic sinus surgery: A comparison with thrombin-soaked gelatin foam. Am J Rhinol. 2003;17:51-5.
5. Chandra RK, Conley DB, Haines GK III, et al. Long-term effects of FloSeal packing after endoscopic sinus surgery. Am J Rhinol. 2005;19:240-3.
6. Kastl KG, Betz CS, Diedek V, et al. Control of bleeding following functional endoscopic sinus surgery using carboxymethylated cellulose packing. Eur Arch Otorhinolaryngol. 2009;266:1239-43.
7. Szczygielski K, Rapiejko P, Wojdas A, et al. Use of CMC foam sinus dressing in FESS. Eur Arch Otorhinolaryngol. 2010;267:537-40.
8. Kim DW, Lee EJ, Kim SW, et al. Advantages of glove finger-coated polyvinyl acetate pack in endoscopic sinus surgery. Am J Rhinol. 2012;26:147-9.
9. Valentine R, Wormald PJ. Nasal dressings after endoscopic sinus surgery: what and why? Cur Opin Otolaryngol Head Neck Surg. 2010;18:44-8.
10. Bugten V, Nordgård S, Skogvoll E, et al. Effects of nonabsorbable packing in middle meatus after sinus surgery. Laryngoscope. 2006;116:83-8.
11. Weber R, Keerl R, Hochapfel F, et al. Packing in Endonasal Surgery. Am J Otolaryngol Head Neck Surg. 2001;22:306-20.
12. Chaaban M, Illing E, Riley KO, et al. Spontaneous cerebrospinal fluid leak repair: a five-year prospective evaluation. Laryngoscope. 2014;124:70-5.
13. Shaw CL, Dymock RB, Cowin A, et al. Effect of packing on nasal mucosa of sheep. J Laryngol Otol. 2000;114:506-9.
14. Jacobson JA, Kasworm EM. Toxic shock syndrome after nasal surgery. Case reports and analysis of risk factors. Arch Otolaryngol Head Neck Surg. 1986;112:329-32.
15. Jacobson JA, Stevens MH, Kasworm EM. Evaluation of single-dose cefazolin prophylaxis for toxic shock syndrome. Arch Otolaryngol Head Neck Surg. 1988;114:326-7.
16. Cote DWJ, Wright ED. Triamcinolone-impregnated nasal dressing following endoscopic sinus surgery: a randomized, double-blind, placebo-controlled study. Laryngoscope. 2010;120:1269-73.
17. Rudmik L, Mace J, Mechor B. Effect of a dexamethasone Sinu-Foam middle meatal spacer on endoscopic sinus surgery outcomes: a randomized, double-blind placebo-controlled trial. Int Forum Allergy Rhinol 2011;2(3):248-51.
18. Pletcher SD, Goldberg AN. Treatment of recurrent sinonasal polyposis with steroid-infused carboxymethylcellulose foam. Am J Rhinol Allergy. 2010;24(6):451-3.
19. Chaudhry AL, Chaanban MR, Woodworth BA. Topical Triamcinolone Acetonide/Carboxymethylcellulose Foam for Acute Exacerbations of Chronic Rhinosinusitis/Nasal Polyposis. Vancouver, BC, Canada: American Academy of Otolaryngology Head and Neck Surgery International Meeting; 2013.
20. Han JK, Marple BF, Smith TL, et al. Effect of steroid-releasing sinus implants on postoperative medical and surgical interventions: an efficacy meta-analysis. Int Forum Allergy Rhinol. 2012;2(4):271-9.
21. Bolger WE, Kuhn FA, Kennedy DW. Middle turbinate stabilization after functional endoscopic sinus surgery: the controlled synechiae technique. Laryngoscope. 1999;109:1852-3.
22. Friedman M, Schalch P. Middle turbinate medialization with bovine serum albumin tissue adhesive (BioGlue). Laryngoscope. 2008;118:335-8.
23. Moukarzel N, Nehmé A, Mansour S, et al. Middle turbinate medialization technique in functional endoscopic sinus surgery. J Otolaryngol. 2000;29:144-7.
24. Thornton. Middle turbinate stabilization technique in endoscopic sinus surgery. Arch Otolaryngol Head Neck Surg. 1996;122:869-72.
25. Dutton JM, Hinton MJ. Middle turbinate suture conchopexy during endoscopic sinus surgery does not impair olfaction. Am J Rhinol Allergy. 2011;25(2):125-7.
26. Bhalla RK, Kaushik V, de Carpentier J. Conchopexy suture to prevent middle turbinate lateralisation and septal haematoma after endoscopic sinus surgery. Rhinology. 2005;43(2):143-5.
27. Perloff JR, Palmer JN. Evidence of bacterial biofilms on frontal recess stents in patients with chronic rhinosinusitis. Am J Rhinol. 2004;18:377-80.
28. Rudmik L, Soler ZM, Orlandi RR, et al. Early postoperative care following endoscopic sinus surgery: an evidence-based review with recommendations. Int Forum Allergy Rhinol. 2011;1(6):417-30.

29. Rudmik L, Smith TL. Evidence-based practice: postoperative care in endoscopic sinus surgery. Otolaryngol Clin North Am. 2012;45:1019-32.
30. Wright ED, Agrawal S. Impact of perioperative systemic steroids on surgical outcomes in patients with chronic rhinosinusitis with polyposis: evaluation with the novel perioperative sinus endoscopy (POSE) scoring system. Laryngoscope. 2007;117:1-28.
31. Al-Shemari H, Abou-Hamad W, Libman M, et al. Bacteriology of the sinus cavities of asymptomatic individuals after endoscopic sinus surgery. J Otolaryngol. 2007;36:43-8.
32. Nadel DM, Lanza DC, Kennedy DW. Endoscopically guided cultures in chronic sinusitis. Am J Rhinol. 1998;12:233-41.
33. Tomooka LT, Murphy C, Davidson TM. Clinical study and literature review of nasal irrigation. Laryngoscope. 2000;110:1189-93.
34. Liang KL, Su MC, Tseng HC, et al. Impace of pulsatile nasal irrigation on the prognosis of functional endoscopic sinus surgery. J Otolaryngol Head Neck Surg. 2008;37:148-53.
35. Wormald PJ, Cain T, Oates L, et al. A comparative study of three methods of nasal irrigation. Laryngoscope. 2004;114:2224-7.
36. Singhal D, Weitzel EK, Lin E, et al. Effect of head position and surgical dissection on sinus irrigant penetration in cadavers. Laryngoscope. 2010;120:2528-31.
37. Lewenza S, Charron-Mazenod L, Cho JJ, et al. Identification of bacterial contaminants in sinus irrigation bottles from chronic rhinosinusitis patients. J Otolaryngol Head Neck Surg. 2010;39:458-63.
38. Lee JM, Nayak JV, Doghramji LL, et al. Assessing the risk of irrigation bottle and fluid contamination after endoscopic sinus surgery. Am J Rhinol Allergy. 2010;24:197-9.
39. Dijkstra MD, Ebbens FA, Poublon RM, et al. Fluticasone propionate aqueous nasal spray does not influence the recurrence rate of chronic rhinosinusitis and nasal polyps 1 year after functional endoscopic sinus surgery. Clin Exp Allergy. 2004;34:1395-400.
40. Jorissen M, Bachert C. Effect of corticosteroids on wound healing after endoscopic sinus surgery. Rhinology. 2009;47:280-6.
41. Rowe-Jones JM, Medcalf M, Durham SR, et al. Functional endoscopic sinus surgery: 5 years follow up and results of a prospective, randomised, stratified, double-blind, placebo controlled study of postoperative fluticasone propionate aqueous nasal spray. Rhinology. 2005;43:2-10.
42. Stjarne P, Olsson P, Alenius M. Use of mometasone furoate to prevent polyp relapse after endoscopic sinus surgery. Arch Otolaryngol Head Neck Surg. 2009;135:296-302.
43. Kanowitz SJ, Batra PS, Citradi MJ. Topical budesonide via mucosal atomization dvice in refractory postoperative chronic rhinosinusitis. Otolaryngol Head Neck Surg. 2008;139:131-6.
44. Lavigne F, Cameron L, Renzi PM, et al. Intrasinus administration of topical budesonide to allergic patients with chronic rhinosinusitis following surgery. Laryngoscope. 2002;112:858-64.
45. Bhalla RK, Payton K, Wright ED. Safety of budesonide in saline sinonasal irrigations in the management of chronic rhinosinusitis with polyposis: lack of significant adrenal suppression. J Otolaryngol Head Neck Surg. 2008;37:821-5.
46. Welch KC, Thaler ER, Doghramji LL, et al. The effects of serum and urinary cortisol levels of topical intranasal irrigations with budesonide added to saline in patients with recurrent polyposis after endoscopic sinus surgery. Am J Rhinol Allergy. 2010;24:26-8.
47. Bugten V, Nordgård S, Steinsvag S. The effects of debridement after endoscopic sinus surgery. Laryngoscope. 2006;116:2037-43.
48. Kemppainen T, Seppä J, Tuomilehto H, et al. Repeated early debridement does not provide significant symptomatic benefit after ESS. Rhinology. 2008;46:238-42.
49. Lee JY, Byun JY. Relationship between the frequency of postoperative debridement and patient discomfort, healing period, surgical outcomes, and compliance after endoscopic sinus surgery. Laryngoscope. 2008;118:1868-72.
50. Nilssen EL, Wardrop P, El-Hakim H, et al. A randomized control trial of post-operative care following endoscopic sinus surgery: debridement versus no debridement. J Laryngol Otol. 2002;116:108-11.
51. Bugten V, Nordgård S, Steinsvag S. Long-term effects of postoperative measures after sinus surgery. Eur Arch Otorhinolaryngol. 2008;265:531-7.
52. Kuhnel T, Hosemann W, Wagner W, et al. How traumatising is mechanical mucous membrane care after interventions on paranasal sinuses? A histological immunohistochemical study. Laryngorhinootologie. 1996;75:575-9.
53. Vaiman M, Eviatar E, Segal S. Effectiveness of second-generation fibrin glue in endonasal operations. Otolaryngol Head Neck Surg. 2002;126:388-91.
54. Shrime MG, Tabaee A, Hsu AK, et al. Synechia formation after endoscopic sinus surgery and middle turbinate medialization with and without FloSeal. Am J Rhinol. 2007;21:174-9.
55. Franklin JH, Wright ED. Randomized, controlled, study of absorbable nasal packing on outcomes of surgical treatment of rhinosinusitis with polyposis. Am J Rhinol. 2007;21:214-7.
56. Miller RS, Steward DL, Tami TA, et al. The clinical effects of hyaluronic acid ester nasal dressing (Merogel) on intranasal wound healing after functional endoscopic sinus surgery. Otolaryngol Head Neck Surg. 2003;128:862-9.
57. Wormald PJ, Boustred RN, Le T, et al. A prospective single-blind randomized controlled study of use of hyaluronic acid nasal packs in patients after endoscopic sinus surgery. Am J Rhinol. 2006;20:7-10.
58. Woodworth B, Chandra RK, LeBenger, JD, et al. A gelatin-thrombin matrix for hemostasis after endoscopic sinus surgery. Am J Otolaryngol Head Neck Surg. 2009;30:49-53.
59. Shi R, Zhou, J, Wang, B, et al. The clinical outcomes of new hylauronan nasal dressing: a prospective, randomized, controlled study. Am J Rhinol Allergy. 2013;27:71-6.

60. Shinkwin C, Beasley, N, Simo, R, et al. Evaluation of surgicel Nu-knit, Merocel and Vasolene gauze nasal packs: a randomized trial. Rhinology. 1996;34:41-3.
61. Karkos P, Thinakararajan, T, Goodyear, P, et al. Day-case endoscopic sinus surgery using dissolvable haemostatic nasal packs: a pilot study. Eur Arch Otorhinolaryngol. 2007; 264:1171-4.
62. Weber R, Mai R, Hosemann W, et al. The success of 6-month stenting in endosnasal frontal sinus surgery. Ear Nose Throat J. 2000;79:930-2, 934, 937, 938, 940, 941.
63. Freeman SB, Blom ED. Frontal sinus stents. Laryngoscope. 2000;110:1179-82.
64. Orlandi RR, Knight J. Prolonged stenting of the frontal sinus. Laryngoscope. 2009;119:190-2.
65. Neel H, Whicker, JH, Lake, CF. Thin rubber sheeting in frontal sinus surgery: animal and clinical studies. Laryngoscope. 1976;86:524-36.
66. Beule AG, Scharf C, Biebler KE, et al. Effects of topically applied dexamethason on mucosal wound healing using a drug-releasing stent. Laryngoscope. 2008;118:2073-7.
67. Annys E, Jorissen M. Short term effects of antibiotics (Zinat) after endoscopic sinus surgery. Acta Otorhinolaryngol Belg. 2000;54:23-8.
68. Jiang RS, Liang KL, Yang KY, et al. Postoperative antibiotic care after functional endoscopic sinus surgery. Am J Rhinol. 2008;22:608-12.
69. Albu S, Lucaciu R. Prophylactic antibiotics in endoscopic sinus surgery: a short follow-up study. Am J Rhinol Allergy. 2010;24:306-9.

Section 2

Management of Inflammatory Sinus Disease

Chapters

CHAPTER

9 Basic Functional Endoscopic Sinus Surgery

Spencer C Payne

PHILOSOPHY AND APPROACH

As we have discussed previously, chronic sinusitis and other disorders of the nose and paranasal sinuses exist along a spectrum of severity and difficulty. It would thus be unreasonable to expect that any one method of surgery or extent of dissection could be proscribed for all patients. The functional part of endoscopic sinus surgery requires that efforts are made to preserve as much of the natural structure of the sinuses as can be while ensuring that the anatomy that either obstructs the sinus or prevents adequate debridement or topical application of medication is removed. In the next chapters, we will discuss the options for the patient who has failed primary surgery (Chapter 10) and when minimal surgery can be effective through balloon dilation (Chapter 11). In this chapter, the focus will be on performing complete, but logical dissections of the paranasal sinuses and it is the expectation that the surgeon will reduce or expand the extent of dissection as mandated by the underlying disease.

What is important for any surgery, especially endoscopic sinus surgery, is that a preoperative plan be established based on patient factors and anatomical issues identified on the CT scan and that this plan be executed in an organized fashion. Essential to this goal is the identification of landmarks on the CT scan that can be translated to the patient's endoscopic exam such that they can be referred to often during the procedure. It is important preoperatively to note the location and status (dehiscent or not) of the ethmoidal arteries, the presence of Haller or Onodi cells, the slope of the skull base (both in the AP and lateral dimensions) and the complexity of the ethmoid pneumatization. Once these points have been established and a plan has been created, the surgery can begin.

O.R. SETUP AND PATIENT POSITIONING

The operating table should be turned at least 90°–180° away from the anesthesia cart to provide sufficient room for the surgeon and the equipment (Fig. 9.1). The right handed surgeon will find it easiest to be on the patient's right side with the scrub and back table across the patient on their left side. The video cart should be positioned at around the 1 or 2 o'clock position to facilitate an ergonomic view. The IGS tower, if being used, can be positioned either to

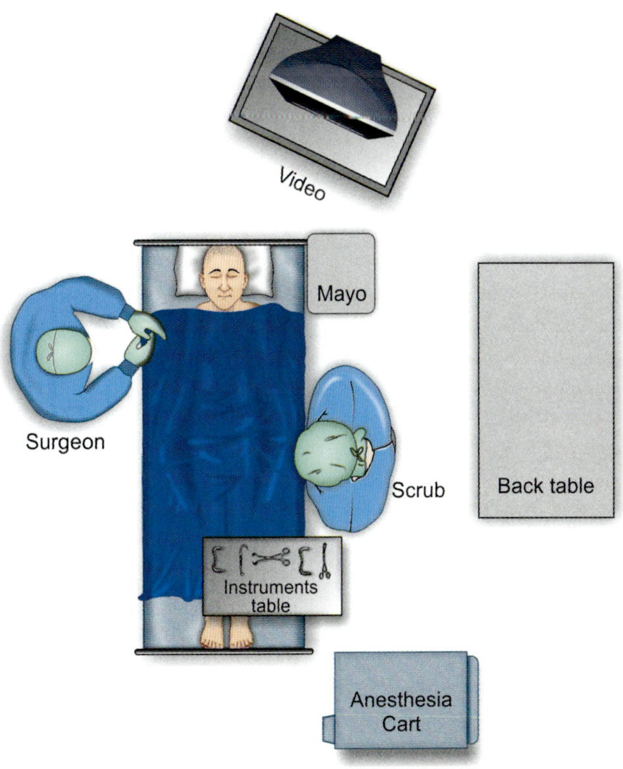

Fig. 9.1: Room positioning.

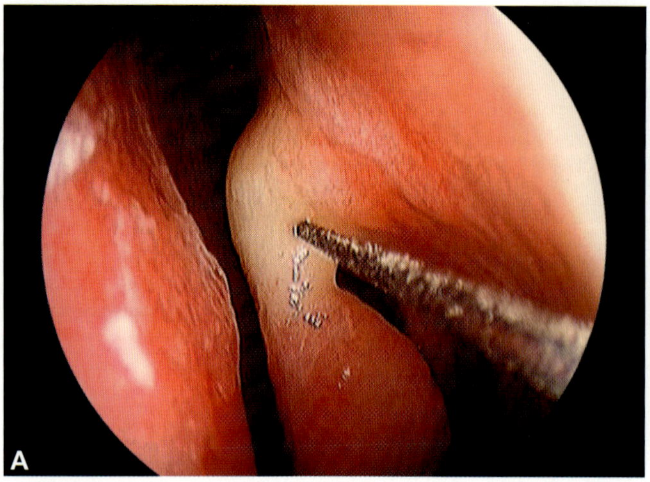

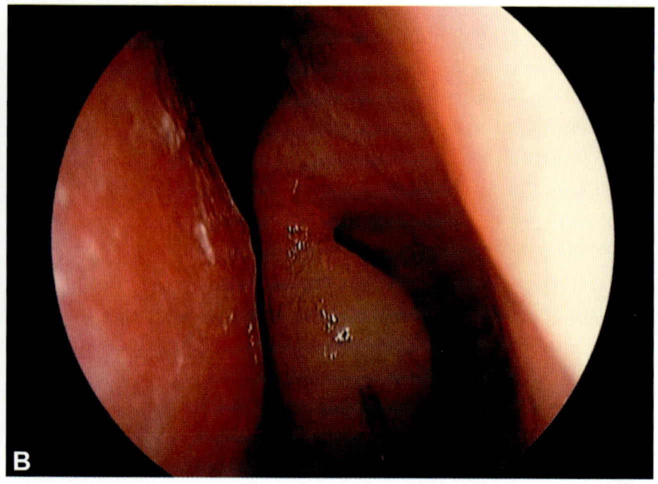

Figs. 9.2A and B: Injection sites for basic endoscopic sinus surgery. (A) At the root of the middle turbinate; (B) inferomedially on the head of the middle turbinate. If possible, a third injection can be placed posteriorly near the edge where the sagittal component of the turbinate transitions to the axial.

the left or right of the video tower depending on room size and surgeon preference. Appropriate reversal of this setup can be utilized for the left-handed surgeon.

Before draping, any anesthetic monitoring cables are elevated off the floor and secured to the bed to minimize discomfort and optimize the operative area for standing or sitting. Once draped, the various cables (light, endoscope, and powered instrumentation) and suction tubes are secured to the bed. This prevents movement during the case, which can often limit the maneuverability of the surgeon's hand as the cables can be weighty.

As was noted in Chapter 6, positioning of the patient can greatly improve visualization of the sinuses by decreasing blood loss.[1] Either the head of bed can be elevated or the patient is placed in a reverse trendelenburg position of about 20°–30° in order to reduce central venous pressure and subsequent venous and capillary bleeding.

BEFORE THE SURGERY

Nasal Preparation

Preparation of the nose begins in the preoperative suite with three applications, separated by 5–10 min, of oxymetazoline sprays. In the operating room, once general anesthesia has been induced, the nose is packed with oxymetazoline-soaked pledgets under direct inspection. It is unlikely to be able to place these in the middle meatus primarily at this point and so effort is made to atraumatically place them in the anterior nasal cavity. This enhances the decongestant effect on the septum and turbinates, which had previously been initiated in the preoperative suite. There is debate regarding the appropriate vasoconstrictor in sinus surgery.[2] The safest overall is oxymetazoline which is why we generally use it preferentially and phenylephrine should be avoided. Topical epinephrine, used 1:1,000 to 1:5,000 can be employed for better hemostasis but the surgeon is cautioned to avoid in patients with cardiac history and to employ mechanisms and/or protocols to guarantee against accidental injection (such as coloring with fluorescein). After draping, the nose is injected with a focus on the middle turbinate in three locations:

- Over the axilla at the junction of the turbinate and the lateral wall with medial positioning to help guide any bleeding from the injection site away from the middle meatus (Fig. 9.2A).
- Inferomedially on the head of the middle turbinate and (Fig. 9.2B).
- Posteriorly along the inferior aspect of the turbinate (not shown).

Additionally, if the uncinate is visible direct injection of the uncinate can be accomplished, otherwise gentle medialization and placement of a vasoconstrictor-soaked pledget is performed. The vestibular vibrissae are then trimmed. This helps minimize collection of blood at the nostril, which can stain the endoscope during removal and reinsertion throughout the case.

Effective Nasal Cleaning and Suctioning

After sufficient time has elapsed, usually upon completion of equipment setup and a time-out where the surgical plan and patient specific concerns are discussed amongst members of the operative suite team, the nose should be suctioned and the procedures commenced. As simple an act as nasal suctioning can play a large role in minimizing trauma to the nose. At this early point and throughout the case, care should be taken to enter the nose carefully without applying any suction and proceed first to the nasopharynx, which often serves as the reservoir for saliva, mucous and blood. Suction is then applied and blood is cleared from the nose from posterior to anterior. In this manner, the often times sharp edge of the suction is less likely to cause inadvertent trauma. It is also important to not dwell on cut surfaces throughout the case but focus only on removing blood pools and not areas where coagulation has already occurred as this may disrupt the clot and reinitiate bleeding. Instead warm saline irrigation (104°F) can be a miraculous adjunct for the surgeon to deal with areas of persistent oozing.

Nasal Inspection

After the nasal preparation is complete, the nose is inspected and the need for a septoplasty is further assessed. For optimal surgery, good access to the middle meatus is essential, especially if frontal sinus exploration is to be performed. Pay close attention to whether superior dorsal deflection, often at the superior most portion of the bone-cartilaginous junction of the turbinate, prevents access or visualization of the axilla of the middle turbinate (Fig. 9.3). Consider as well that the appearance of the nose after such significant decongestant during the preparatory phase may underrepresent the access in the postoperative nasal cavity for inspection and/or debridement. If necessary, an endoscopic septoplasty can be performed (*see* Chapter 13). Otherwise, note is made of the presence of purulence, polyps, or other anatomical issues that may require addressing.

FESS BASIC CONCEPT

As we learned in Chapter 3, the ethmoid complex derives from a numbered series of ethmoturbinals (ETs), which despite some variability, result in several consistent landmarks. For a complete unilateral sinus surgery, we subscribe to the anterior–posterior, posterior–anterior approach given its orderly progression and demonstrated safety.[3] If followed from anterior to posterior, in order, the identification and dissection of these ET derivatives creates an organized and orderly progression for surgery and forces the surgeon to consider the next step in terms

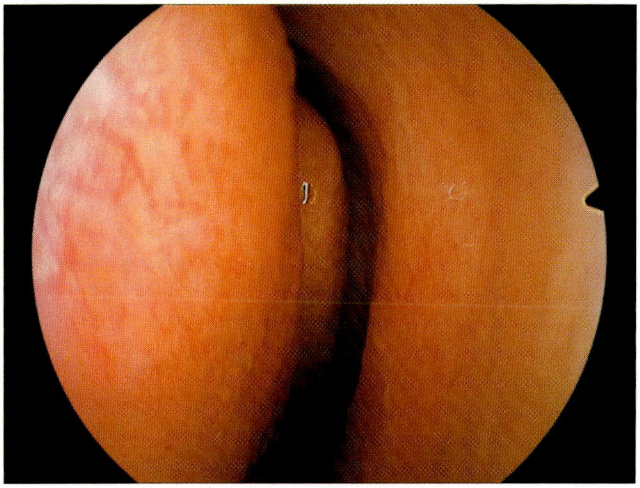

Fig. 9.3: Septal deflection prevents access to the middle meatus. Consider an endoscopic septoplasty to address.

of defined anatomy. The first of these derivatives is the uncinate process (ET1). From there, we move on to the identification and dissection of the ethmoid bulla (ET2), basal lamella of the middle turbinate (ET3), and finally the superior turbinate and posterior ethmoids (ET4). The sphenoid sinus is then opened, if necessary, and the skull base is identified. A posterior-to-anterior approach is then performed and septations are removed superiorly along the ethmoid roof as we work our way back towards the frontal sinus.

The use of powered instrumentation for sinus surgery was introduced in the mid 1990s. The benefits are continuous suctioning and a consistently sharp instrument, but with the significant drawback of substantial iatrogenic injury occurring quickly due to its standard 3,000–5,000 rpms. As a result, several methods of integrating its use into sinus dissection have evolved including restricting it to polypectomy alone, using it to clean up the "mucosal soup" left over from nonpowered dissection (to borrow a phrase from Richard Harvey), or as the primary means of dissection. It is our practice to utilize it as the primary means of dissection. The reader is cautioned, however, as this is often difficult for the beginning surgeon as this requires "intimate" knowledge of the best angles, directionality of force application, and tip manipulations in order for the microdebrider to take the place of multiple instruments that have all been specially designed for distinct purposes. As such, the basic steps for the dissections will be described and where appropriate, pointers for powered and nonpowered options provided.

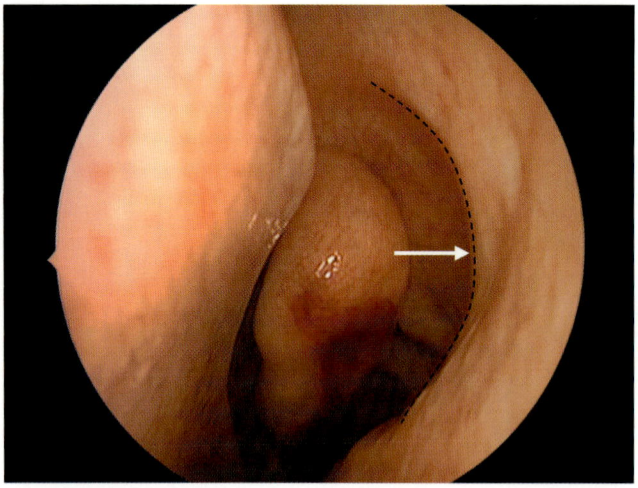

Fig. 9.4: The maxillary line. The dashed line corresponds to the maxillary line, the junction of the uncinate to the ascending process of the maxilla and denotes the underlying lacrimal suture. It serves as the absolute anterior border of any uncinectomy. Also note the "shaded" trough posterior to this (arrow), which is likely the anterior most extent of the ethmoid infundibulum.

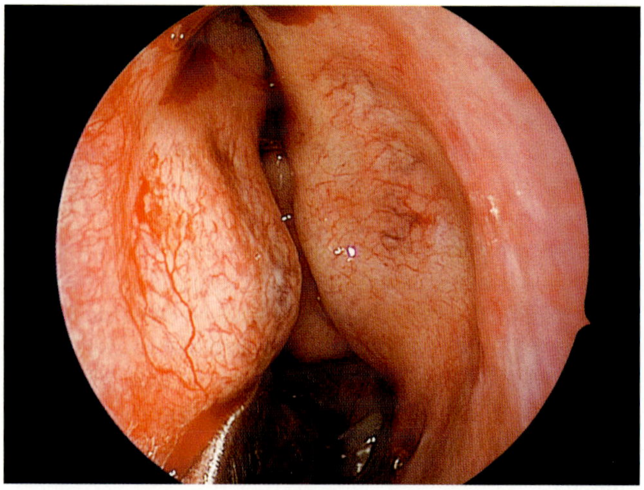

Fig. 9.5: Middle turbinate medialization. The convex side of an elevator is used to displace the turbinate such that the ethmoid bulla and uncinate process can be easily identified.

UNCINECTOMY AND MIDDLE MEATAL ANTROSTOMY

Given the variability of the pneumatization of the ethmoid sinuses and frontal sinus outflow configurations, the maxillary sinus, along with the sphenoid, is one of the most important consistencies in sinus surgery. Its roof can lead you to the lamina and serve as a guide for the appropriate trajectory to the sphenoid sinus. As such, its opening at the beginning of most sinus cases serves an important role. Original descriptions of maxillary antrostomies included starting in the posterior fontanelle or using sickle knives to incise the uncinate anteriorly. We, however, prefer to utilize a back-biter to incise the uncinate in a retrograde fashion as this is less likely to result in either the secondary-ostium/recirculation phenomenon or accidental injury to the orbit or lacrimal sac seen with these older techniques.

The procedure starts with identifying the maxillary line that helps to identify the attachment of the uncinate to the maxilla and the location of the lacrimal suture (Fig. 9.4).[4] Along with the anterior head of the middle turbinate, these landmarks denote the anterior most extent of any uncinectomy such that iatrogenic injury to the lacrimal sac and duct can be avoided. In reality, the deepest portion of the trough often apparent just posterior to this line and also noted in Figure 9.4 is usually the anterior most extent of the ethmoid infundibulum and a good reference for how far anterior one can incise the uncinate.

Surgical Steps

- Use Freer or blunt side of Cottle elevator to medialize the middle turbinate and visualize the uncinate and ethmoid bulla (Fig. 9.5).
- Optionally a vertical relaxing incision can then be made in the posterior aspect of the meatus medial to the inferior aspect of the ethmoid bulla in the basal lamella of the middle turbinate as this has been shown to improve access and reduce trauma in cases where limited anterior surgery is to be performed (Fig. 9.6).[5]
- A pediatric or microbackbiter (Fig. 9.7) is then inserted into the middle meatus while closed, opened superiorly, and rotated into position behind the uncinate at a level approximately even with the inferior aspect of the ethmoid bulla, which will roughly divide the uncinate into its superior 2/3rd and inferior 1/3rd. This division typically represents the level at which the natural ostium can be found anteriorly (Fig. 9.8). This technique may require modification in the setting of differently positioned uncinate processes (Figs. 9.9 and 9.10).
- Gentle medial traction is placed on the uncinate before each bite to gauge its mobility and anterior attachment in order to minimize iatrogenic injury to the lacrimal apparatus while maximizing uncinate removal.
- The backbiter is serially closed, opened, advanced anteriorly, and closed again until the anterior aspect of the infundibulum is reached (Fig. 9.11).
- The area is suctioned to ensure a full three-layer incision was created and then a maxillary ball probe

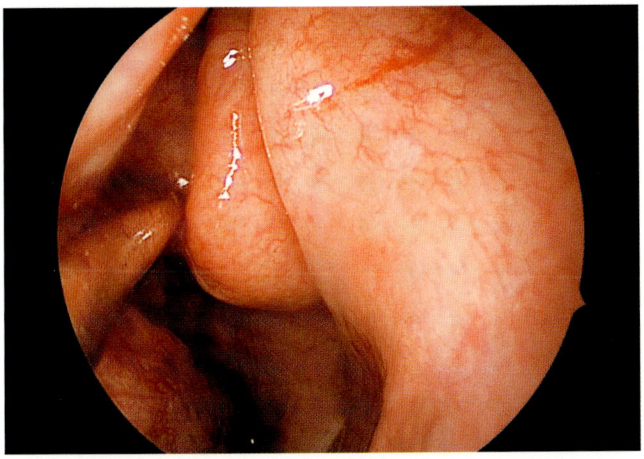

Fig. 9.6: Site of basal lamella relaxing incision. This is an optional step that may be necessary if gentle medialization does not allow for persistent displacement of the turbinate.

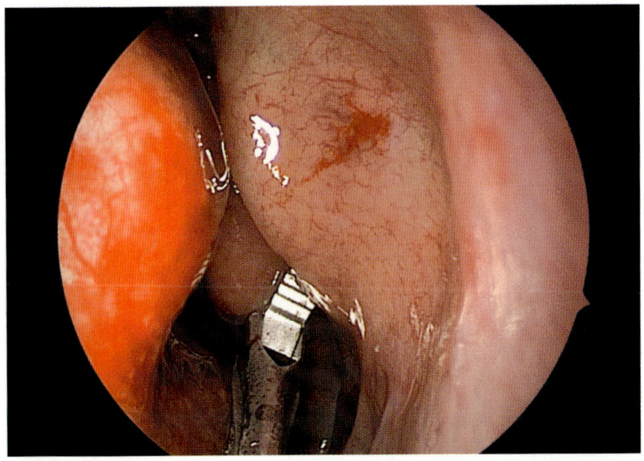

Fig. 9.7: Backbiter positioned behind the uncinate process.

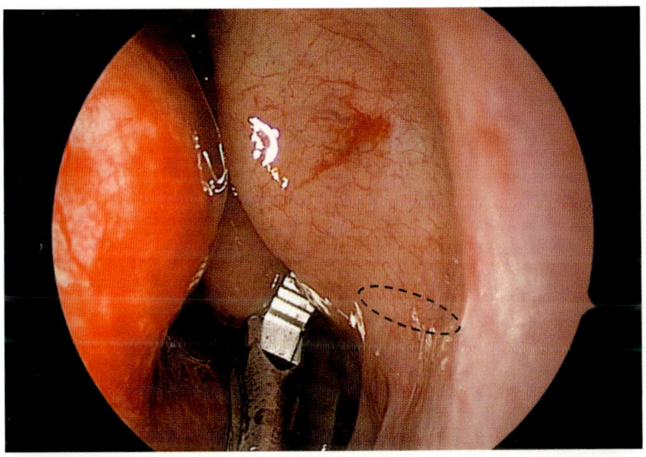

Fig. 9.8: Location of maxillary ostium behind the uncinate process (drawing).

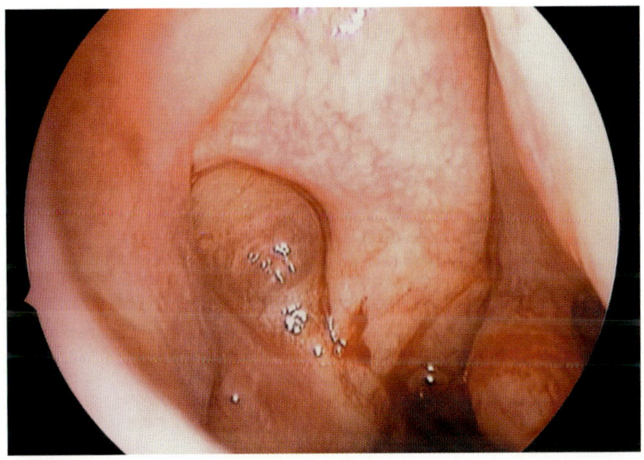

Fig. 9.9: Atelectatic uncinate. Seen often in the case of silent sinus syndrome, it may be helpful to first use the hook end of a frontal seeker to gently medialize the uncinate before removal.

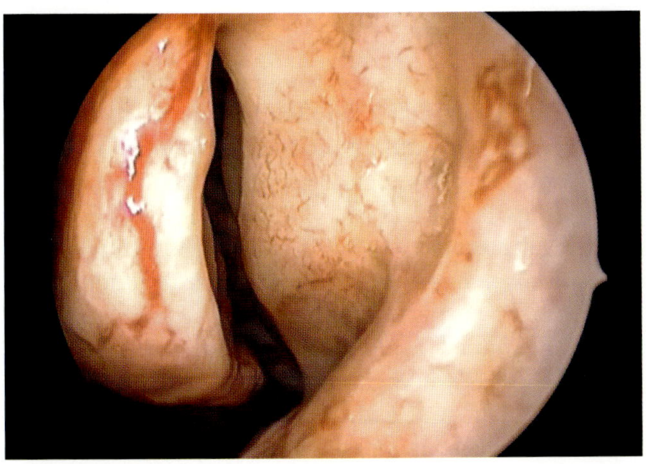

Fig. 9.10: Broad coronal uncinate. The uncinate exists in the coronal plane and use of backbiter may be difficult. Up-biting thru-cuts or Kerrison Rongeurs may work better depending on the actual angle.

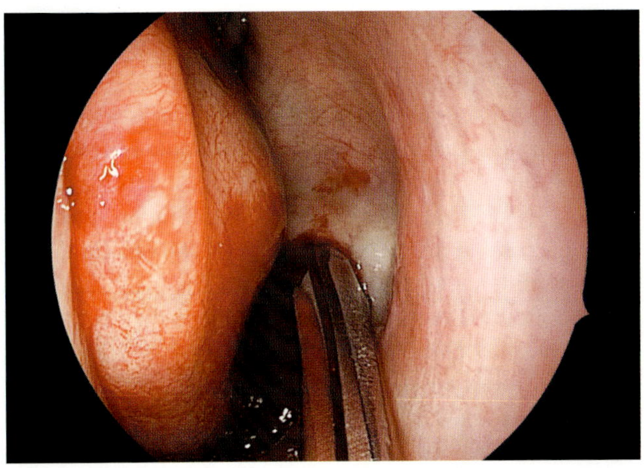

Fig. 9.11: Backbiter at anterior aspect of infundibulum. Note blanching where cutting tine is about to bite posterior to maxillary line.

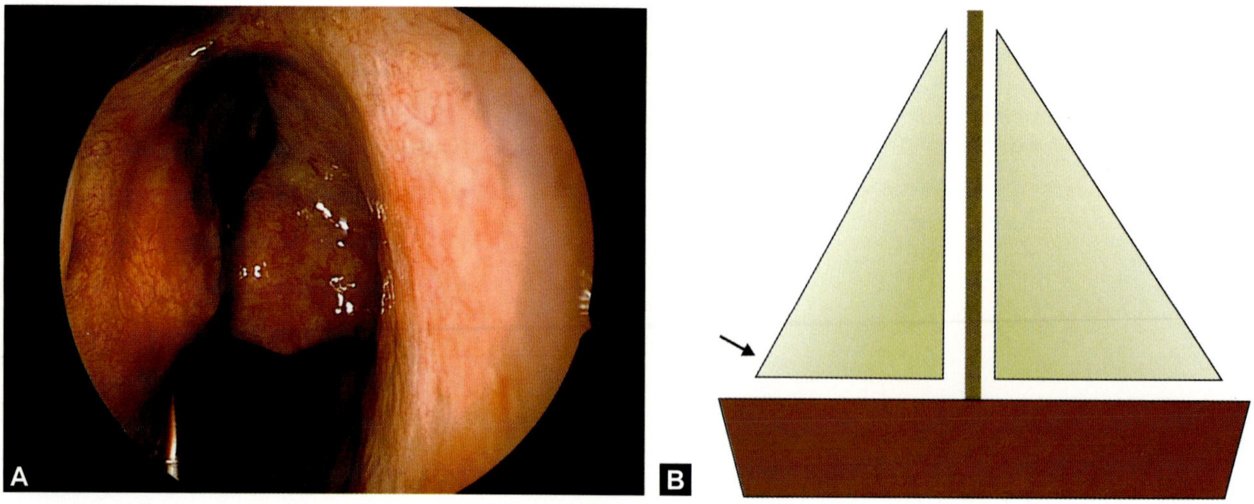

Figs. 9.12A and B: The (A) incised uncinate process resembles an (B) aft sail. The arrow points to the clew of the aft sail.

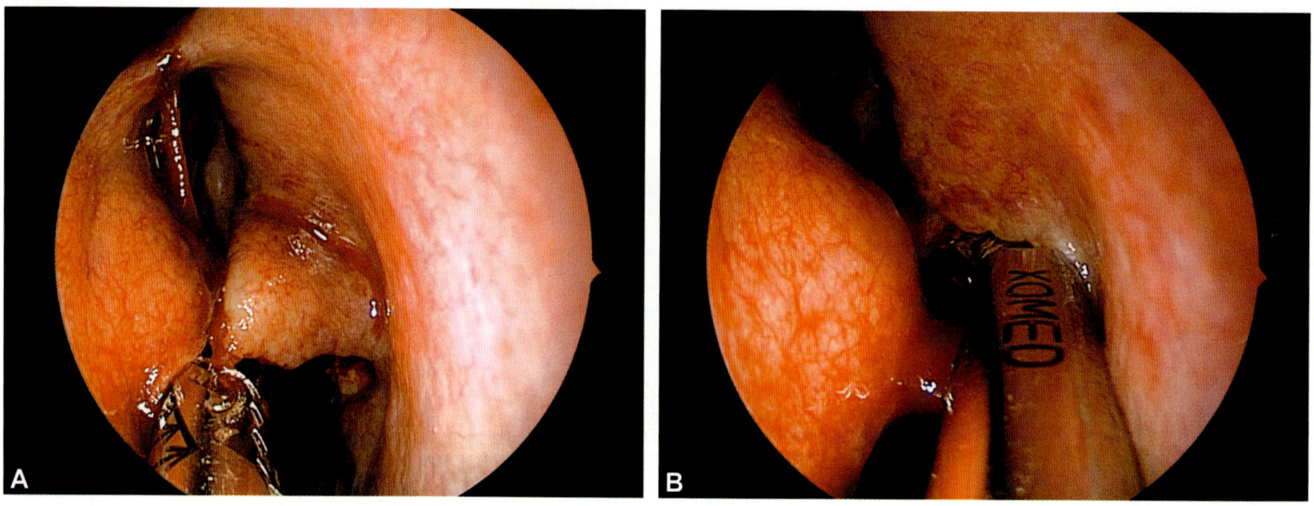

Figs. 9.13A and B: Powered removal of the uncinate. (A) The "clew" of the uncinate is engaged first and the excision follows the; (B) lateral attachment of the uncinate superiorly.

seeker is placed into the infundibulum, directed superiorly and with medial traction along the anterior attachment of the uncinate, the uncinate is prolapsed such that its plane of projection is converted from its more typical sagittal to a coronal orientation. To a certain extent, it now resembles the aft sail of a boat with its mobile clew posteromedially (Figs. 9.12A and B).

- The superior portion of the uncinate is then removed. We employ either of two options for this:
  - Powered dissection: a closed, straight or gently angled (15°) microdebrider is introduced in to the middle meatus and directed towards the now inferior medial aspect of the uncinate. Starting at this "clew" the inferior portion is removed laterally and the microdebrider gradually turned superiorly such that it may skim the attachment to the lateral wall without producing undue injury to the mucosa of the lateral aspect of the infundibulum (Figs. 9.13A and B).
  - Nonpowered: Using an up-biting thru-cutting forcep, the uncinate is engaged at its anterolateral inferior aspect with the lateral cutting surface of the forcep against the lateral wall attachment (Fig. 9.14). Recognizing the crescentic shape of the uncinate, and with the operative wrist in radial-flexion, sequential bites are made superiorly until the uncinate transitions back into a primarily sagittal orientation. At this point, either rotation of

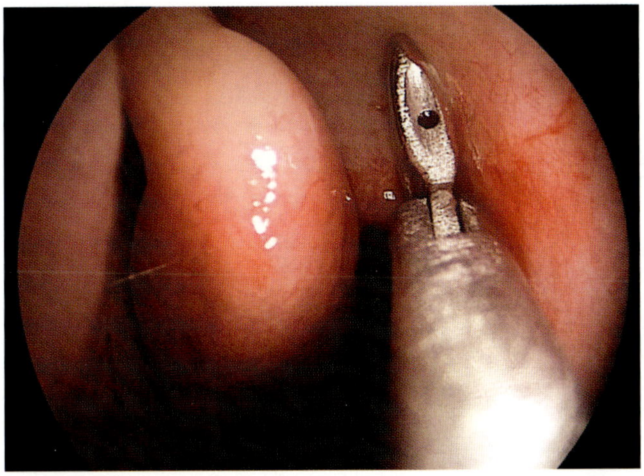

Fig. 9.14: Nonpowered removal of the uncinate. An up-biting thru-cutting forcep engages the uncinate attachment laterally and incision proceeds superiorly.

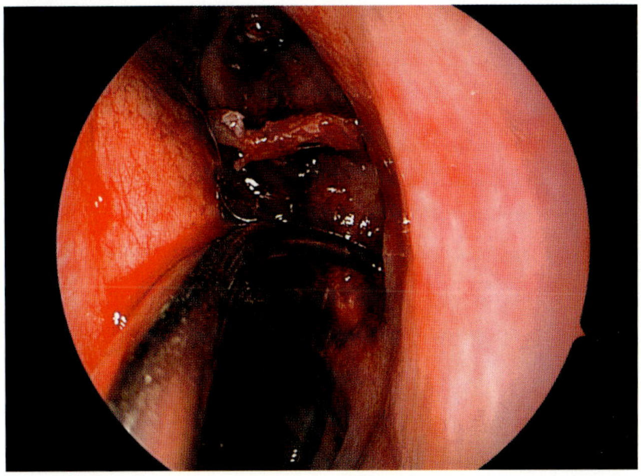

Fig. 9.15: Maxillary probe in normal location of ostium. Gently medialize the inferior aspect of the uncinate and dilate the ostium to make room for cutting instrument.

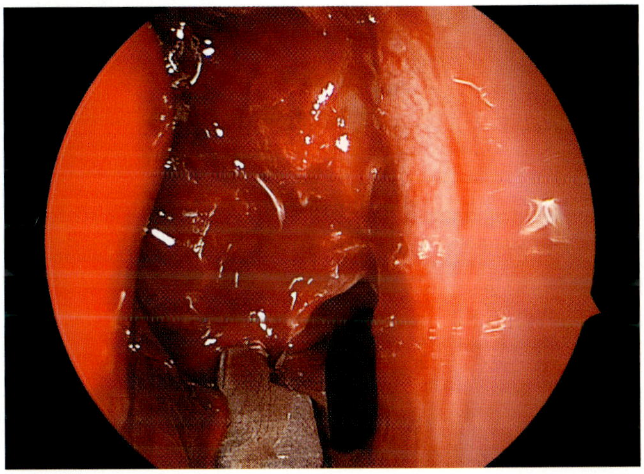

Fig. 9.16: Straight thru-cut extending antrostomy posteriorly. This cut is angled inferiorly and does not need to extend to the posterior maxillary wall.

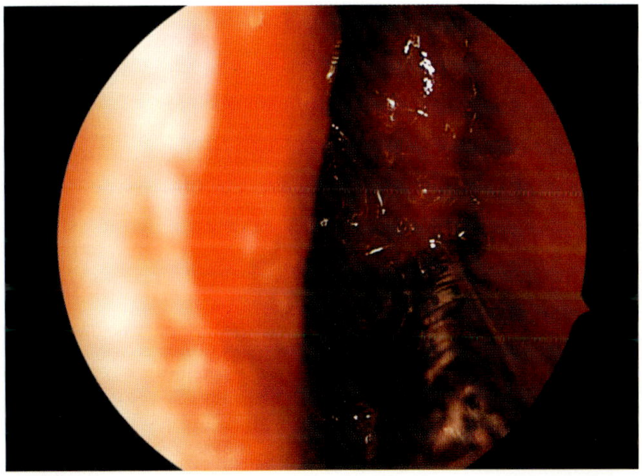

Fig. 9.17: Microdebrider is positioned to remove the "car door" of tissue.

the up-biting forcep medially or a straight cutting forcep is used to complete the excision. The area is then cleaned with microdebrider.

- The maxillary probe is again used to explore the infundibulum inferiorly, identify the maxillary ostium and then gently medialize the inferior portion of the uncinate to make room for cutting instruments (Fig. 9.15). An angled, 30° endoscope is often helpful at this point to fully visualize the ostium.
- A Stammberger down biting forcep is carefully inserted and the anterior aspect of the uncinate is excised in 2–3 cuts, advancing each subsequent cut slightly posteroinferiorly along the superior aspect of the inferior turbinate.
- A straight thru-cut is then inserted and the opening extended posteriorly to the desired size (Fig. 9.16). It is not often necessary to take the opening all the way to the posterior sinus wall, especially as branches of the sphenopalatine artery may be found in this area.
- This uncinate/medial maxillary wall complex can be thought of as a "car door" hinged posteriorly. After displacing the "door" medially, a microdebrider can then be used to remove it superiorly up to the orbital floor (Fig. 9.17) and subsequently cleanly trim the edges along the inferior turbinate, taking care to use the proximal cutting surface of the debrider opening in order to avoid abrasions along the turbinate.

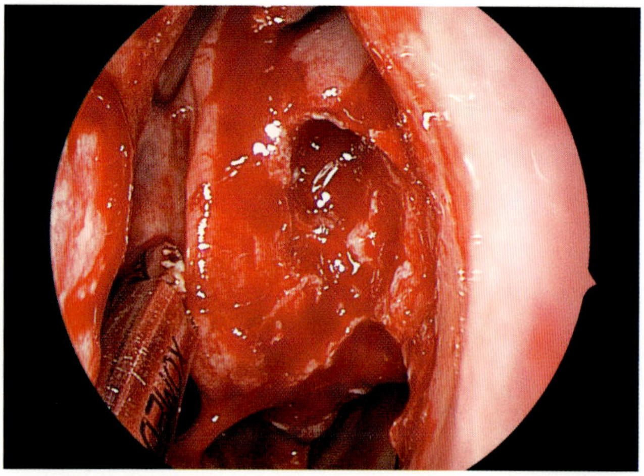

Fig. 9.18: Microdebrider positioned in the hiatus semilunaris superioris—The bulla is opened from medial to lateral.

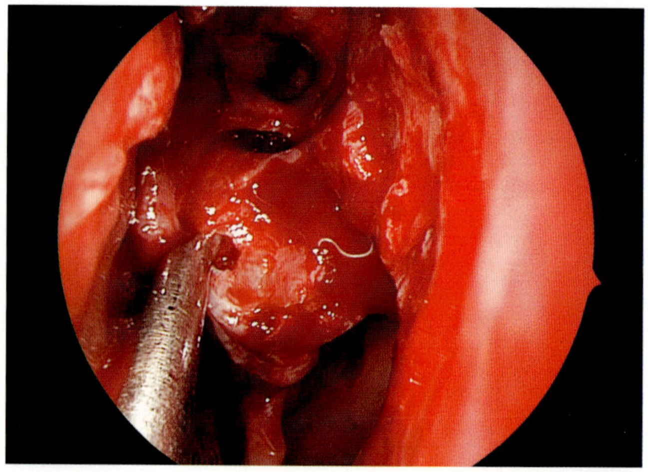

Fig. 9.19: Complex pneumatization of anterior ethmoid—Dissection has continued well posterior to the plane of the middle turbinate basal lamella without having breached it. An infrabullar cell is noted inferiorly (suction).

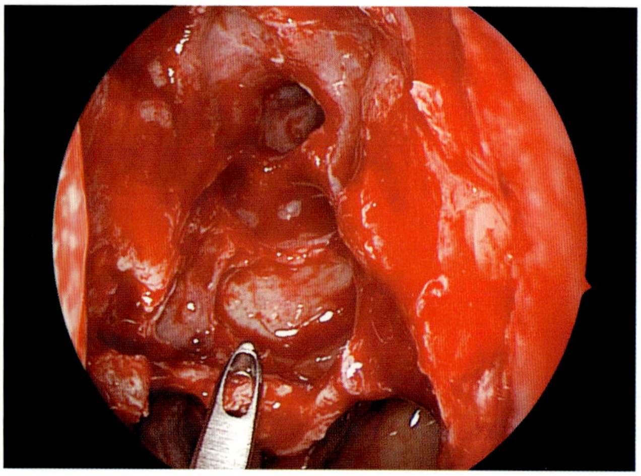

Fig. 9.20: Removal of inferior wall of infrabullar cell—The inferior portion of a bullar or infrabullar cell is often best removed with straight thru-cuts.

- Any intrasinus polyps are removed, biopsies or cultures taken, and the sinus then fully irrigated. An angled (40° or 60°) debrider can be helpful in removing any clearly mobile polyps within the sinus.

ETHMOIDECTOMY

Dissection of the ethmoid complex can be difficult because of its highly variable anatomy. Inspection of the CT scan preoperatively will help identify the presence of numerous suprabullar cells, variable pneumatization of the basal lamella of the middle turbinate resulting in apparent "middle-ethmoid" cells, and the slope of the transition of middle turbinate's coronal to axial component (seen best on sagittal imaging) which will better define the area to best transgress its basal lamella.

Anterior Ethmoidectomy

Steps:

- Following completion of the maxillary antrostomy, if performed, the middle meatus is thoroughly irrigated so that the next landmark (ethmoid bulla, ET2) can be identified.
- Starting medially in the hiatus semilunaris superioris (that space between the medial aspect of the bulla and the sagittal component of the middle turbinate), the bulla is opened. This can be completed with either a j-currette or microdebrider (Fig. 9.18).
- Once the space is opened, focus is paid to the anterior wall, which is opened from medial to lateral and from inferior to superior. Typically, a small ostium can be noted posteromedially and any tissue bridge spanning this should be removed.
- Otherwise complex pneumatization of the anterior ethmoid region may be present and dissection continues posteriorly to the area where the middle turbinate basal lamella would have originally suggested (Fig. 9.19).
- Identification of the orbital lamina is critical at this stage and bullar removal continues laterally until it is encountered. This can be facilitated laterally using a small 2-mm Kerrison Rongeur or mushroom punch.
- The inferior wall can be removed with straight thru cutting forceps (Fig. 9.20) or alternatively with the microdebrider aimed inferiorly. When using the

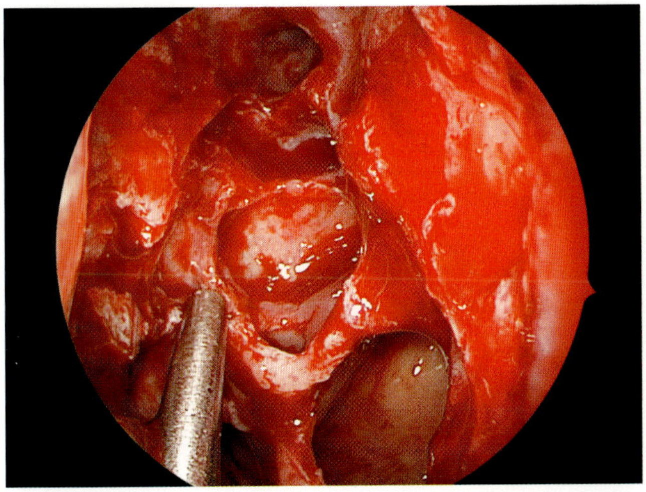

Fig. 9.21: Optimal site of middle turbinate basal lamella transgression. This is at the level of the roof of the maxillary sinus and approximately at the transition point between the coronal and axial segments of the middle turbinate.

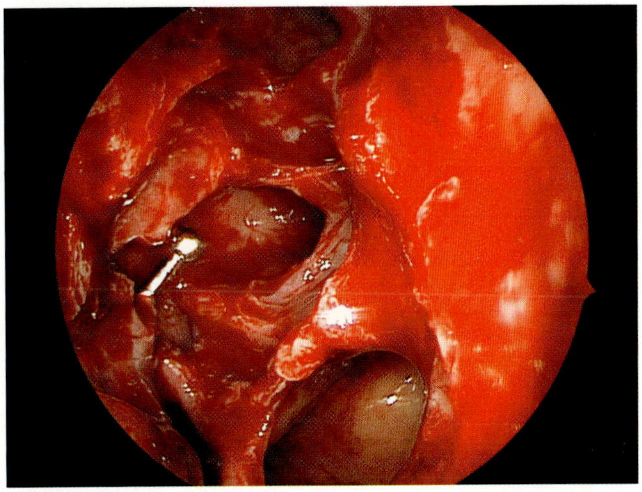

Fig. 9.22: Ball tip probe entering ethmoid complex through superior meatus.

microdebrider to cut in an inferior direction, it is important to move the endoscope to a more medial or lateral position than the debrider itself so that visualization of the cutting surface is not obfuscated by absolute coaxial positioning.

- The removal of the superior aspect of the bullar face continues superiorly to a level below the cut surface of the uncinate. This is important regardless of whether a frontal exploration is to be performed. Maintaining different levels of dissection of these two structures will minimize postoperative scarring or later difficulty with the dissection if a frontal exploration is to be completed.

Posterior Ethmoidectomy

Steps:

- If a posterior ethmoidectomy is to be performed, the meatus is again copiously irrigated and any bleeding controlled either with warm irrigation or repeat vasoconstrictor-soaked packing.
- The third ET deriviative is identified, the basal lamella of the middle turbinate, and its slope is examined in relation to the roof of the maxillary sinus. The optimal point to transgress the turbinate is medially at a level consistent with the maxillary roof which is often where the coronal component of the turbinate transitions to an axial orientation (Fig. 9.21).
- The basal lamella is punctured either with curette or the microdebrider and the lamella opened up from medial to lateral following any cell tracts that can be identified.
- If the superior turbinate is not visible additional dissection medially at the level the basal lamella was transgressed should be performed. A ball tip probe can be slid past the middle turbinate medially and directed into the superior meatus to help identify this location if it is not readily apparent (Fig. 9.22).
- Once identified, and either through the middle meatus or the medial corridor, the inferior aspect of the superior turbinate is incised from anterior to posterior to the face of the sphenoid (Figs. 9.23A and B).
- Additional dissection of the inferior aspect of the posterior ethmoid complex can then be performed.
- If a sphenoidotomy is to be performed, follow the steps in the next section and establish the posterior skull base; otherwise confirm with image guidance or CT scan whether the posterior most ethmoid cell extends to the ethmoid roof. If it does not, consider a sphenoidotomy in order to safely establish this landmark.
- After completion of the sphenoidotomy, we find it easiest to dissect remaining ethmoid partitions with a reverse post 30° scope and angled microdebrider attachment. Be careful not to blind members of the operative team with the light cable while switching between endoscopes.
- Using a curved suction or angled curettes, the ethmoid roof is explored and the location of septations is noted. If the tissue is hypertrophied or polypoid in nature, a short curved 90° suction is most helpful in compressing this tissue and defining the anatomy (Fig. 9.24).

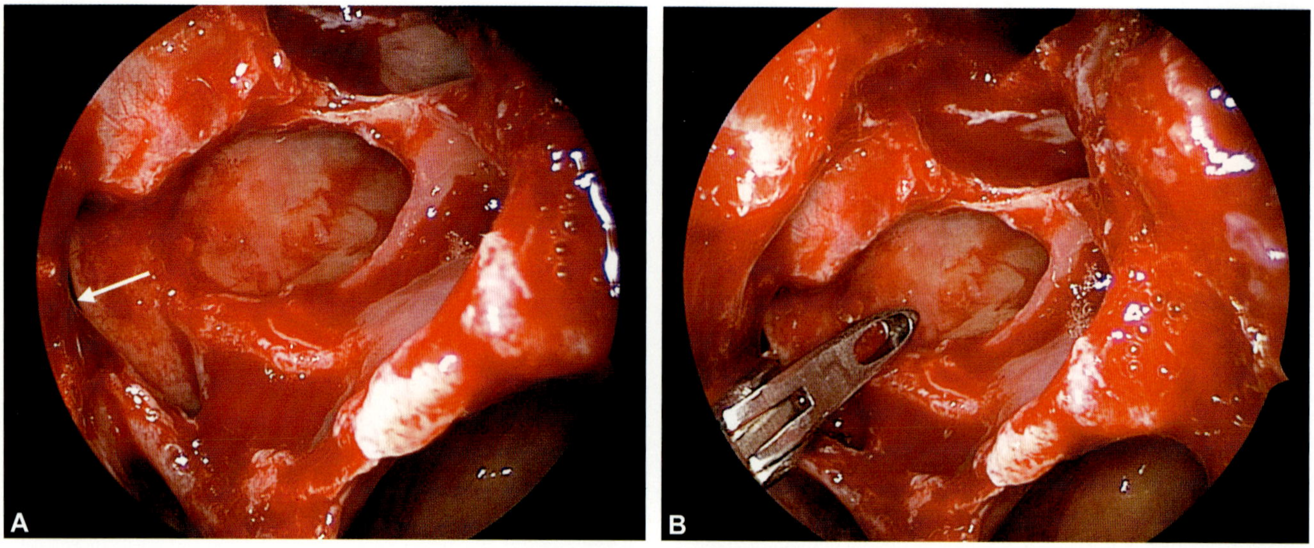

Figs. 9.23A and B: Superior turbinate being incised. (A) The edge of the superior turbinate can be seen (arrow) and the; (B) inferior aspect can be removed without concern for loss of smell as this area does not have olfactory neurons.

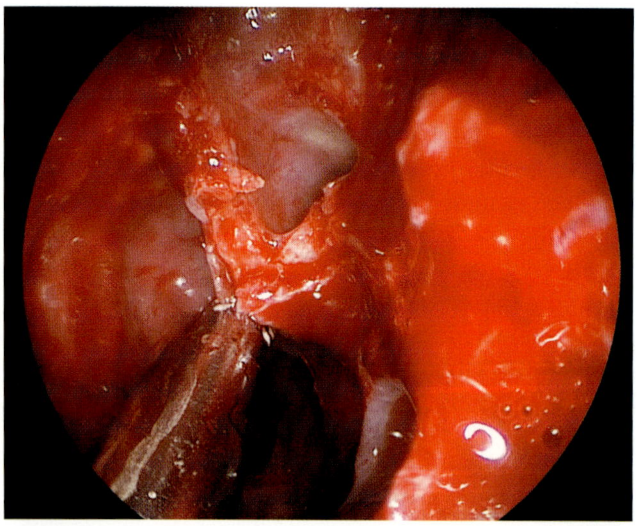

Fig. 9.24: Removal of ethmoid septations along the roof—This can be performed with microdebrider after first gentle fracturing with suction or curette or incising with thru-cutting forceps.

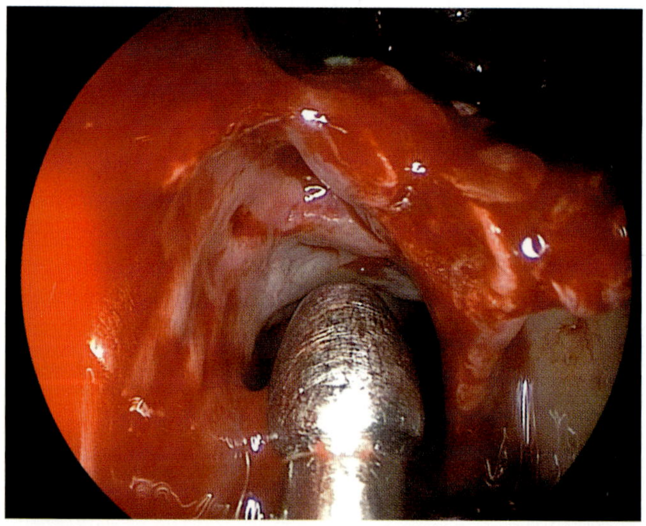

Fig. 9.25: Anterior ethmoid artery in mesentery of skull base. This prevents complete removal of septations to the ethmoid roof without placing the artery at risk and/or forcing the surgeon to clip and/or bipolar the artery.

- Up-biting thru-cutting forceps, giraffe forceps, or angled microdebrider are then used to take down the septations to the ethmoid roof. We progress from posterior to anterior. Take note of the location of the anterior ethmoid artery and whether it courses the skull base or below it in a mesentery. This is often just anterior to the attachment of the basal lamella of the middle turbinate to the ethmoid roof and dissection in this area should proceed cautiously (Fig. 9.25).

SPHENOIDOTOMY

After Initial AP Portion of Ethmoidectomy

Steps:

- After removal of the superior turbinate and dissection of the posterior ethmoid cells, the area is again copiously irrigated and bleeding controlled as necessary.

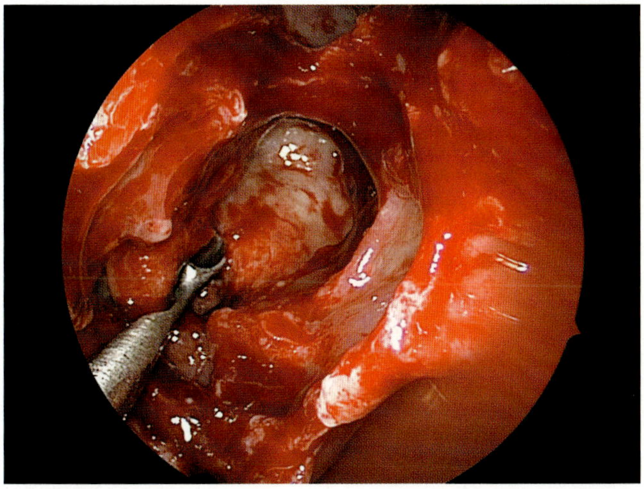

Fig. 9.26: Opening of sphenoid sinus—A cottle elevator or j-currette are placed within the ostium and the sphenoid face opened laterally.

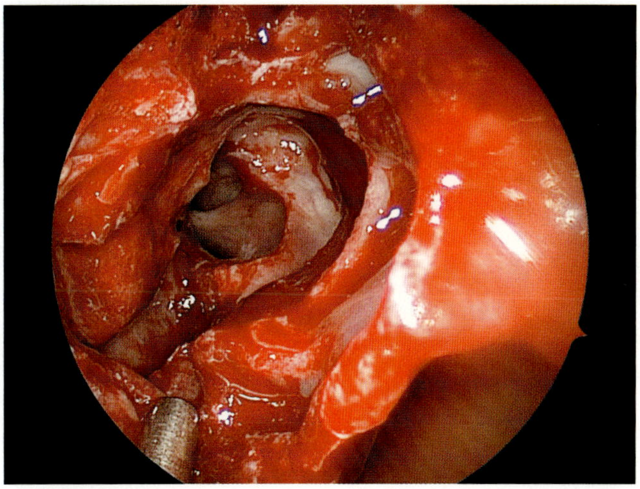

Fig. 9.27: Final sphenoid opening—The sphenoid has been extended maximally laterally and superiorly to minimize risk of postoperative scarring.

- A j-currette or Cottle elevator is then inserted into the sphenoid ostium and force is applied laterally and inferiorly to fracture the sphenoid face (Fig. 9.26).
- 2-mm Kerrison rongeurs can then be inserted and used to expand the opening laterally and superiorly. If the bone of the sphenoid face is rather thick and unable to be fractured as noted in Step 2, the Kerrison itself can be used initially. Inserting it upside-down will align the 45° tip perfectly with the orientation of the sphenoid ostium. Once through the ostium with the tip, it can then be rotated to face superolaterally and the ostium expanded as noted.
- The opening is cleaned with the microdebrider and further work with up-biting thru-cutting forceps expands the opening to the lamina and skull base working to create a square shaped opening which will minimize postoperative scarred closure (Fig. 9.27).
- Care is taken not to open the ostium inferiorly so as to not inadvertently disrupt the posterior septal artery. Additionally, we do not extend the opening inferomedially so as to preserve a small portion of intact mucosa of the ostium. It is felt that this will further reduce complete closure of the sphenoidotomy postoperatively.
- The ethmoidectomy is then completed if further work is necessary.

Isolated Sphenoid Disease; No Ethmoidectomy Completed

The reader is referred to Chapter 24: Steps 1–8.

FRONTAL SINUS EXPLORATION

Given the variability of the frontal sinus outflow tract, no one set of instructions can substitute for proper analysis of imaging and preoperative planning. As we learned in Chapter 3, the outflow tract is defined by the variations in the derivatives of the first and second ETs which exist, respectively, anterior and posterior to its course. Note must be made of the presence, or lack thereof, of Kuhn Type I, II, or III frontal cells as well as the existence and lateral extent of any suprabullar and/or, more specifically, supraorbital cells. Further, it is important to note the location of the uncinate attachment. If attaching laterally to the orbital lamina, as is present in 85% of patients, the outflow tract is directed medially. If it attaches medially or superiorly to the middle turbinate or ethmoid roof respectively then the tract is directed laterally. Superior attachment of the uncinate can also result in a secondary pneumatization in to the frontal bone medial to this site resulting in what has been termed an "intersinus septal cell." The net effect of the presence of this cell is an increased difficulty in obtaining an optimally sized opening as the septations between the frontal sinus and this cell can often be quite thick. In any event, repetitive cleaning of the dissection cavity with warm saline irrigations and reapplication of vasoconstrictor could not be more aggressively advocated as the dissection progresses.

Steps:

- A reverse post 30° or 45° endoscope is then utilized if it had not been in use already.

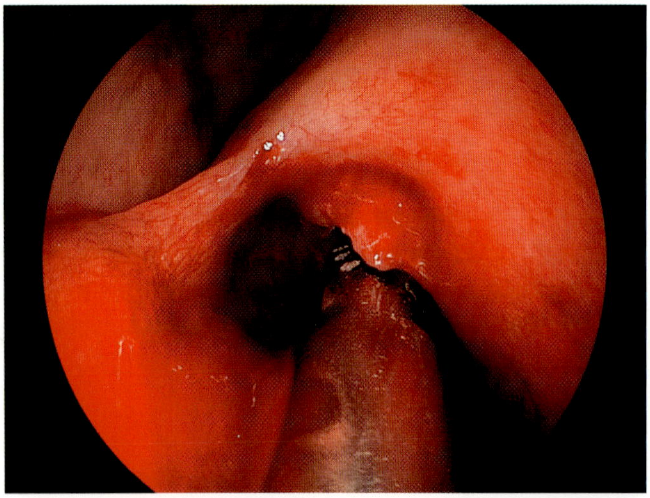

Fig. 9.28: Anterior opening of agger nasi cell. The bone is first cut with up-biting thru-cuts, standard or articulated Kerrison Rongeurs, and then the soft tissue cleaned with microdebrider.

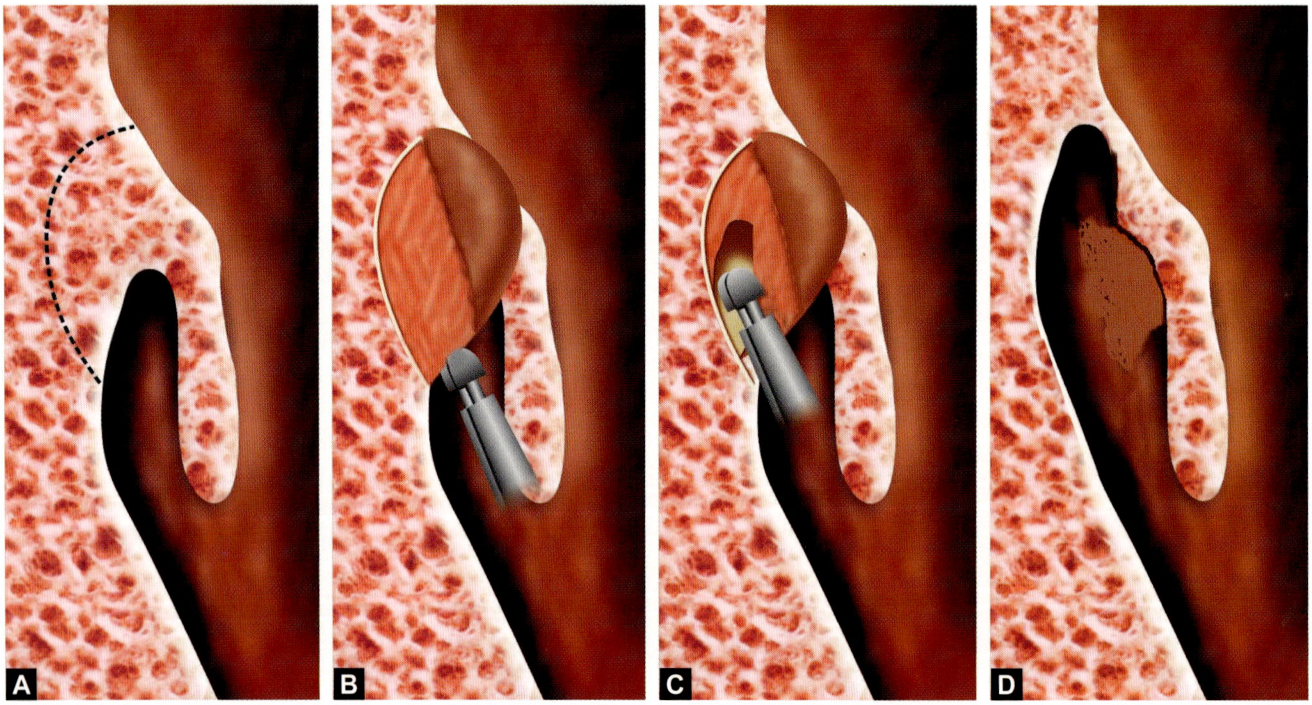

Figs. 9.29A to D: Anterior opening of the agger nasi cell (alternate)—A tissue flap can be harvested from lateral to the axilla (A) before bone removal is performed (B and C) and then folded back down (D) to prevent scarring in this area.

- Any remaining uncinate tissue is resected as superiorly as possible to the undersurface of the agger nasi cell. This can be accomplished with angled microdebrider or, sometimes more quickly, with an angled punch such as a Frontal/Curved Kerrison or Hosemann punch.
- The floor of the agger nasi cell is punctured with curette or the microdebrider and opened anteriorly. Often this will involve removal of bone and mucosa just lateral to the attachment of the middle turbinate superiorly. Care must be taken to minimize trauma to the middle turbinate at this stage to prevent post-operative lateralization (Fig. 9.28). Mucosa from the caudal face of the agger may be harvested prior to the bone removal and folded posteriorly along the lateral aspect of the middle turbinate attachment after bone removal to prevent such "zippering" afterwards (Figs. 9.29A to D).
- The medial and posterior walls of the agger are then identified and are removed from inferior to superior

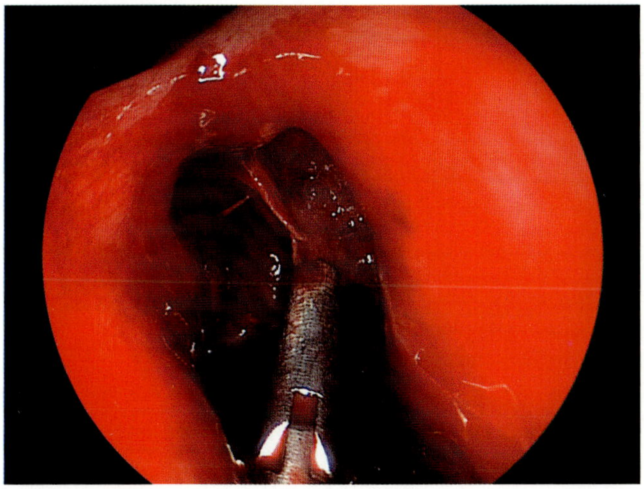

Fig. 9.30: Removal of posterior wall of the agger. With anterior agger wall removed, the posterior wall comes into view and can be removed, here with articulate Kerrison Rongeurs.

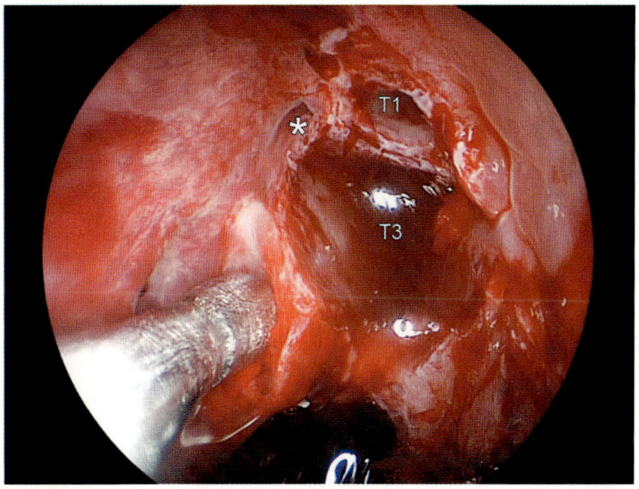

Fig. 9.31: Additional recess exploration—Removal of the superior portion of the agger nasi reveals opening to Type I cell laterally (T1), large opening to the type 3 cell inferiorly (T3) with the frontal outflow tract medially (asterisk).

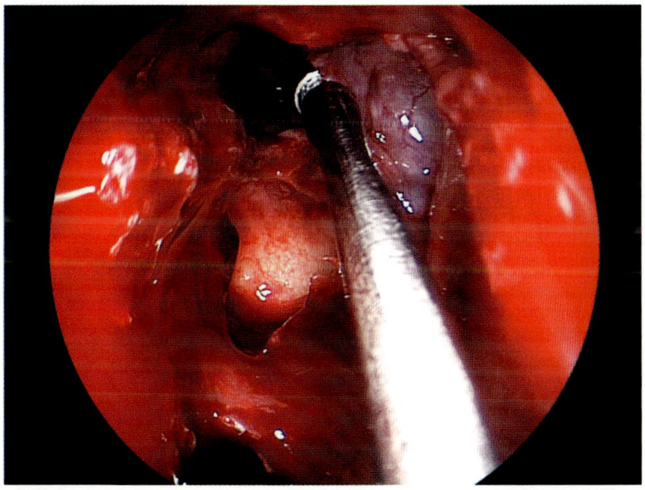

Fig. 9.32: Removal of the basal lamella of the ethmoid and roof of type 3 cell. Curved mushroom punch removing superior extension of ethmoid bulla lamella and roof of type 3 cell.

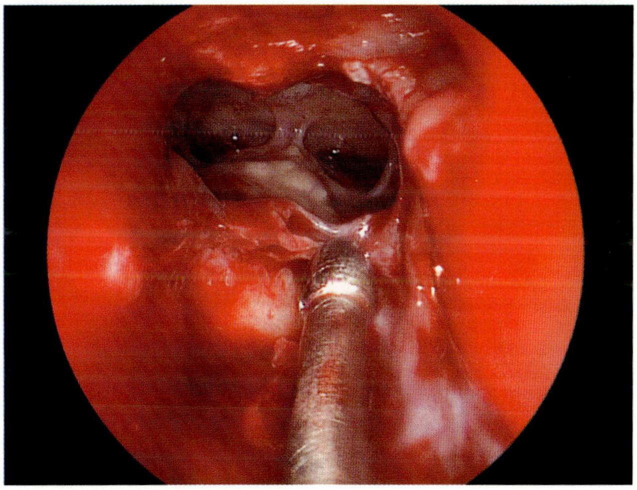

Fig. 9.33: Final opening of frontal sinus.

as well. This is often easiest with thru-cutting giraffe instruments followed by angled microdebriding to clean the edges (Fig. 9.30).

- With the agger cell removed inspection of the frontal recess continues. If this final "uncapping" opened the recess, the dissection is complete. Otherwise, as in this patient, dissection continues superiorly to open additional obstructing anatomy (Fig. 9.31).
- Removal of superior Kuhn Type Frontal cells is performed sequentially, using angled or articulating giraffe thru-cutting forceps.
- With removal of the medial and posterior walls of these cells the frontal sinus comes in to view and final removal of the basal lamella of the ethmoid (posterior aspect of outflow tract) and the roof of any remaining frontal cells is accomplished (Figs. 9.32 and 9.33).
- The frontal sinus is copiously irrigated to remove all mucous and/or infectious contents; this will further aid in hemostasis as well.
- A sheet of 0.20" silastic cut in a modified "liberty bell" configuration (Fig. 9.34) is then rolled and placed in the frontal opening with side grabbing giraffe

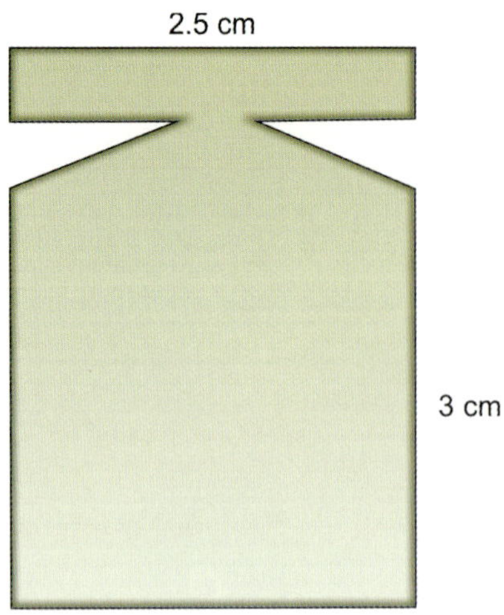

Fig. 9.34: Modified "Liberty bell" configuration of silastic sheet dressing.

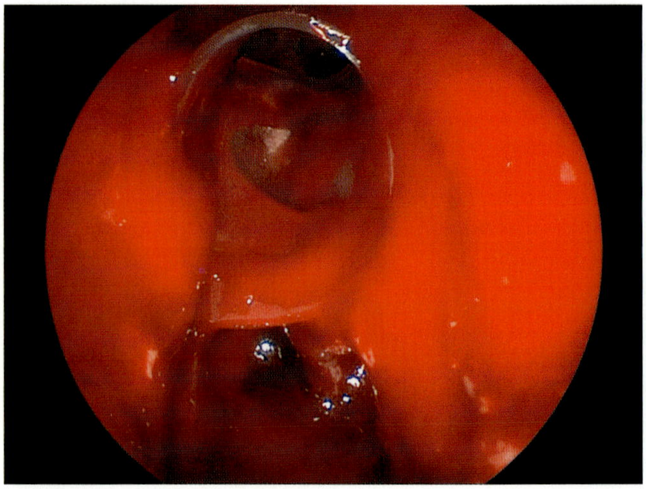

Fig. 9.35: Rolled silastic sheet dressing in place in frontal sinus opening.

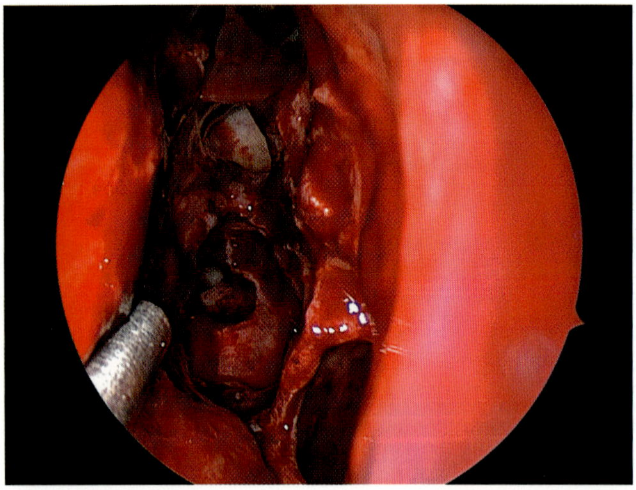

Fig. 9.36: Final common spheno-frontal-ethmoid cavity. The sphenoid sinus is seen in the distance with the maxillary opening laterally (right) and the rolled silastic visible in the frontal recess superiorly.

forceps (Fig. 9.35). This is only a temporary dressing to minimize fibrinous or sanguinous debris in this. It is to be removed at the first postoperative visit and greatly facilitates, more so eliminates, debridement in this area.

NASAL INSPECTION, CLEANING, AND DRESSING PLACEMENT

Steps:

- Following the completion of the operative plan, the nose is copiously irrigated with warm saline and the final cavity (Fig. 9.36) is inspected.
- Any residual sites of significant bleeding are identified. Consider expanding any mucosal or bone removal in areas of persistent oozing as a clean mucosal-to-mucosal coaptation will often solve the problem.
- Otherwise bipolar cautery is to be utilized as monopolar cautery will result in significant "collateral" damage.
- Any number of dressing materials is available to the surgeon at this point and a debate on their merits is beyond the scope of this chapter. We prefer to use a half-piece of a 4 cm Nasopore® dressing in each middle meatal cavity. It is positioned anteriorly between the head of the middle turbinate to help prevent lateralization or significant airflow through the ethmoid cavity so that healing can occur unabated by dried crusting.
- The nasal cavity, nasopharynx, oral cavity, and oropharynx are then suctioned and the patient allowed to emerge from anesthesia; it is preferable if in agreement with the anesthesiology colleagues for the patient to be extubated deep to prevent excessive coughing or straining due to irritation from the endotracheal tube or LMA on emergence.

CONCLUSIONS

Thorough sinus surgery requires careful preoperative planning and significant attention to the subtleties of instrument handling to prevent inadvertent trauma to the nasal cavity. No one surgery will be the most appropriate for all patients and the operative plan must be tailored to the anatomy and the disease. Attention to the ET derivatives in order will maintain an orderly progression through the sinus cavities and when paired with identification of specific landmarks such as the maxillary roof, orbital lamina, and sphenoid sinus will optimize patient safety.

REFERENCES

1. Timperley D, Harvey RJ. Perioperativ and intraoperative techniques to improve surgical outcomes in skull base surgery. Otolaryngol Clin North Am. 2010;43:699-730.
2. Higgins TS, Hwang PH, Kingdom TT, et al. Systematic review of topical vasoconstrictors in endoscopic sinus surgery. Laryngoscope. 2011;121:422-32.
3. Schaefer SD, Li JC, Chan EK, et al. Combined anterior-to-posterior and posterior-to-anterior approach to paranasal sinus surgery: an update. Laryngoscope. 2006;116:509-13.
4. Chastain JB, Cooper MH, Sindwani R. The maxillary line: anatomic characterization and clinical utility of an important surgical landmark. Laryngoscope. 2005;115:990-2.
5. Getz AE, Hwang PH. Basal lamella relaxing incision improves endoscopic middle meatal access. Int Forum Allergy Rhinol. 2013;3:231-5.

CHAPTER

10 Revision Sinus Surgery

Mohamad R Chaaban, Bradford A Woodworth

The overall success rate for primary endoscopic sinus surgery (ESS) ranges in the literature from 80% to 97%.[1-8] Since chronic rhinosinusitis (CRS) is a medical disease, surgery is often performed to help medical treatments work more effectively. As such, persistent CRS can be evaluated as either medical or surgical failure. Sinus disease can persist despite excellent surgery because of other management failures including patient noncompliance with medications (e.g., topical nasal steroids), poor allergy management, severe inflammatory or granulomatous disease, or undiagnosed genetic or immunologic defect (e.g., cystic fibrosis, immunoglobulin deficiency). However, persistent problems in disease management may also develop because of the technical failures at the initial surgery. Patients who have persistent disease despite appropriate and aggressive medical management (*see* Chapter 4) may require revision sinus surgery.

Before proceeding with surgical revision, risk factors that led to persistent disease should be evaluated. Patient risk factors may include allergies, tobacco use, gastroesophageal reflux disease, previous open sinus procedures, severe mucosal disease, inadequate postoperative care, scarred ostia, nasal synechiae, and inadequate surgery.[9-12] It is critical to assess the extent of the inflammatory disease by objective measures (e.g., nasal endoscopy and CT scan) and the subjective symptoms of the patient. An individual with an excellent quality of life and minimal symptoms despite persistent mucosal disease on nasal endoscopy typically requires no intervention except in the case of impending problem (e.g., mucocele). A thorough evaluation of the constellation of symptoms should be completed to avoid further unnecessary surgery. Some symptoms such as postnasal drip (PND) and headache may not be aided with another procedure if secondary to another underlying cause. PND has been found to be associated with acid reflux at the level of the nasopharynx and hypopharynx regardless of whether or not the patients had CRS.[13] Furthermore, up to 90% of patients who present with headaches and normal CT scan had the diagnosis of migraine in one study.[14] Patients had resolution or reduction of their symptoms following triptan treatment.

Physical examination should always be accompanied by a nasal endoscopy to assess possible mechanical problems or scarring that could be blocking sinus ostia. Recirculating mucus secondary to a posteriorly placed maxillary surgical antrostomy is a common mistake during the initial surgery and is best seen with an angled 30° or 45° endoscope. Frontal or ethmoid sinusitis from a lateralized middle turbinate, scarring of the sphenoid ostia, and scarred residual ethmoid partitions can also be observed with nasal endoscopy that will be missed with an anterior speculum examination. A CT scan should be acquired to determine the location and extent of the sinus disease that needs to be addressed. Acquisition in a format compatible with the surgeon's computer-assisted navigation system is necessary for image guided surgery. The indications for the utilization of image guidance as reported by the American Academy of Otolaryngology—Head and Neck Surgery[15] include revision sinus surgery, distorted sinus anatomy, extensive polyposis, involvement of the sphenoid and frontal sinus, pathology abutting the skull base/orbit/optic nerve or carotid artery, presence of CSF rhinorrhea, and benign or malignant sinonasal neoplasms. Magnetic resonance imaging (MRI) scans may be helpful in select patients when there is concern of tumor, dehiscence of the skull base with adjacent opacification (possible encephalocele), or to differentiate inspissated mucus from tumors (e.g., inverted papilloma). MRI also confirms the diagnosis of allergic fungal rhinosinusitis when there is bony wall erosion and characteristic T2 weighted signal drop out. Mucoceles have variable intensities on MRI, but usually are bright on T1 and T2 weighted images depending on the water content.

Disease factors that influence consideration of revision sinus surgery may include polyposis, ciliary dysmotility, advanced Lund-MacKay scores, hyperostosis, asthma, and aspirin exacerbated respiratory disease. Polyposis, regardless of the etiology, predisposes the patient to the likelihood of having revision surgeries. In addition to mucosal inflammation causing sinonasal obstruction, polyps may also inhibit normal mucociliary clearance.[16] There is also an established relationship between the presence of polyps and the requirement for sinus surgery.[17-20] A higher degree of nasal obstruction[21] and more severe disease on CT and endoscopy postoperatively after sinus surgery are seen with nasal polyposis.[22]

To perform adequate and safe revision sinus surgery, a thorough understanding of the anatomy is required with attention to landmarks remaining after previous surgery. Triplanar CT image guidance is helpful in such instances when scarring obscures the anatomic structures or there is a loss of landmarks.[15] The primary purpose of revision sinus surgery is to achieve widely patent sinuses to enable clinical nasal endoscopy visualization, access for topical medical delivery (e.g., topical intranasal steroids), and facilitate mucus clearance.[23-25]

This chapter will focus on revision surgery of the maxillary, ethmoid, and sphenoid sinuses. Revision frontal sinus surgery will be discussed in Chapter 12.

FESS FAILURES: CAUSES

Reasons for revision sinus surgery could include patient or surgical factors. Patient factors include both the recalcitrant nature of the disease process such as those patients with polyposis or recurrent bacterial or fungal infections. Surgical factors include incomplete surgical intervention, stenosis or areas of mucus recirculation, complications of prior surgery, or the presence of neoplasia on histology. In a study by Musy and Kountakis,[26] the most common surgical reasons for revision ESS included (in descending order); lateralization of the middle turbinate, incomplete anterior ethmoidectomy, scarred frontal recess, retained agger nasi cell, incomplete posterior ethmoidectomy, retained uncinate, middle meatal antrostomy stenosis, and recurrent polyposis.

PREOPERATIVE CONSIDERATIONS

Endoscopic visualization in the office coupled with careful review of the CT scan of the sinuses is crucial in making sure adequate and complete surgery is performed. Removing all residual partitions while preserving sinus mucosa is critical in preventing osteitis following surgery. Mucus recirculation is one of the most common reported reasons for revision surgery.[18]

CT scans may demonstrate findings such as the presence of Haller (infundibular) cells, residual uncinate process, polyposis recurrence, and stenosis of the surgical sinus openings. Since one of the risk factors for revision is the presence of inhalant allergies, allergy testing and immunotherapy may be instituted prior to surgery. Reducing the reactivity of the sinus and nasal mucosa should be a routine part of long-term management of CRS and will assist with lessening inflammation perioperatively. In addition, some symptoms may be related to allergic rhinitis which could have been missed from the patient's initial presentation.

The septum can decrease access to the sinuses during revision surgery. Indeed, the presence of a deviated septum may represent the underlying reason why further revision sinus surgery is required. Limited visualization during the previous surgery could have resulted in incomplete surgery or shortcuts that cause complications (e.g., middle turbinate resection resulting in subsequent lateralization of the remnant).

Thorough evaluation of the preoperative CT scan to check for orbital or skull base dehiscence is critical to avoid intraoperative violation of the boundaries. Previous orbital decompression surgery for Grave's disease, congenital dehiscence of the orbital wall, and an uncinate process that is adhered to the medial orbital wall are set ups for injury (Figs. 10.1A to C). Skull base dehiscence can be secondary to previous ESS or trauma, neurosurgical procedures, and natural bony defects secondary to polyp expansion or allergic fungal sinusitis (Figs. 10.2A to C).[27-29] In addition, preoperative imaging should be reviewed for any bony dehiscence of the carotid artery or optic nerve within the sphenoid sinus prior to sphenoidotomy (Fig. 10.3).

SURGICAL LANDMARKS IN REVISION SINUS SURGERY

Following initial ESS, landmarks may be distorted. In addition to image guidance, stable landmarks that are usually unaltered by previous surgery should be identified. The bulge or convexity of the lateral nasal wall representing the nasolacrimal duct is helpful to identify the maxillary sinus ostium and the anterior aspect of the frontal sinus recess. Residual uncinate may be present

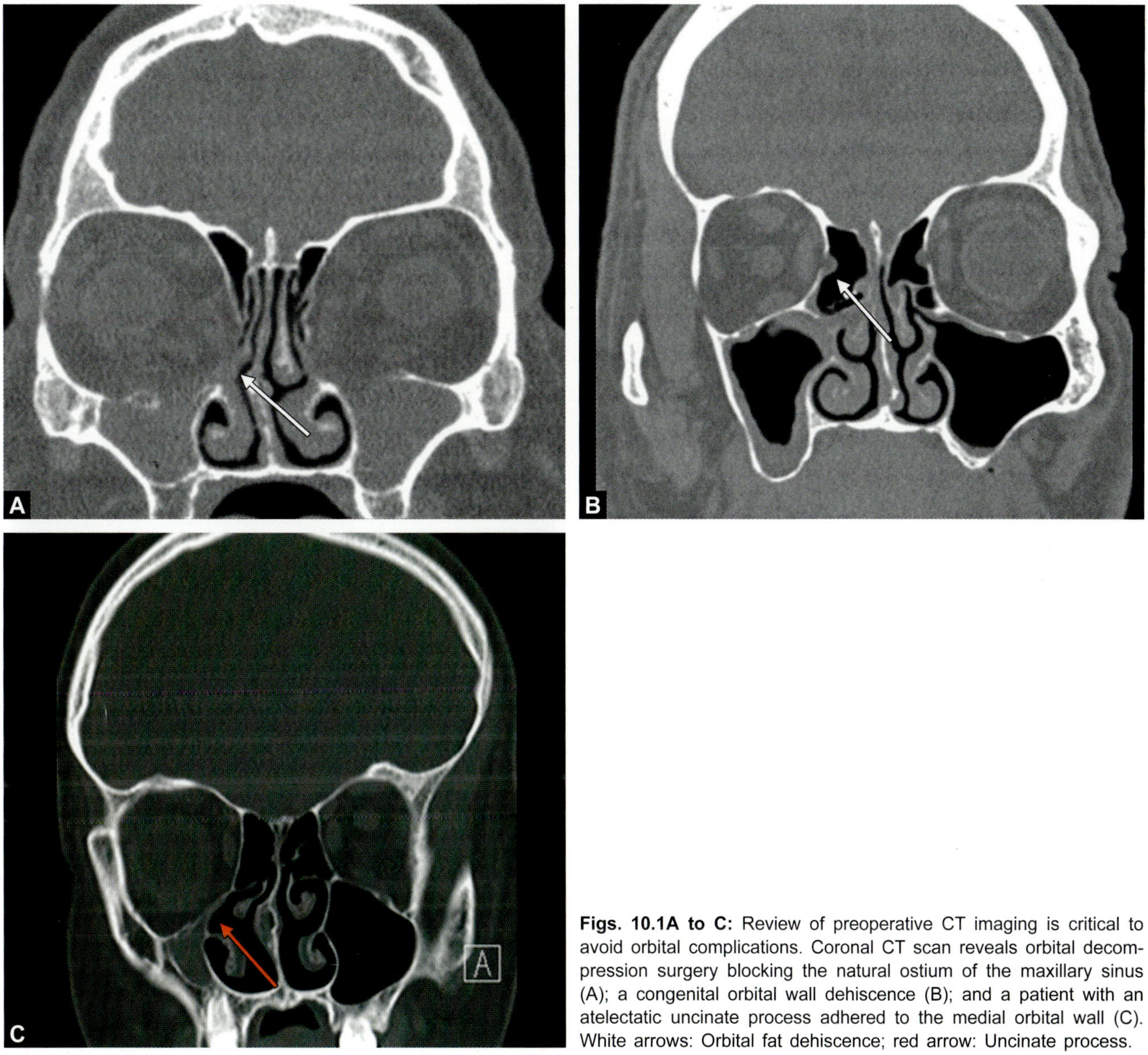

Figs. 10.1A to C: Review of preoperative CT imaging is critical to avoid orbital complications. Coronal CT scan reveals orbital decompression surgery blocking the natural ostium of the maxillary sinus (A); a congenital orbital wall dehiscence (B); and a patient with an atelectatic uncinate process adhered to the medial orbital wall (C). White arrows: Orbital fat dehiscence; red arrow: Uncinate process.

and can form the border of the agger nasi. Landmarks for the middle meatus during surgical revision include the posterior fontanelle of the maxillary sinus located superior to the posterior attachment of the inferior turbinate as well as the sphenopalatine foramen, which is located slightly superior to the end of the horizontal portion of the middle turbinate basal lamella (if present).[30,31] It is necessary to note the relationship between the orbital floor and the lateral attachment of the inferior turbinate during revision maxillary antrostomy. Following revision maxillary sinus antrostomy, identifying the posterior maxillary sinus wall assists with perceptual depth as it represents the level of the anterior sphenoid sinus wall. For completion sphenoethmoidectomy, identifying a scarred superior turbinate may be difficult and the natural sinus ostium is usually medial to its tail.[32] The safest approach in this situation to the sphenoid sinus is through its natural ostium, which can be located at the level of the posterior medial orbital floor and adjacent to the nasal septum close to the midline. The anterior wall of the sphenoid is around 7 cm from the collumella and at a 30° angle from the nasal floor. Following identification

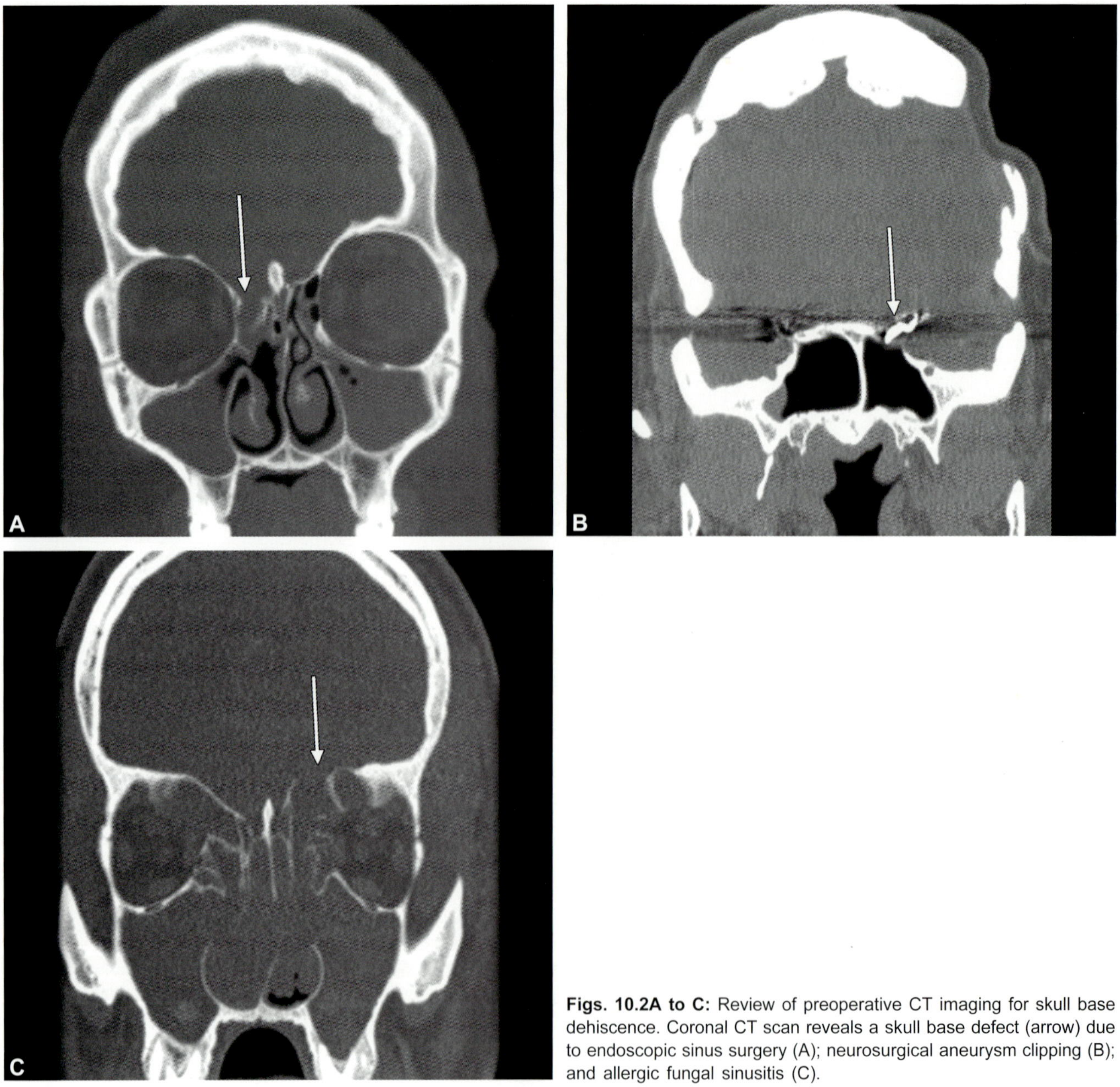

Figs. 10.2A to C: Review of preoperative CT imaging for skull base dehiscence. Coronal CT scan reveals a skull base defect (arrow) due to endoscopic sinus surgery (A); neurosurgical aneurysm clipping (B); and allergic fungal sinusitis (C).

of the sphenoid sinus, completion ethmoidectomy is performed from posterior to anterior. The skull base is identified and care should be taken in the sphenoid to avoid injury to critical structures particularly a dehiscent carotid artery or optic nerve. Revision ethmoidectomy is completed by removing residual partitions laterally to the level of the medial orbital wall. Revision frontal sinus surgery, if required, will require angled endoscopes and frontal sinus dissection instruments. Details regarding revision frontal sinus surgery will be discussed in a separate chapter.

SURGICAL TECHNIQUES

Step 1

After decongestant with topical vasoconstrictor of choice (1:1,000 epinephrine or oxymetazoline), identify remaining landmarks (e.g., nasolacrimal convexity, arch of choana, superior turbinate). If the middle meatus is sealed by a lateralized middle turbinate (or remnant), incise with a sickle knife or freer parallel to the orbit (Figs. 10.4A to C).

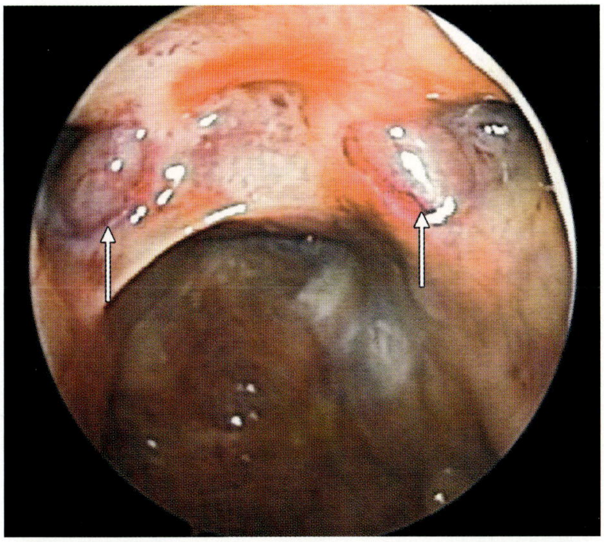

Fig. 10.3: Transnasal endoscopic view of a common sphenoid sinus in a gentleman with bilateral dehiscent carotid arteries (arrows).

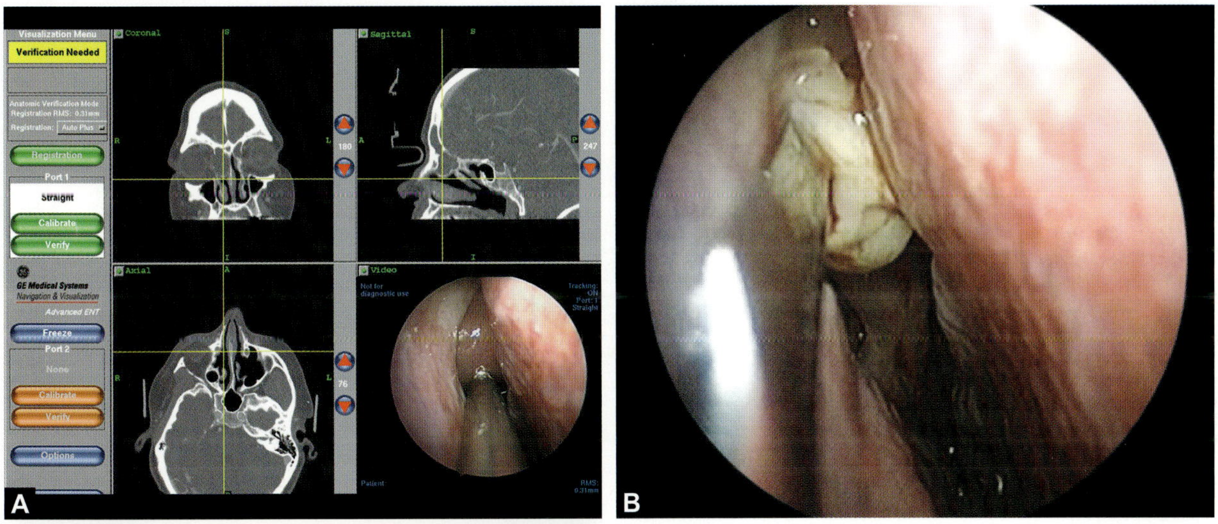

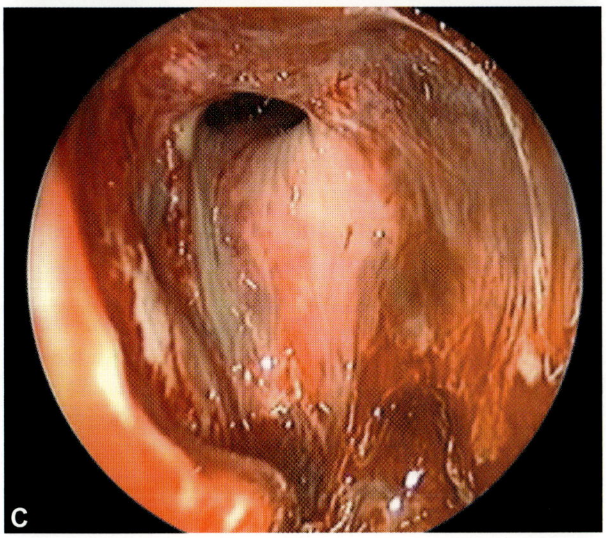

Figs. 10.4A to C: A patient with a history of previous endoscopic sinus surgery presents with bilateral frontoethmoidal mucoceles secondary to lateralized middle turbinate remnant (A—triplanar imaging with endoscopic view). A sickle knife is used to incise the turbinate medial and parallel to the orbit with immediate extravasation of mucus (B). The expansile cavity is revealed after resection of the middle turbinate remnant (C).

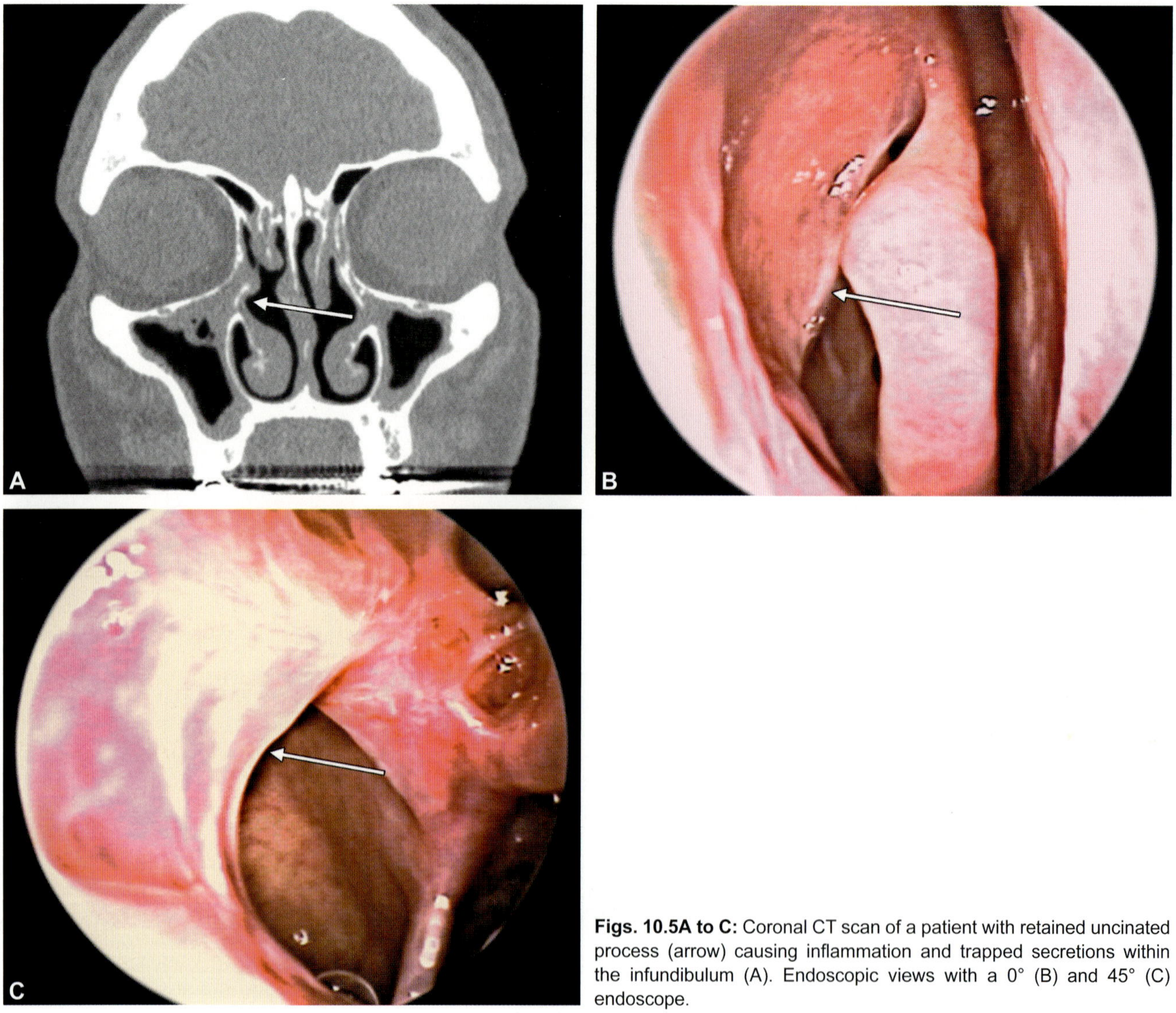

Figs. 10.5A to C: Coronal CT scan of a patient with retained uncinated process (arrow) causing inflammation and trapped secretions within the infundibulum (A). Endoscopic views with a 0° (B) and 45° (C) endoscope.

Step 2

Identify any residual uncinate process posterior to the nasolacrimal prominence (Figs. 10.5A to C). If there is a posterior antrostomy, reflect the uncinate away from the orbit with a ball tip probe and use a backbiting forceps to remove it in a safe fashion (Fig. 10.6). Scar bands causing recirculating mucus can be resected using similar methods (Fig. 10.7).

Step 3

Take down the posterior portion of the medial maxillary wall to identify the level of the posterior maxillary wall. Penetrate the basal lamella of the middle turbinate with a j curette at the junction of the horizontal and vertical portions (Fig. 10.8). This will keep your dissection inferior and away from the skull base. A short posterior ethmoid recognized on preoperative imaging will caution you to keep the dissection inferior and avoid penetration of the skull base (Figs. 10.9A and B).

Step 4

Identify any remnant of the superior turbinate and establish the relationship to the arch of the choana and the

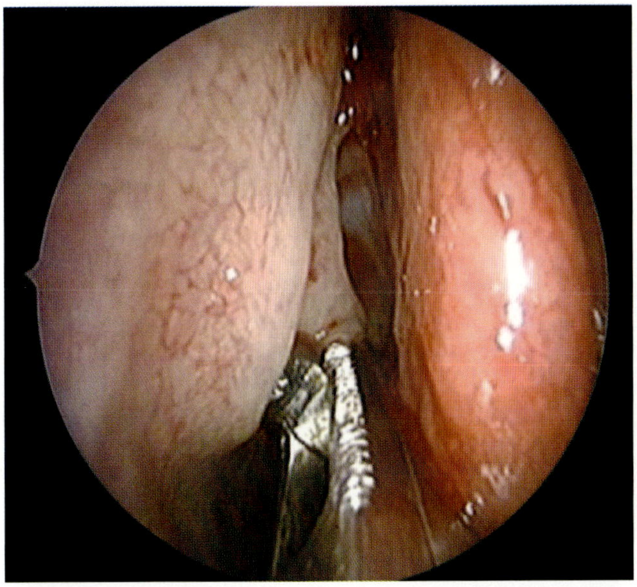

Fig. 10.6: A backbiting forceps is used to take down the uncinate process.

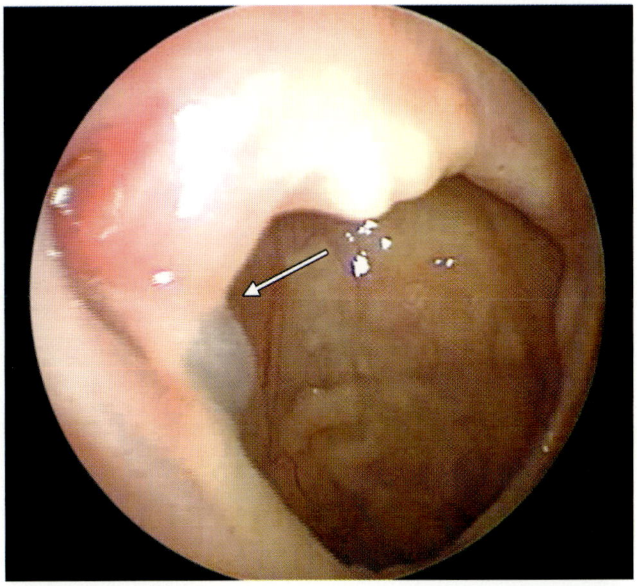

Fig. 10.7: A 70° endoscopic view of recirculating mucus (arrow) within the maxillary ostia and scar band from previous surgery.

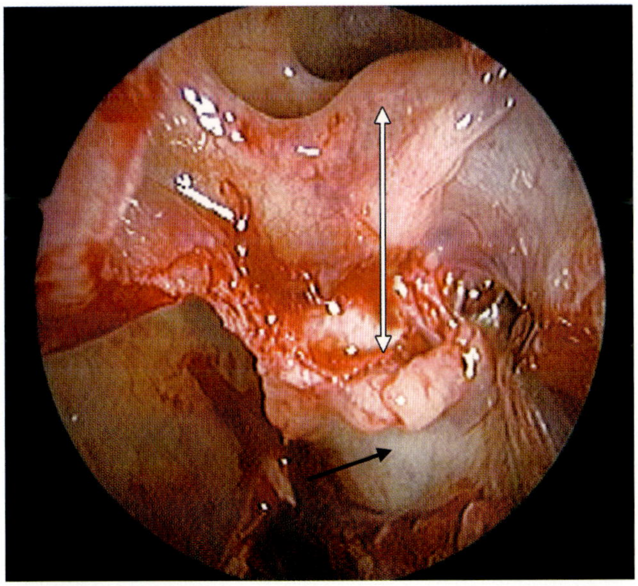

Fig. 10.8: A j curette is inserted through the basal lamella at the inferomedial junction of the vertical (white arrow) and horizontal (black arrow) portions of the basal lamella.

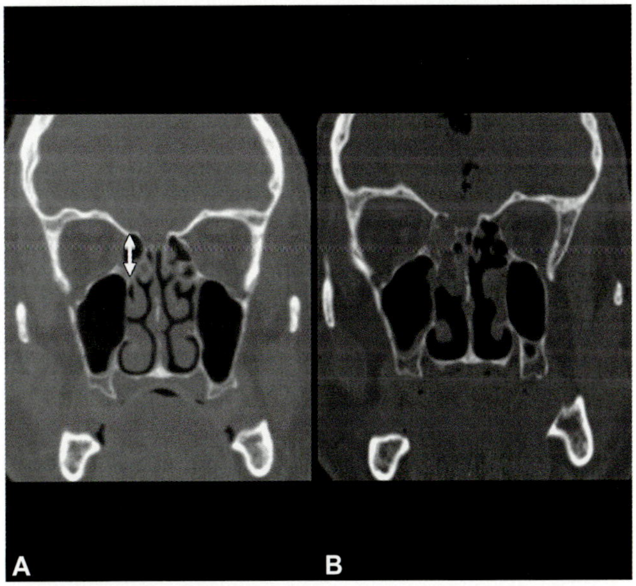

Figs. 10.9A and B: Failure to recognize a short posterior ethmoid on preoperative image (A: white arrow) resulted in a skull base defect, pneumocephalus, and cerebrospinal fluid leak (B).

posterior maxillary wall. Resect the inferior third of the turbinate if still present and identify the natural ostium of the sphenoid sinus (Figs. 10.10A and B). If the posterior ethmoid has already been dissected or there is a prior sphenoidotomy, go directly to widening the sphenoidotomy with a Kerrison punch or sphenoid ostium punch to definitively identify skull base in the sphenoid sinus (Fig. 10.11).

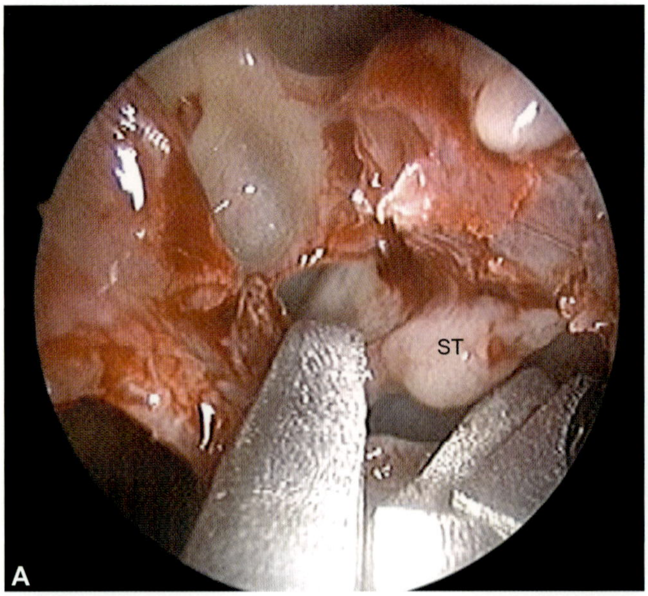

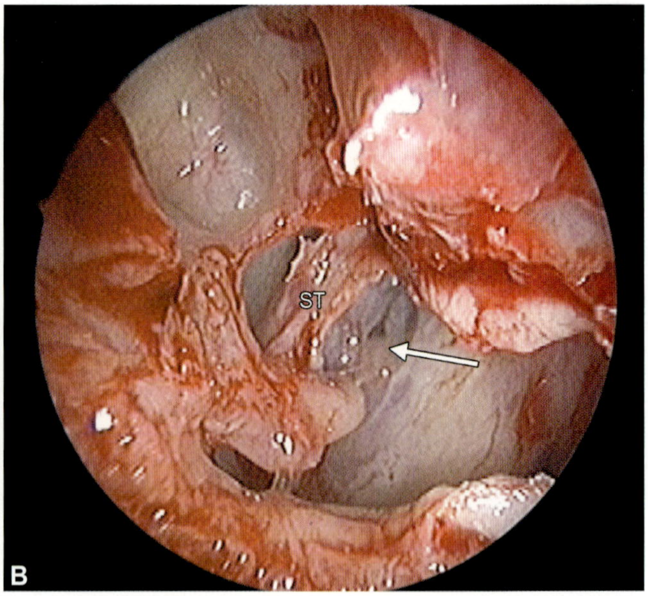

Figs. 10.10A and B: Endoscopic view of resection of the inferior third of the superior turbinate (ST) (A) to identify the natural ostia (arrow) of the sphenoid sinus (B).

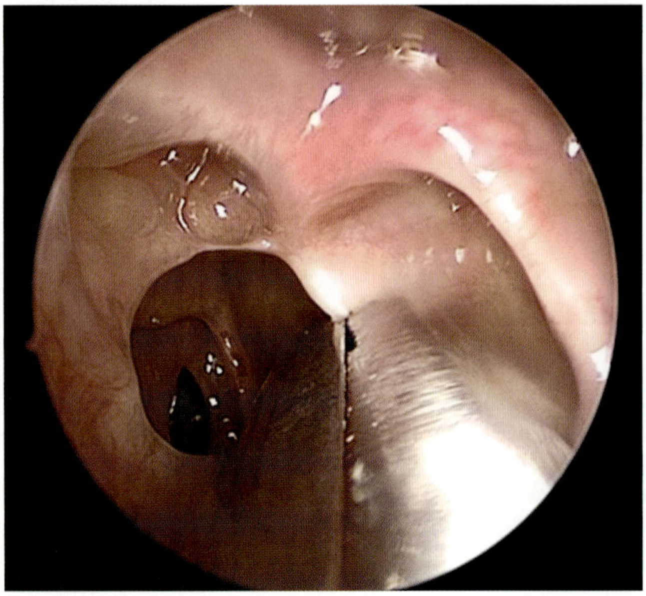

Fig. 10.11: A patient with previous sinus surgery and sphenoidotomy has multiple residual ethmoid partitions. Revising the sphenoid sinus to visualize the skull base provides the basis for skeletonizing the ethmoid cavity partitions.

Step 5

Once skull base is identified, remove the remaining partitions of the ethmoid cavity with an up-biting thru-cut forceps by feeling behind each partition for depth and marching forward in a posterior to anterior direction (Figs. 10.12A and B). Keep parallel to the middle turbinate and lateral lamella during removal. CT imaging should be evaluated for a low-lying or asymmetric skull base/cribriform plate (Fig. 10.13). In addition, make certain to avoid the anterior ethmoid artery if it presents within an ethmoid partition below the skull base (Figs. 10.14A and B).

Step 6

Once the ethmoid cavity partitions are resected to the frontal recess, switch to angled endoscopes (70° is preferred) and frontal dissection instruments (e.g., thru-cut forceps, frontal Kerrison, and frontal curettes). Resect residual partitions of the frontal recess with mucosal preservation to open the natural drainage pathway (Figs. 10.15A to C). Extended frontal sinus techniques are discussed in Chapter 12.

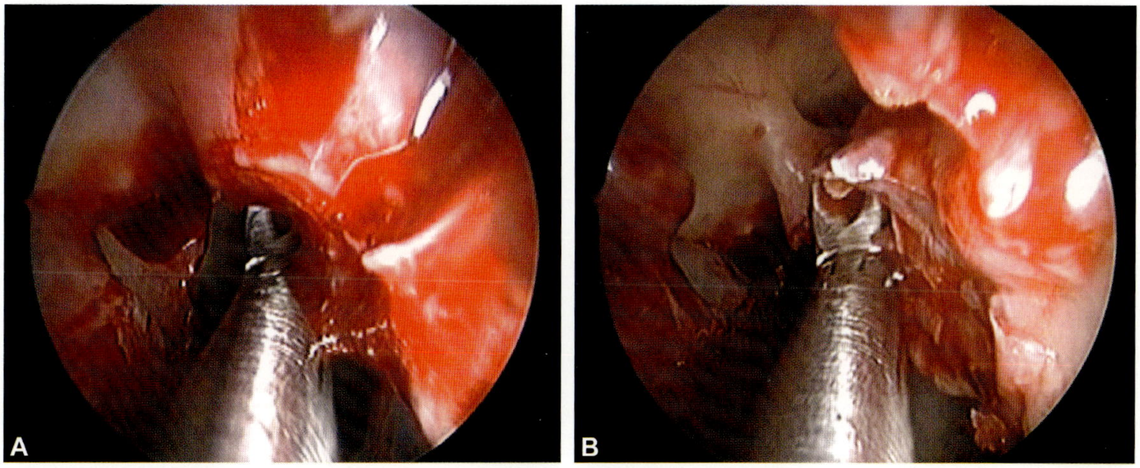

Figs. 10.12A and B: An up-biting thru-cut forceps is placed behind the partition to feel the skull base and measure the depth (A) and then the partition is removed (B).

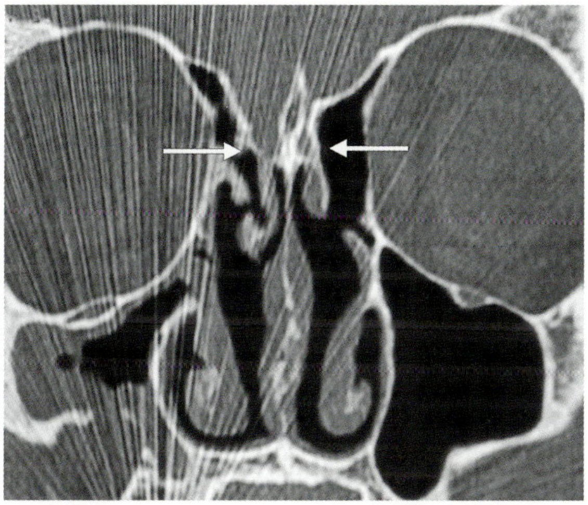

Fig. 10.13: Coronal CT scan of an asymmetric skull base (arrows) representing a set up for injury during revision surgery.

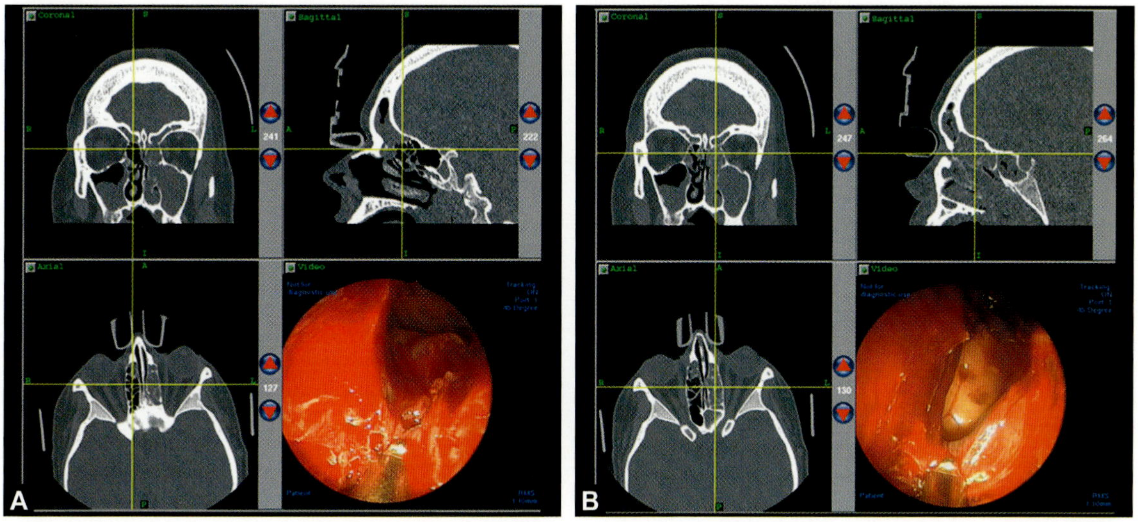

Figs. 10.14A and B: Triplanar CT images and 70° endoscopic view of a right (A) and left (B) anterior ethmoid artery positioned 5 mm below the skull base.

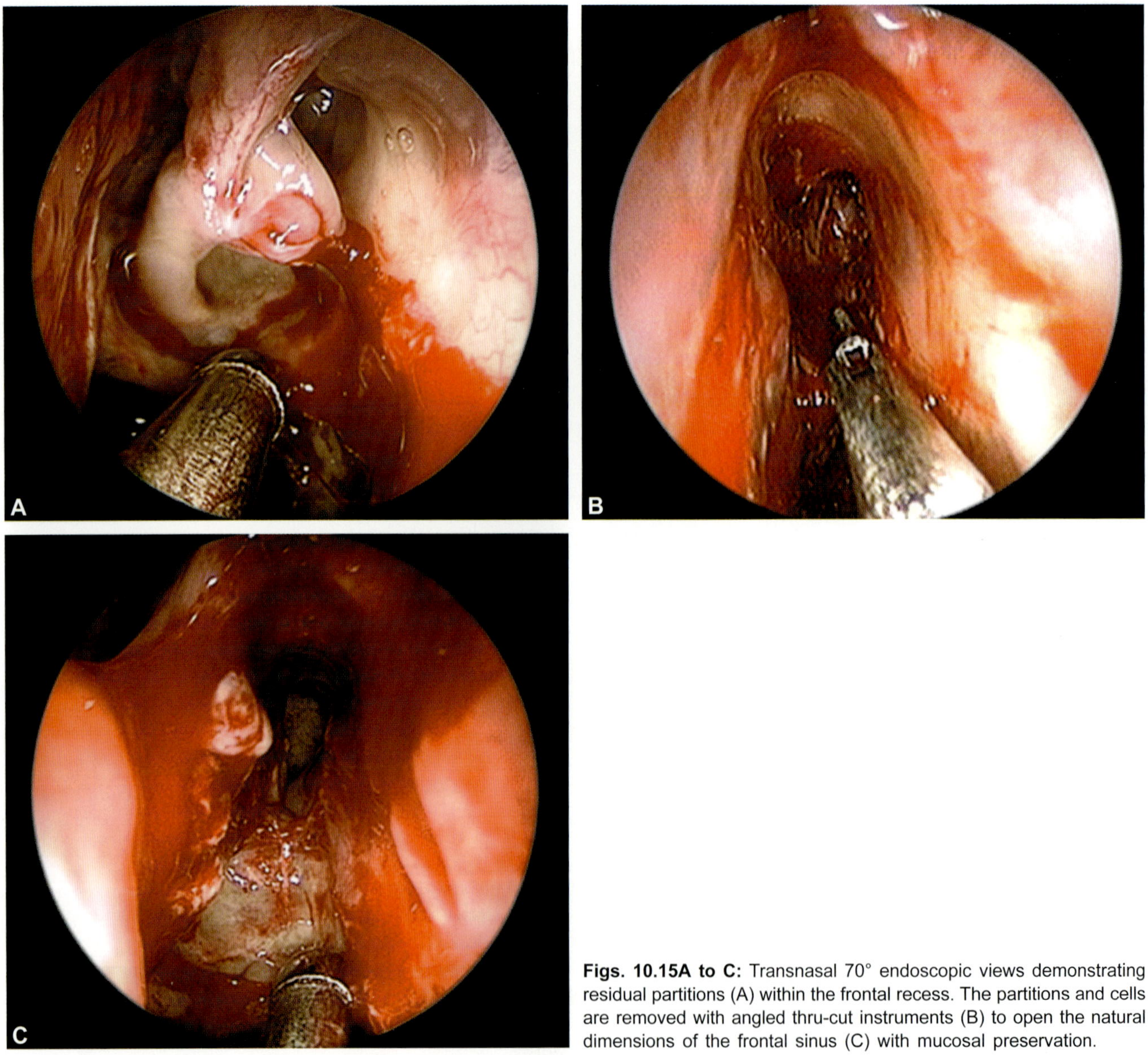

Figs. 10.15A to C: Transnasal 70° endoscopic views demonstrating residual partitions (A) within the frontal recess. The partitions and cells are removed with angled thru-cut instruments (B) to open the natural dimensions of the frontal sinus (C) with mucosal preservation.

REFERENCES

1. Davis WE, Templer JW, Lamear WR, et al. Middle meatus anstrostomy: patency rates and risk factors. Otolaryngol Head Neck Surg. 1991;104:467-72.
2. Hoffman SR, Dersarkissian RM, Buck SH, et al. Sinus disease and surgical treatment: a results oriented quality assurance study. Otolaryngol Head Neck Surg. 1989;100:573-7.
3. Hoffman SR, Mahoney MC, Chmiel JF, et al. Symptom relief after endoscopic sinus surgery: an outcomes-based study. Ear Nose Throat J. 1993;72:413-4, 419-20.
4. Levine HL. Functional endoscopic sinus surgery: evaluation, surgery, and follow-up of 250 patients. Laryngoscope. 1990; 100:79-84.
5. Schaefer SD, Manning S, Close LG. Endoscopic paranasal sinus surgery: indications and considerations. Laryngoscope. 1989;99:1-5.
6. Schaitkin B, May M, Shapiro A, et al. Endoscopic sinus surgery: 4-year follow-up on the first 100 patients. Laryngoscope. 1993;103:1117-20.
7. Smith LF, Brindley PC. Indications, evaluation, complications, and results of functional endoscopic sinus surgery in 200 patients. Otolaryngol Head Neck Surg. 1993;108: 688-96.
8. Stammberger H. Endoscopic endonasal surgery—concepts in treatment of recurring rhinosinusitis. Part II. Surgical technique. Otolaryngol Head Neck Surg. 1986;94:147-56.

9. Chambers DW, Davis WE, Cook PR, et al. Long-term outcome analysis of functional endoscopic sinus surgery: correlation of symptoms with endoscopic examination findings and potential prognostic variables. Laryngoscope. 1997;107:504-10.
10. Senior BA, Kennedy DW, Tanabodee J, et al. Long-term results of functional endoscopic sinus surgery. Laryngoscope. 1998;108:151-7.
11. Kennedy DW. Prognostic factors, outcomes and staging in ethmoid sinus surgery. Laryngoscope. 1992;102:1-18.
12. Briggs RD, Wright ST, Cordes S, et al. Smoking in chronic rhinosinusitis: a predictor of poor long-term outcome after endoscopic sinus surgery. Laryngoscope. 2004;114:126-8.
13. Skedros DG, Cass SP, Hirsch BE, et al. Sources of error in use of beta-2 transferrin analysis for diagnosing perilymphatic and cerebral spinal fluid leaks. Otolaryngol Head Neck Surg. 1993;109:861-4.
14. Schlosser RJ, Bolger WE. Management of multiple spontaneous nasal meningoencephaloceles. Laryngoscope. 2002; 112:980-5.
15. Surgery A-HPoI-OUoC-A. American Academy of Otolaryngology-Head Neck Surgery. http://www.entlink.met/practice/rules/image-guiding.cfm; 2005.
16. Waguespack R. Mucociliary clearance patterns following endoscopic sinus surgery. Laryngoscope. 1995;105:1-40.
17. Jiang RS, Hsu CY. Revision functional endoscopic sinus surgery. Ann Otol Rhinol Laryngol. 2002;111:155-9.
18. King JM, Caldarelli DD, Pigato JB. A review of revision functional endoscopic sinus surgery. Laryngoscope. 1994; 104:404-8.
19. Lawson W. The intranasal ethmoidectomy: an experience with 1,077 procedures. Laryngoscope. 1991;101:367-71.
20. liu CM YT, Hsu MM. Clinical evaluation of maxillary diffuse polypoid sinusitis after functional endoscopic sinus surgery in the management of chronic rhinosinusitis. An objective assessment. J Laryngol Otol. 1994;105:832-5.
21. Deal RT, Kountakis SE. Significance of nasal polyps in chronic rhinosinusitis: symptoms and surgical outcomes. Laryngoscope. 2004;114:1932-5.
22. Toros SZ, Bolukbasi S, Naiboglu B, et al. Comparative outcomes of endoscopic sinus surgery in patients with chronic sinusitis and nasal polyps. Eur Arch Otorhinolaryngol. 2007;264:1003-8.
23. Chaaban MR, Walsh EM, Woodworth BA. Epidemiology and differential diagnosis of nasal polyps. Am J Rhinol Allergy. 2013;27:473-8.
24. Chaaban MR, Kejner A, Rowe SM, et al. Cystic fibrosis chronic rhinosinusitis: a comprehensive review. Am J Rhinol Allergy. 2013;27:387-95.
25. Virgin FW, Rowe SM, Wade MB, et al. Extensive surgical and comprehensive postoperative medical management for cystic fibrosis chronic rhinosinusitis. Am J Rhinol Allergy. 2012;26:70-5.
26. Musy PY, Kountakis SE. Anatomic findings in patients undergoing revision endoscopic sinus surgery. Am J Otolaryngol. 2004;25:418-22.
27. Chaaban MR, Illing E, Riley KO, et al. Spontaneous cerebrospinal fluid leak repair: A five-year prospective evaluation. Laryngoscope. 2014;124:70-5.
28. Jones V, Virgin F, Riley K, et al. Changing paradigms in frontal sinus cerebrospinal fluid leak repair. Int Forum Allergy Rhinol. 2012.
29. Chaaban MR, Conger B, Riley KO, et al. Transnasal endoscopic repair of posterior table fractures. Otolaryngol Head Neck Surg. 2012;147:1142-7.
30. Holly LT, Foley KT. Three-dimensional fluoroscopy-guided percutaneous thoracolumbar pedicle screw placement. Technical note. J Neurosurg. 2003;99:324-9.
31. Bolger WE, Brown CL, Church CA, et al. Safety and outcomes of balloon catheter sinusotomy: a multicenter 24-week analysis in 115 patients. Otolaryngol Head Neck Surg. 2007;137:10-20.
32. Brown SM, Sadoughi B, Cuellar H, et al. Feasibility of near real-time image-guided sinus surgery using intraoperative fluoroscopic computed axial tomography. Otolaryngol Head Neck Surg. 2007;136:268-73.

CHAPTER 11

Balloon Dilation of the Sinuses

Spencer C Payne

BACKGROUND

Brief History

The use of balloon-based catheters in the management of sinonasal disease dates back a few decades. Case reports on the use of balloons to reduce sinus fractures or to provide local drug delivery can be found as early as the 1980s and 1990s. It was in 2005 though that the use of balloon dilation of sinus ostia for the management of chronic rhinosinusitis truly came in to being. At that time, Acclarent, Inc. introduced their Balloon Sinuplasty™ system that utilized a nonconformable balloon, which was capable of creating microfractures in the bone surrounding the drainage pathways of the frontal, maxillary, and sphenoid sinus. Shortly thereafter articles began appearing in the literature regarding its safety, and efficacy.[1,2] The original procedure, performed with fluoroscopy in the operating room under general anesthetic, has evolved into simple procedure utilizing lighted guides that can often be performed in the office under topical and local anesthetic. Since the introduction of balloon technology by Acclarent, companies such as Entellus and Entrigue have also developed their own products with slightly different takes.

Safety and Efficacy

Since the introduction of balloon catheter technology, numerous articles have been published ranging from case reports and case series to prospective trials. Most of these demonstrate efficacy of balloon dilation systems in the management of sinus disease. One year data from a prospective trial (CLEAR)[3] indicated a 91.6% patency rate based on endoscopic or radiographic examination. Additionally, Sino-Nasal Outcome Test 20 (SNOT-20) quality of life scores were noted to decrease significantly (2.14–0.91) and these results were consistent with radiographic improvement as well, even if patients receiving hybrid surgery in which ethmoidectomies were also performed were removed from the analysis. The 2-year[4] results published separately showed durability of symptomatic and radiographic improvement and indicated an overall revision rate of close to 10%. Around the same time, these results were published, data from a prospective registry of cases were also released indicating that of 1,036 patients on whom balloon dilation was performed there were two patients with cerebrospinal fluid (CSF) leaks and another six cases where postoperative bleeding required packing or cautery; all complications were seen in hybrid cases however, so the role of the balloon in these circumstances remains uncertain.[5]

One published prospective randomized study in the US literature evaluates the use of balloon dilation in management of the frontal sinus compared with standard frontal sinus exploration. Plaza et al.[6] noted that balloon dilation was at least comparable in efficacy with frontal sinus exploration in managing sinus disease with an overall resolution of disease of 81% in the balloon group. The article suffers from some statistical reporting errors thus it can only be concluded that balloon dilation is effective but direct comparison with standard FESS is difficult.

In addition to the CLEAR study, three other prospective cohort studies have noted benefit from balloon dilation. The BREATHE[7] study looked at transantral infundibular dilation using an Entellus system and found radiographic patency of 95.8% and significant reduction of SNOT-20 scores to below 1. Additional office-based dilation studies by Albritton et al.[8] and Karanfilov et al.[9] have further echoed the feasibility and success of balloon dilation in the office setting.

Controversy

Since its introduction, and despite reports of its efficacy, controversy has shrouded the use of balloon dilation in managing sinus disease. The technology and its utilization remain in a continuous evolution with literature reflecting these changes. Initial concerns with the use of flouroscopy[10,11] were allayed as the lighted guides and guidewires were introduced with instrument iterations. However, reports have also noted where the technology tends to fail, either with false dilations[12], failed access[13], barosinusitis[14], and severe frontal inflammation.[15] Some of the controversy appears to be generated by a swinging pendulum in the recognition of inflammation as the primary issue in the pathogenesis of chronic rhinosinusitis (CRS) with less emphasis on anatomical obstruction and ostial occlusion. It must however be noted that the recognition of CRS as an inflammatory condition connotes, in truth, that it is a spectrum of diseases with a myriad of causative and exacerbatory conditions including ostial narrowing or closure and the resultant difficulty in effective mucociliary clearance of the sinus. The bridging thought process is that for any sinus condition for which anatomy is the primary etiology, balloon dilation should be reasonably able to effect a positive outcome and that for any condition in which ostial-occlusion prevents adequate drug delivery to manage an inflammatory condition, balloon dilation may be helpful in effecting a positive outcome. What remains to be completely settled is for which inflammatory conditions this technology may be best suited.

INDICATIONS

Adult

Given the numerous studies evaluating the efficacy of balloon dilation, some general guidelines can be applied such that the proper patient is selected. The most conservative recommendation is that this technology is best used on patients with at most mild to moderate disease. The application of this categorization may be up for debate but would generally apply to patients with scattered mucosal thickening, mild polyp disease, or isolated "dependent" sinus disease such that the likelihood that anatomical obstruction is the primary etiology is increased. Further, one case report indicates the usefulness of the procedure in managing acute frontal sinusitis[16] and the author has also used it in this scenario multiple times with good result. Chronic maxillary atelectasis, whether in the setting of hypoplastic or silent sinus syndrome, is also an optimal situation where an anatomical cure can be effected.[17] Two other publications have indicated that office or OR management of frontal ostium stenosis after more traditional procedures may be amenable to balloon technology. Melroy[18] and Luong et al.[19] have both noted a benefit in this situation with 13 patients combined having patent frontals after a revision procedure with balloon dilation.

Pediatric

Several studies have suggested an important role of balloon dilation in the management of pediatric CRS. Ramadan first reported in 2009 that balloon sinuplasty was at least successfully performed in 91% of attempted sinuses noting however that, unlike in adults, hypoplastic sinuses were not amenable to the procedure. Follow-up studies evaluating symptomatic improvement in the pediatric population found that the addition of balloon dilation with irrigation to adenoidectomy in children failing to improve on medical therapy increased success from around 50% to around 80%.[20,21]

Selection for the Office Setting

To ensure a successful dilation and patient experience, there are several key factors that should be evaluated before selecting a patient to undergo office dilation. The nervous or jittery patient is a definite contraindication. Should the patient appear to not tolerate straight-forward endoscopy, they will not make a good candidate for an office procedure. Additionally, anatomical concerns may limit your access. Extent of septal deviation and the presence of middle turbinate variants must also be carefully assessed. The more experienced surgeon may be able to deal with a septal deviation but this may not be optimal for the novice. Additionally, given the need to manipulate and rotate devices within the middle meatus, deviations in addition to turbinate variants will necessitate addressing the middle turbinate in the same setting (e.g., concha bullosa resection).

TECHNIQUE

Analgesia for the Office Setting

Preparation of the nose begins with alternating doses of oxymetazoline and 4% topical tetracaine or lidocaine. Utilization of an atomizer as discussed in Chapter 5 is recommended. Five minutes are allowed between dosings, with three doses applied of each drug. Following this, cotton balls soaked in a "preparatory mixture" of 50:50 oxymetazoline and tetracaine are placed strategically medial and lateral to the middle turbinate as well as the over the axilla of the middle turbinate. After 5 min,

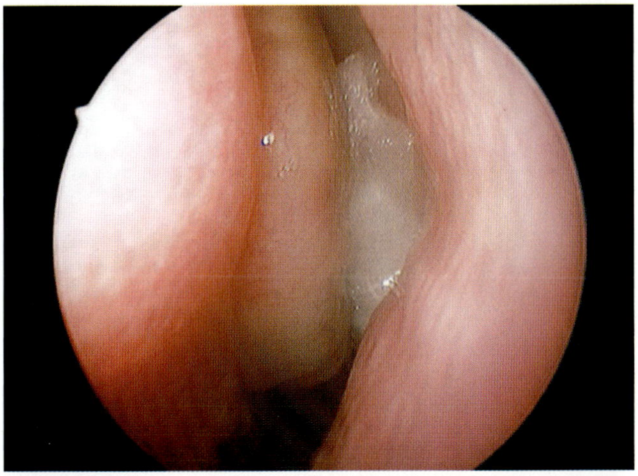

Fig. 11.1: Middle meatal analgesia: Cotton soaked in oxymetazoline and lidocaine or tetracaine is packed into middle meatus to ready the area for instrumentation.

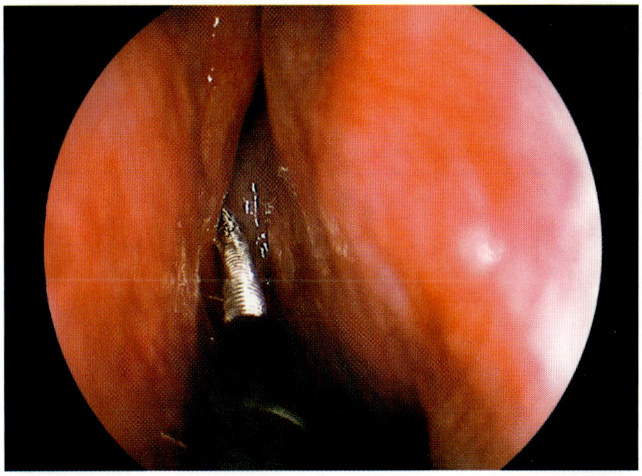

Fig. 11.2: Wiring of right sphenoid sinus: A guide wire is seen being thread into the right sphenoethmoidal recess behind the inferior aspect of the superior turbinate.

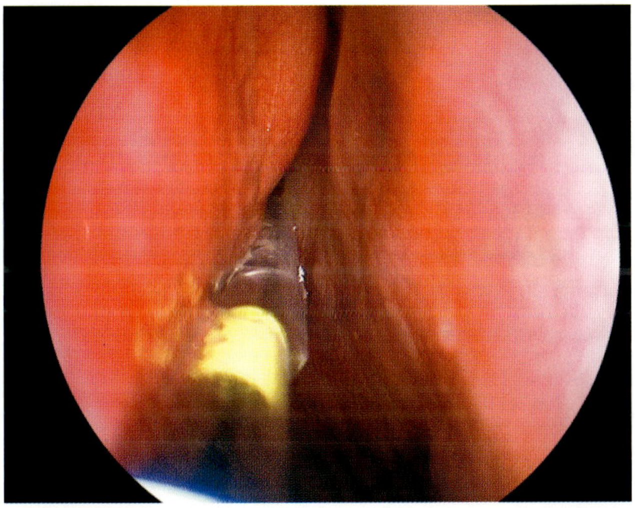

Fig. 11.3: Sphenoid balloon placement: A balloon is thread over the guidewire; the catheter is marked such that the proximal portion of the balloon is seen to be outside the sinus.

injection of the middle turbinate as described in Chapter 9 can be performed. If frontal or maxillary dilation is to be performed, the middle turbinate can be medialized with a freer and placement of additional cotton soaked in the "preparatory mixture" high and deep in the middle meatus is completed (Fig. 11.1).

Sphenoid Sinus

When dilating multiple sinuses in one setting, the author prefers to dilate the sphenoid sinus first. Given its posterior location and the need to often gently lateralize the middle turbinate, addressing this sinus first helps avoid problems with successive dilation of the more anterior sinuses to follow. Optimally, a small 2.7 or 3 mm endoscope is used. Gentle lateralization of the middle turbinate can be performed with a freer elevator along its inferior edge, and progressing posteriorly until the superior turbinate is visualized. Care is taken to maintain a 30° trajectory, often along the inferior aspect of the middle turbinate, to avoid dissection too superiorly and inadvertent skull base injury. Frequently, the sphenoid ostium can be visualized directly, just medial to the posterior edge of the superior turbinate in the sphenoethmoidal recess. In the setting of recurrent or chronic sinusitis, this landmark may be obscured however. Using a straight guide, a guidewire is thread through the inferior aspect of the sphenoethmoidal recess (Fig. 11.2). One should quickly check the nasal cavity and nasopharynx to ensure inadvertent "misfiring" into the wrong area. Usually, the sinus is cannulated with minimal difficulty and the balloon is then extended over the wire through the sphenoid os (Fig. 11.3). The balloon is then inflated per manufacture instructions (Fig. 11.4). Serial dilations may need to be performed to adequately dilate the os as well as gently lateralize the superior turbinate. If irrigation of the sinus is to be performed, this can be done at this point. As it is a straight trajectory, threading an irrigating catheter over the wire may not be necessary. Upon completion of the procedure the opening is inspected to ensure adequacy (Fig. 11.5).

Frontal Sinus

Many surgeons have found this to be one of the more straightforward sinuses to dilate and it was this ease, compared with formal dissection of the frontal recess,

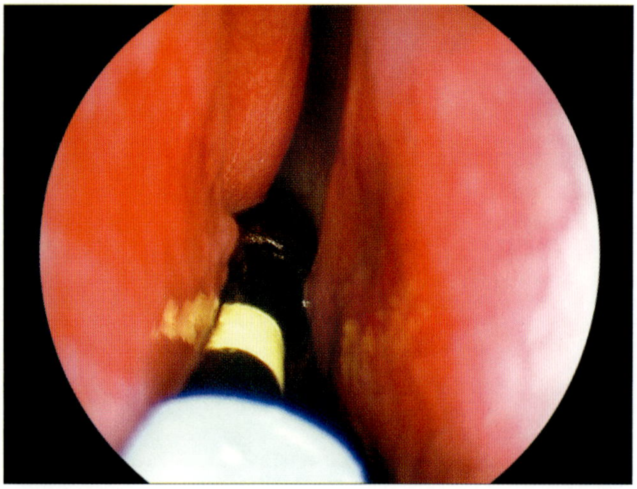

Fig. 11.4: Sphenoid balloon inflation.

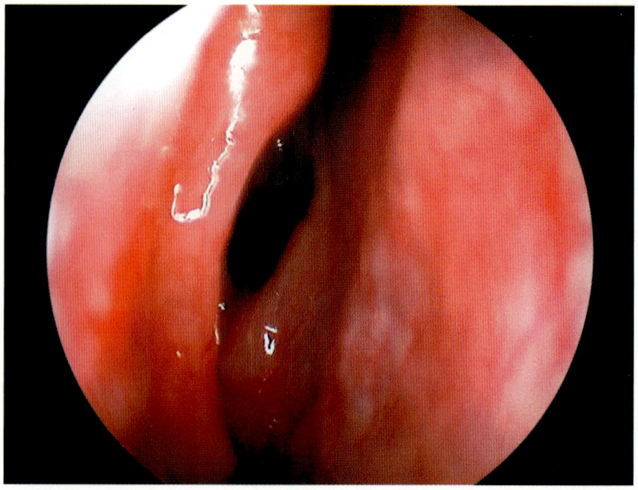

Fig. 11.5: Postdilation view of sphenoid: The dilated right sphenoid ostium is readily visible.

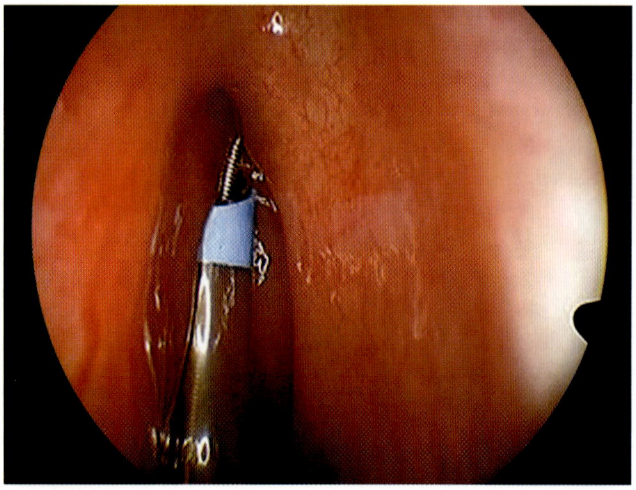

Fig. 11.6: Wiring the left frontal: The frontal guide is seen here placed just medial to the uncinate process and directed superolaterally as the guidewire is noted to extend beyond the tip in a similar trajectory.

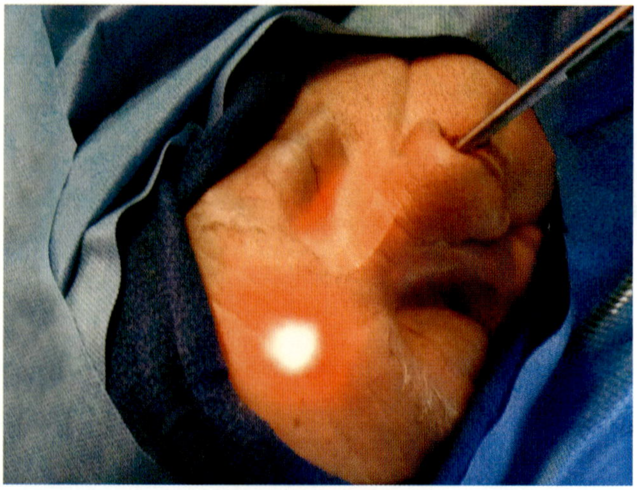

Fig. 11.7: Confirmation of frontal access: Visualization of a bright, well-defined illumination of the frontal sinus is key to confirming access to the sinus.

that made sinus dilation so attractive initially. However, difficulty with accessing the sinus has been described.[22] It is thought that difficulty with this sinus can be minimized if performing dilation before any additional ethmoid dissection. Doing so avoids issues with false tracts between mucosa and bone.

After medialization of the middle turbinate, the guide or device is brought into the middle meatus and aimed superiorly. Careful inspection of the preoperative radiology can indicate whether the frontal outflow tract is expected to be medial or lateral depending on the attachment of the uncinate superiorly to the lamina or skull base respectively. Slipping just posterior to the uncinate and aiming as predicted by radiology, a guide wire is thread superiorly in to the sinus (Fig. 11.6). If using a lighted wire, the forehead is inspected to discern a sharp circle of illumination (Fig. 11.7). Cannulation of a supraorbital cell or incomplete access of the frontal sinus is more often seen as a diffuse illumination of the forehead as opposed to a more focal brightness that moves with guidewire manipulation. The balloon is then thread over the wire into the sinus and inflated as suggested for the device used. If using a shorter, less than 20 mm balloon, multiple dilations along the outflow tract are performed

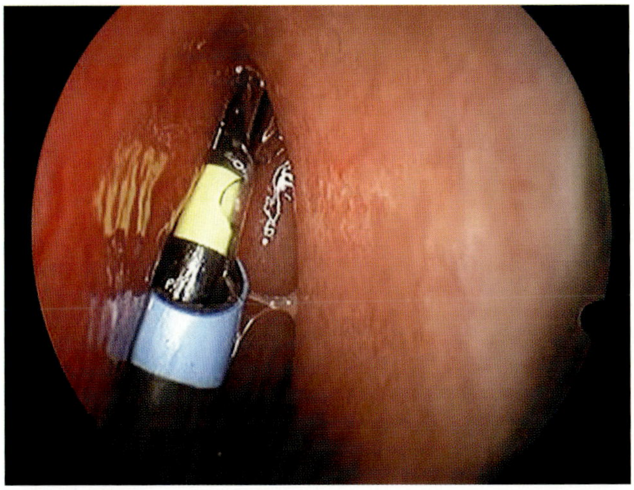

Fig. 11.8: Balloon placement during frontal dilation: When using smaller length balloons, multiple dilations along the outflow tract may be necessary. Seen here the balloon marker indicates the proximal portion of the balloon is below the uncinate.

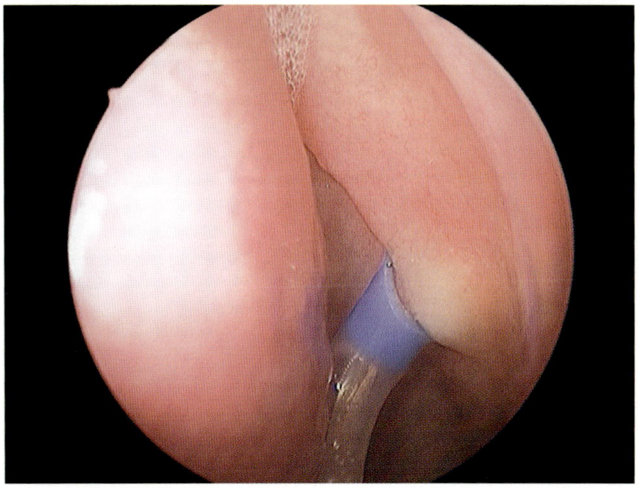

Fig. 11.9: Tip up approach: Accessing the ethmoid infundibulum is often easiest with a tip-up approach with the guide seen here aimed up as It slides behind the uncinate.

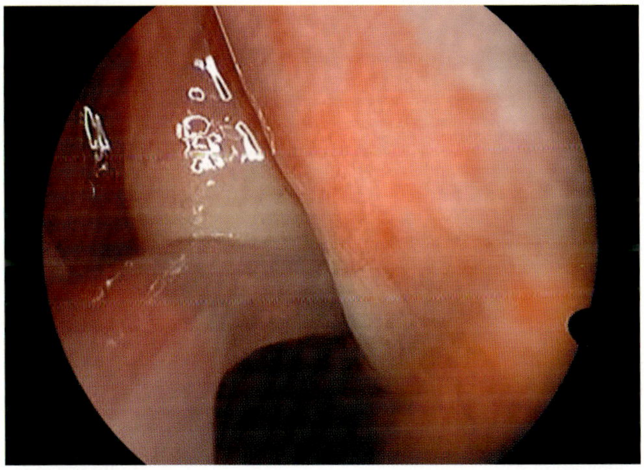

Fig. 11.10: Maxillary guide rotation: After accessing the infundibulum, the guide is rotated superiorly to better aim the wire toward the natural ostium.

to ensure patency from frontal infundibulum through to the middle meatus. Usually, the initial dilation is superior in the outflow tract followed by dilation with the tip of the balloon exposed (Fig. 11.8).

Difficulty accessing the sinus can be addressed with incremental dilations. In this setting, an inability to advance a wire along the known/obvious tract (such may be the case with a very pneumatized agger or type III cell) and be achieved. The wire is threaded as far as allowed followed by the balloon and limited dilation. The wire and balloon are then serially advanced and inflated along the outflow tract superiorly until the entire tract has been addressed.

Maxillary Sinus

Despite the ease with which this sinus can be accessed through traditional methods, its posteriorly directed transition space can make its dilation via balloon at times very difficult. One has to carefully inspect the preoperative imaging and the endoscopic appearance of the uncinate to determine the proper orientation and placement of the guide/device. After medialization of the middle turbinate, the guide is brought into the middle meatus. An angulation of the device/guide greater than 90° is often necessary (M-110 in the case of the Acclarent device). The end of the device is brought below the ethmoid bulla in to the inferior aspect of the ethmoid infundibulum in a "tip-up" orientation (Fig. 11.9). The uncinate is "hooked" and gently medialized as the device is then rotated superiorly (Fig. 11.10) such that the trajectory of the device then aims towards the natural ostium of the sinus, which is located anteriorly in the infundibulum at the junction of the lower and middle thirds of the uncinate (Fig. 11.10). The guidewire is then thread into the sinus, often requiring multiple attempts. Advancement of the wire should proceed with minimal resistance and placement can be confirmed with inspection of the maxilla under the upper lip if using a lighted guide. Similar to the other sinuses, the balloon is then thread over the wire or device into the sinus with the proximal balloon edge left outside the infundibulum (Fig. 11.11) and inflated as directed which usually results in significant displacement of the uncinate (Fig. 11.12). Irrigation can then be performed (Fig. 11.13)

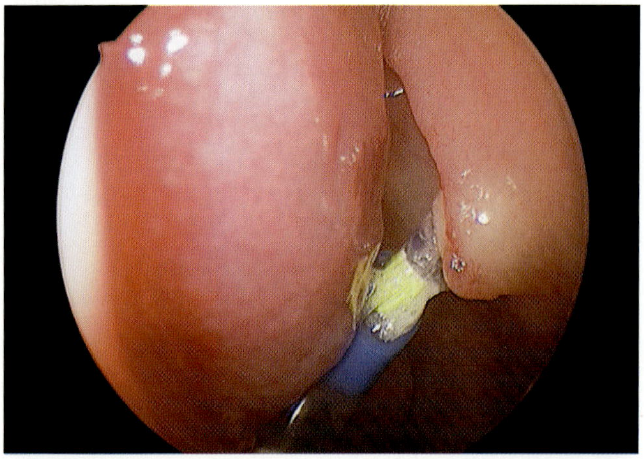

Fig. 11.11: Maxillary balloon placement: After insertion, the guide and proximal edge of the balloon are directed posteriorly allowing the balloon to follow the natural trajectory of the transition space.

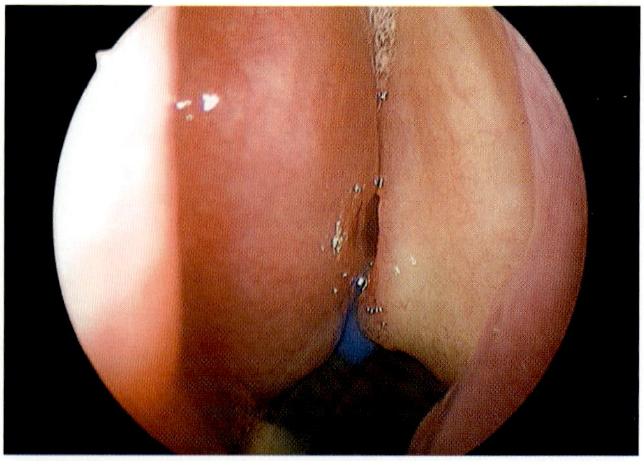

Fig. 11.12: Maxillary balloon inflation: The uncinate process is noted to medialize with inflation of the infundibulum.

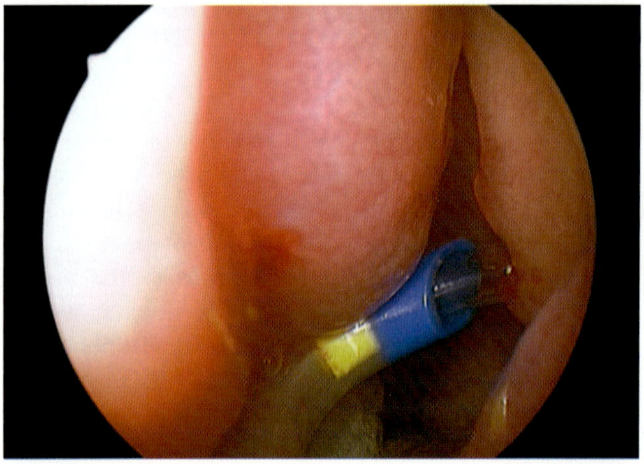

Fig. 11.13: Maxillary irrigation: An irrigation catheter is seen thread into the ostium; this often does not require a guidewire after dilation has been achieved.

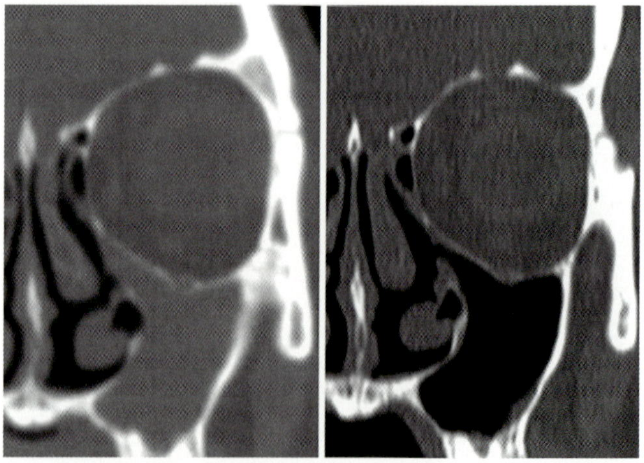

Fig. 11.14: Maxillary ballon patient radiology: Pre- and postoperative CT scans of maxillary balloon dilation patient showing resolution of silent sinus syndrome.

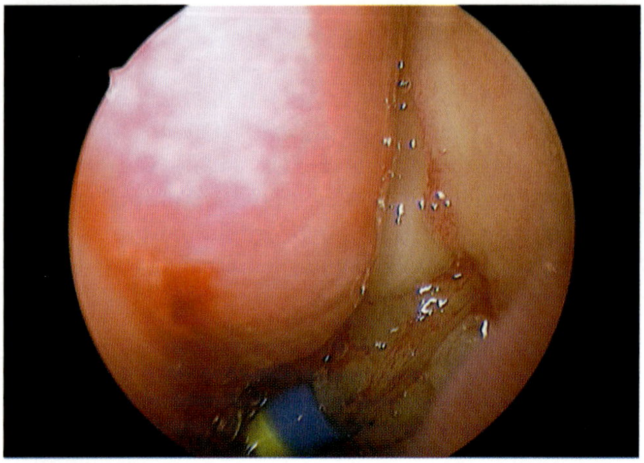

Fig. 11.15: Maxillary sinus irrigation: Mucoid debris is noted to be expelled from the sinus during irrigation.

and in the case of this patient with silent sinus syndrome (Fig. 11.14), significant mucoid material can be evacuated (Fig. 11.15).

CONCLUSIONS

Balloon dilation remains a controversial technology in the treatment of sinus disease. Multiple studies indicate that in a variety of situations its efficacy is comparable to FESS in mild to moderate disease. Proper patient selection and postoperative medical therapy similar to traditional procedures will optimize success for the novice and experienced surgeon.

Its migration to the office setting and ease of performance will likely firmly anchor the technology amongst the armamentarium of otolaryngologists.

REFERENCES

1. Brown CL. Bolger WE. Safety and feasibility of balloon catheter dilation of sinus ostia: A preliminary investigation. Ann Otol Rhinol Laryngol. 2006;115:293-9.
2. Bolger WE, Vaughan WC. Catheter-based dilation of the sinus ostia: initial safety and feasibility analysis in a cadaver model. Am J Rhinol. 2006;20:290-4.
3. Kuhn FE, Church CA, Goldberg AN, et al. Balloon catheter sinusotomy: One-year follow-up - Outcomes and role in functional endoscopic sinus surgery. Otolaryngol Head Neck Surg. 2008;139:S27-37.
4. Weiss RL, Church CA, Kuhn FA, et al. Long-term outcome analysis of balloon catheter sinusotomy: Two-year follow-up. Otolaryngol Head Neck Surg. 2008;139:S38-46.
5. Levine HL, Sertich AP, Hoisington DR, et al. Multicenter registry of balloon catheter sinusotomy outcomes for 1,036 patients. Ann Otol Rhinol Laryngol. 2008;117:263-70.
6. Plaza G, Eisenberg G. Montojo J, et al. Balloon dilation of the frontal recess: a randomized clinical trial. Ann Otol Rhinol Laryngol. 2011;120:511-8.
7. Stankiewicz J, Truitt T, Atkins J Jr. One year results: transantral balloon dilation of the ethmoid infundibululm. Ear Nose Throat J. 2010;89:72-7.
8. Albritton FDt, Casiano RR, Sillers MJ. Feasibility of in-office endoscopic sinus surgery with balloon sinus dilation. Am J Rhinol All. 2012;26:243-8.
9. Karanfilov B, Silvers S, Pasha R, et al. Office-based balloon sinus dilation: a prospective, multicenter study of 203 patients. Int Forum Allergy Rhinol. 2013;3:404-11.
10. Chandra RK. Estimate of radiation dose to the lens in balloon sinuplasty. Otolaryngol Head Neck Surg. 2007;137:953-5.
11. Church CA, Kuhn A, Mikhail J, et al. Patient and surgeon radiation exposure in balloon catheter sinus osteal dilation. Otolaryngol Head Neck Surg. 2008;138:187-91.
12. Brenner PS, Abadie WM, Weitzel EK, et al. Unexpected consequences of transnasal balloon dilation of the maxillary ostium. Int Forum Allergy Rhinol. 2011; 1:466-70.
13. Tomazic PV, Stammberger H, Braun H, et al. Feasibility of balloon sinuplasty in patients with chronic rhinosinusitis: the Graz experience. Rhinology. 2013;51:120-7.
14. Andrews JN, Weitzel EK, Eller R, et al. Unsuccessful frontal balloon sinuplasty for recurrent sinus barotrauma. Aviat Space Environ Med. 2010;81:514-6.
15. Catalano PJ, Payne SC. Balloon dilation of the frontal recess in patients with chronic frontal sinusitis and advanced sinus disease: an initial report. Ann Otol Rhinol Laryngol. 2009;118:107-12.
16. Hopkins C, Noon E, Roberts D. Balloon sinuplasty in acute frontal sinusitis. Rhinology. 2009;47:375-8.
17. Sun DQ, Dubin MG. Treatment of chronic maxillary atelectasis using balloon dilation. Otolaryngol Head Neck Surg. 2013 Aug 19. [Epub ahead of print]
18. Melroy CT. The balloon dilating catheter as an instrument in sinus surgery. Otolaryngol Head Neck Surg. 2008;139: S23-6.
19. Luong A, Batra PS, Fakhri S, et al. Balloon catheter dilatation for frontal sinus ostium stenosis in the office setting. Am J Rhinol. 2008;22:621-4.
20. Ramadan HH, Terrell AM. Balloon catheter sinuplasty and adenoidectomy in children with chronic rhinosinusitis. Ann Otol Rhinol Laryngol. 2010;119:578-82.
21. Ramadan HH, McLaughlin K, Josephson G, et al. Balloon catheter sinuplasty in young children. Am J Rhinol Allergy. 2010;24:e54-6.
22. Tomazic PV, Stammberer H, Braun H, et al. Feasibility of balloon sinuplasty in patients with chronic sinusitis: the Graz experience. Rhinology. 2013:51:120-7.

CHAPTER 12

Extended Frontal Techniques

Mohamad R Chaaban, Bradford A Woodworth

INTRODUCTION

Management of inflammatory frontal sinus disease has improved dramatically over the last several decades. Open procedures, such as the osteoplastic flap, were performed routinely for refractory frontal sinusitis prior to the development of endoscopic sinus surgery.[1] As techniques, instrumentation, and expertise continued to evolve, the endoscopic frontal sinusotomy eventually became the gold standard approach for the majority of disease because of the absence of external incisions and reduced morbidity. At the same time, extended endoscopic frontal sinus procedures were developed as a necessity to alleviate disease not amenable to standard endoscopic techniques.[2] Furthermore, these extended procedures facilitated management of complex frontal sinus disease (e.g., neoplasms, cerebrospinal fluid leaks) that required improved exposure.[3-7] This chapter will highlight advanced endoscopic frontal sinus surgery techniques including the Draf IIB and Draf III (modified endoscopic Lothrop) procedures.

PREOPERATIVE CONSIDERATIONS

In general, the indications for extended frontal sinus techniques include patients with recalcitrant chronic frontal sinusitis, mucocele or mucopyocele, osseous lesions, failed obliteration, trauma, and significant comorbidities such as cystic fibrosis, ciliary dyskinesia, and aspirin-exacerbated respiratory disease. Choosing the best approach to the frontal sinus pathology depends upon multiple factors, but most importantly on the type and extent of the patient's frontal sinus disease, anatomical barriers, and the expertise of the surgeon. Assessment of the patient's symptoms, endoscopic findings, and associated signs of disease on the CT scan are also critical to proper patient selection.

A thorough review of the sinus CT scan is crucial for surgical planning. Coronal images should be evaluated for remnant agger nasi cells, superior remnant of the uncinate process, frontal cells, supraorbital ethmoid cells, and intersinus septal cells. The sagittal and axial views permit assessment of the anterior and posterior dimensions of the frontal recess and further identification of a supraorbital ethmoid, frontal recess, and intersinus septal cells. Iatrogenic frontal sinus disease may be present following previous attempts at frontal sinusotomy. This may result from incomplete surgery with scarring of frontal recess partitions, mucosal damage or stripping, or lateralization of the middle turbinate. The presence of neo-osteogenesis ensures more difficulty during revision surgery. Mucoceles may also develop in the years following iatrogenic closure of the frontal sinus, resulting in dehiscence or thinning of the anterior/posterior tables of the frontal sinuses and/or orbital roof.

Image guidance is recommended for all frontal sinus surgeries and is even more helpful for revisions when the anatomy may be obscured by scarring from previous surgeries as well as loss of surgical landmarks. In addition, the use of angled instruments and scopes is important when surgically managing frontal sinus disease. These include frontal sinus dissection instruments as well as angled 70° diamond burrs, which may be used in the various approaches. Care must always be exercised when dealing with the frontal sinus mucosa to prevent stripping and/or circumferential removal of tissue that may lead to scarring.

THE DRAF IIB PROCEDURE

As noted in the previous chapter on endoscopic frontal sinusotomy (Draf IIA), surgery to the frontal sinus involves at least an anterior if not a total ethmoidectomy. Wolfgang Draf recommended a Draf IIB when an intraoperative frontal sinus ostium created by the Draf IIA technique was less than 5 × 7 mm^2.[8,9] However, the size of the frontal ostium opened to the natural dimensions with mucosal sparing techniques should be at the discretion and expertise/experience of the surgeon. A Draf IIA procedure requires the removal of the floor of the frontal sinus to the boundaries of the natural dimensions (ethmoid roof, medial orbital wall, nasofrontal beak, and middle turbinate). The Draf IIB extends the opening by removing the top portion of the middle turbinate to extend the medial boundary to the septum and removal of the nasofrontal beak with a drill. It has been suggested to use frontal sinus punches instead of drills during extension to the Draf IIB to limit the amount of trauma to the surrounding mucosa.[10] However, thick bone necessitates use of the drill. The frontal sinus intersinus septal cell can also be opened during this procedure. This cell is not present in all patients, but has been reported to exist in 34% of scans (101 of 300 reviewed).[11] Removing the common wall that separates it from the frontal recess may provide more space in enlarging the frontal sinus recess.

A technical variation of the Draf IIA or IIB for individuals with a lateralized middle turbinate is the frontal sinus rescue procedure.[12] When the middle turbinate is scarred to the lateral nasal wall, the anterior aspect of the turbinate is partially removed up to the level of the skull base preserving the mucosa on the lateral surface. The preserved mucosa, in this technique, is rotated medially and superiorly to the skull base.

THE DRAF III PROCEDURE

Because of the anatomic complexity of the frontal sinus, Lothrop[13] indicated that an intranasal approach to the frontal sinus is not safe because of its close proximity to the lamina papyracea and the anterior skull base. For this reason, he described an external approach to the frontal sinus that included an external ethmoidectomy, removal of the frontal sinus floor, large superior nasal septectomy, as well as removal of a portion of the lamina papyracea and lacrimal bone. The Draf III is an endoscopic version of this approach (hence modified endoscopic Lothrop).[8] The indications for Draf III are similar to those of Draf IIB except that it is favored for far lateral disease (e.g. tumors) that can be approached from the contralateral nostril. In addition, this is an excellent salvage procedure for failed frontal sinus obliteration. A relative contraindication to this procedure is a narrow anterior-posterior (AP) depth of the frontal sinus of less than 1.5 cm.[14] The AP diameter includes the thickness of the frontal beak (not more than 1 cm) as well as the distance from the beak to the anterior skull base.[14,15] The decision for performing the procedure for smaller diameters is dependent on the experience and expertise of the surgeon. Potential complications include cerebrospinal fluid leak, orbital injury, smell loss, epistaxis, and pneuomocephalus.[16,17] The frontal sinus neo-ostium may also narrow with time after surgery with patency rates ranging from 82%[18] to 100%. The healing of this frontal sinus neostium may lead to neo-osteogenesis and further narrowing of the combined ostium. Methods to improve the patency and stenosis have included coverage with expandable polyvinyly acetate,[19] placement of iodinated gauze until granulation tissue has completely covered the exposed bone,[20] and the use of mucosal grafts to cover exposed bone of the frontal sinus cavity.[21] Mucosal grafts harvested from the superior septum during septectomy (or posterior aspect of the inferior turbinate) and positioned on the drilled bone of the anterior nasofrontal beak had 100% patency during the duration of clinical follow up with no AP Draf III diameter less than 50% of its original size.

ADJUNCTIVE PROCEDURES

Lateral disease inaccessible with a Draf IIB or Draf III may be addressed using an above and below approach with an endoscopic procedure and either a frontal sinus trephination or osteoplastic flap. Trephinations can also be stented with an irrigating device to administer saline flushes or topical steroids/antibiotics as indicated.

Surgical Technique: Draf IIB

Step 1

Preparation of the patient is similar to standard frontal sinusotomy. The nasal mucosa is decongested and the image guidance calibrated.

Step 2

A total ethmoidectomy or sphenoethmoidectomy are performed as previously described with removal of all ethmoid partitions to the frontal recess.

Step 3

The frontal recess is inspected using a 70° endoscope and residual partitions and cells of the frontal recess are removed with 60° and 90° thru-cut frontal instruments, frontal Kerrison punch, frontal curettes, and Hosemann punch as previously described.

Step 4

The attachment of the middle turbinate is removed utilizing a side to side through-cutting frontal instrument (Fig. 12.1A).

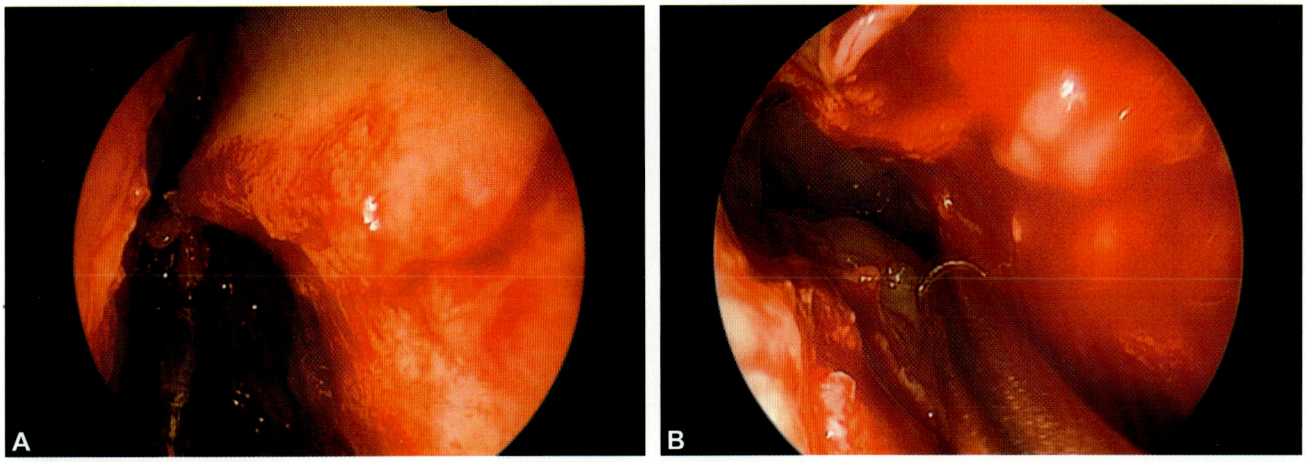

Figs. 12.1A and B: Following a Draf IIA, the anterosuperior aspect of the middle turbinate is removed with a 60° frontal thru-cut instrument (A). The opening is enlarged medially to the level of the nasal septum after removal of the anterior middle turbinate attachment (B).

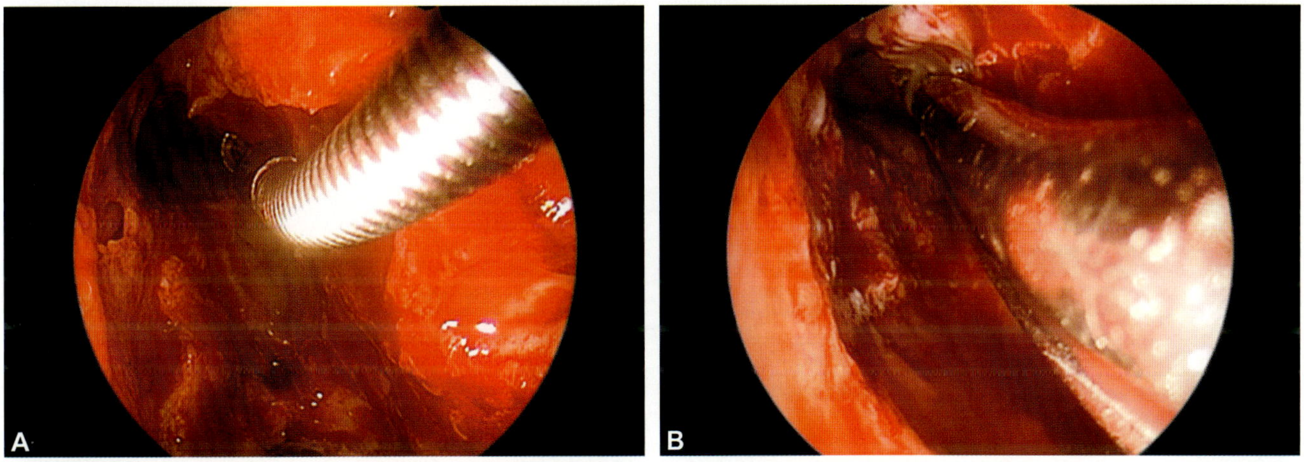

Figs. 12.2A and B: The ostium is enlarged further by removal of the nasofrontal beak with a Hosemann punch (A) and a 70° 4 mm drill (B). This completes the Draf IIB frontal sinusotomy.

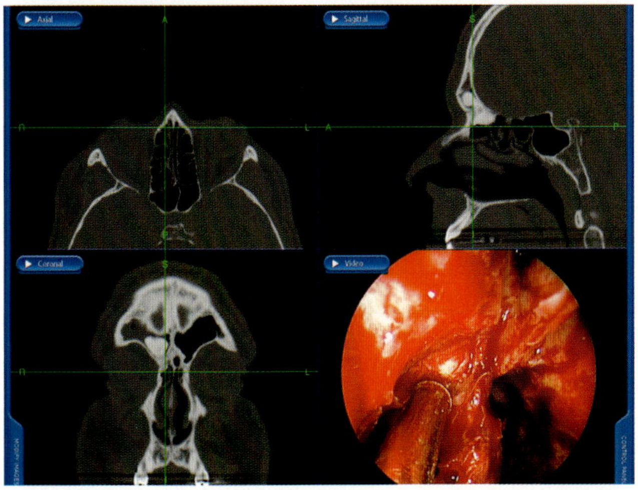

Fig. 12.3: A Draf IIB has been performed on the patient's left side and a frontal osteoma exposed on the right following a superior septectomy.

Step 5

The frontal sinusotomy is extended anteromedially to the level of the septum with a Hosemann or frontal mushroom punch (Fig. 12.1B).

Step 6

The size of the sinusotomy is enlarged by removing the nasofrontal beak using Hosemann punch (Fig. 12.2A), frontal Kerrison, or 70° diamond bur (Fig. 12.2B). Bone is removed at the discretion of the surgeon with the limits including the periosteum and periorbita, but usually leaving a thin layer of bone.

Surgical Technique: Draf III

Steps 1–4

Same as mentioned above.

Step 5

Frontal sinusotomy as previously described at least on one side (Fig. 12.3).

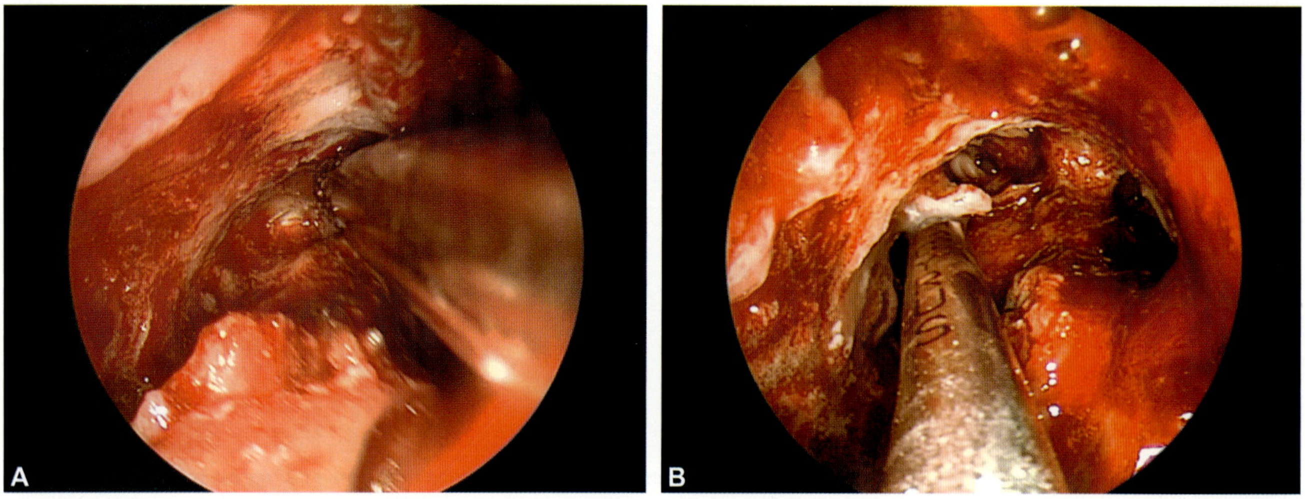

Figs. 12.4A and B: A common frontal ostium is formed by removing the intersinus septum with 70° drills and/or with frontal sinus thru-cutting instruments and removal of the right nasofrontal beak (A). The osteoma is drilled to a thin layer and removed from the frontal sinus (B).

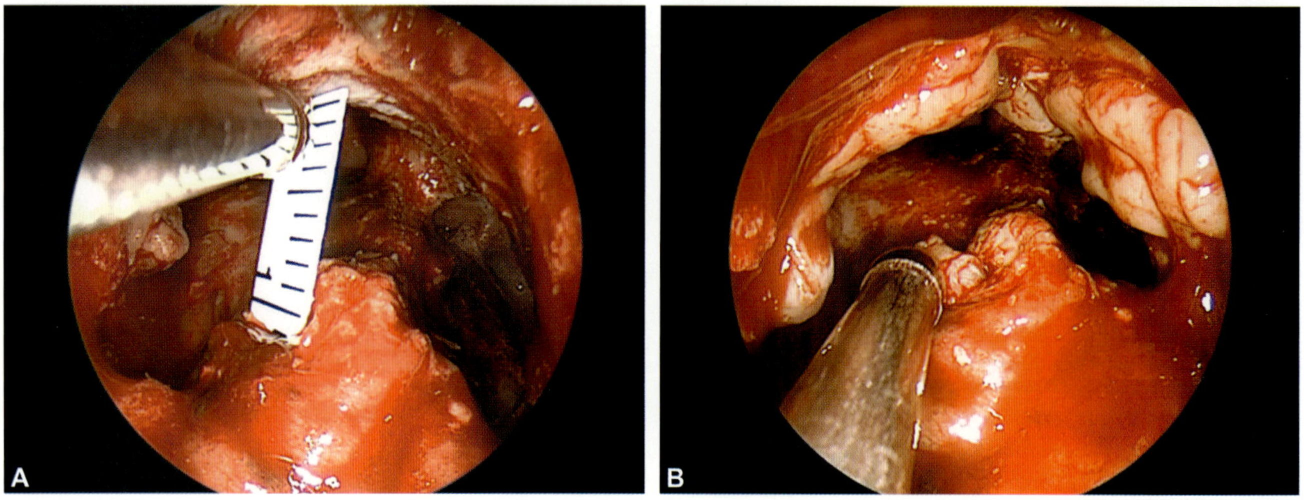

Figs. 12.5A and B: The final Draf III is horseshoe shaped due to the anterior position of the cribriform plate. The anterior–posterior diameter is approximately 9 mm (A). The septal mucosal free grafts are used to cover the raw bone anteriorly in the common frontal sinus cavity (B).

Step 6

A curved beaver blade is used to make the incisions in the septal mucosa for the superior septectomy. Mucosal grafts are harvested on each side and placed on the back table in saline and on ice. The cartilage and bone are then removed. The size of the septectomy should be 2×2 cm^2. This is particularly important to allow for instruments to reach the far lateral frontal sinus on the opposing side.

Step 7

Using 70° diamond burrs, the nasofrontal beak is drilled off bilaterally (Figs. 12.4A and B). The anterior "horseshoe" of the cribriform plate is left alone. If possible, posterior table and anterior ethmoid roof mucosa is left intact.

Step 8

The ostium should be widened maximally to a thin shell of bone over the periosteum anteriorly and laterally.

Step 9

Septal mucosal free grafts are then inserted over the exposed bone anteriorly (Figs. 12.5A and B). These may be fixed in place with fibrin glue if necessary. Bilateral thin silastic stents are cut to fit and unfurled within the Draf III opening so that the grafts are covered anteriorly (Figs. 12.6A and B).

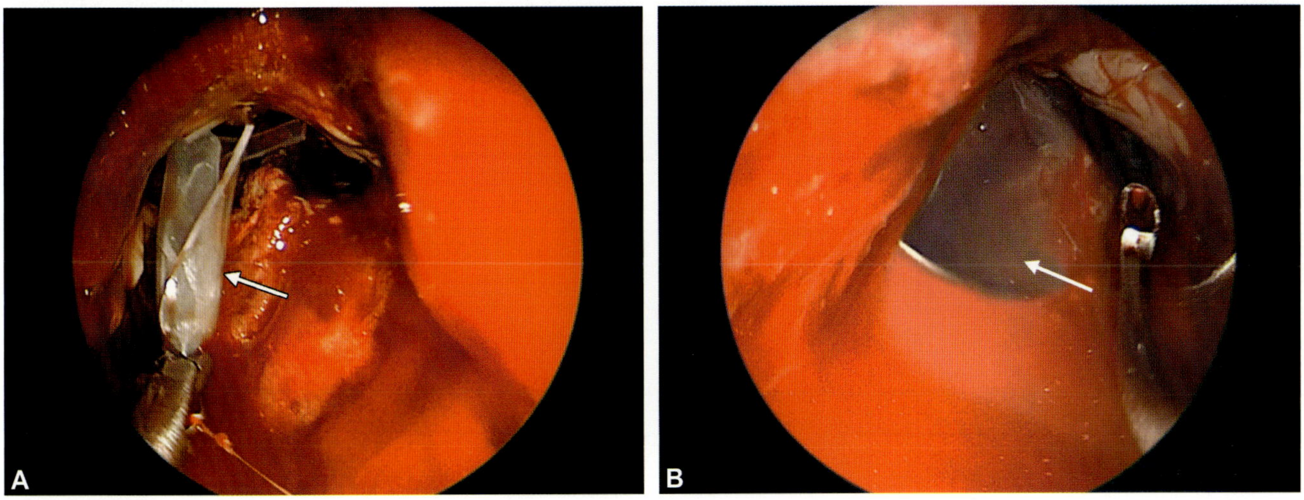

Figs. 12.6A and B: A rolled thin silastic frontal sinus stent is placed on either side (A) and unfurled so that the grafts will be covered (B). Arrows: Silastic.

REFERENCES

1. Hardy. Osteoplastic frontal sinusotomy: An analysis of 250 operations. Ann Otol Rhinol Laryngol. 1976;85:253-32.
2. Weber R, Draf W, Keerl R, et al. Long-term results of endonasal frontal sinus surgery. HNO. 1996;44(9):503-9.
3. Illing E, Chaaban MR, Riley KO, et al. Porcine small intestine submucosal graft for endoscopic skull base reconstruction. Int Forum Allergy Rhinol. 2013;3(11):928-32.
4. Chaaban MR, Illing E, Riley KO, et al. Spontaneous cerebrospinal fluid leak repair: A five-year prospective evaluation. Laryngoscope. 2013;124:70-5.
5. Jones V, Virgin F, Riley K, et al. Changing paradigms in frontal sinus cerebrospinal fluid leak repair. Int Forum Allergy Rhinol. 2012;2:227-32.
6. Virgin F, Baranano CF, Riley K, et al. Frontal sinus skull base defect repair using the pedicled nasoseptal flap. Otolaryngol Head Neck Surg. 2011;145:338-40.
7. Woodworth BA, Schlosser RJ, Palmer JN. Endoscopic repair of frontal sinus cerebrospinal fluid leaks. J Laryngol Otol. 2005;119(9):709-13.
8. Draf W. Endonasal micro-endoscopic frontal sinus surgery: the Fulda concept. Oper Tech Otolaryngol-Head Neck Surg. 1991;2:234-40.
9. Draf W. Endonasal frontal sinus drainage type I-III according to Draf. In: The Frontal Sinus. Berlin: Springer-Verlag. 2005:219-32.
10. Dubin MG KF. Endoscopic modified Lothrop (Draf III) with frontal sinus punches. Laryngoscope. 2005;115(9):1702-3.
11. Merrit R BJ, Kuhn FA. The intersinus septal cell. Am J Rhinol. 1996;10:299-302.
12. Citardi MJ, Javer AR, Kuhn FA. Revision endoscopic frontal sinusotomy with mucoperiosteal flap advancement: the frontal sinus rescue procedure. Otolaryngol Clin North Am. 2001;34(1):123-32.
13. Lothrop HA. XIV. Frontal sinus suppuration: The establishment of permanent nasal drainage; the closure of external fistulae; epidermization of sinus. Ann Surg. Jun 1914; 59(6):937-57.
14 Gross CW HS. The modified Lothrop procedure: indications, results, and complications. Otolaryngol Clin North Am. 2001;34(1):133-7.
15. Kountakis S. The Frontal Sinus. Berlin: Springer-Verlag; 2005. pp. 233-41.
16. Kuhn FA, Javer AR, Nagpal K, et al. The frontal sinus rescue procedure: early experience and three-year follow-up. Am J Rhinol. 2000;14(4):211-6.
17. Chaaban MR, Woodworth BA. Complications of skull base reconstruction. Adv Otorhinolaryngol. 2013;74:148-62.
18. Schlosser RJ, Zachmann G, Harrison S, et al. The endoscopic modified Lothrop: long-term follow-up on 44 patients. Am J Rhinol. 2002;16(2):103-8.
19. Kang IG, Jung JH, Woo JH, et al. The effect of expandable polyvinyl acetate packing for preventing stenosis of the frontal sinus ostium. Am J Rhinol Allergy. 2010;24(5):392-5.
20. Chin D, Snidvongs K, Kalish L, et al. The outside-in approach to the modified endoscopic Lothrop procedure. Laryngoscope. 2012;122(8):1661-9.
21. Conger BT, Jr., Riley K, Woodworth BA. The Draf III mucosal grafting technique: A prospective study. Otolaryngol Head Neck Surg. 2012;146(4):664-8.

CHAPTER

13

Endoscopic Septoplasty

Brian A Fishero, Spencer C Payne

INTRODUCTION

Anatomy

The nasal septum is the midline structure dividing the two nasal cavities into left and right. It serves to provide support to the external structure of the nose and assists in laminar airflow through the nose. It is composed of the quadrangular cartilage anterior. Posteriorly, bony contributions come from the perpendicular plate of the ethmoid and the vomer primarily. It is stabilized by fixation to the nasal spine of the frontal bone and the crests of the maxillary and palatine bones. The mucosal lining is made of pseudostratified columnar respiratory epithelium. Blood supply to the septum comes from both the internal and external carotid arteries. The posterior blood supply is primarily from the sphenopalatine, posterior ethmoid, and greater palatine arteries. The anterior blood supply is from the anterior ethmoid arteries as well as the superior labial artery. Innervation is supplied by the ophthalmic and maxillary divisions of the trigeminal nerves.

History of the Procedure

Septoplasty has evolved as we have come to better understand the anatomy and physiology of the nose. In the 19th century, the operation consisted of identifying the convex surface of the septum and resecting both cartilage and mucosa. The more modern mucosal sparing procedure, performed with a headlight and nasal speculum, was first described by Freer[1] and Killian.[2] This was again modified by Cottle in 1948 when he described a more conservative approach which involved sparing cartilage where possible.[3] Little changed in septoplasty technique until the introduction of the nasal endoscope to the procedure. Endoscopic septoplasty (ES) is a relatively new technique. It was first described in 1991 by Lanza et al.[4] and Stammberger et al.[5]

ADVANTAGES AND LIMITATIONS OF ENDOSCOPIC SEPTOPLASTY

With open septoplasty, the surgeon employs a headlight and nasal speculum to assess the septum. This affords excellent visualization of the caudal septum with a more limited view posteriorly. In performing an open septoplasty, only one individual, the surgeon, can see at any given time. This makes both engaging operating room staff and training resident surgeons more challenging.

The primary advantage of ES is superior posterior visualization. Both lighting and magnification allow for precise assessment of the septum and prevention of unintentional violations of the septal mucosa. Angled endoscopes allow for examination of the nasal vault and other areas not visible on anterior rhinoscopy. The video tower has the added advantage of showing the surgery to the rest of the team so that the scrub nurse can anticipate needs and surgeons in training can appreciate finer technical points.

Many patients who undergo septoplasty also require endoscopic sinus surgery (ESS). With ES, the operation can transition seamlessly from septoplasty to ESS without a change in instrumentation or setup. When septoplasty is performed in conjunction with ESS, it can potentially lead to better outcomes as lateralization of the middle turbinate can be prevented, nasal obstruction can be addressed, and postoperative debridement can be more easily performed in clinic.

In terms of speed, there is no significant difference in operative time between ES and open septoplasty. In a series of 1,035 endoplastic septoplasties, Hwang et al.[6] proved that ES could be done on average in under 14 min.

TECHNIQUE

Preoperative Evaluation

Preoperative evaluation and documentation is critical when determining both the necessity of a septoplasty and which technique is more appropriate, be it open or endoscopic. A history of unilateral nasal obstruction may or may not be elicited. If the patient does have subjective obstruction, this should be confirmed with objective findings. Narrow internal nasal valves with a severe caudal deflection may be better served with an open septoplasty or functional rhinoplasty. Endoscopic septoplasty may be indicated if deviation exists further posteriorly. Indications for ES include deviations in the bony or cartilaginous septum causing obstruction or the need for improved access to the osteomeatal complex (OMC) during planned ESS. Intraoperative assessment is almost as important as the preoperative physical exam. Decongestion may show an adequate view of the OMC, obviating the need for ES.

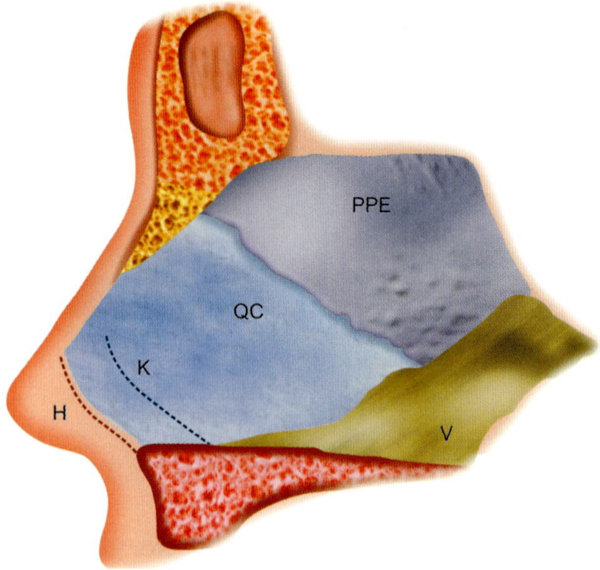

Fig. 13.1: Septal anatomy—Anatomy and components of nasal septum demonstrating location of Killian incision (K dashed line) (K: Killian incision; H: Hemitransfixion incision; QC: Quadrangular cartilage; PPE: Perpendicular plate of the ethmoid; V: Vomer).

Patient Preparation

The procedure begins in the preoperative holding area with topical decongestion. Three doses of 0.05% oxymetazoline are applied to each nasal cavity spaced over 15 min. The patient is brought to the operative room and placed in a supine position. The patient is orotracheally intubated and the endotracheal tube is secured with tape to the left lower lip to keep it out of the operative field. After this, the nose is packed with two cottonoids soaked with 0.05% oxymetazoline on either side. This should be done under direct visualization with a nasal speculum and light source to prevent unintentional trauma. If ESS is also being performed, it is preferable to place one pledget within the middle meatus. This is often not possible on one side if the deviation is severe. If ESS is not being performed, one pledget is lodged medial to the middle turbinate and the other medial to the inferior turbinate. The bed is then lowered and the patient reclined in a beach-chair position with the head elevated. The room is set up in a similar manner as detailed in Chapter 9.

The cottonoids are then removed and the nose is inspected with a 0° endoscope to assess the degree of deviation. One percent lidocaine with 1:100,000 epinephrine is then injected at the site of the planned Killian incision in a submucoperichondrial plane with a 25 gauge needed. This injection results in both vasoconstriction as well as hydrodissection to assist in locating the correct plane. The nasal vibrissae are then trimmed with curved iris scissors. This serves both to improve visualization as blood will collect on the vibrissae and to force the surgeon to delay the incision as the vasoconstrictive effects of the epinephrine take effect.

Incision

A Killian incision (Fig. 13.1) is preferable for ES. While making the incision, the endoscope is rested against the ala at a 30°–45° angle to the septum. A curvilinear incision is placed 1–2 mm posterior to the mucocutaneous junction. It is made with a #15 blade scalpel positioned with the cutting surface facing superiorly. The incision arcs from just anterior to the maxillary crest at the nasal sill to just posterior to the caudal border of the upper lateral cartilage (Fig. 13.2). To prevent inadvertently avulsing the superior aspect of the flap, care must be taken to extend the incision far enough superiorly by gently displacing the upper lateral cartilage with the scalpel. The mucosa overlying the upper lateral cartilage will not be damaged provided a sawing motion is avoided. While various alterations to this incision have been described, the key to is make the incision long enough so that the flap can be raised easily.

The incision can be placed on either side of the septum. The authors generally prefer to place the incision on the same side as the handedness of the surgeon. For instance, a right-handed surgeon would find it easier to

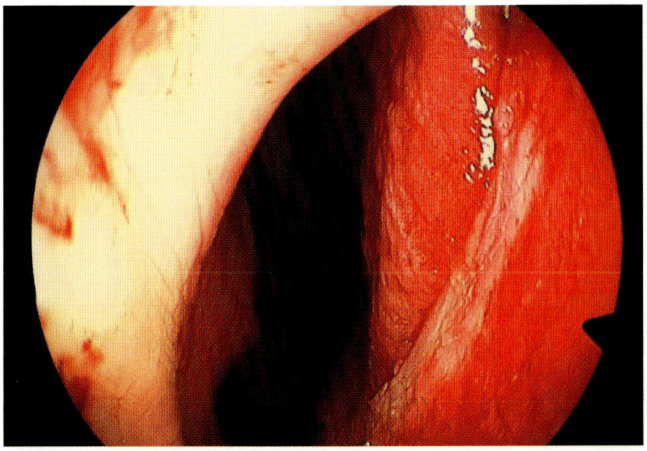

Fig. 13.2: Killian incision—An incision has been made in the respiratory mucosa of the caudal septum inferiorly from the maxillary crest, just posterior to pyriform aperture to the upper lateral cartilage.

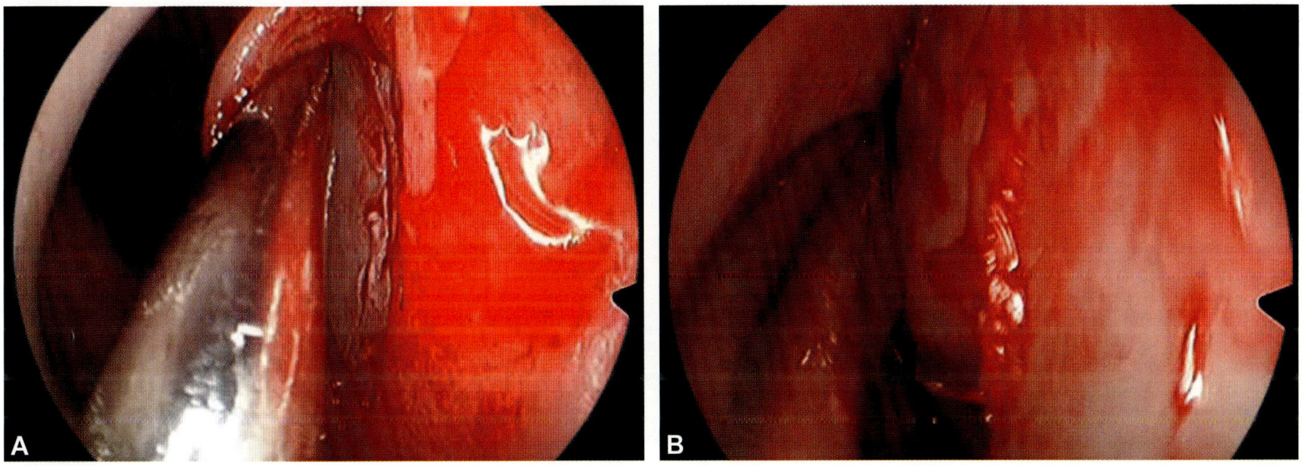

Figs. 13.3A and B: Flap elevation—(A) Flap elevation starts anteriorly in a submucoperichondrial plane and continues initially to (B) just posterior to the bony–cartilaginous junction, which is often denoted by a lateral bowing and curvature back toward midline just distal to junction as seen here.

perform the dissection from the right side of the septum provided there are no anatomic variants that would dictate placing the incision on the left side. If there is a prominent septal spur, we prefer to place the incision on the ipsilateral side as the deviation. This allows for dissection in tunnels inferior and superior to the spur so that it can be removed without lacerating the overlying mucosa. If ESS is being performed concomitantly, the incision can be made on the less obstructed side at the beginning of the operation. The sinuses can be addressed on the contralateral side first if there is bleeding from the incision.

Flap Elevation and Septal Resection

After the incision has been made through the mucosa and perichondrium, a submucoperichondrial flap is raised (Figs. 13.3A and B). While Cottle or Freer elevators could be used, the authors prefer a suction elevator (Fig. 13.4) as this dual purpose instrument can speed dissection. Care must be taken to identify the correct plane. Using the edge of the suction Cottle, the cartilage's pearly color with rough texture is identified. Dissection is carried posteriorly. As the flap is raised, the endoscope can be placed medial to the flap to allow for both good visualization as well as lateral retraction to assist in flap elevation. Dissection is carried past the deviation. The cartilage is scored and incised anterior to any deviation. Using a blunt instrument to make the cartilage incision prevents inadvertent perforation of the contralateral flap. The contralateral submucoperichondrial plane is identified and dissection carried posteriorly to the bony cartilaginous junction. Care is taken in this area and the dissection carried posteriorly over the bone in a submucoperiosteal plane. The deviated cartilage is removed with a combination of

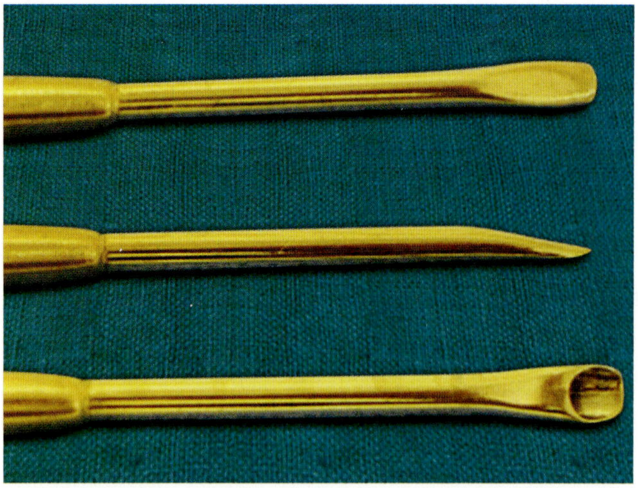

Fig. 13.4: Suction elevator—Cottle or Freer elevators can be used; the authors prefer to use a modified Stamm suction elevator which can cut and elevate as necessary.

a Ballenger swivel knife and Blakesley forceps. As with traditional open septoplasty, care is taken to preserve an L-strut for nasal structural support. Any bony deviations can then be removed with Jansen-Middleton forceps. This double action instrument allows for bone removal without a rocking motion that could transmit energy to the cribriform and result in a cerebrospinal fluid (CSF) leak. Attention is then turned to any spurs in the maxillary crest or vomer. If cartilage remains on the superior aspect of the bone, it is incised horizontally approximately 2 mm superior to the spur. Anteriorly, near the posterior septal angle, a vertical incision is made with a #15 blade through the cartilage and down onto the maxillary crest. This strip of cartilage is dissected off of the spur with a Cottle or suction elevator. For large spurs, a separate dissection plane can be made inferior to the spur. This inferior tunnel is connected to the superior dissection plane taking care not to perforate the flap over the spur. The spur can be removed with a rongeur or osteotome. Care is taken to conservatively remove bone from the maxillary crest to prevent nasopalatine nerve or arterial injury and resulting postoperative dental anesthesia and intraoperative bleeding, respectively.

The submucoperiosteal space is irrigated with warm saline to remove any residual bone or cartilage chips. The warm irrigant also helps with hemostasis. The endoscope is placed back into the nasal cavity and the septum is inspected. If the axilla of the middle turbinate is not visible on one side from residual deviation, the problem is usually with the septal process of the frontal bone. Even if all deviated cartilage and bony spurs are removed, a persistent deviation here will cause the mucosal flaps to rest off of midline. The septal process of the frontal bone can be trimmed or fractured with impunity as it rests anterior to the cribriform plate. Provided no significant manipulation of the superior cartilaginous septum or upper lateral cartilages has taken place, there should be minimal if any concern for cosmetic issues with this maneuver.

If a rent was not made in the mucosal flap, a controlled incision is made on one side to prevent a septal hematoma. A cottonoid is placed between the flaps and 2 cm horizontal incision is made with a #15 blade approximately 1 cm above the nasal floor posteriorly. The cottonoid is removed, and the flaps are coapted.

Septal Suturing

Although it is not necessary to close the Killian incision, we have found that doing so reduces early postoperative congestion and crusting. A 4-0 chromic gut suture is used on a tapered needle. The sutures can be placed in interrupted or continuous fashion (Figs. 13.5A and B). A transseptal quilting stitch is then placed using 4-0 plain gut on a straight needle. This further reduces the risk of hematoma collection. The endoscope is used to both apply counterpressure and provide visualization to prevent inadvertent trauma to the turbinates. Any unintentional mucosal tears can be reapproximated by incorporating them into the quilting stitch. Areas with bilateral perforations can be addressed by placing crushed cartilage or bone within the flaps to prevent a permanent perforation.[7] Splints and packing are almost never necessary.[8,9]

TECHNIQUE MODIFICATIONS

Every septum is different. As such, the surgeon should have several tools available to allow for an individualized operation. By careful preoperative examination, the precise problematic area can be identified and surgical planning can proceed accordingly.

Isolated Septal Spur

In the case of an isolated septal spur with an otherwise reasonably straight septum (Fig. 13.6), a more tailored approach can be used. The overlying mucosa is injected with local anesthetic as with the Killian incision. A horizontal incision is made over the crest of the spur with a 15-blade. Superior and inferior submucosal flaps are raised with a Cottle or suction elevator to expose the

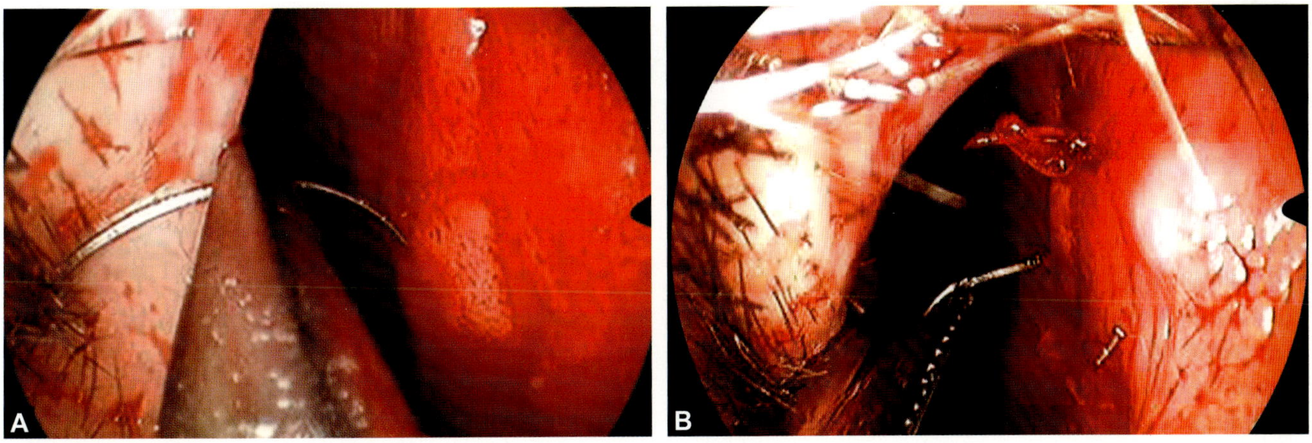

Figs. 13.5A and B: Septal suturing—A tapered needle (RB-1) is used to prevent unnecessary tearing and is (A) held in a "back-handed" manner to drive it through the anterior flap (B) often in two steps; two interrupted stitches are placed.

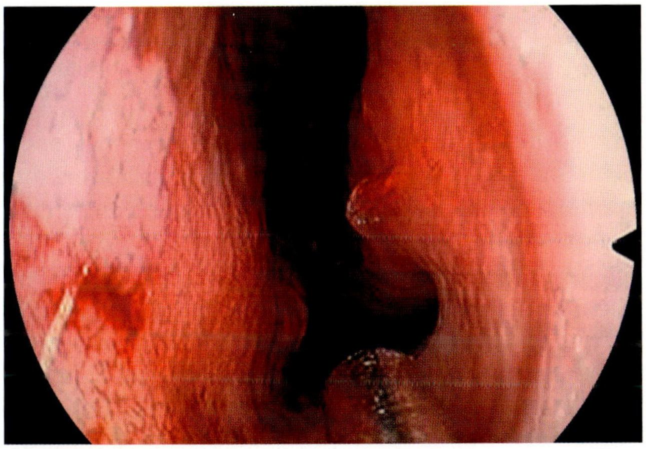

Fig. 13.6: Isolated septal spur—An alternative method can be used to address these spurs when the septum is otherwise straight from anterior to posterior.

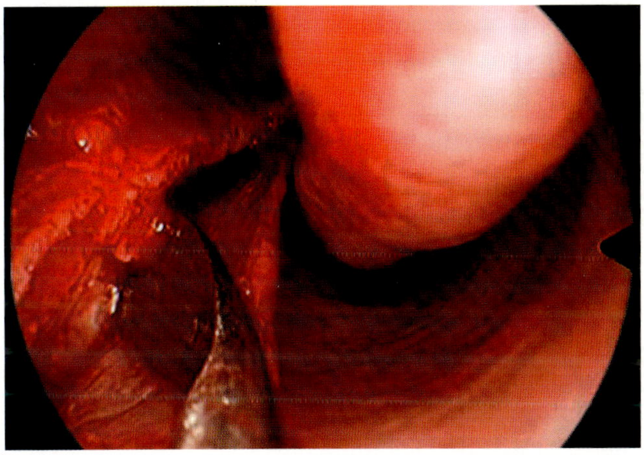

Fig. 13.7: Spur flap elevation—Superior and Inferior flap elevation occurs after horizontal incision over the spur has been completed. This is often easily accomplished with the sharp end of a Cottle elevator.

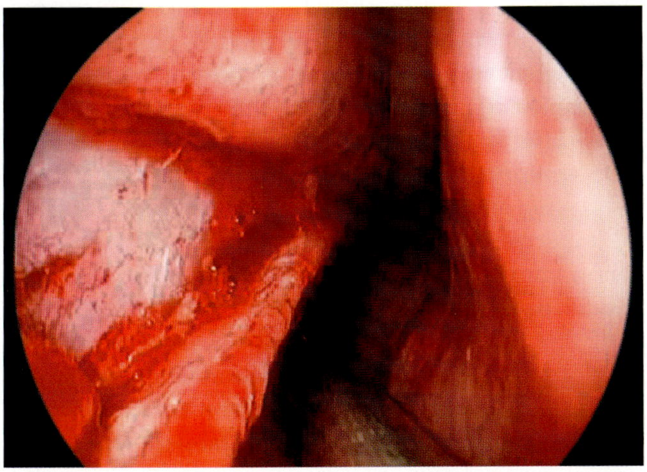

Fig. 13.8: Flap reapproximation—Following resection of the spur the airway is much more patent and the flaps are laid back down; packing is usually not necessary but absorbable material can be used.

bony spur (Fig. 13.7). The bone can then be addressed using one of several techniques. We prefer using a septoplasty burr (Medtronic Xomed, Inc., Jacksonville, FL). Alternatively, using a 4 mm microdebrider has been proven to be a safe and effective alternative.[10] This may be the more practical choice if it is already set up for an ensuing ESS. As the spur is removed, care must be taken to preserve the contralateral mucosa to prevent a septal perforation. Once the bony deviation is removed, the flaps are reapproximated (Fig. 13.8) with either a modified quilting suture or absorbable packing.

Isolated Deviation of the Bony Septum

Deviations may be limited to the bony septum with an otherwise straight cartilaginous septum. In this case, a

Killian incision is not necessary as the incision could be placed further posteriorly. By doing so, the risk of associated morbidity including worsened edema and septal perforation can be limited.[11] With the endoscope, the incision is made just anterior to the bony cartilaginous junction. Dissection is carried in a submucoperichondrial, then submucoperiosteal plane past the deviation. As described earlier, the cartilage is transgressed at the bony-cartilaginous junction and contralateral flaps are raised. The bony deviation is removed with Jansen-Middleton and pituitary forceps. The flaps are then reapproximated. The endoscope provides an obvious advantage over open septoplasty in terms of visualization, which may translate into lower risk of perforation. Clearly, by making the incision posterior to the cartilage, risk of a cartilaginous septal injuy is eliminated.

Revision Surgery

In cases of prior septoplasty, the bony and cartilaginous framework may be absent. As the mucosal flaps have healed to each other without intervening rigid support, the risk of perforation is higher in revision septoplasty. The endoscopic approach provides the advantage of being able to limit dissection over the residual deviation and avoid areas where the framework no longer exists. This helps limit the risk of perforation as the septum can be inspected and palpated with a ball tipped probe.[6] If small perforations do occur, they will be easily identified and can be treated appropriately.

POSTOPERATIVE CONSIDERATIONS

Whether nasal packing or splints are effective in preventing hematoma formation, perforations, or infections has been a topic of debate. Packing options include Gelfoam, Merocel, Surgicel, Nasopore, silastic sheets, Vaseline gauze, or glove finger. In a study of 105 patients undergoing septoplasty, Ardehali divided patients into two groups. One group received nasal packing postoperatively and the other group was treated with a quilting stitch only. None of the patients in either group developed a hematoma. Two of the patients with packing and one without packing suffered a septal perforation and mucosal adhesions. The no packing group had significantly less postoperative pain as measured by the visual analog scale.[8] It is our practice to not use packing.

Patients should be counseled regarding postoperative expectations and appropriate care to promote healing. Small amounts of oozing are expected through the second day. Saline sprays and irrigations are important to keep the nose moist and hasten healing. We instruct patients to irrigate with saline (¼ teaspoon kosher salt, ¼ teaspoon baking soda in 8 oz. of distilled or tap water) twice daily beginning the day after surgery.

COMPLICATIONS

Postoperative complications after ES are rare. They are the same as traditional septoplasty: dental numbness, postoperative hemorrhage, septal perforation, synechiae, CSF leak, and no improvement of nasal obstructive symptoms. The likelihood of encountering a complication with endoscopic techniques is similar to traditional, open septoplasty.[12]

Dental hypesthesia over the four maxillary incisors may result from injury to the nasopalatine nerve with aggressive dissection over the maxillary spine and anterior maxillary crest. Chung et al.[9] found a 4.3% incidence of transient dental numbness in his series of endoscopic septoplasties. This is comparable to traditional open techniques.[9] If patients are not counseled regarding this risk preoperatively, this can lead to considerable distress. Fortunately, his bothersome problem is often self limited and resolves after several weeks.[9] The risk is reduced when the septoplasty is limited to posterior deviations.

There is a less than 1% risk for postoperative hemorrhage or hematoma after septoplasty.[6,9,10,13] In our experience of over 300 endoscopic septoplasties performed without either nasal packing or quilting sutures, only two postoperative hematomas occurred. Both were identified and treated without further complication. Epistaxis and septal hematomas can be prevented by identifying patients at risk for postoperative bleeding. This includes patients on both pharmacological and herbal anticoagulants. Anticoagulation should be held before and after surgery if possible and activity should be limited through at least 7 days after surgery to prevent blood pressure elevation. With appropriate counseling, patients can be educated to identify concerning symptoms and to distinguish the expected minor postoperative bleeding from a more concerning hemorrhage. Septal hematomas are often painful, particularly during an endoscopic exam. If identified, they should be drained via needle aspiration or incision to prevent a subsequent perforation or deviation.

Despite making every attempt to repair mucosal perforations at the time of surgery, septal perforations can result if bilateral mucosal tears are approximated. Patients may be asymptomatic from small posterior perforations. If large enough, the perforation can disrupt laminar airflow, causing turbulence and resulting subjective nasal obstruction. The turbulent flow results in crusting, dryness, pain, and a whistling noise. This is a particular problem with small, anterior perforations. The rate of septal perforation after ES ranges from 1% to 6.7%. This is similar to open septoplasty.[6,9,12,14-16]

Cerebrospinal fluid leak is an uncommonly encountered yet serious complication of septoplasty. It is often attributed to a twisting motion applied to the superior septum that causes a fracture across the cribriform plate with resulting dural tear. This should be repaired immediately if noted intraoperatively. Postoperatively, patients may complain of headache, clear rhinorrhea, or a salty tasting post nasal drip. If suspicious of a CSF leak, the fluid should be collected and tested for beta tau transferrin to rule out the presence of CSF. Hospital admission and meningitis prophylaxis is indicated while the patient awaits skull base repair.

Perhaps the most common and disappointing adverse outcome is continued nasal obstruction. Ideally, a good preoperative assessment has accurately identified the septum as the culprit prior to septoplasty. Failure to recognize a collapsing nasal valve or hypertrophied inferior turbinates will lead to an unsatisfactory result following septoplasty. Endoscopic septoplasty has a roughly 70% success rate in achieving resolution of nasal obstruction. This is comparable to the 63–85% success rates with open septoplasty.[17] Infrequently, the cause of continued obstruction is residual septal deformity.[7,9]

OUTCOMES

Although the results are quite similar between[18] the two techniques, several studies have shown that ES has an advantage over open septoplasty in terms of outcomes. Nayak et al.[18] showed superior improvement in nasal obstruction with ES over open septoplasty. This was likely because residual deviation was found in 20% of ES patients and 49% of open septoplasty patients. Although none of their ES patients had contact areas postoperatively, 13% of the open septoplasty patients did.[18] Overall, resolution of obstructive symptoms has been reported to range between 70% and 88%.[9,17,18] Objective improvement has been measured with acoustic rhinometry. In a study involving over 1,000 patients, nasal breathing resistance was statistically significantly improved in 98% of their patients. This study also reported that their patients had no complications including septal hematoma or perforation.[19]

Endoscopic septoplasty has been shown to be less painful than traditional septoplasty. In a study measuring pain on a visual analog scale comparing ES to open septoplasty in 50 patients, Gulati et al.[20] found an average pain rating of 7.24 with open septoplasty versus 1.6 with ES ($p < 0.05$). He also showed lower rates of postoperative headache in the ES group.[20]

CONCLUSION

Endoscopic septoplasty is a safe and effective alternative to open septoplasty. The endoscope provides a means of achieving superior visualization, which allows for a more precise dissection that can lead to improved outcomes over traditional septoplasty. When performed concurrently with sinus surgery, it can shorten operative time and keep the rest of the operating room staff engaged in the surgery.

REFERENCES

1. Freer O. The correction of deflections of the nasal septum with minimal traumatism. JAMA. 1902;38:636-42.
2. Killian G. The submucous window resection of the nasal septum. Ann Otolaryngol Rhinol Laryngol. 1905;14:363-93.
3. Cottle MH, Loring RM. Newer concepts of septum surgery; present status. Eye Ear Nose Throat Mon. 1948;27:403-6.
4. Lanza DC, Kennedy DW, Zinreich SJ, eds. Nasal Endoscopy and its Surgical Applications. 7th ed. New York: Appleton & Lange; 1991.
5. Stammberger H. Functional Endoscopic Sinus Surgery. The Messerklinger Technique. Philadelphia: BC Decker; 1991:432-3.
6. Hwang PH, McLaughlin RB, Lanza DC, et al. Endoscopic septoplasty: indications, technique, and results. Otolaryngol Head Neck Surg. 1999;120:678-82.
7. Sousa A, Iniciarte L, Levine H. Powered endoscopic nasal septal surgery. Acta Med Port. 2005;18:249-55.
8. Ardehali MM, Bastaninejad S. Use of nasal packs and intranasal septal splints following septoplasty. Int J Oral Maxillofac Surg. 2009;38:1022-4.
9. Chung BJ, Batra PS, Citardi MJ, et al. Endoscopic septoplasty: revisitation of the technique, indications, and outcomes. Am J Rhinol. 2007;21:307-11.
10. Raynor EM. Powered endoscopic septoplasty for septal deviation and isolated spurs. Arch Facial Plast Surg. 2005; 7:410-2.
11. Kim DW, Egan KK, O'Grady K, et al. Biomechanical strength of human nasal septal lining: comparison of the constituent layers. Laryngoscope. 2005;115:1451-3.
12. Bloom JD, Kaplan SE, Bleier BS, et al. Septoplasty complications: avoidance and management. Otolaryngol Clin North Am. 2009;42:463-81.
13. Sindwani R, Wright ED. Role of endoscopic septoplasty in the treatment of atypical facial pain. J Otolaryngol. 2003; 32:77-80.

14. Chaaban M, Shah AR. Open septoplasty: indications and treatment. Otolaryngol Clin North Am. 2009;42:513-9.
15. Dolan RW. Endoscopic septoplasty. Facial Plast Surg. 2004; 20:217-21.
16. Durr DG. Endoscopic septoplasty: technique and outcomes. J Otolaryngol. 2003;32:6-11.
17. Siegel NS, Gliklich RE, Taghizadeh F, et al. Outcomes of septoplasty. Otolaryngol Head Neck Surg. 2000;122: 228-32.
18. Nayak DR, Balakrishnan R, Murthy KD. An endoscopic approach to the deviated nasal septum—a preliminary study. J Laryngol Otol. 1998;112:934-9.
19. D'Ascanio L, Manzini M. Quick septoplasty: surgical technique and learning curve. Aesthetic Plast Surg. 2009;33: 814-8.
20. Gulati SP, Wadhera R, Ahuja N, et al. Comparative evaluation of endoscopic with conventional septoplasty. Indian J Otolaryngol Head Neck Surg. 2009;61:27-9.

CHAPTER

14 Surgical Management of the Nasal Turbinates

Philip E Zapanta, Devon C Flaherty, Ameet Singh

INTRODUCTION

The nasal turbinates have important roles in the functional milieu of the sinonasal cavity. These roles are critical for ideal airflow, proper air temperature, nasal humidification, olfaction, and filtration. Any pathological process that can affect a patient's sinonasal quality of life may involve the supreme, superior, middle, or inferior turbinates. Inferior turbinate hypertrophy is a common cause of nasal obstruction. Middle turbinate enlargement may play a secondary role in nasal obstruction, sinonasal pressure, rhinosinusitis, and sinogenic headaches. The anatomy and physiology of the turbinates are detailed in Chapters 2 and 3.

MIDDLE TURBINATE SURGICAL MANAGEMENT

The most common surgical indication for the middle turbinate is the presence of a concha bullosa. A concha bullosa is the pneumatization of turbinate bone triggered by development of the ethmoid air cells into the middle turbinate bone[1] (Fig. 14.1). The presence of a concha bullosa (a normal variant) may impair paranasal sinus ventilation and mucociliary clearance in the middle meatus.[2] It is classically identified by imaging of the sinuses (Fig. 14.2), but may identified on nasal endoscopy in some cases.

Surgery of the concha bullosa is usually indicated during endoscopic sinus surgery for chronic rhinosinusitis, air cell disease, or refractory nasal obstruction. In rare cases, it may be indicated for sinus pressure, and/or sinogenic headaches. Usually, the lateral wall of the concha bullosa is resected to improve middle meatal access and ventilation (Fig. 14.3).[2] Theoretical contraindications include risks for, atrophic rhinitis, empty nose syndrome, as well as the risk of osteitis, anosmia or cerebrospinal fluid (CSF) leak resulting in excessive middle turbinate manipulation. Other potential disadvantages of middle turbinate surgery include loss of anatomical landmarks

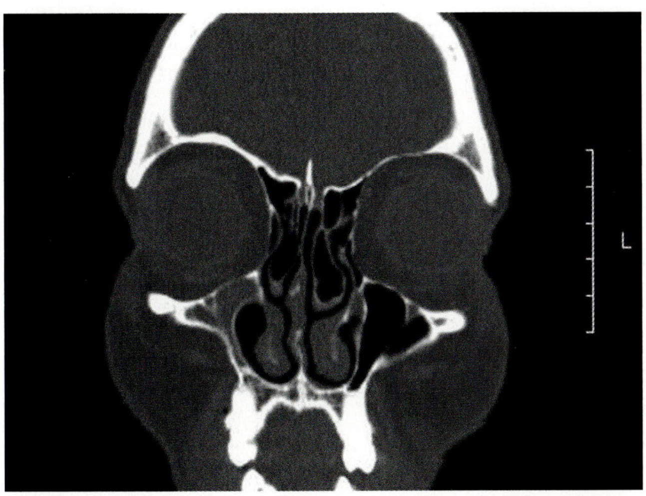

Fig. 14.1: A concha bullosa is the pneumatization of turbinate bone triggered by development of the ethmoid air cells into the middle turbinate bone.

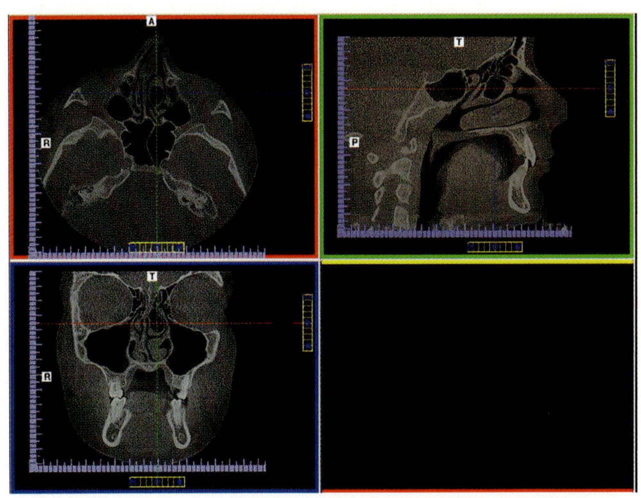

Fig. 14.2: A concha bullosa is classically identified by imaging of the sinuses, but may identified on nasal endoscopy in some cases.

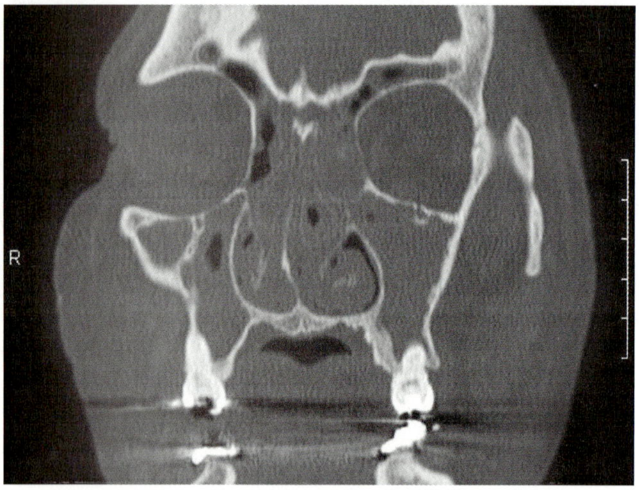

Fig. 14.3: CT scan of diseased concha bullosa.

for future endoscopic sinus surgery, and unintended synechiae of the osteomeatal complex leading to recurrent or chronic rhinosinusitis.

Concha Bullosa Resection

Topical vasoconstriction of the nasal cavity is performed (e.g., 4% cocaine soaked cottonoids) and additional vasoconstriction is performed by injecting local anesthesia (e.g., 1% lidocaine with 1:100,000 epinephrine) into the middle turbinate and axilla of the turbinate (*see* Fig. 9.2). A sickle knife is used to enter the concha bullosa (Fig. 14.4A). If the concha bullosa is more posterior, a tru-cut Blakesley may be used to make a horizontal cut through the middle turbinate until the concha bullosa is encountered. The lateral aspect of the concha bullosa is removed with a combination of endoscopic scissors, Tru-cuts forceps (Fig. 14.4B), or microdebrider (Fig. 14.4C). Excessive manipulation of the medial aspect of the middle turbinate must be avoided to prevent instability and lateralization of the middle turbinate, hyposmia/anosmia, or CSF leak (Fig. 14.4D). The posteromedial ostium of the concha bullosa must be connected to the larger outflow tract to prevent mucous recirculation. Lateralization of the turbinate or synechiae are rare, especially if the medial mucosal surface is intact.

Middle Turbinate Medialization

Synechiae formation between the middle turbinate and lateral nasal wall can occur after endoscopic sinus surgery resulting in persistent chronic rhinosinusitis. Synechiae formation is more likely to occur with lateralization of the middle turbinate after surgery. Two main techniques have been utilized to decrease that risk, namely suture medialization and controlled synechiae formation. One method is to create a controlled scar band between the septum and the medial wall of the middle turbinate called "Bolgerization," named after the surgeon that described the technique.[3] Typically, the surgeon denudes the septal mucosa and medial middle turbinate mucosa at their mutual contact point. A middle meatal spacer or suture may be used to keep the middle turbinate juxtaposed with the septum until the intended synechiae matures. The other technique to keep the middle turbinate medialized is to place a horizontal mattress suture through both middle turbinates and septum (conchopexy). A recent study shows that permanent medialization of the middle turbinate (specifically conchopexy) does not impair olfaction.[4]

Middle Turbinate Flaps

Middle turbinate flaps have been described for closure of septal perforations, frontal sinus surgery as a reconstruction of skull base defects of the fovea ethmoidalis, cribriform plate, and selected sellar, clival, and planum defects. These techniques are covered elsewhere in this textbook.[5,6]

INFERIOR TURBINATE SURGICAL MANAGEMENT

The inferior turbinate is made up of a central bony component with soft erectile tissue covered with mucosa. The turbinate bone attaches to the medial portion of the maxillary and palatine bones. The soft tissue of the inferior turbinate contains seromucinous glands and venous sinusoids. The mucosa is composed of pseudostratified epithelium ciliated columnar epithelium. The inferior turbinates play an important role in warming, filtering, and humidifying inspired air. They also play a dynamic role in determining nasal resistance. Nasal obstruction results when the inferior turbinate enlarges enough to compromise nasal airflow.[7,8] Turbinate hypertrophy may occur secondary to inhalant allergens, airborne particles, infection, or inflammation. The bony and/or soft tissue components of the inferior turbinate may play a significant role in nasal obstruction.[9] If the turbinate hypertrophy does not respond to medical therapy, surgery may be considered to reduce their size. Different surgical techniques may be utilized depending on the location, mucosal, or bony hypertrophy of the inferior turbinate.

The indications for inferior turbinate surgery are usually based on the outcome of improving the nasal

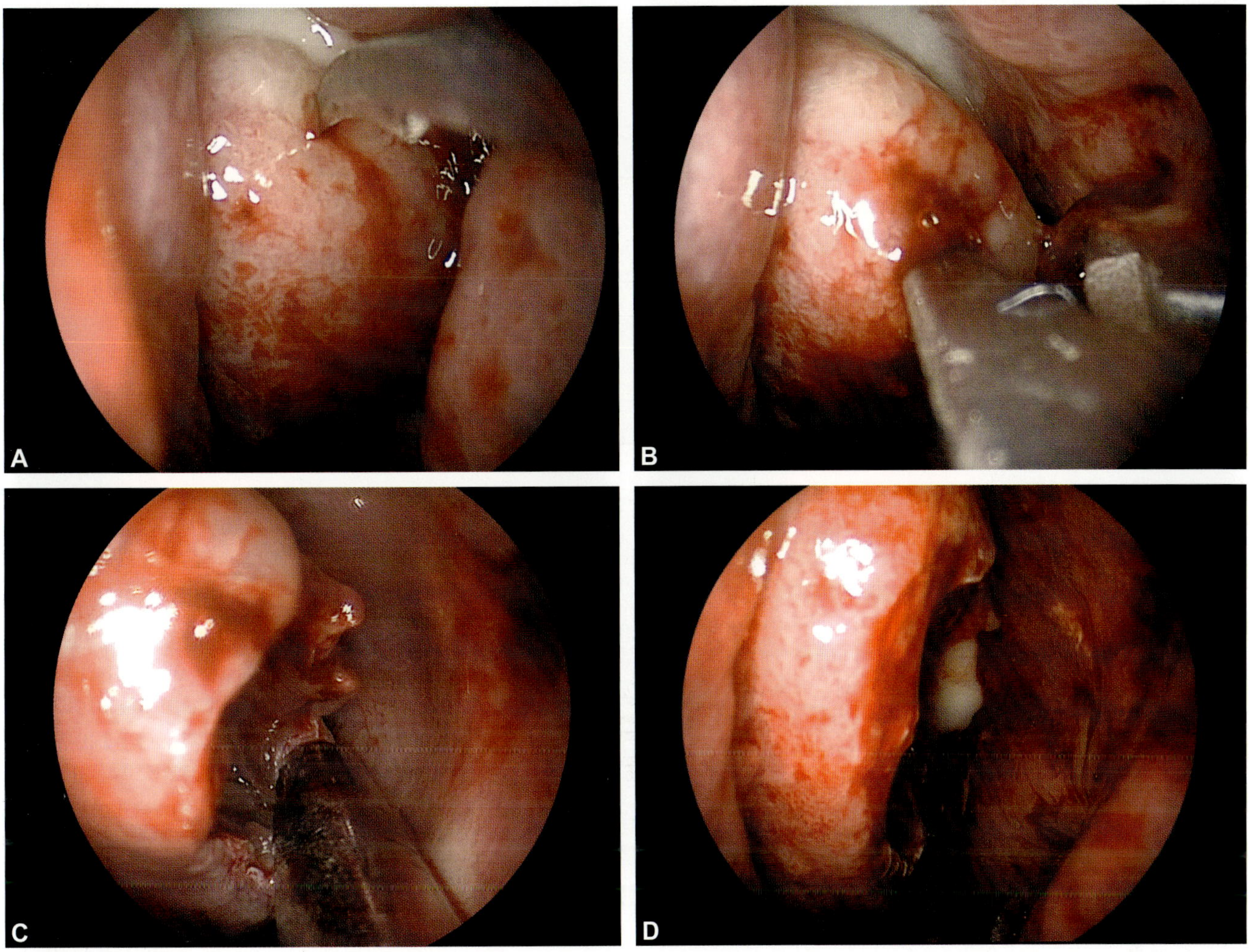

Figs. 14.4A to D: (A) A sickle knife is used to enter the concha bullosa. (B and C) The lateral aspect of the concha bullosa is removed with a combination of endoscopic scissors, tru-cuts forceps (B); or microdebrider (C). (D) Excessive manipulation of the medial aspect of the middle turbinate must be avoided to prevent instability and lateralization of the middle turbinate, hyposmia/anosmia, or CSF leak.

airway. Typical indications include (1): failure of medical therapy for chronic nasal obstruction; (2) multilevel treatment for obstructive sleep apnea; (3) inability to tolerate a continuous positive airway pressure mask; (4) refractive rhinitis medicomentosa; (5) in combination with endoscopic sinus surgery, septoplasty, rhinoplasty, or endoscopic skull base surgery.[10-12] Contraindications include atrophic rhinitis, paradoxical nasal obstruction, and specific device concerns used to address the inferior turbinate (i.e., using radiofrequency ablation in the setting of an electrical implant).

Turbinate Lateralization

In 1904, Killian first described turbinate lateralization as an alternative to the radical total turbinectomy.[13] Lateralization of the inferior turbinate improves the nasal airflow by increasing the area of the internal valve. The internal nasal valve is defined by the superior angle (angle between septum and upper lateral cartilage) and the anterior head of the inferior turbinate. Lateralization of the inferior turbinate improves the angle at which the turbinate attaches to the maxillary and palatine bone, thereby improving the airflow through the nasal valve area. Even minor improvements in the valve area can result in clinically significant improvements in nasal obstruction. This technique's simplicity allows it to be performed easily as an adjunct to other sinonasal procedures.[14]

After decongestion of the nasal cavity, a Boise/Goldman elevator is used to apply inferior and lateral pressure against the attachment of the inferior turbinate.

Endoscopic visualization may be helpful for proper placement of the elevator. The elevator may be marched in an anterior–posterior direction while lateralizing each section of the inferior turbinate. "Infracture" of the turbinate may be performed by placing the elevator in the inferior meatus to fracture the turbinate medially and superiorly. This maneuver promotes a more complete fracture before lateralization of the inferior turbinate.

Lateralization of the inferior turbinates has remained a widely utilized technique due to its technical ease, minimal risks, and low complications rates.[15-17] This technique results in minimal mucosal trauma, and preserves parasympathetic nerve endings and lacrimal function.[14] Lateralization is particularly useful in situations where the bony portion of the inferior turbinate extends into the nasal airway obstructing nasal airflow along the floor.[18] Lateralization is also a good adjunct procedure especially in cases where the inferior meatus is spacious enough accommodate the displaced turbinate tissue.[19]

Some of the literature suggests that lateralization of the inferior turbinates is largely temporary.[10,20] Several authors have contended that the effects of lateralization are short-term since outfracturing does not have any glandular or venous plexus disruption and the turbinates may hypertrophy to occupy the newly opened nasal airway.[15,20] However, a 2010 prospective study demonstrated that patients noted subjective nasal improvement and CT scans demonstrated objective evidence of an improved airway (angle between the inferior turbinate and the lateral nasal fossa wall) of an improved airway ($p < 0.005$) at 1 and 6 months after inferior turbinate lateralization.[21]

Lateralization of the inferior turbinates is a conservative technique for addressing hypertrophy of the inferior turbinates. Although, this procedure is usually insufficient as a stand-alone procedure for addressing the turbinates, it has good benefit with minimal risk of complications.

Inferior Turbinate Soft Tissue Reduction

The soft tissue portion of the inferior turbinate may be reduced using a variety of techniques which include monopolar cautery, bipolar cautery, radiofrequency volumetric reduction (RFVTR), and microdebrider-assisted inferior turbinoplasty (MAIT). The electrocautery and RFVTR techniques cause submucosal thermal injury resulting in soft tissue fibrosis, and reduction in the size of the turbinate. The MAIT technique allows for actual soft tissue removal, reducing the bulk of the submucosal turbinate tissue without damaging the overlying mucosa.

Monopolar/Bipolar Electrocautery

Monopolar or bipolar electrocautery are performed by infiltrating the turbinate with a small amount of local anesthesia with epinephrine and then placing a long needle into the submucosa along the length of the turbinate. As each device has a unique power output, a good rule of thumb is to apply enough energy until the mucosa has blanched in the area of the applied energy.

Radiofrequency Volumetric Tissue Reduction

Radiofrequency volumetric tissue reduction is a relatively newer surgical technique for inferior turbinate reduction. It has been previously used to ablate accessory conduction pathways seen in Wolf–Parkinson–White syndrome.[22] This procedure uses radiofrequency energy to excite ions within the target tissue, which causes an elevation in tissue temperature (between 60 and 90°C) resulting in denaturation of proteins in the deep mucosal and submucosal layers.[23] The result is tissue coagulation and fibrosis over time, which reduces turbinate volume yet preserves nasociliary function of mucosa.[24] Compared with electrocautery, there is reduced thermal collateral damage.[25] Various machines exist to supply the radiofrequency ablation energy. The most common devices are the Coblator II System with the ReFlex Ultra Wand (ArthroCare ENT, Austin, TX) and the Surgitron with the Bayonet RF Turbinate Volume Reduction Electrode (Ellman International, Inc., Hewlett, NY). The procedure is relatively contraindicated in patients with cardiac pacemakers or in patients who have other implantable electronic medical devices.[26]

After decongestion and vasoconstriction of the nasal cavity, the handheld radiofrequency ablation device (Fig. 14.5A) is used to pierce the inferior turbinate and create a submucosal pocket anteriorly to posteriorly. The device is activated and slowly withdrawn to reduce the majority of the turbinate submucosa (Fig. 14.5B). The pierced mucosa is coagulated upon exiting the submucosal pocket to decrease the risk of postoperative bleeding.

Radiofrequency volumetric tissue reduction as well as monopolar and bipolar electrocautery can be performed in the clinic setting with local anesthesia due to their short procedural time, minimally invasive nature, and minimal pain.[11,23] Inferior turbinate soft tissue reduction

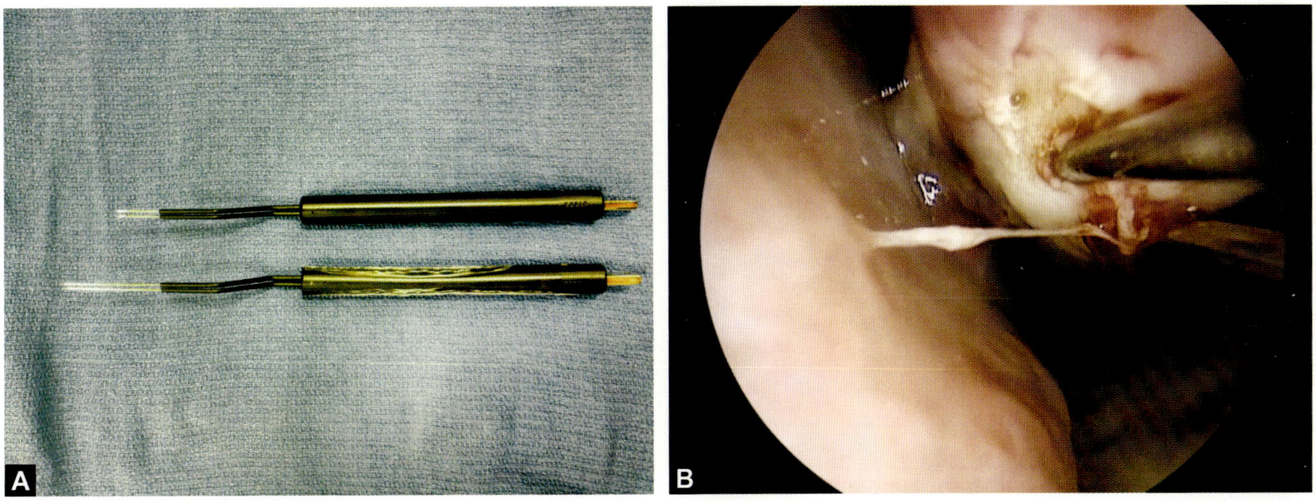

Figs. 14.5A and B: (A and B) After decongestion and vasoconstriction of the nasal cavity, the handheld radiofrequency ablation device (A) is used to pierce the inferior turbinate and create a submucosal pocket anteriorly to posteriorly. The device is activated and slowly withdrawn to reduce the majority of the turbinate submucosa (B).

is cost effective since the operating room is not required, and patients may elect to return to work the same day. Complications are rare although maxillary tooth numbness, mild pain, and tissue edema may be observed in the first postoperative week. Multiple studies in the literature have shown improvements in patients with nasal obstruction after failure of medical therapy after RFVTR using visual analog scores, rhinomanometry, and NOSE scores in the short and long term.[11,24,27]

Microdebrider Assisted Inferior Turbinoplasty

Microdebrider-assisted inferior turbinoplasty is another technique used for submucosal turbinate reduction. Like other submucosal reduction techniques, this method allows for reduction of submucosal turbinate soft tissue over the turbinate bone using specialized microdebrider blades.[28] A more aggressive modification called microdebrider-assisted inferior turbinoplasty with bone removal (MAITBR) involves removal of inferior turbinate bone as well as submucosal tissue. MAIT is associated with a better nasal mucociliary transport time when compared with RFVTR.[29]

After decongestion and vasoconstriction of the nasal cavity, the inferior turbinate is infiltrated with a local anesthetic containing epinephrine. Using endoscopic guidance, a small stab incision in the anterior head of the turbinate is made and a submucosal flap is created using a Freer or Cottle elevator. Alternatively, many microdebrider blades have a sharp dissecting tip which may be used to make the stab incision (Medtronic Xomed, Jacksonville, FL) (Fig. 14.6A). The tip of the blade may be used to create a submucosal flap in a subperiosteal plane. The flap elevation is performed in the medial and inferior portions of the turbinate bone. With the microdebrider blade facing the bone and toward the overlying mucosa, the device is activated to allow controlled resection of submucosal tissue. Attention is most often directed to the anterior head of the inferior turbinate which contributes to narrowing of the nasal valve. Submucosal dissection may be directed to the posterior and medial portions of the inferior turbinate using the same or different stab incision. Inferior turbinate bone may also be removed with more aggressive microdebrider turbinate blades (e.g., 3.5 mm inferior turbinate blade; Medtronic Xomed, Jacksonville, FL) (Fig. 14.6B). To minimize trauma to the branches of sphenopalatine artery, the dissection should be limited to the anterior 2/3 of the inferior turbinate.

Inferior Turbinate Bone Resection

Submucosal resection/reduction (SMR) of the inferior turbinate was first described by Spielberg in the early 1920s.[30] This technique focused on removing the inferior turbinate bone while leaving the overlying mucosal flaps intact. As with the other surgical techniques, preserving a functional overlying mucosa is critical to the success of SMR and to decrease the risk of atrophic rhinitis and empty nose syndrome. A microdebrider assisted SMR technique has also been used to address the submucosal and bony hypertrophy of the inferior turbinate (MASMR).

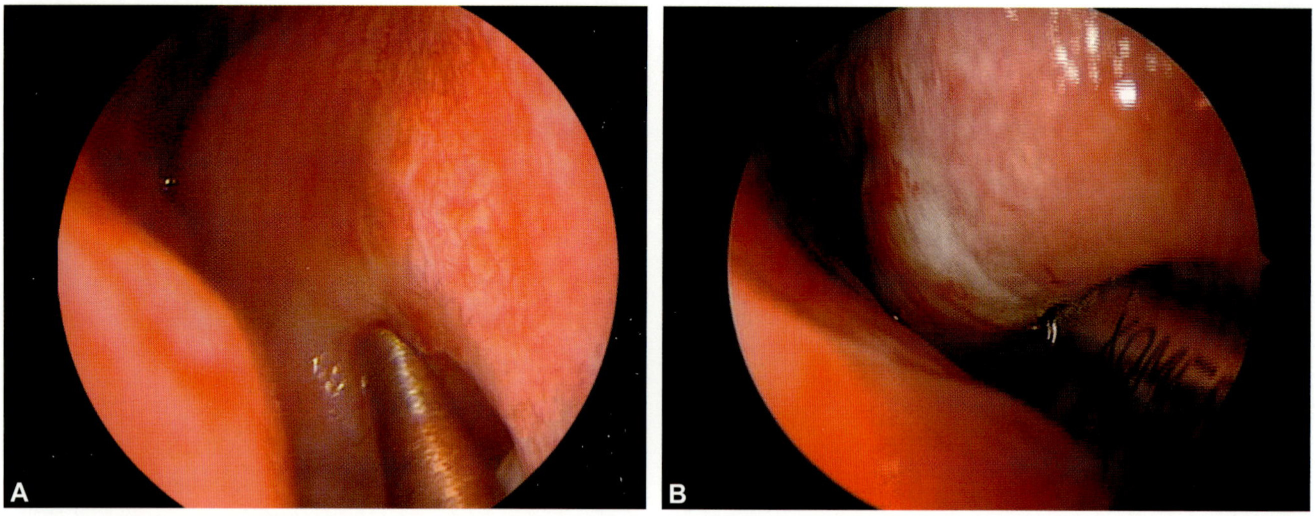

Figs. 14.6A and B: (A) Many microdebrider blades have a sharp dissecting tip which may be used to make the stab incision (Medtronic Xomed, Jacksonville, FL). (B) Inferior turbinate bone may also be removed with more aggressive microdebrider turbinate blades (e.g., 3.5 mm inferior turbinate blade, Medtronic Xomed, Jacksonville, FL).

A mucosal incision is made in the middle of the anterior head of the inferior turbinate (Fig. 14.7A) and often carried posteriorly along its inferior edge. Medial and lateral subperiosteal flaps are created to isolate the bony component of the turbinate (Fig. 14.7B). The inferior turbinate bone is removed using a Metzenbaum scissors (Figs. 14.7C and D). The remaining mucosal flaps are rolled over to cover any exposed bone (Fig. 14.7E). Packing may be placed to ensure flap healing and control bleeding.

Complete Turbinate Resection

With the advent of all the above-mentioned techniques, complete turbinate resection is rarely used. Total inferior turbinate resections have been associated with paradoxical nasal obstruction and/or atrophic rhinitis. Complete turbinate resections are now usually performed in cases of malignancy. Limited resection of the inferior turbinate may be performed in patients undergoing maxillary mega-antrostomy for recalcitrant chronic maxillary sinusitis or for endoscopic medial maxillectomy for treatment of sinonasal tumors (e.g., inverted papilloma).

Complete turbinate resections may be performed by medializing the inferior turbinate and using heavy scissors to amputate the inferior turbinate from the attachment to the maxillary and palatine bones (Fig. 14.8). Partial turbinate resection usually involves preserving the anterior head of the inferior turbinate and posterior attachment of the inferior turbinate to the lateral nasal wall. Great care should be taken to control the inferior turbinate artery, a branch of the sphenopalatine artery, to prevent significant postoperative bleeding.

POSTOPERATIVE CARE

Packing is generally not required for the majority of surgical procedures for the inferior turbinate. Submucous resection techniques with or without microdebrider assistance may require some packing to ensure flap healing and reduce postoperative oozing. Patients are usually managed with nasal saline sprays and irrigation to reduce crusting, mucous, and crusting. Pain is generally well managed with over the counter medications (e.g., acetaminophen, NSAIDs). As the risk of postoperative bleeding is low, the use of aspirin and NSAIDs is usually not contraindicated.

DISCUSSION

There are several advantages to using a microdebrider-assisted SMR technique (MASMR). Since turbinate mucosa is spared, there are decreased rates of crusting and atrophic rhinitis. When compared with traditional turbinate resection, MASMR has a low incidence of postoperative bleeding as there is minimal free mucosal edges.[15] MAITBR is very effective in reducing bony turbinate hypertrophy commonly seen in compensatory changes associated with a deviated septum.[31]

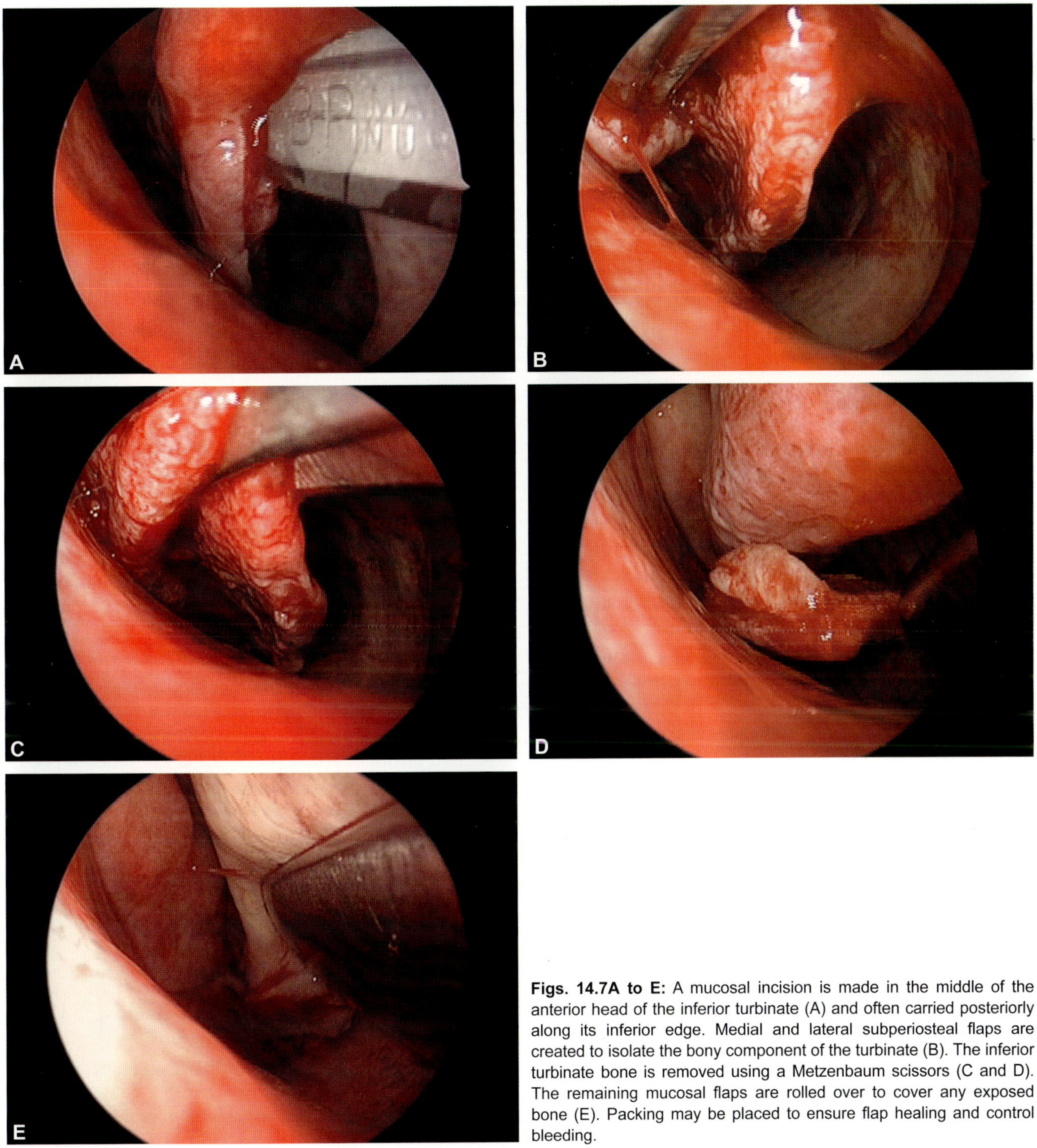

Figs. 14.7A to E: A mucosal incision is made in the middle of the anterior head of the inferior turbinate (A) and often carried posteriorly along its inferior edge. Medial and lateral subperiosteal flaps are created to isolate the bony component of the turbinate (B). The inferior turbinate bone is removed using a Metzenbaum scissors (C and D). The remaining mucosal flaps are rolled over to cover any exposed bone (E). Packing may be placed to ensure flap healing and control bleeding.

A major disadvantage of MASMR is its relative technical difficulty. Even in experienced hands, there is a chance of shredding the mucosa. This can potentially lead to bleeding and impaired physiological function.[10] Another drawback of this technique is the potential need for postoperative packing.[32] Lastly, the preservation of mucosa can also have a unintended effect. Over time, the preserved mucosa may allow for a postoperative recurrence of obstruction, rhinorrhea, and postnasal drip.[32,33]

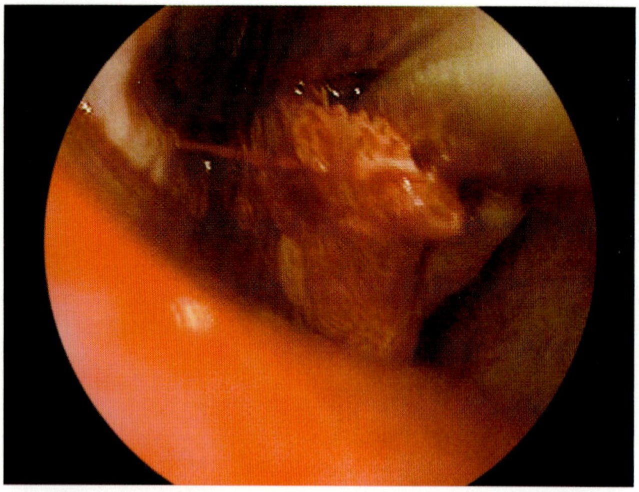

Fig. 14.8: Complete turbinate resections may be performed by medializing the inferior turbinate and using heavy scissors to amputate the inferior turbinate from the attachment to the maxillary and palatine bones.

Long-term outcomes are favorable for MASMR. In one randomized control study, 60 patients underwent MASMR.[29] At 3 years postoperatively, there was a reported decrease in nasal obstruction ($p<0.0001$), sneezing ($p<0.0001$), rhinorrhea ($p<0.0001$), and snoring ($p<0.0001$). There was also a relatively low rate of complications one year after surgery. Only 1/60 of the patients developed transient nasal dryness and 7/60 patients developed postoperative crusting. No patients developed atrophic rhinitis, postoperative bleeding, synechiae, or loss of mucosa.

This same study compared two popular techniques of inferior turbinate reduction: radiofrequency-assisted inferior turbinoplasty to MAIT.[29] Although MAIT may have higher complication rates of mucosal tearing, syncytia, and crusting, it is more effective at decreasing symptoms of nasal obstruction, sneezing, rhinorrhea, snoring while maintaining a lower mucociliary transit time at three year follow up.

Yanez and Mora[34] performed a long-term prospective study of patients who had a modified MAITBR. After making a submucosal pocket with cold instrumentation, they used a standard microdebrider to remove the stroma and reshape the bone of the inferior turbinate. This created both a decrease in overall volume as well as decreased the ability of the inferior turbinate to engorge in response to the environmental triggers. Only one patient (0.29%) had postoperative bleeding (classified as minimal), and the rest of the operated group (340) had no complications (99.7%). At 10-year follow up, 91% were still symptom free.

Obviously, the MAITBR is a more aggressive procedure, but it does remove a significant portion of the obstructing inferior turbinate bone. In theory, preserving the medial mucosa will help prevent some of the complications of a turbinectomy and the more aggressive soft tissue removal will help prevent stromal hypertrophy. Gupta and colleagues examined the long-term outcomes of this technique with a postoperative questionnaire.[35] With a mean follow up time of 24 months (range 6–40 months), the majority experienced significant improvement in their nasal obstructive symptoms. One patient (4%) complained of nasal dryness.

While inferior turbinate surgery is not commonly done for allergic rhinitis induced turbinate hypertrophy, Huang and Cheng[36] addressed this issue with a prospective study. Fifty patients with perennial allergic rhinitis due to *Dermatophagoides farinae* and *Dermatophagoides pteronyssinus* had their inferior turbinates reduced with a 2.0 mm microdebrider inferior turbinate blade. Nasal obstruction, rhinorrhea, sneezing, and postnasal drip improved. It was theorized that the microdebrider damages a branch of the postnasal nerve, which plays a role in sneezing and hypersecretion. Its disruption may have led to symptomatic improvement.

The most feared and discussed complication of inferior turbinate reduction surgery is empty nose syndrome that is distinct from atrophic rhinitis. Empty nose syndrome was fairly common with radical turbinectomies.[37] Atrophic rhinitis may also present later in patients who have had turbinate resections.[38] The studies mentioned in this chapter reported no cases of this in association with the newer techniques of turbinate surgery: outfracturing of the inferior turbinate, radiofrequency ablation, microdebrider-assisted SMR, and cold knife removal of the inferior turbinate bone.

SUMMARY

A comprehensive preoperative evaluation, appropriate technique selection, and meticulous surgical and postoperative care are important for the success of turbinate surgery. A wide spectrum of techniques is available to the otolaryngologist to address turbinate hypertrophy. Mucosal preservation of the turbinate, regardless of the turbinate reduction technique, is critical to the success of the procedure.

REFERENCES

1. Hatipoglu HG, Cetin MA, Yuksel E. Concha bullosa types: their relationship with sinusitis, ostiomeatal and frontal sinus disease. Diagn Interv Radiol. 2005;11:145-9.

2. Lal D, Stankiewicz JA. Primary sinus surgery. In: Flint PW, Haughey BH, Lund VJ, et al. (Eds). Cummings Otolaryngology - Head and Neck Surgery. Philadelphia: Mosby Elsevier; 2010.
3. Bolger WE, Kuhn FA, Kennedy DW. Middle turbinate stabilization after functional endoscopic sinus surgery: the controlled synechiae technique. Laryngoscope. 1999; 109:1852-3.
4. Dutton JM, Hinton MJ. Middle turbinate suture conchopexy during endoscopic sinus surgery does not impair olfaction. Am J Rhino Allergy. 2011;25:125-7.
5. Chen PG, Bassiouni A, Wormald PJ. Incidence of middle turbinate lateralization after axillary flap approach to the frontal recess. Int Forum Allergy Rhinol. 2014;4:333-8.
6. Prevedello DM, Barges-Coll J, Fernandez-Miranda JC, et al. Middle turbinate flap for skull base reconstruction: cadaveric feasibility study. Laryngoscope. 2009;119:2094-8.
7. Leong SC, Eccles R. Inferior turbinate surgery and nasal airflow: evidence-based management. Curr Opin Otolaryngol Head Neck Surg. 2010;18:54-9.
8. Hol MK, Huizing EH. Treatment of inferior turbinate pathology: a review and critical evaluation of the different techniques. Rhinology. 2000;38:157-66.
9. Hanif J, Jawad SS, Eccles R. The nasal cycle in health and disease. Clin Otolaryngol Allied Sci. 2000;25:461-7.
10. Nurse LA, Duncavage JA. Surgery of the inferior and middle turbinates. Otolaryngol Clin N Amer. 2009;42:295-309.
11. Porter MW, Hales NW, Nease CJ, et al. Long-term results of inferior turbinate hypertrophy with radiofrequency treatment: A New Standard of Care? Laryngoscope. 2006;116:554-7.
12. Coste A, Yona L, Blumen M, et al. Radiofrequency is a safe and effective treatment of turbinate hypertrophy. Laryngoscope. 2001;111:894-9.
13. Aksoy F, Yıldırım YS, Veyseller B, et al. Midterm outcomes of outfracture of the inferior turbinate. Otolaryngol Head Neck Surg. 2010;143:579-84.
14. Chhabra N, Houser SM. The surgical management of allergic rhinitis. Otolaryngol Clin N Am. 2011;44:779-95.
15. Jackson RLE, Koch J. Controversies in the management of inferior turbinate hypertrophy: a comprehensive review. Plast Reconstr Surg. 1999;103:300-12.
16. Salam MA, Wengraf C. Concho-antropexy or total inferior turbinectomy for hypertrophy of the inferior turbinates? A prospective randomized study. J Laryngol Otol. 1993; 107:1125-8.
17. Passali D, Biagini C, Pedace E. Presumed physiopathology of the nasal wall surgery and contemporary techniques of the inferior turbinates surgery. Acta Otorhinolaryngol Ital. 1996;16:202-10.
18. Moche JA, Palmer O. Surgical management of nasal obstruction. Oral Maxillofac Surg Clin of North Am. 2012;24: 229-37.
19. Goode R. Surgery of the turbinates. J Otolaryngol. 1978; 7:262-8.
20. O'Flynn PE, Milford CA, Mackay IS. Multiple submucosal out-fractures of interior turbinates. J Laryngol Otol. 1990; 104:239-40.
21. Aksoy F, Yildirim YS, Veyseller B, et al. Midterm outcomes of outfracture of the inferior turbinate. Otolaryngol Head Neck Surg 2010;143:579-84.
22. Jackman WM, Wang XZ, Friday KJ, et al. Catheter ablation of accessory atrio-ventricular pathways (Wolf Parkinson White syndrome) by radiofrequency current. N Engl J Med. 1991;324:1605-11.
23. Cavaliere M, Mottola G, Iemma M. Comparison of the effectiveness and safety of radiofrequency turbinoplasty and traditional surgical technique in treatment of inferior turbinate hypertrophy. Otolaryngol Head Neck Surg. 2005; 133:972-8.
24. Garzaro M, Pezzoli M, Landolfo V, et al. Radiofrequency inferior turbinates reduction: long-term olfactory and functional outcomes. Otolaryngol Head Neck Surg. 2012; 146:146-50.
25. Sapci T, Usta C, Evcimik F, et al. Evaluation of radiofrequency thermal ablation results in inferior turbinate hypertrophies by magnetic resonance imaging. Laryngoscope. 2007;117:623-7.
26. Donohue JH, Anderson MT, Mayo-Smith WW. Pacemaker reprogramming after radiofrequency ablation of a lung neoplasm. AJR. 2007;189:890-2.
27. Lin HC, Lin PW, Friedman M, et al. Long-term results of radiofrequency turbinoplasty for allergic rhinitis refractory to medical therapy. Arch Otolaryngol Head Neck Surg. 2010;136:892-5.
28. Chen YL, Tan CT, Huang HM. Long-term efficacy of microdebrider-assisted inferior turbinoplasty with lateralization for hypertrophic inferior turbinates in patients with perennial allergic rhinitis. Laryngoscope. 2008;118:1270-4.
29. Liu CM, Tan CD, Lee FP, et al. Microdebrider-assisted versus radiofrequency-assisted inferior turbinoplasty. Laryngoscope. 2009;119:414-8.
30. Spielberg W. The treatment of nasal obstruction by submucous resection of the inferior turbinate bone. Report of cases. Laryngoscope. 1924;34:197-203.
31. Ozcan KM, Gedikli Y, Ozcan I, et al. Microdebrider for reduction of inferior turbinate: evaluation of effectiveness by computed tomography. J Otolaryngol Head Neck Surg. 2008;37:463-8.
32. Mabry RL. Inferior turbinoplasty: patient selection, technique, and long-term consequences. Otolaryngol Head Neck Surg. 1988;98:60-6.
33. Katz S, Schmelzer B, Cammaert T, et al. Our technique of partial inferior turbinoplasty: long-term results evaluated by rhinomanometry. Acta Otorhinolaryngol. 1996;50:13.
34. Yanez C, Mora N. Inferior turbinate debriding technique: ten-year results. Otolaryngol Head Neck Surg. 2008;138: 170-5.
35. Gupta A, Mercurio E, Bielamowicz S. Endoscopic inferior turbinate reduction: an outcomes analysis. Laryngoscope. 2001;111:1957-9.
36. Huang TW, Cheng PW. Changes in nasal resistance and quality of life after endoscopic microdebrider assisted inferior turbinoplasty in patients with perennial allergic rhinitis. Arch Otolaryngol Head Neck Surg. 2006;132:990-3.
37. Houser SM. Surgical treatment for empty nose syndrome. Arch Otolaryngol Head Neck Surg. 2007;133:858-63.
38. Passali D, Lauriello M, Anselmi M, et al. Treatment of the inferior turbinate: long-term results of 382 patients randomly assigned to therapy. Ann Otol Rhinol Laryngol. 1999;108:569-75.

Section 3

Adjunctive Surgical Procedures

Chapters

CHAPTER

15

Endoscopic Dacryocystorhinostomy

Brian A Fishero, Spencer C Payne

INTRODUCTION

History of the Procedure

The goal of a dacryocystorhinostomy (DCR) is to create a fistula between the nasolacrimal apparatus and the nasal cavity to allow for the egress of tears into the nose. The procedure is indicated for patients with epiphora due to obstruction of the lacrimal outflow tract from the level of the lacrimal sac through the valve of Hasner and can be performed via either an external or endonasal approach.

Endonasal DCR was first described in 1893 by Caldwell.[1] This approach provided limited exposure and suboptimal results. External DCR was described a decade later by Toti.[2] This technique remained the standard of care because of the success rates of roughly 90% in the hands of experienced surgeons.[3] It was not until the 1980s, with the adoption of the endoscope for sinus surgery, that an endonasal approach was again described.[4]

Initially, endoscopic success rates were lower than those for the external approach as exposure of the lacrimal sac was insufficient. Early endoscopic techniques involved removal of the frontal process of the maxilla with a rongeur up to the axilla of the middle turbinate.[5] Wormald et al.[6] showed that the lacrimal sac is in fact located superior to the axilla of the middle turbinate instead of anterior and inferior as is the common misperception. By using a curette or powered drill to remove additional bone that is beyond the limits of a rongeur, success rates have improved to become comparable to those of the external approach.[3,5,7]

The endoscopic technique has several advantages over the more traditional external approach. Most obviously, there is no incision on the face. This results in superior cosmetic outcomes. The incision and dissection with the external approach also necessitate division of the medial insertion of the orbicularis oculi muscle. By avoiding this step, there is less disturbance of the lacrimal pump mechanism.[7,8] The endoscopic approach also allows the surgeon to address other sinonasal pathology including septal deviation.

Pathophysiology

Nasolacrimal duct obstruction can be either functional or anatomic in nature. The type of obstruction is important to delineate for patient counseling as DCR success rates for anatomic and functional obstruction have been reported at 97% and 84%, respectively.[9] Anatomic obstruction is more common than functional obstruction. The level of obstruction can be inferred from punctal irrigation and confirmed with dacryocystogram. The lacrimal sac or nasolacrimal duct is the site of obstruction in more than 70% of cases of physical obstruction of the lacrimal outflow system.[10] Functional obstruction is caused by a narrowed lacrimal system, a poor pump mechanism, or a combination of the two. It is characterized by normal punctal irrigation and dacryocystogram results in conjunction with abnormal lacrimal scintillogram results. With the scintillogram, a radioactive tracer is placed in the conjunctiva and tracked as it moves naturally through the nasolacrimal apparatus. Failure to empty normally into the nose indicates a functional cause of obstruction.

Anatomy

The lacrimal excretory system begins with the two punctae located at the medial portion of each eyelid. Each punctal opening widens into an ampulla, which is oriented perpendicular to the lid margin. Then, there is a sharp turn into the canaliculus. When palpating with lacrimal probes preoperatively, knowledge of this orientation is helpful as the probe should first be aimed perpendicular to the lid margin then turned medially. The individual canaliculi are generally just under one centimeter in length before they merge to become the common canaliculus. Fewer than 10% of individuals will not have a common canaliculus and instead have canaliculi that drain to the sac individually.[11] The common canaliculus moves posteriorly to the medial canthal tendon before turning into the lacrimal sac.

The lacrimal sac and nasolacrimal duct are contiguous structures. The sac rests within the nasolacrimal fossa, which is defined by the anterior lacrimal crest of the frontal process of the maxilla and the posterior crest of the lacrimal bone. The sac measures approximately 10 mm from the fundus to the duct. It rests just anterior to the middle turbinate's attachment to the lateral nasal wall. The superior extent of the fundus rests 8–10 mm above the axilla of the middle turbinate. The duct descends within the thick bone of the frontal process of the maxilla and lacrimal bone for roughly 12 mm before reaching the inferior meatus.[12] The valve of Hasner sits at the duct's opening to the inferior meatus.

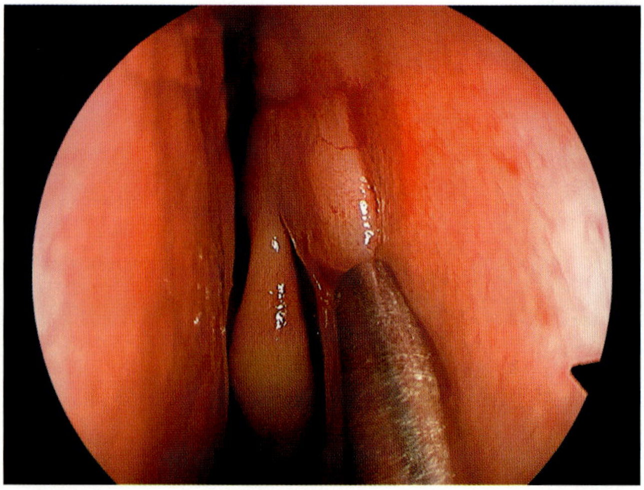

Fig. 15.1: Mucosal incisions—A posterior-based mucosal flap is fashioned with the base including and extending superior to the axilla of the middle turbinate.

TECHNIQUE

Patient Evaluation

As there is a wide differential diagnosis for epiphora, the surgeon must be precise with the etiology before embarking on DCR. Preoperatively, the patient should be carefully examined for causes of epiphora other than nasolacrimal obstruction. This determination should be made in conjunction with an ophthalmologist. Other causes of epiphora include ectropion, punctual malposition, blepharitis, or corneal irritation among others. While watching the punctae for discharge suggestive of distal obstruction, the medial canthal region is massaged. A lacrimal probe should be used to dilate and probe both punctae. As the probe is directed medially through the common canaliculus, the area of obstruction may be palpable. If the probe slides easily through the canaliculus until the probe rests firmly on bone, it is likely that the canaliculi are patent to the lacrimal sac.[5] This can be tested by irrigating the punctum with saline and observing for reflux or normal drainage through the nose and confirmed with a dacryocystogram.[5] Once the etiology of the epiphora has been defined, the patient can be appropriately counseled preoperatively regarding expectations after surgery.

Patient Preparation

The procedure begins in the preoperative holding area with topical decongestion. Three doses of 0.05% oxymetazoline are applied to each nasal cavity spaced over 15 min. The patient is brought to the operative room and placed in a supine position. The patient is orotracheally intubated and the endotracheal tube is secured with tape to the left lower lip to keep it out of the operative field. After this, the nose is packed with two cottonoids soaked with 0.05% oxymetazoline on either side. This should be done under direct visualization with a nasal speculum and light source to prevent unintentional trauma. The bed is then lowered and the patient reclined in a beach-chair position with the head elevated. The room is set up in a similar manner as detailed in Chapter 9.

The cottonoids are then removed and the nose is inspected with a 0° endoscope to assess the nose. If exposure to the axilla of the middle turbinate is limited, a septoplasty as described in Chapter 13 may be indicated. Otherwise, 1% lidocaine with 1:100,000 epinephrine is then injected the head and axilla of the middle turbinate as well as the lateral nasal wall anterior to the middle turbinate. The nasal vibrissae are then trimmed with curved iris scissors.

Surgical Steps

Step 1

Make mucosal incisions. Start with a horizontal incision on the lateral nasal wall superior and posterior to the insertion of the middle turbinate. This is carried anteriorly over the frontal process of the maxilla 1 cm anterior to the axilla. This is connected to a vertical incision, which is carried inferiorly to the junction of the inferior turbinate with the lateral nasal wall. Inferiorly, the vertical incision is connected to a horizontal incision extended posteriorly to the anterior attachment of the uncinate process (Fig. 15.1).

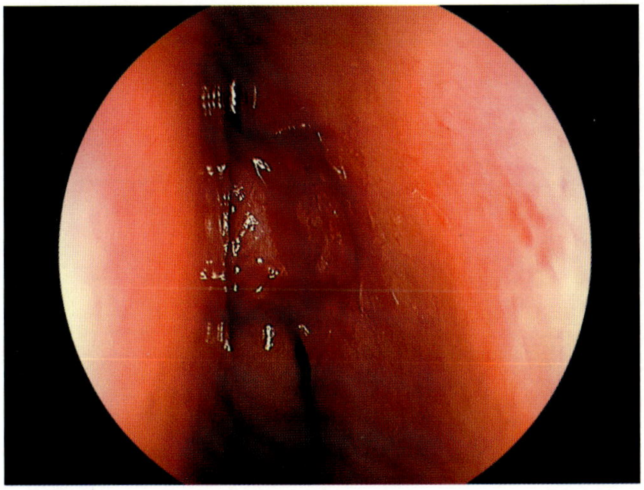

Fig. 15.2: Flap elevation—The flap is elevated and placed medially, tucked behind the middle turbinate to keep it out of the way during the remainder of the dissection.

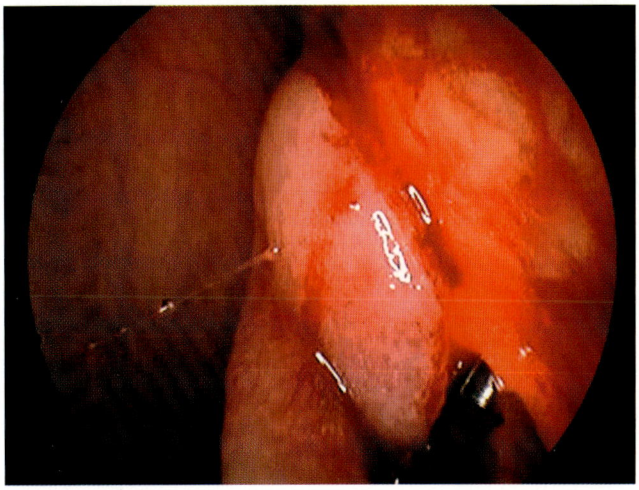

Fig. 15.3: Bone removal—Kerrison rongeurs of a Hajek-Kofler punch can be used to remove bone beginning posteriorly where the thin lacrimal bone meets the thicker ascending process of the maxilla. This is followed by drilling.

Step 2

Elevate a posteriorly based mucosal flap. Use a 30° endoscope for superior visualization. A suction elevator is used to elevate from anterior to posterior in a submucoperiosteal plane. Bleeding should be minimal provided dissection is kept in the correct plane. Dissection is taken to the attachment of the uncinate process (Fig. 15.2).

Step 3

Identify and remove overlying lacrimal bone. Palpate the lateral nasal wall beginning superior to the attachment of the inferior turbinate. The lacrimal bone is soft in contrast to the thick frontal process of the maxilla. Using a cottle, fracture and elevate the thin lacrimal bone on the posterior aspect of the nasolacrimal duct. Using a Kerrison rongeur, engage the lacrimal bone taking care to protect the underlying duct. Remove bone superiorly until the instrument can no longer engage the bone (Fig. 15.3).

Step 4

Remove overlying frontal process of the maxilla. Thin the residual exposed bone using a 15° endoscopic burr. Take care to not injure the underlying sac as dissection is carried superiorly. At the posterior and superior extent of the exposed bone, the mucosa of the agger nasi cell will be encountered posterior to the sac (Fig. 15.4). Anterior to the sac, the deep surface of the dermis may be exposed. This should completely define the nasolacrimal sac as it transitions into the nasolacrimal duct.

Step 5

Open the nasolacrimal sac. Place a lacrimal probe through the inferior punctum and advance medially until the tip of the probe can be seen making an impression on the sac intranasally. Make a vertical incision from superior to inferior along the sac with a spear knife or ophthalmologic beaver blade (#66) (Fig. 15.5).

Step 6

Create nasolacrimal sac mucosal flaps. Make anterior releasing incisions superiorly and inferiorly with the sickle knife to allow for an anteriorly based nasolacrimal sac mucosal flap. Make the posterior releasing incisions with microscissors to create a posteriorly based mucosal flap. These are optional and studies have indicated creation of flaps does not improve outcome. Many surgeons recommend removal of as much of the medial portion of the sac as possible to prevent shifting of the flaps and resultant stenosis.

Step 7

Lay down lateral nasal wall mucosal flap. Trim the posteriorly based mucosal flap raised in step 5 so that the central portion of it will not overly the new stoma. The superior and inferior limbs of the flap, if still available can be laid over any exposed bone.

Step 8

Insert silicone tubing. Crawford lacrimal intubation tubes are then passed through both the superior and inferior punctum. Gently guide each end of the tube through the lacrimal canaliculi and thread them into the nose. Join the two free ends intranasally by tying a knot. Take care to tie the knot such that it rests within the nasal cavity and not directly within the rhinostomy (Fig. 15.6). Place small pieces of gelfoam around the tubing to prevent undue trauma and keep the mucosal flaps in place.

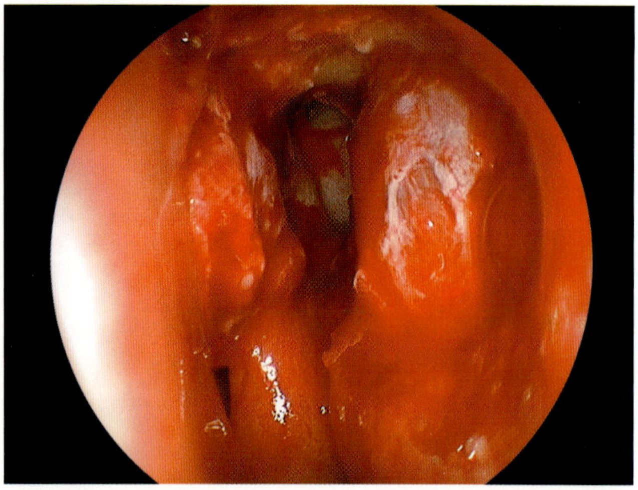

Fig. 15.4: Sac Exposure—Full exposure of the sac may require opening of the anterior wall of the agger nasi cell (seen here in the middle of the photo).

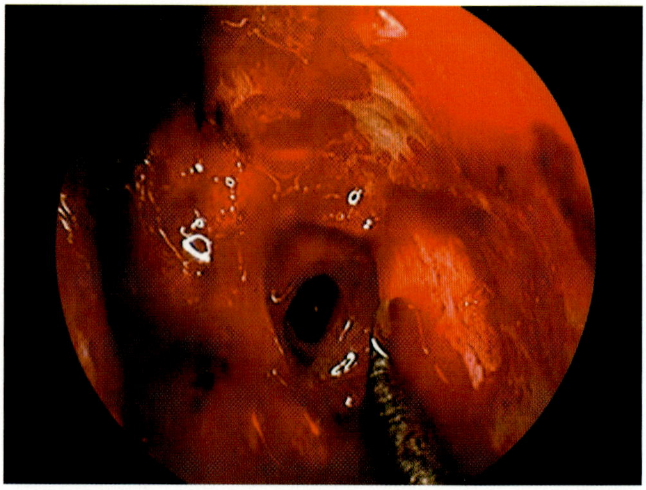

Fig. 15.5: Sac Incision—A round knife (seen here) or #66 beaver blade incises the sac vertically. A more posterior incision may facilitate creation of an anterior flap.

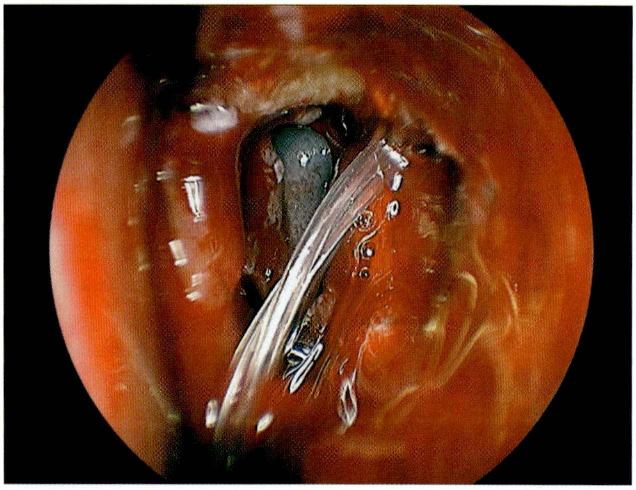

Fig. 15.6: Lacrimal intubation tubes—Crawford tubing seen coming through common canaliculus into the lacrimal sac. These are tied together with the knot resting outside the middle meatus.

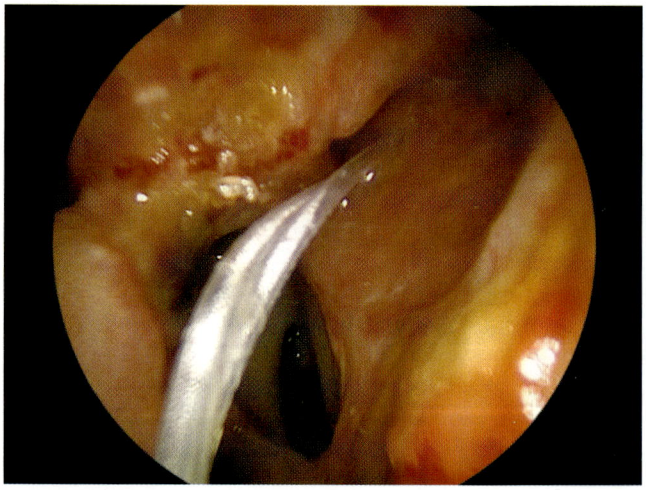

Fig. 15.7: Postoperative appearance—Two week postoperative appearance showing marsupialization of the sac with some fibrinous debris over exposed bone. The agger nasi can be seen just lateral to the tubing.

Postoperative Management

Patients are maintained on systemic antibiotics (cephalexin or amoxicillin/clavulanic acid) for 7 days postoperatively. Ophthalmic antibiotic drops (neomycin/polymyxin B/dexamethasone) are used over the same duration. Saline nasal irrigations are started on the evening of surgery or the following day. This helps to prevent accumulation of debris with resulting inflammation and granulation tissue around the ostium. At follow up appointments, care is taken to debride any crusting or debris. Increased granulation tissue can be expected around the third week with scarring around week six.[8] With that in mind, we leave the silicone tubes in place until at least week four. A typical appearance of the postoperative healing is seen in Figure 15.7.

Preventing Restenosis

Successful outcome is dependent upon the creation of a large ostium and prevention of reclosure. Cukurova et al.[8] reported that granulation tissue formation was the most frequent cause of failure in his case series of 126 patients who underwent endoscopic DCR. Adhesions can also form due to trauma to the middle turbinate or septum. By positioning a local mucosal flap over the exposed bone, healing occurs by primary instead of secondary intent. Granulation tissue formation and subsequent scarring with reclosure of the ostium is thus minimalized. While several variances in technique have been describe, all entail marsupializing the duct into the nose and laying mucosa over the exposed bone. Factors that predict failure include postoperative scarring, intraductal stones, and tumor causing obstruction. Preoperative computed tomography and dacryocystography is helpful in identifying some of these factors.[8]

We prefer to place bicanalicular silicone stents at the conclusion of the procedure. This is done to stent the wound and prevent closure of the rhinostomy. The tubing itself can cause a foreign body reaction resulting in inflammation and granulation of the wound. While postoperative irrigations and nasal debridements can help prevent this complication, granulation tissue formation can be minimalized if the knot that is tied in the tubing does not rest at the ostium but instead lies further within the nasal cavity to avoid trauma to the surgical site.[8]

CONCLUSION

Successful DCR is defined by both resolution of symptoms and a patent rhinostomy on postoperative examination.[13] In the hands of an experienced surgeon, success rates of endoscopic DCR should be over 90%.[9] As the technique has been refined, one can expect to reach the same high rate of success as the more traditional external approach.

REFERENCES

1. Caldwell G. Two new operations for obstruction of the nasal duct, with preservation of the canaliculi, and with an incidental of a new lacrymal probe. Am J Ophthalmol. 1893;10:189-93.
2. Toti A. Nuovo metodo conservatore di cura radicale delle suppurazioni croniche del sacco lacrimale. Clinica Moderna. 1904;10:385.
3. Feretis M, Newton JR, Ram B, et al. Comparison of external and endonasal dacryocystorhinostomy. J Laryngol Otol. 2009;123:315-9.
4. McDonogh M, Meiring JH. Endoscopic transnasal dacryocystorhinostomy. J Laryngol Otol. 1989;103:585-7.
5. Wormald PJ. Powered endoscopic dacryocystorhinostomy. Otolaryngol Clin North Am. 2006;39:539-49, ix.
6. Wormald PJ, Kew J, Van Hasselt A. Intranasal anatomy of the nasolacrimal sac in endoscopic dacryocystorhinostomy. Otolaryngol Head Neck Surg. 2000;123:307-10.
7. Pittore B, Tan N, Salis G, et al. Endoscopic transnasal dacryocystorhinostomy without stenting: results in 64 consecutive procedures. Acta Otorhinolaryngol Ital. 2010; 30:294-8.
8. Cukurova I, Caner Mercan G, Cetinkaya E, et al. Endoscopic dacryocystorhinostomy: outcomes using mucosal flap preserving technique. Eur Arch Otorhinolaryngol. 2013; 270:1661-6.
9. Wormald PJ, Tsirbas A. Investigation and endoscopic treatment for functional and anatomical obstruction of the nasolacrimal duct system. Clin Otolaryngol Allied Sci. 2004;29:352-6.
10. Kashkouli MB, Parvaresh M, Modarreszadeh M, et al. Factors affecting the success of external dacryocystorhinostomy. Orbit. 2003;22:247-55.
11. Yazici B, Yazici Z. Frequency of the common canaliculus: a radiological study. Arch Ophthalmol. 2000;118:1381-5.
12. Whitnall SE. The Anatomy of the Human Orbit and Accessory Organs of Vision. New York: Oxford University Press; 1932.
13. Wormald PJ, Tsirbas A. Chapter 21: Powered endoscopic dacryocystorhinostomy. In: Cohen AJ, Mercandetti M, Brazzo BG (Eds). The Lacrimal System: Diagnosis, Management, and Surgery. New York: Springer Science+Business Media, Inc.; 2006. pp. 223-35.

CHAPTER

16

Endoscopic Orbital Surgery

Madeleine R Schaberg

INTRODUCTION

Given the proximity of the paranasal sinuses to the orbit, certain pathologies of the orbit are amenable to surgical correction through an endonasal endoscopic approach. The orbit and the orbital apex share their medial wall with the lateral wall of the ethmoid and sphenoid sinuses. Thus, medially located pathologies of the orbit and orbital apex can be addressed using endoscopic orbital surgery techniques.

The most common endoscopic orbital approach is surgical decompression of the orbit for the treatment of exophthalmos and optic neuropathy. Orbital decompression, originally described by Walsh and Ogura in the early 1950s,[1] was transformed in the 1980s by the introduction of the endoscope. First described by Kennedy et al.,[2] endoscopic orbital decompression has become the preferred approach for specific pathologies of the orbit. Endoscopic orbital decompression avoids facial incisions and allows excellent visualization of the medial and inferior orbital walls. In addition, various diseases and lesions of the orbital apex can also be approached endoscopically.

Multiple open approaches have traditionally been used to approach the orbit and orbital apex including transconjunctival, transcranial, medial approaches via a lynch incision, and orbitotomy (medial, superior or lateral).[3,4] Many lesions in this area however are amenable to an endoscopic approach though the transethmoidal transsphenoidal corridor. This approach allows excellent exposure as well as visualization, allowing excision, biopsy, and decompression of the optic nerve. This chapter will detail the anatomy, pathology and surgical approaches.

ANATOMY

The orbit is essentially a compartment with three bony boundaries, medially, laterally and posteriorly, and a tarsoligamentous diaphragm anteriorly. Anteriorly, it is a four-sided pyramid, which becomes three sided as the apex is approached. Seven different bones contribute to its structure; frontal, lacrimal, sphenoid, ethmoid, maxillary, palatine, and zygomatic. The medial orbital wall is largely made up of the quadrangular orbital plate of the ethmoid bone. The lateral orbital wall is composed of the greater wing of sphenoid and the zygomatic bone. The orbital floor's main contribution is the orbital plate of the maxilla and it slopes posteriorly and medially at a 45° angle. The orbital roof is contributed to by the frontal bone and the lesser wing of sphenoid. The orbit rests superior to the maxillary sinus, adjacent to the ethmoid sinuses, and anterior to the sphenoid sinus (Fig. 16.1). The orbital apex is the narrowest portion and coursing through this apex is the optic nerve and its associated neurovascular structures. There are three foramina through which critical structures enter. Cranial nerves III, IV and VI as well the lacrimal, frontal, and nasociliary nerves enter the orbit through the superior orbital fissure. The superior orbital fissure is the largest communication between the orbit and the middle cranial fossa. The orbital branch of the middle meningeal artery, the recurrent branch of the lacrimal artery, and the associated superior orbital and superior ophthalmic veins also enter via this large conduit. The inferior orbital fissure allows passage of the infraorbital and zygomatic nerve as well as parasympathetics traveling to the lacrimal gland, the infraorbital artery and vein, and the inferior ophthalmic vein going to the pterygoid plexus. The optic canal houses the ophthalmic artery, the central retinal vein, and the optic nerve. The optic nerve is encased in pia, arachnoid and dura, and thus is considered an extension of the brain. It is generally divided into four segments; intracranial (15 mm), intracanalicular (5–11 mm), intraorbital (25–35 mm), and intraocular (1 mm). Because of the rigid buttresses of the orbit, pathology within the orbit can cause a "compartment syndrome" causing compression of the vasculature and optic nerve.

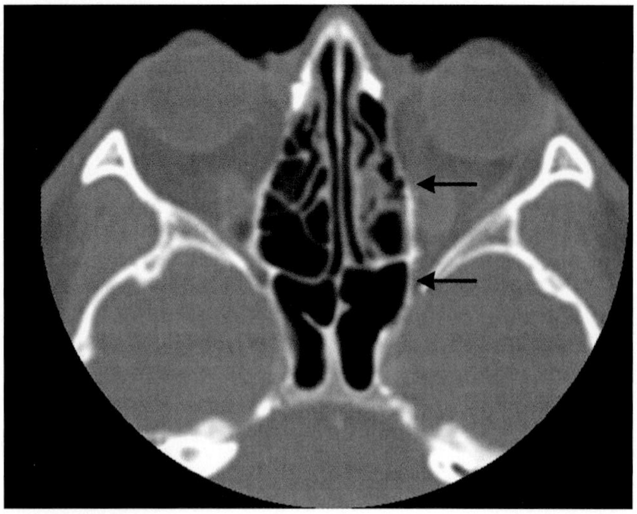

Fig. 16.1: Axial computed tomography (CT) scan with bone windows. Black arrows indicate common wall between orbit and ethmoid and sphenoidal sinuses.

The major blood supply to the orbit is from the ophthalmic artery, the first branch of the internal carotid artery. The ophthalmic artery passes over the optic nerve in 85% of cases and then heads for the medial orbital wall. It branches into multiple branches, the most critical of which are the anterior and posterior ethmoid arteries. These arteries then exit the medial wall of the orbit and supply the ethmoid cavity. It is important to note the exact location of the anterior and posterior ethmoid foramina through which the anterior and posterior ethmoid arteries pass. The distance from the orbital rim to the anterior ethmoid artery is roughly 25 mm, from the anterior to posterior ethmoid artery is 12 mm, and then to optic nerve is 6 mm.

There are a total of six extraocular muscles responsible for moving the globe. All four rectus muscles (medial, lateral, superior, and inferior) originate from the fibrous annulus of Zinn (a continuation of the dura of the middle cranial fossa). The annulus of Zinn surrounds the optic nerve as it enters the orbit. The superior and inferior oblique, however, originate from the posterior orbital wall.

PATHOLOGY

A wide and varied group of pathologies affect the orbit (Table 16.1). Bacterial infections within the orbit, which are amenable to endoscopic surgical drainage, are generally an orbital complication of ethmoidal sinusitis (Figs. 16.2 and 16.3). These were described by Chandler and include subperiosteal abscesses. The management of subperiosteal abscesses remains controversial and depending on size and location a trial of nonsurgical management is often indicated.[5] The most common bacteria isolated are Staphylococci, Streptococci, and Bacteroides (Fig. 16.4).[6]

Table 16.1: Orbital pathologies

Neoplasms	Schwannoma, meningioma, glioma, pleomorphic adenoma, lymphoma, adenoid cystic carcinoma, squamous cell carcinoma, rhabdomyosarcoma, metastatic disease
Infectious	Bacterial-subperiosteal abscess, orbital abscess fungal
Inflammatory	Wegener's, sarcoidosis, Churg–Strauss, pseudotumor
Traumatic	MVA, falls

Ophthalmopathy associated with thyroid dysfunction is the most common extrathyroidal sequelae of Graves disease, an autoimmune disease of the thyroid gland, which primarily affects the thyroid gland and the orbit. Autoantibodies to the thyrotropin receptor (TSH) result in hyperthyroidism. The orbital complications that develop secondarily are not fully understood but result in enlargement of the extraocular muscles and fat due to the deposition of glycosaminoglycan and infiltration with T-cells. The final common pathway is an increase in the intraconal volume. This increased orbital volume causes proptosis and optic nerve compression. Optic nerve compression from either vascular compromise and/or stretching of the nerve itself leads to the development of optic neuropathy. Orbital complications of Graves occur in 40–75% of those affected by the disease.[7] These manifestations range from exophthalmos to subluxation of the globe with exposure keratitis, corneal abrasions, and blindness (Fig. 16.5). Visual loss has been shown in 2–7% of Graves patients with long-term follow-up.[8,9]

Inflammatory granulomatous disease affecting the orbit include Wegener's granulomatosis, sarcoidosis, and Churg–Strauss. These can present with acute optic neuropathy and require decompression while awaiting medical treatment. Vascular lesions include lymphangioma as well as arteriovenous malformations. Neoplasms of the orbit are varied and extremely rare. Those of neural origin are neurofibromas, gliomas, schwannomas, and meningiomas. Malignant tumors, while uncommon, have varied pathologies: lymphoma, adenoid cystic carcinoma, squamous cell carcinoma, rhabdomyosarcoma (the most prevalent orbital malignancy in children), liposarcoma, leiomyosarcoma and metastases. Fibro-osseous lesions include osteomas, fibrous dysplasia, and ossifying fibromas.

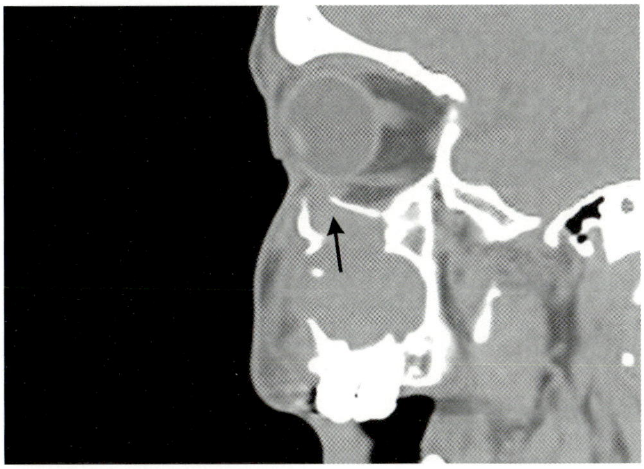

Fig. 16.2: Sagittal CT scan demonstrating opacified maxillary sinus with extension of infectious process into orbit proper. Black arrow demonstrates loss on bone in orbital floor.

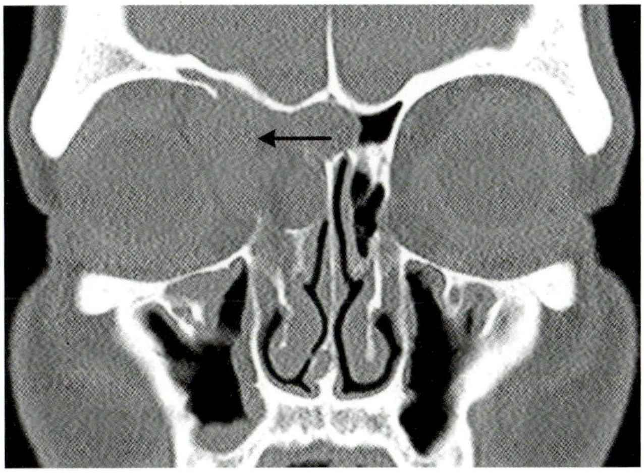

Fig. 16.3: Coronal CT scan showing right ethmo-orbital mucocele. Black arrow points to loss of medial orbital wall.

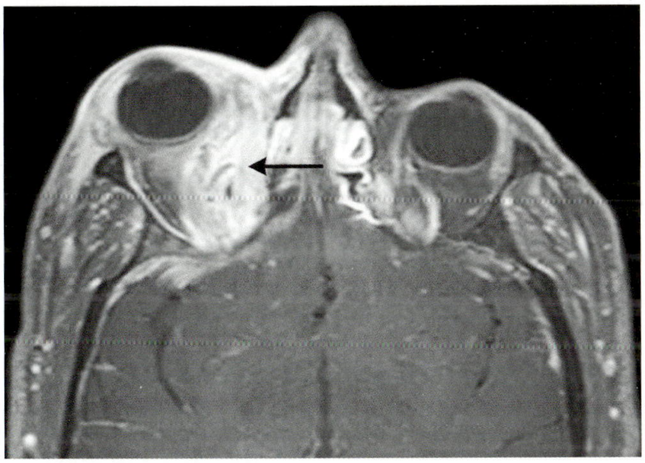

Fig. 16.4: Axial magnetic resonance image (MRI) with arrow demonstrating methicillin-resistant *Staphylococcus aureus* (MRSA) orbital abscess.

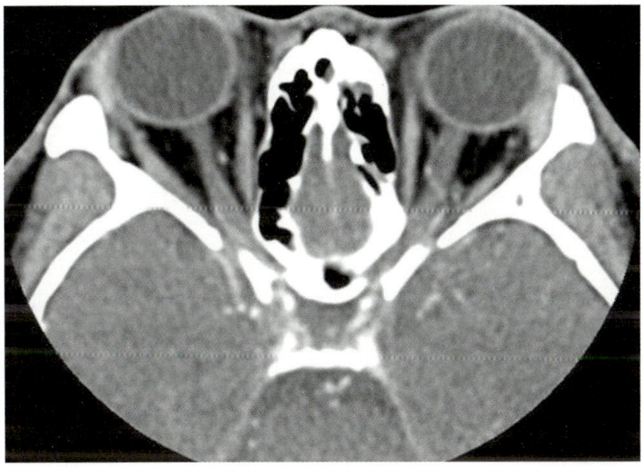

Fig. 16.5: Axial CT scan showing significant proptosis in patient with Graves disease.

ENDOSCOPIC ORBITAL DECOMPRESSION

Preoperative Evaluation

All patients should undergo thin-cut computed tomography (CT) scan as well as magnetic resonance imaging (MRI). MRI is preferred for assessing soft tissue structures such as extraocular muscles, in particular the medial rectus, and optic nerve. CT is critical for evaluation of the bony architecture and pneumatization pattern of the paranasal sinuses. The CT must be carefully inspected for anatomical variations, such as Haller cells, Onodi cells, prolapsed uncinate, dehiscent carotid artery or optic nerves, dehiscent anterior ethmoidal artery, and low-hanging skull base. A Haller cell is an infraorbital cell, which encroaches on the natural maxillary sinus ostium. An Onodi cell, which is a posterior ethmoidal cell that pneumatizes superiorly and posteriorly beyond the anterior wall of the sphenoid sinus, may contain the optic nerve in 12–25% of people.[10] The optic nerve is dehiscent in 4% of patients and twice as many will have a dehiscent carotid artery.[11] An ophthalmologic consultation is paramount for a preoperative evaluation. In addition, a multidisciplinary approach with the ophthalmologist is preferred for any endoscopic orbital surgery.

Technique

General anesthesia is generally utilized for all endoscopic orbital surgery. The operating room setup and patient positioning is akin to that used for endoscopic sinus surgery. Image-guided surgery may be considered to verify relevant anatomy. The patient is placed supine on the operating room table and decongested with 4% cocaine soaked pledgets for 5–7 min. The patient's CT scan is reviewed in the coronal, axial and sagittal planes, and image guidance is calibrated to within 1 mm of accuracy. The zero degree endoscope is the placed on the appropriate side and the middle turbinate is medialized. The uncinate and lateral nasal walls are then injected with 1% lidocaine with epinephrine (1:100,000). An uncinectomy is performed followed by a wide maxillary sinus antrostomy. A wide maxillary sinusotomy allows the use of the posterior maxillary wall and superior maxillary wall as landmarks as well as preventing occlusion of the ostium after herniation of orbital fat. A complete ethmoidectomy is then performed, including exenteration of all cells to the face of sphenoid posteriorly and superiorly to the skull base. This can be accomplished using straight and up biting through cutting instruments as well as powered instrumentation. Removal of the middle turbinate is usually unnecessary and it should be left in place for maximal preservation of normal nasal architecture and physiology.

The medial orbital wall can then be addressed endoscopically though the ethmoid cavity. The lamina papyracea is identified and skeletonized. This bone is usually quite thin and can be removed using elevators, curettes and Blakesley forceps. Once the underlying periorbita is exposed, no powered instrumentation should be used. Once the bone is removed posteriorly the orbital apex is exposed 2 mm anterior to the face of the sphenoid. The thick bone of the optic strut is much harder than the thin bone of the lamina and defines the posterior limit of the dissection. Care should be taken to preserve the underlying periorbita, as it protects the orbital contents (Fig. 16.6). If it is violated, orbital fat will begin to herniate into the surgical field.

If the medial orbital floor is removed, it is carried out by fracturing the bone medial to the infraorbital nerve in a downward fashion. This can often be performed with a curette in one move since there is a natural plane medial to the infraorbital nerve. The fragmented bone is then removed. The superior maxillary roof is best visualized with the 30° endoscope.

Next the periorbita is incised allowing the fat to herniate into the ethmoid cavity. This is generally done by making multiple parallel incisions. These incisions are carried out from posterior to anterior to prevent the herniating fat from obscuring the surgeon's view (Fig. 16.7). The protected tip sickle knife is used to prevent injury to orbital contents. Great care must be taken to avoid injury

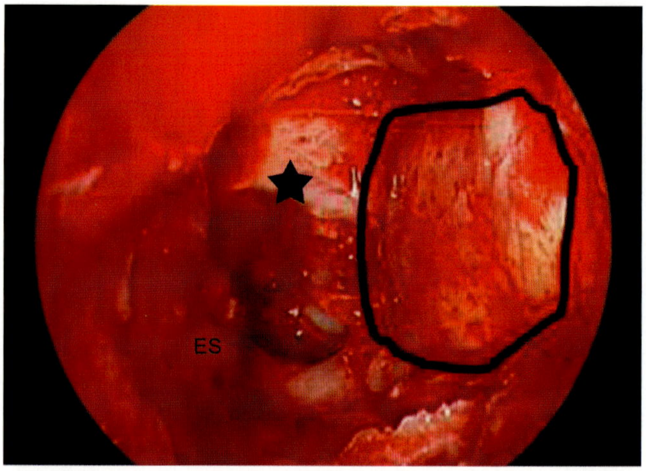

Fig. 16.6: Endoscopic view of ethmoid cavity, medial wall (ES), face of sphenoid (*), and removed lamina papyracea with periorbita exposed (black circle).

to the medial rectus muscle which lies just millimeters below the periorbita. Some authors recommend leaving a "fascial sling" over the medial rectus muscle to minimize the risk of diplopia.[7,12] Fat is allowed to herniate into the ethmoid cavity (Fig. 16.8). A hemostatic foam is then placed in the middle meatus and no intranasal packing is used.

A team approach with the addition of a lateral decompression by an oculoplastics surgeon is indicated for maximal decompression. A combined transconjunctival approach for additional inferior wall decompression has also been described. These approaches are best accomplished with a team of surgeons from both otolaryngology and ophthalmology.

Outcomes

The degree of exophthalmos, as measured by the distance between the orbital rim and the corneal apex, is the primary objective measurement of success. The reduction in exophthalmos was found to be 3.5 mm on average with a solely endoscopic medial wall decompression.[13] The addition of external approaches increases this reduction to 7.4 mm.[14]

Less commonly reported in the literature is the change in visual acuity. This is likely due to the varied indications for surgery and is more difficult to evaluate since a patient with cosmetically deforming proptosis may not have a significant compromise to visual acuity thus leading to little change in pre- and postoperative Snellen testing. All techniques result in improved Snellen measurements with the greatest improvements seen in the combined endoscopic and transantral approach.[13]

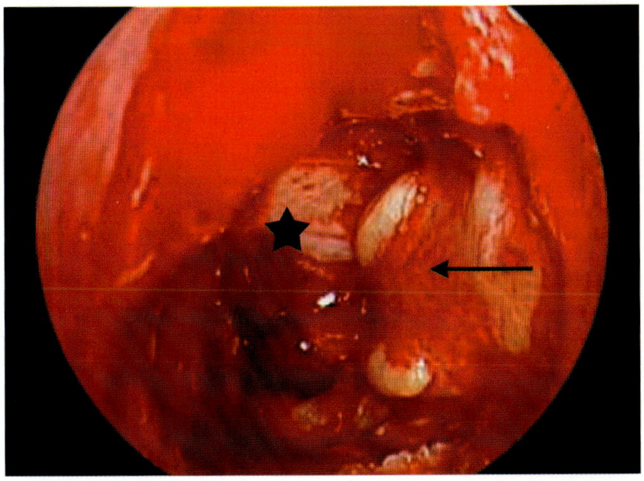

Fig. 16.7: Endoscopic view of prolapsing orbital fat after parallel incisions in the periorbita have been carried out (black arrow points to intervening periorbita). Face of sphenoid (*).

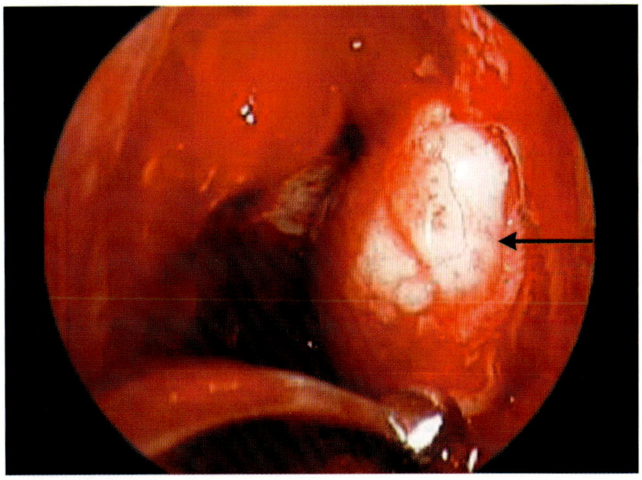

Fig. 16.8: Black arrow points to orbital fat prolapsing into ethmoid cavity. The protected sickle knife is in the foreground.

Overall improvement rates vary widely in the literature, ranging from 20% to 90%,[15,16] most likely due to nonuniformity of disease severity and diversity of patient population.

Complications

Diplopia is the most common complication, ranging from 15% to 60% in the literature, of worsening or new diplopia.[16,17] Other complications of sinusitis and epiphora have been reported in the literature at less than 5%.[18] Rare incidents of cheek paresthesia and cerebrospinal fluid (CSF) leak have been reported.[19]

OPTIC NERVE DECOMPRESSION

Indications

Compressive nontraumatic optic neuropathy occurs in 2–8% of patients with Graves ophthalmopathy and nerve decompression is often indicated to preserve vision, especially when steroids have been ineffective.[20] Decompression in the setting of traumatic optic neuropathy (TON), however, is a more controversial area and occurs in 0.5–1.5% of those with head injury.[21] The mode of injury is hypothesized to be a combination of direct injury followed by secondary injury. The initial trauma causes direct damage to the nerve, causing swelling, resulting in a reduction in blood flow and hypoxia to the nerve with resultant apoptosis and subsequent blindness. The goal of treatment in TON is prevention of secondary injury. Surgical intervention has not been shown to have better results than steroids alone.[22,23] Some studies demonstrated a statistically significant difference in improvement of vision with surgery if performed within 7 days of injury.[23,24] These studies remain difficult to compare because of the fact that baseline visual acuity is the best predictor of outcome.[25]

Technique

Similar to the description for orbital decompression, a wide maxillary sinusotomy followed by a complete ethmoidectomy is performed. A wide transethmoidal sphenoidotomy is performed, and the anterior face of sphenoid is removed using the Kerrison rongeurs. The lateral opticocarotid recess along with the optic canal and carotid artery are identified in the lateral wall of the sphenoid sinus. The lamina is removed 1.5 cm anterior to the junction with the lesser wing of the sphenoid. Once the hard bone of the optic strut is encountered, a self-irrigating diamond burr on a high speed drill is used to thin this bone until it can be removed using a curette or Kerrison rongeur. Bone should be removed for 1 cm posterior to the sphenoid face for maximal decompression.[28] Once the bone is adequately removed, hemostasis can be achieved using the bipolar electrocautery and/or hemostatic agents. For maximal decompression, the optic nerve sheath should be incised; hemostatic foam without packing is then placed in the sphenoid and ethmoid cavities.

Outcomes

In the setting of compressive non-TON, significant improvement is generally seen immediately following decompression, and continued improvement may be realized in the subsequent months. A large study of over 150 patients demonstrated no worsening of vision in any patients postoperatively after endoscopic optic nerve decompression.[23]

Complications

Reported complications have included infection, ophthalmic artery injury, and CSF leak.[23,24,7]

Conclusion

The transnasal endoscopic approach allows superior access and visualization. This procedure has been shown to be effective in compressive optic neuropathy. This is a safe procedure and in the setting of the more controversial TON, the suggested guidelines by multiple authors for intervention are progressive visual loss on high dose steroids (>72 h), and/or CT evidence of bony or hematoma impingement.[24,26]

ENDOSCOPIC ORBITAL APEX APPROACH

Technique

This approach also begins with a complete ethmoidectomy as previously described. A wide transethmoidal sphenoidotomy is performed, and the anterior face of sphenoid is removed using the Kerrison rongeurs or high speed drill to expose the lateral wall of the sphenoid sinus. If additional visualization is required, a posterior septectomy can be performed to allow for a bi-nostril technique. Endoscope placement in the contralateral nare and approaching the lesion from the ipsilateral side can often improve access and prevent scissoring of instruments. If a cerebrospinal fluid leak is anticipated, a vascularized nasoseptal flap may harvested prior to the sphenoidotomy or posterior septectomy. This ensures preservation of the pedicle supplied by the posterior septal branch of the sphenopalatine artery, which crosses the anterior face of the sphenoid 10 mm below the sphenoid ostium. If additional exposure is needed, the middle turbinate may also be removed. The lamina papyracea is identified and removed in a anterior to posterior direction, approximately 1 cm anterior to the sphenoid bone. The location of the optic nerve and carotid artery must be identified with the neuronavigation and Doppler. The lamina papyracea is removed to expose the periorbita of the orbit. The bone of the orbital apex is much thicker than that of the lamina and requires thinning with a diamond burr on a high speed drill for adequate removal. Copious irrigation should be used to avoid damage to the nerve secondary to thermal injury. The periorbita is then incised, and the medial orbital mass is exposed. If necessary, depending on location of lesion, the medial rectus can be isolated and retracted using silk sutures.

The entire intracanalicular portion of the optic nerve should be addressed if optic nerve decompression is necessary, extending to the posterior wall of the sphenoid as described above.

The closure required is dependant on necessity of closure of a cerebrospinal fluid leak and size of defect. This can be accomplished with a multilayer closure including fascia, possible rigid buttress, and a vascularized flap. Tissue sealants such as Duraseal (Covidien, Mansfield, MA) may be placed, followed by a hemostatic agent and light packing.

Outcomes

In one study, endoscopic endonasal approaches to the orbital apex were successful in 18 patients with varying sizes and pathology of tumor, ranging from idiopathic orbital inflammatory syndrome to metastatic renal cell carcinoma, to cavernous hemangioma.[27]

Complications

Cerebral contusion as well as damage to surrounding nerves including the oculomotor, trochlear, abducens, and trigeminal may occur. Blindness can result from iatrogenic injury to the optic nerve. Injury to the carotid artery and CSF leaks have also been reported. A complication rate of 22% was reported by one of the largest series published to date.[27] Minor sinonasal complications include synechiae and acute or chronic sinusitis.

Conclusion

Because of the diversity of pathology, the endonasal endoscopic approach to the orbital apex, must be highly individualized and varies greatly. It is critical that a multidisciplinary team consisting of all three specialties, otolaryngology, neurosurgery, and ophthalmology be involved.

SUMMARY

Because of the proximity of the orbit and paranasal sinuses, endonasal endoscopic approaches to the orbit were a natural extension beyond the paranasal sinuses after the introduction of the endoscope. The advantages of the endoscope include a panoramic view, excellent visualization, angled vision, and the ability to advance the scope into the surgical field for magnification. These approaches eliminate external incisions, decrease postoperative morbidity and hospital stay, and in many instances actually provide improved visualization and access with less disruption of normal tissue. The addition of image guidance to our armamentarium has additionally proved invaluable in this area with such complex and critical anatomy.

Patient selection is critical and not all lesions are amenable to an endoscopic approach. While endoscopic approaches are applicable for many different disease processes, open approaches such as craniotomy or orbitotomy are still necessary for some lesions. A multidisciplinary team approach is imperative to successful management of orbital and orbital apex pathology.

REFERENCES

1. Walsh TE, Ogura JH. Transantral orbital decompression for malignant exophthalmos. Laryngoscope. 1957;67:544-68.
2. Kennedy DW, Goodstein ML, Miller NR, et al. Endoscopic transnasal orbital decompression. Arch Otolaryngol Head Neck Surg. 1990;116:275-82.
3. Kirath H, Bulur B, Bigic S. Transconjunctival approach for retrobulbar intraconal orbital cavernous hemangiomas. Orbital surgeon's perspective. Surg Neurol. 2005;64:71-4.
4. Leone CR, Wissinger JP. Surgical approaches to disease of the orbital apex. Ophthalmology. 1988;95:391-7.
5. Garcia GH , Harris GJ. Criteria for nonsurgical management of subperiosteal abscess of the orbit: analysis of outcomes 1988–1998. Ophthalmology. 2000;107:1454-6.
6. Fakhri S, Pereira K. Endoscopic management of orbital abscesses. Otolaryngol Clin North Am. 2006;39:1037-47.
7. Pletcher SD, Sindwani R, Metson R. Endoscopic orbital and optic nerve decompression. Otolaryngol Clin North Am. 2006;39:943-58.
8. Warren JD, Spector JG, Burde R. Long term follow-up and recent observations on 305 cases of orbital decompression for dysthyroid orbitopathy. Laryngoscope. 1989;99:35-40.
9. Garrity JA, Fatourechi V, Bergstralh EJ, et al. Results of transantral orbital decompression in 428 patients with severe Graves'ophthalmopathy. Am J Ophthalmol. 1993; 116:533-47.
10. Weinberger DG, Anand VK, Al-Rawi M, et al. Surgical anatomy and variations of the Onodi cell. Am J Rhinol. 1996; 10:365-70.
11. Fujii K, Chambers SM, Rhoton AL. Neurovascular relationships of the sphenoid sinus. A microsurgical study. J Neurosurg. 1979;50:31-9.
12. Metson R, Samaha M. Reduction of diplopia following endoscopic orbital decompression: the orbital sling technique. Laryngosocpe. 2002;112:1753-7.
13. Leong SC, White PS. Outcomes following surgical decompression for dysthyroid orbitopathy (Graves' disease). Curr Opin Otolaryngol Head Neck Surg. 2010;18:37-43.
14. Chu EA, Miller NR, Grant MP, et al. Surgical treatment of dysthyroid orbitopathy. Otolaryngol Head Neck Surg. 2009; 141:39-45.
15. Schaefer SD, Soliemanzadeh P, Della Rocca DA, et al. Endoscopic and transconjunctival orbital decompression for thyroid-related orbital apex compression. Laryngoscope. 2003;113:508-13.
16. Metson R, Dallow RL, Shore JW. Endoscopic orbital decompression. Laryngoscope. 1994;104:950-7.
17. Eloy P, Trussart C, Jouzdani E, et al. Transnasal endoscopic orbital decompression and Graves' ophthalmopathy. Acta Otorhinolaryngol Belg. 2000;54:165-74.
18. Wee DT, Carney AS, Thorpe M, et al. Endoscopic orbital decompression for Graves' ophthalmopathy. J Laryngol Otol. 2002;116:6-9.
19. Leong SC, White PS. Outcomes following surgical decompression for dysthyroid orbitopathy (Graves' disease). Curr Opin Otolaryngol Head Neck Surg. 2010;18:37-43.
20. Chu EA, Miller NR, Lane AP. Selective endoscopic decompression of the orbital apex for dysthyroid optic neuropathy. Laryngoscope. 2009;119:1236-40.
21. Steinsapir KD, Goldberg RA. Traumatic optic neuropathy. Surv Ophthalmol. 1994;38:487-518.
22. Levin LA, Beck RW, Joseph MP, et al. The treatment of traumatic optic neuropathy: the International Optic Nerve Trauma Study. Ophthalmology. 1999;106:1268-77
23. Li H, Zhou B, Shi J, et al. Treatment of traumatic optic neuropathy: our experience of endoscopic optic nerve decompression. J Laryngol Otol. 2008;122:1325-29.
24. Rajiniganth MG, Gupta Ak, Gupta A, et al. Traumatic optic neuropathy: visual outcome following combined therapy protocol. Arch Otolaryngol Head Neck Surg. 2003;129: 1203-6.
25. Yu-Wai-Man P, Griffiths PG. Steroids for traumatic optic neuropathy. Cochrane Database Syst Rev. 2007;CD006032.
26. Robinson D, Wilcsek G, Sacks R. Orbit and orbital apex. Otolaryngol Clin North Am. 2011;44(4):903-22.
27. Murchison AP, Rosen MR, Evans JJ, et al. Endoscopic approach to the orbital apex and periorbital skull base. Laryngoscope. 2011;121:463-7.
28. Luxenberger W, Stammberger H, Jebeles JA, et al. Endoscopic optic nerve decompression: the Graz experience. Laryngoscope. 1998;108:873-82.

CHAPTER

17

Endoscopic Medial Maxillectomy

Alexandra Kejner, Bradford A Woodworth

HISTORY

The technical aspects of the medial maxillectomy procedure have continued to evolve since its introduction in 1826 by Lazars. The original surgical approach was plagued by hemorrhage and infection and it was not until 1927 when the sublabial approach was adopted that it began to gain more popularity. This obviated the large facial incisions that had been used previously. Improvements in technology and anesthetic allowed for further variations on the approach to a medial maxillectomy including the lateral rhinotomy, Weber Ferguson incision, and midfacial degloving.[1] Following the adoption of endoscopic sinus surgery in the 1980s, there was a paradigm shift toward endoscopic resection in select cases of both benign and malignant tumors and even combining endoscopic techniques with open incisions or midfacial degloving procedures.[2-5] There are now a number of modifications of the endoscopic medial maxillectomy, including leaving a remnant of the inferior turbinate and the entire nasolacrimal duct (when possible) to avoid empty nose syndrome and chronic epiphora.[6,7]

INDICATIONS

- Neoplastic processes including inverted papillomas and select malignant neoplasms including squamous cell carcinoma involving the maxilla and lateral nasal wall.
- Invasive fungal sinusitis
- Chronic granulomatous diseases involving the nose and sinuses (the authors prefer postponing this surgery until the patient's granulomatous process is under maximum control in order to maximize healing).
- Chronic maxillary sinusitis refractory to maximum medical management and standard maxillary antrostomy for improved access for topical medications (the authors prefer this technique for recalcitrant cystic fibrosis sinusitis). This is typically in the setting of a "failed maxillary sinus" with chronic mucociliary dysfunction.
- Chronic maxillary sinusitis/mucoceles caused by prolapsed orbital fat from previous medial orbital decompression surgery.[7]

ANATOMY

- The lateral nasal wall includes the inferior turbinate, infundibulum (with maxillary ostium), uncinate process, and nasolacrimal duct.
- The boundaries for a modified medial maxillectomy are the nasolacrimal duct anteriorly, the posterior maxillary wall posteriorly, the nasal floor and inferior turbinate medially, the lateral maxillary wall laterally, the agger nasi and lamina papyracea superiorly and the maxillary sinus floor inferiorly.
- The nasolacrimal duct runs anteriorly in the bony lateral nasal wall and empties into the inferior meatus (Hasner's valve) just below the attachment of the inferior turbinate.
- The inferior turbinate spans the length of the nasal cavity. The majority of the maxillary sinus cavity lies inferior to the superior attachment of the inferior turbinate to the lateral nasal wall. Removing a portion of the inferior turbinate significantly improves exposure of the maxillary sinus.[8]

SURGICAL TECHNIQUES

Preoperative Medical Clearance

Aspirin and Plavix are held at least 7 days prior to surgery if medically allowable. If patients are anticoagulated chronically, medical consultation is warranted prior to surgery. Hypertension issues should be addressed prior to surgery as should any cardiac disease. Underlying chronic rhinosinusitis can be addressed at the first preoperative visit with aggressive medical therapy, including culture-directed antibiotics, steroid taper when appropriate, and topical medications/irrigations. Total intravenous anesthesia has been suggested as a method for decreasing intraoperative blood loss, although evidence is varied in the literature.[9,10]

Imaging

Preoperative imaging is obtained to use in conjunction with the stereotactic surgical navigation system. This consists of computed tomography with fine cuts (0.65–1 mm cuts) of the face/sinuses without contrast. The location of the nasolacrimal duct, dehiscences of the lamina papyracea, and tumor extension/erosion into the nose or through the anterior wall of the maxillary sinus should be noted on preoperative imaging as the anatomy/location of these areas may affect the approaches utilized during surgical intervention and help with patient counseling. Tumor origin and extension should be identified such that the approach matches the exposure required (transseptal, Caldwell-Luc, etc.).

Equipment

- 0°, 30°, and 70° rigid endoscopes
- Stereotactic surgical navigation system[11]
- Curved and straight beaver blades
- J curette
- Suction Freer elevator or Cottle elevator
- Turbinate scissors
- Thru-cut instruments (Blakesley, back-biting, side-biting)
- 15° diamond drill
- Small curved hemostat
- Suction bovie
- Kennedy pack
- Small latex-free glove
- 2-O Prolene suture
- Endoscrub II (Medtronic®, Jacksonville, Fla.).

Medications

- 1:1,000 topical epinephrine is our decongestant/hemostatic agent of choice intraoperatively.[12]
- We do not typically utilize injectable lidocaine with epinephrine unless a septoplasty is performed.

Positioning

- Surgeon is at the right side of the patient
- Video monitor and surgical navigation monitor are on the left of the patient, facing the surgeon.
- The patient is placed in reverse Trendelenburg position to decrease blood loss and improve endoscopic view.[13]
- The endotracheal tube is taped at the left lower lip with the circuit extending down the side of the patient and away from the surgeon's workspace to decrease incidence of unintended extubation.

Intraoperative Technique

Step 1

Orotracheal intubation is undertaken by anesthesia and the tube is secured along the left lower lip. The eyes are protected and topical epinephrine pledgets are placed in the nose. The surgical navigation system is then registered.

Step 2

A rigid 0° endoscope is used to examine the nose and paranasal sinuses. Septoplasty is performed if necessary for improved access. We prefer the endoscopic approach given the ease of visualization with the 0° endoscope and the suction Freer.

Step 3

Uncinectomy or revision of the existing middle meatal antrostomy is then completed.

Step 4

A Freer elevator is used to medialize the inferior turbinate. A small, curved hemostat is clamped to the turbinate posterior to the anterior one third in preparation for cutting the turbinate. By leaving this remnant in place, we decrease the risk of atrophic rhinitis.[14] The clamp is left in place for 30 seconds to improve hemostasis prior to division. A turbinate scissor is used to incise the inferior turbinate several millimeters posterior to the nasolacrimal opening (Fig. 17.1). The remaining posterior stump is cauterized using suction cautery.

Step 5

Incise the mucosa of the nasal floor with a curved beaver blade (Figs. 17.2A and B). This cut extends from the attachment of the inferior turbinate medially toward the septum. The posterior cut begins at the level of the posterior maxillary wall adjacent to the posterior remnant of the inferior turbinate and this is carried to the base of the septum. The flap is elevated using either a Cottle elevator or a suction Freer to tent the mucosa up to allow

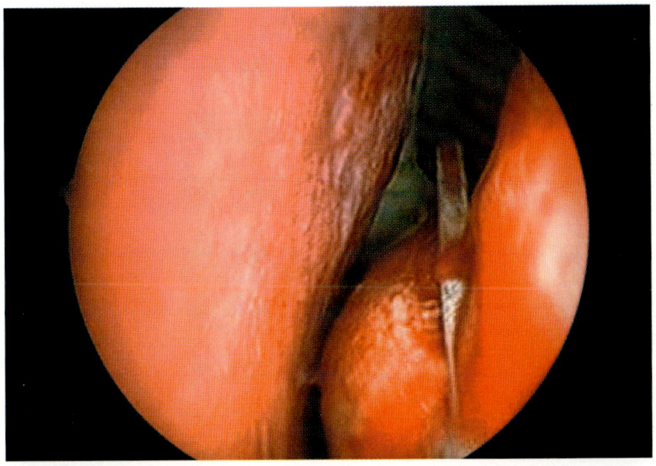

Fig. 17.1: A modified medial maxillectomy is performed for a patient with severe recalcitrant chronic maxillary sinusitis from cystic fibrosis. The inferior turbinate is first clamped then incised with a turbinate scissors just posterior to the anterior third and nasolacrimal duct.

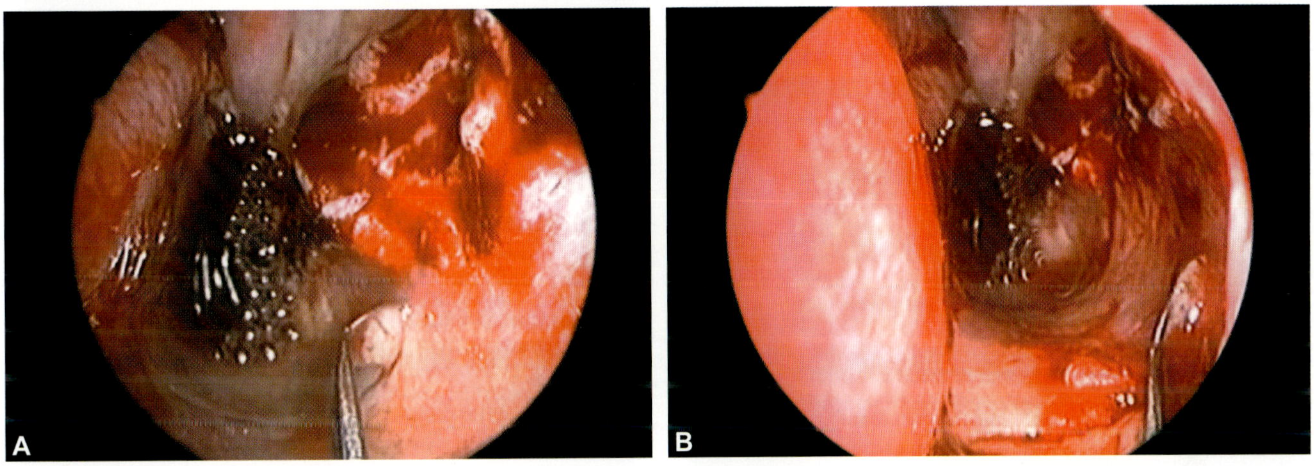

Figs. 17.2A and B: A posterior (A) and anterior (B) incision is made in the nasal floor using a curved beaver blade.

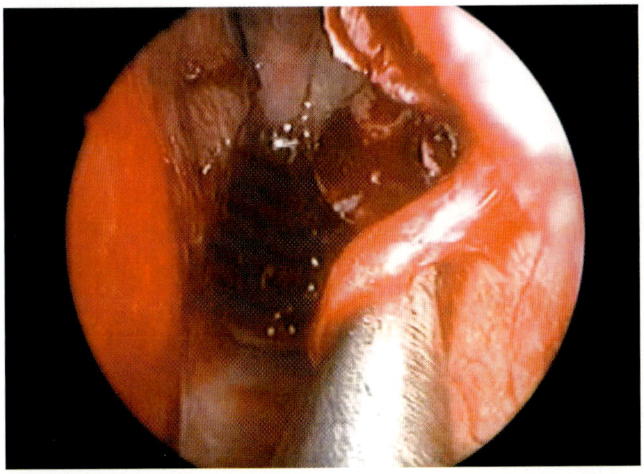

Fig. 17.3: An elevator is used to raise the medially based nasal mucosal floor flap.

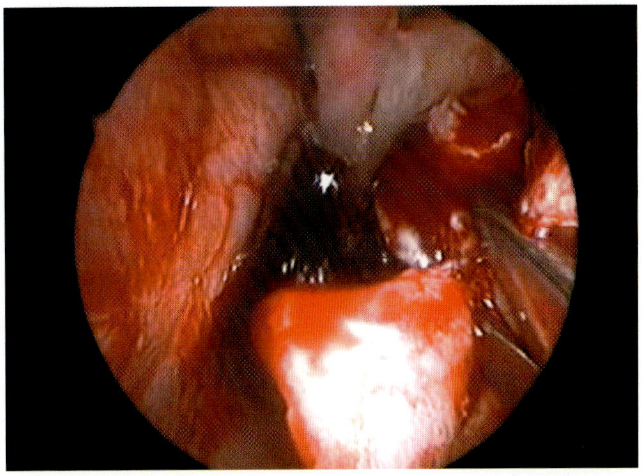

Fig. 17.4: The flap is incised along the wall to provide maximal length.

for the superomedial cut (Fig. 17.3). A turbinate scissor is inserted with the tines straddling the tented mucosa, thus incising the mucosa inferior to the attachment of the inferior turbinate (Fig. 17.4). A longer flap will ultimately

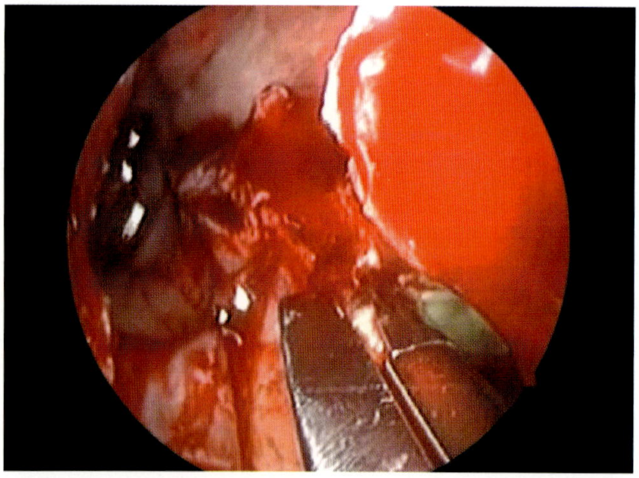

Fig. 17.5: The maxillary wall is opened with a j curette and then taken down with thru-cut forceps.

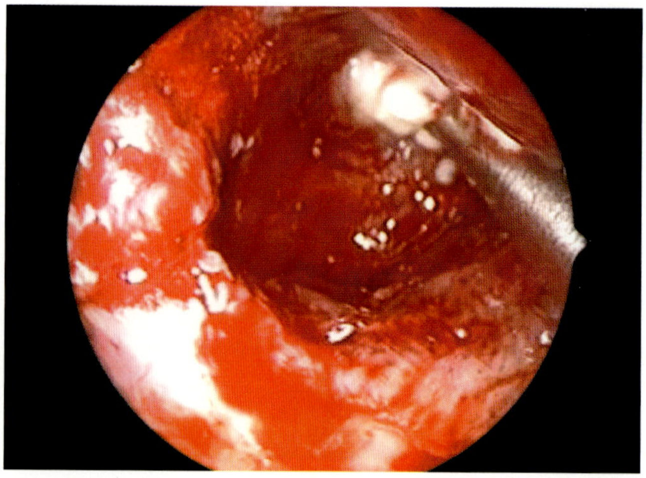

Fig. 17.6: Trapped purulent cystic fibrosis secretions are removed with the curved suction and visualized with a 70° endoscope.

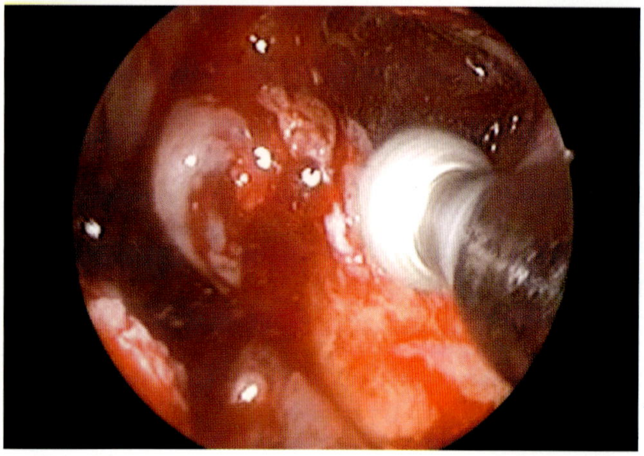

Fig. 17.7: The inferior maxillary wall is drilled flush to the maxillary sinus floor.

allow for more flexibility of the flap itself. Preservation of the mucosal integrity is paramount.

Step 6

After identification of Hasner's valve (inferior to the anterior 1/3 of the inferior turbinate remnant), use a J curette to enter the medial maxillary wall into the maxillary sinus. A backbiter thru-cut forcep extends the opening anteriorly (and inferiorly to Hasner's valve) until the opening is level with the anterior maxillary wall. The nasolacrimal duct is preserved. The posterior aspect is opened using sharp dissection. A Freer reflects the wall medially and an angled thru-cut forcep is used to extend the maxillectomy so that it is flush with the posterior wall (Fig. 17.5).

Step 7

The inferior turbinate and the medial maxillary wall can now be removed en bloc, or, if the inferior turbinate were removed earlier, then the medial maxillary wall and any tumor/inflammatory disease can be removed from the sinus (Fig. 17.6). The posterior inferior turbinate remnant carries the posterolateral nasal artery which should be cauterized to ensure no further bleeding.

Step 8

Drill down the remaining inferior ridge of the medial maxillary wall with a 15 degree diamond bur so that it is flush with the nasal floor (take care to preserve the previously raised mucosal flap) (Fig. 17.7). The mucosal graft is then laid back in place, covering any exposed bony areas (Fig. 17.8) to promote healing (Fig. 17.9). Any remaining tumor/mass is removed. See below for adjuvant approaches.

Special Considerations/ Adjuvant Approaches

- *Dacryocystorhinostomy (DCR)*: This does not have to be performed on every patient. While included in a classical endoscopic medial maxillectomy, this can be avoided unless the duct is directly involved with tumor or additional exposure is required. Surgical technique is described below.
- Many areas of the maxillary sinus can be accessed using angled (70°) endoscopes and instrumentation. When an expansile process such as an odontogenic cyst is encountered, the shift in bony walls of the sinus can increase access to the anterior and inferior maxillary walls (Figs. 17.10A to E).
- *Caldwell-Luc*: Depending on the extent/invasion/attachment of the tumor, it may be necessary to remove the anterior wall via standard Caldwell-Luc approach.

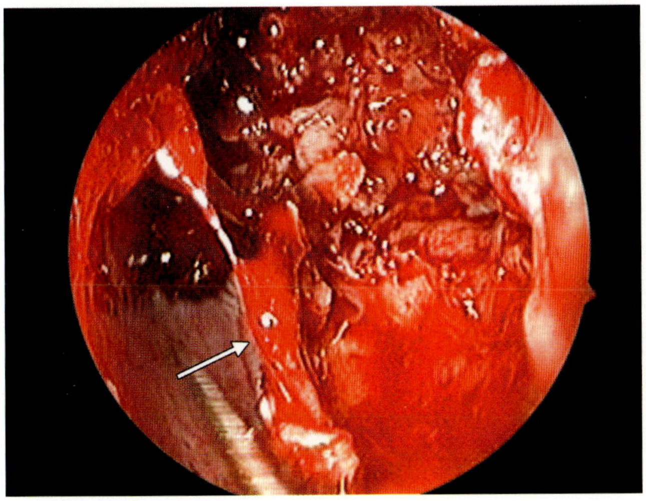

Fig. 17.8: The nasal floor mucosal flap (arrow) is placed over the exposed bone of the inferior maxillary ridge.

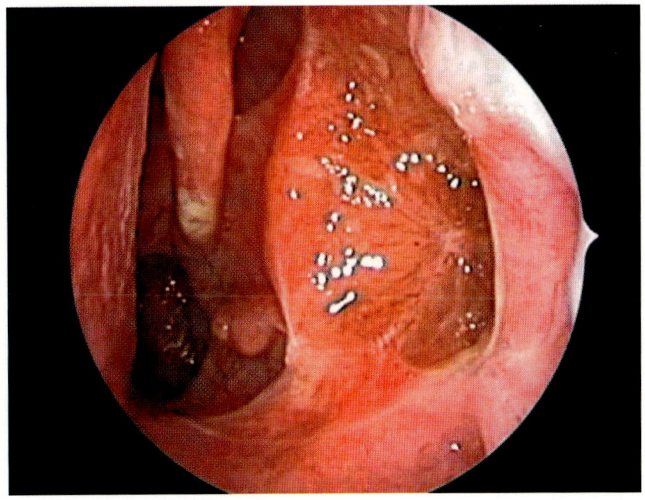

Fig. 17.9: Angled endoscopic view just past the preserved head of the inferior turbinate and nasolacrimal valve shows well healed mucosa with no trapped mucopurulent secretions.

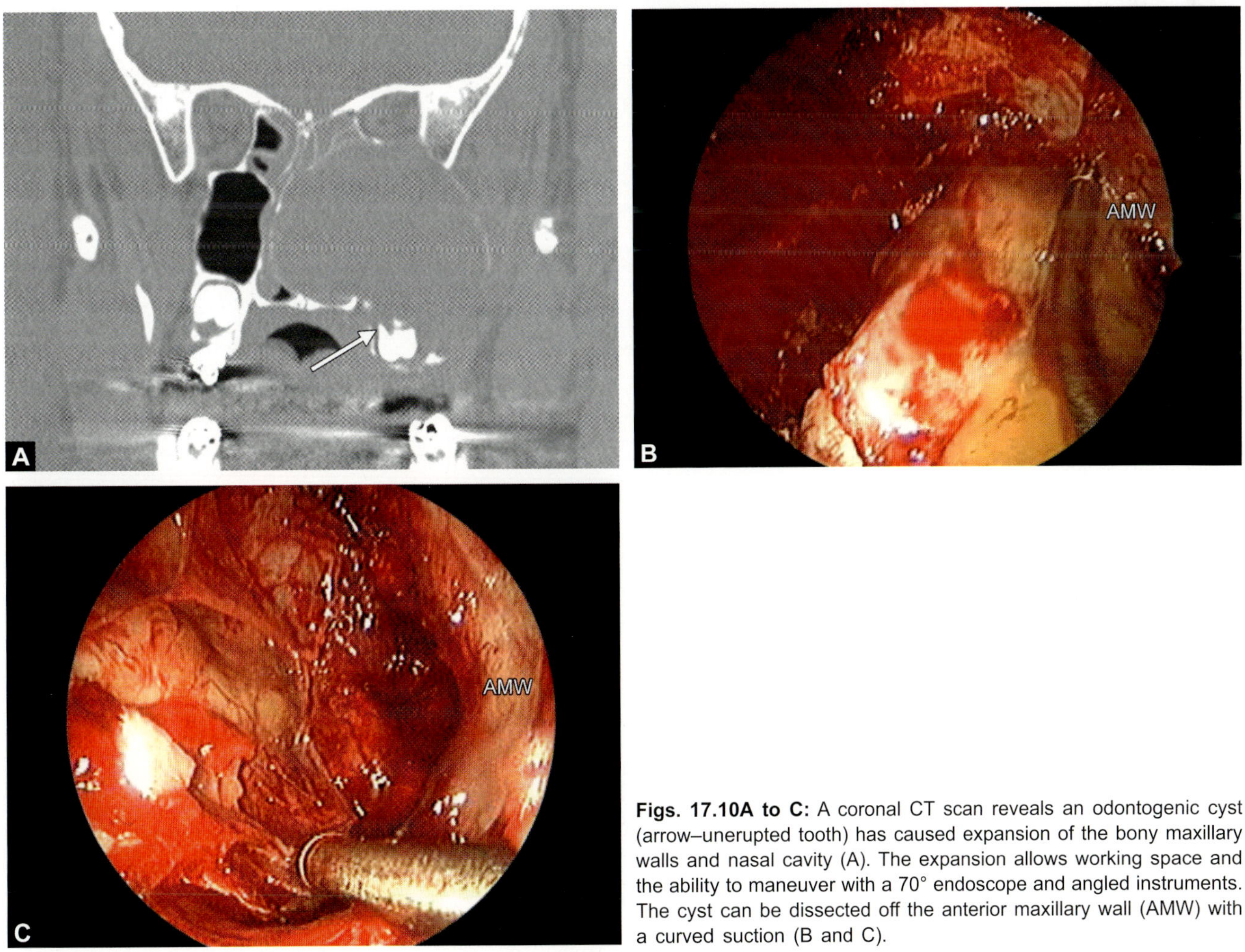

Figs. 17.10A to C: A coronal CT scan reveals an odontogenic cyst (arrow–unerupted tooth) has caused expansion of the bony maxillary walls and nasal cavity (A). The expansion allows working space and the ability to maneuver with a 70° endoscope and angled instruments. The cyst can be dissected off the anterior maxillary wall (AMW) with a curved suction (B and C).

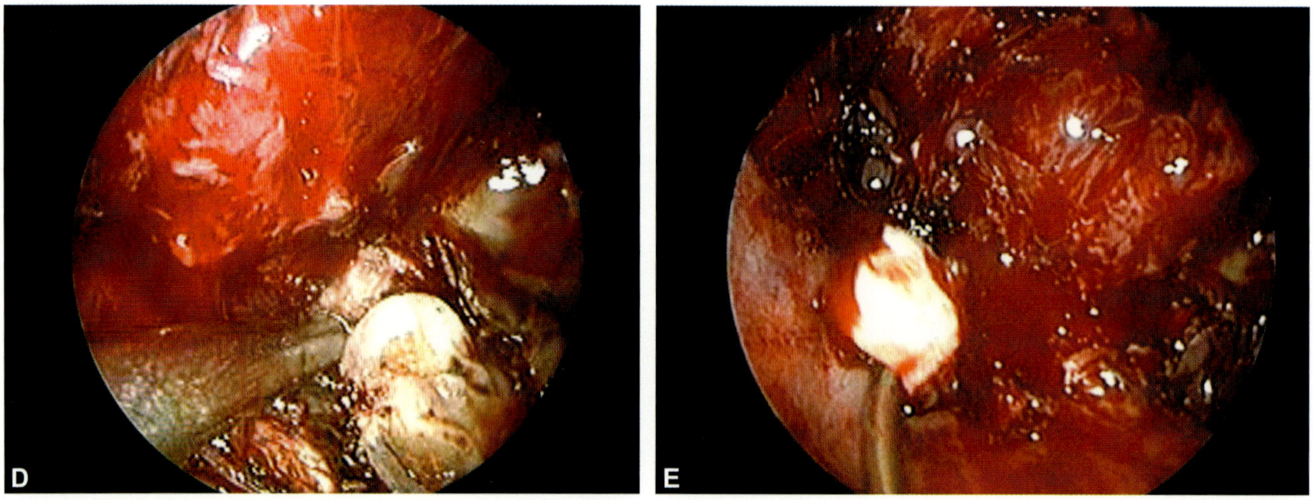

Figs. 17.10D and E: Even the impacted tooth is removed transnasally without an open procedure.

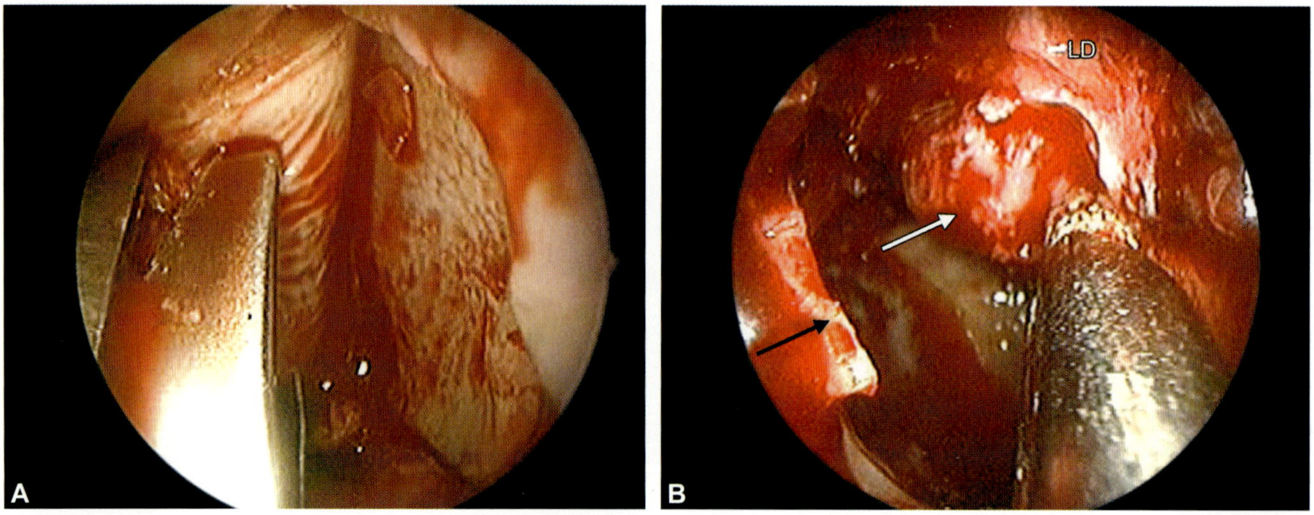

Figs. 17.11A and B: A posteriorly based nasoseptal flap is raised on the right (contralateral) side (A). A cartilage window (black arrow) is incised with intact mucosa on the ipsilateral side allowing complete visualization of the anterior maxillary wall where an inverted papilloma (white arrow) is pedicled (LD-lacrimal duct) (B).

- Multiple variations of the endoscopic medial maxillectomy can increase access to difficult areas of the maxillary sinus, for example, lateral maxillary wall and anterior maxillary wall.
- Anteriorly, the medial buttress of the medial maxillary wall may be completely removed and if needed, the nasolacrimal duct sacrificed. Postoperatively, these patients should undergo DCR +/- stenting in order to prevent stenosis and epiphora.
- If necessary, the inferior turbinate can be completely resected to allow for improved visualization. Patients may have an increased risk of empty nose syndrome (loss of the sensation of air movement causing paradoxical sensation of nasal obstruction[6]) or atrophic rhinitis.
- A canine fossa puncture can create an auxiliary site through which to pass an endoscope or other instruments (microdebriders, etc.).[15]
- For better visualization, a transseptal approach improves access. This is useful for resection of tumors located on the anterior and lateral maxillary wall.

Transseptal Approach

- Lidocaine 1% with epinephrine is infiltrated into the contralateral nostril. A hemitransfixion incision is made.
- A posteriorly based nasoseptal flap is then elevated off of the septal cartilage (Fig. 17.11A).

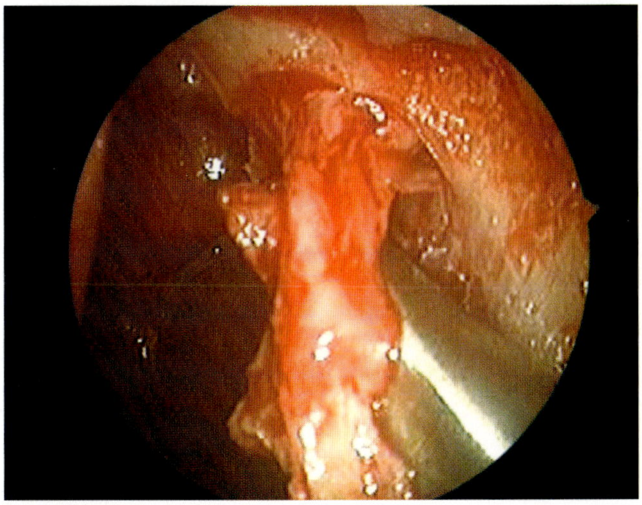

Fig. 17.12: The nasolacrimal duct is completely mobilized up to the lacrimal sac to allow a reliable superior margin for pathology.

- A septal window is incised in a fashion large enough to accommodate two instruments at one time at the level of the contralateral head of the inferior turbinate (Fig. 17.11B). The resulting composite cartilage/mucosal flap is within the border of the nasoseptal flap so that no incisions are in opposition. The nasoseptal flap is stitched anteriorly and flaps quilted with a chromic suture at the completion of the resection.[16]

Dacryocystorhinostomy

- After obtaining exposure of the lacrimal area, the bone is removed with a drill, a rongeur or a Kerrison around the entire length of the duct and sac.
- Once the bone has been removed, the lacrimal sac is then identified and incised. The medial portion is then removed. With tumors, it is useful to skeletonize the entire duct up to the sac so that a reliable margin may be sent to pathology (Fig. 17.12).Removal is confirmed by flooding the eye with saline and checking for free flow into the dacryocystorhinostomy.
- Silicone stents may be placed according to surgeon's preference.[17]

REFERENCES

1. McGuirt W. Maxillectomy. Otolaryngol Clin North Am. 1995;28:1175-89.
2. Day TA, Beas RA, Schlosser RJ, et al. Management of paranasal sinus malignancy. Curr Treat Options Oncol. 2005;6:3-18.
3. Woodworth BA, Bhargave GA, Palmer JN, et al. Clinical outcomes of endoscopic and endoscopic-assisted resection of inverted papillomas: a 15-year experience. Am J Rhinol. 2007;21:591-600.
4. Kostrzewa JP, Sunde J, Riley KO, et al. Radiofrequency coblation decreases blood loss during endoscopic sinonasal and skull base tumor removal. ORL J Otorhinolaryngol Relat Spec. 2010;72:38-43.
5. Blount A, Riley KO, Woodworth BA. Juvenile nasopharyngeal angiofibroma. Otolaryngol Clin North Am. 2011;44:989-1004, ix.
6. Scheithauer M. Surgery of the turbinates and "empty nose" syndrome. GMS Curr Top Otorhinolaryngol Head Neck Surg. 2011;9.
7. Woodworth BA PR, Schlosser RJ. Modified endoscopic medial maxillectomy for chronic maxillary sinusitis. Am J Rhinol. 2006;20:317-9.
8. Tanna N, Edwards JD, Aghdam H, et al. Transnasal endoscopic medial maxillectomy as the initial oncologic approach to sinonasal neoplasms: the anatomic basis. Arch Otolaryngol Head Neck Surg. 2007;133:1139-42.
9. Ragab SM, Hassanin MZ. Optimizing the surgical field in pediatric functional endoscopic sinus surgery: a new evidence-based approach. Otolaryngol Head Neck Surg. 2010;142:48-54.
10. Chaaban MR, Baroody FM, Gottlieb O, et al. Blood loss during endoscopic sinus surgery with propofol or sevoflurane: a randomized clinical trial. JAMA Otolaryngol Head Neck Surg. 2013;139:510-4.
11. Gunkel AR, Freysinger W, Thumfart WF. Experience with various 3-dimensional navigation systems in head and neck surgery. Arch Otolaryngol Head Neck Surg. 2000;126:390-5.
12. Higgins TS, Hwang PH, Kingdom TT, et al. Systematic review of topical vasoconstrictors in endoscopic sinus surgery. Laryngoscope. 2011;121:422-32.
13. Hathorn IF, Habib AR, Manji J, et al. Comparing the reverse Trendelenburg and horizontal position for endoscopic sinus surgery: a randomized controlled trial. Otolaryngol Head Neck Surg. 2013;148:308-13.
14. Virgin F, Rowe SM, Wade MB, et al. Extensive surgical and comprehensive postoperative medical management for severe, recalcitrant cystic fibrosis chronic rhinosinusitis. Am J Rhinol Allergy. 2012;26.
15. Wormald PJ, Ooi E, van Hasselt CA, et al. Endoscopic removal of sinonasal inverted papilloma including endoscopic medial maxillectomy. Laryngoscope. 2003;113:867-73.
16. Harvey RJ, Sheehan PO, Debnath NI, et al. Transseptal approach for extended endoscopic resections of the maxilla and infratemporal fossa. Am J Rhinol Allergy. 2009;23:426-32.
17. Syed MI, Head EJ, Madurska M, et al. Endoscopic Primary dacryocystorhinostomy: Are silicone tubes needed? Clin Otolaryngol. 2013;38:406-10.

CHAPTER

18

Endoscopic Control of Epistaxis

Dane M Barrett, Spencer C Payne

PHILOSOPHY AND APPROACH

Epistaxis is one of the most common otolaryngologic emergencies. In the majority of circumstances, the source of the bleeding is anterior and can be easily managed by direct pressure alone, or through various methods and maneuvers in the clinic or emergency department. Rarely does epistaxis require management beyond these settings.

Failure of these conservative measures often suggests a more posterior source, which occurs in about 5% of cases.[1] In these scenarios, the goal shifts from one of definitive management to that of patient stabilization and temporization of bleeding. This is typically accomplished via placement of temporary nasal packing. The patient may then be transferred to the operating room or interventional radiology suite for definitive control of epistaxis. Traditional practice consisted of inpatient admission and observation; however, this approach has fallen out of favor because of the disadvantages of prolonged hospital stays and increased morbidity.

Definitive interventions generically fall into nonsurgical, endoscopic, or open surgical approaches. The definitive nonsurgical approach consists of percutaneous transarterial embolization of the major feeding vessels. Open approaches consist of the Caldwell-Luc approach to the internal maxillary artery and lynch incision for access to the anterior and posterior ethmoid arteries. Both of these approaches, as with conservative management are associated with increased patient morbidity.[2,3] Enhancements in endoscopic instrumentation and techniques offer excellent visualization with minimal surgical dissection and associated morbidity. As most sources of posterior epistaxis are supplied by branches of the sphenopalatine artery, endoscopic sphenopalatine artery ligation has become a first line therapy.

This chapter will focus on both endoscopic ligation of the sphenopalatine artery and the external approach to the anterior and posterior ethmoid arteries. These are the most common approaches to the major nasal vessels responsible for refractory epistaxis. For discussion on management strategies and algorithms for epistaxis, the reader should refer to other texts.

PREOPERATIVE CONSIDERATIONS

Initial efforts should be focused on ensuring adequate control of bleeding. This should be accomplished prior to bringing the patient to the operating room and can usually be achieved by placement of nasal packing. There are several types of packs available and discussion of the merits of each is beyond the scope of this chapter. Once hemostasis is achieved, the patient should be appropriately stabilized prior to transport to the operating room. Special attention should be given to correcting coagulopathy or hypertension if present.

Once in the operating room, setup and patient positioning is identical to the basic functional endoscopic sinus surgery (FESS) setup discussed in Chapter 9. Bipolar cautery should be part of the standard setup, although it is up to the surgeon to ensure it is available. Hemostatic clip appliers are often necessary to ligate the sphenopalatine artery and its branches. These should also be immediately available if the need arises.

Appropriate patient positioning is crucial to improving the surgical field and reducing intraoperative blood loss. As previously noted, elevating the head of bed or reverse Trendelenburg to an angle of 20-30 degrees decreases central venous pressure. Keeping the central venous pressure low can reduce both venous and capillary bleeding.[4]

Discussion with anesthesia to avoid general anesthetic in favor of total intravenous anesthesia may decrease intraoperative blood loss and improve the surgical field.[5,6] The benefits for TIVA in favor of inhalational agents, however, remain controversial.[7,8] Regardless, clear communication with anesthesiology personnel regarding the operative plan is important.

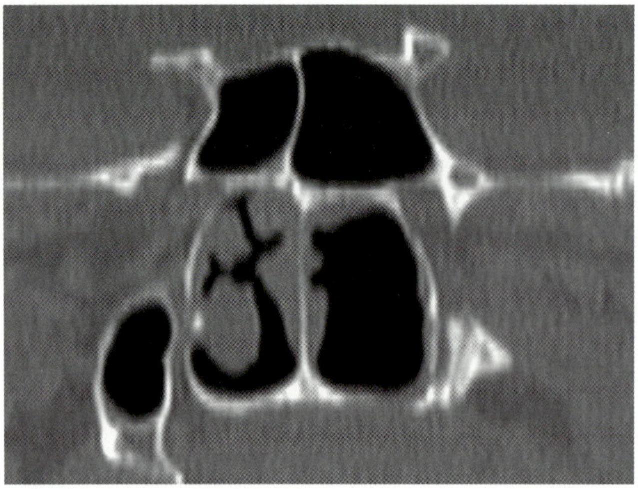

Fig. 18.1: Greater palatine foramen—The foramen can be seen here on the right side of the picture exiting just medial to the alveolus.

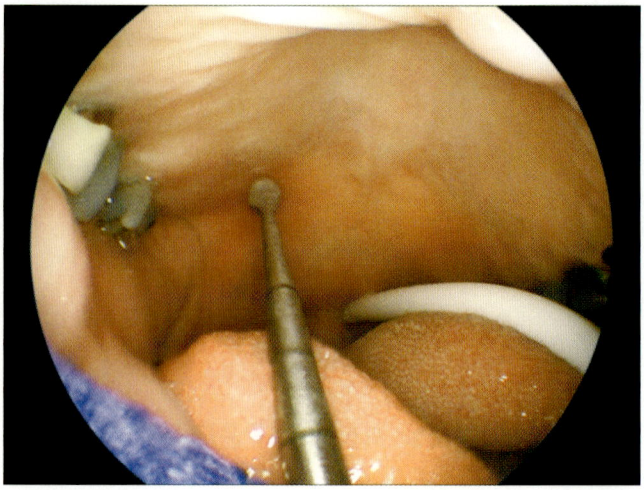

Fig. 18.2: Greater palatine foramen, oral view—Palpation medial to the third molar site anterior to the posterior portion of the hard palate will generally locate a depression, which indicates the site of the foramen (seen just lateral to the head of the elevator).

One maneuver that has been shown to significantly reduce intraoperative bleeding and improve visualization is the infiltration of the pterygopalatine fossa with a vasoconstricting agent.[9] The greater palatine foramen is posteromedial to the third maxillary molar and anteromedial to the maxillary tuberosity and pterygoid hamulus (Fig. 18.1). Practically, the foramen can be found by finger palpation. The junction of the hard and soft palate is found, then the finger is slid anteriorly along the midpoint between the teeth and midline until a depression is felt (Fig. 18.2).

Once the foramen is palpated, a 27 ga spinal needle is inserted through the mucosa and into the greater palatine foramen advancing the needle up the greater palatine canal into the inferior aspect of the pterygopalatine fossa. Maintaining the needle low in the pterygopalatine fossa reduces the risk of intraarterial injection into the internal maxillary artery or anesthesia of the V2. To avoid complication the needle is bent to an angle of 45° 25 mm from the tip and inserted until the bend is reached. Two milliliters of 1% lidocaine with 1:100,000 epinephrine is infiltrated. The distance of the bend is based on the average length of the greater palatine canal in the adult white population as determined in prior studies.[10,11]

If a Lynch incision is planned to control the anterior ethmoid artery, a vasoconstrictive agent should be infiltrated where the incision is planned. Corneal protection should be ensured with an ophthalmic lubricating ointment. Tarsorraphy or steristrips to tape the upper lid to the cheek after sterile preparation can be used to prevent inadvertent corneal abrasion.

If possible, the nasal cavity should also be decongested with nasal pledgets soaked in oxymetazoline. This may not be possible prior to the initiation of the procedure as removal of the nasal packing may result in the reinitiation of profuse bleeding before the surgeon is prepared for definitive management.

ENDOSCOPIC LIGATION OF THE SPHENOPALATINE ARTERY

Basic Concept and Anatomic Considerations

The sphenopalatine artery is a terminal branch of the internal maxillary artery and is the dominant source of posterior nasal blood flow supplying 90% of the nasal mucosa.[12] The sphenopalatine artery emerges from the sphenopalatine foramen to enter the nose. The sphenopalatine foramen is located between the basal lamella of the middle turbinate and the basal lamella of the superior turbinate in the superior meatus. The artery divides into a number of smaller branches. These include the posterior septal nasal artery and the lateral nasal artery. The posterior septal nasal artery travels medially across the sphenoid rostrum inferior to the sphenoid ostium. The lateral nasal artery courses along the lateral nasal wall and is its major blood supply. The sphenopalatine artery may branch prior to exiting the sphenopalatine foramen in up to 16–42% of cases resulting in branches exiting through a separate bony foramina.[13,14] This should be recognized and addressed intraoperatively.

The crista ethmoidalis is an important landmark for identifying the sphenopalatine foramen. The crista ethmoidalis is the fibrous attachment of the middle turbinate basal lamella to the ascending palatine bone. It is a small crest of bone that lies just anterior to the sphenopalatine artery (SPA) and is located within 1 mm of the foramen.[15] It is a useful aid to help identify the sphenopalatine foramen.

Endoscopic ligation of the sphenopalatine artery has distinct advantages over other approaches. It is minimally invasive, targeted, and effective. In a series of 127 patients, endoscopic SPA ligation resulted in control of epistaxis in 98% of patients with no significant complication.[16] It allows for interruption of nasal vasculature at a distal point, preventing retrograde and anastomotic blood flow from ipsilateral or contralateral carotid systems.[17] It also avoids complications associated with manipulation of the pterygopalatine fossa, which may be seen in the Caldwell-Luc approach to the internal maxillary artery (IMAX).[18] Endoscopic SPA ligation also reduces the potential for intraorbital and intracranial complications, which may be seen with angiographic embolization or Caldwell-Luc approach.[19]

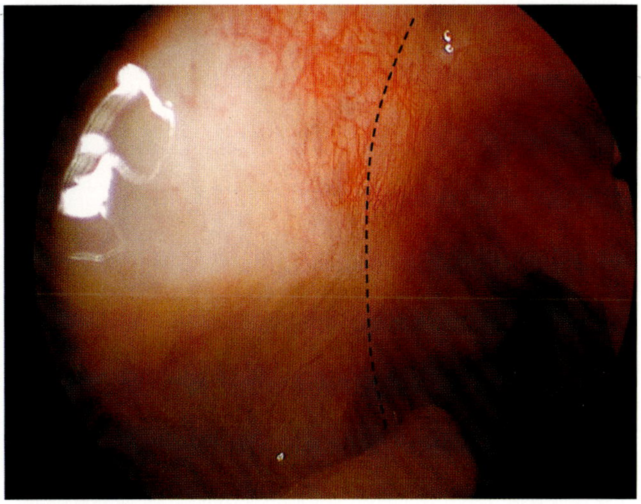

Fig. 18.3: Incision on lateral wall—A posterior-based flap via a curvilinear incision is made (broken line) to allow for dissection on the posterior medial maxillary sinus wall.

Surgical Steps

- The nasal packing is removed if present and pledgets soaked in oxymetazoline are placed into the nasal cavity. This may be done once the airway is established prior to patient positioning and preparation to allow time for full decongestive effect.
- The lateral nasal wall is infiltrated with 1% lidocaine with 1:100,000 epinephrine along the inferoposterior aspect of the middle turbinate. The posterior septum should also be infiltrated where the septum meets the inferior sphenoid rostrum. This should enhance vasoconstriction of the posterior nasal septal branch of the SPA.
- The middle turbinate may be medialized with the blunt end of a freer to improve visualization and access to the posterior nasal cavity.
- The membranous posterior fontanelle of the maxillary sinus is palpated with a sinus seeker or right-angled suction tip. The tip is advanced posteriorly until the junction between the fontanelle and palatine bone is located.
- An incision is made with a #15 blade beginning at the inferior surface of the horizontal portion of the basal lamella to just above the insertion of the inferior turbinate. The incision should be carried down through periosteum with posterior limbs at the inferior and superior aspects of the flap. This allows for the creation of a posteriorly based flap (Fig. 18.3).
- Uncinectomy and/or maxillary antrostomy may improve exposure and are performed if necessary.
- Cottle or suction elevator is used to raise a posteriorly based flap from the insertion of the inferior turbinate onto the sphenoid rostrum. It is important to maintain the elevator hard on bone during the dissection to ensure the flap is raised in a subperiostial plane. Staying low during flap elevation reduce the risk of inadvertent injury to the SPA.
- The crista ethmoidalis should be identified anterior/anteroinferior to the sphenopalatine artery at the sphenopalatine foramen (Figs. 18.4A and B). This crest may need to be taken down with a Kerrison rongeur or curette to access the sphenopalatine foramen. The SPA can usually be seen tenting up during the course of the flap elevation.
- The SPA pedicle is identified and freed from the surrounding mucosa circumferentially. This should be done with a blunt instrument such as a maxillary seeker or other ball-tip probe (Fig. 18.5).
- Once the SPA is adequately exposed, two hemoclips should be placed on the artery with care to ensure that the clips are placed around the entire pedicle (Fig. 18.6).
- The area should be inspected to ensure there is not another branch of the SPA leaving through a separate foramen. This may require a hemoclip, but can usually be cauterized with bipolar (Fig. 18.7).
- The flap is gently replaced and can be bolstered with an absorbable dressing.

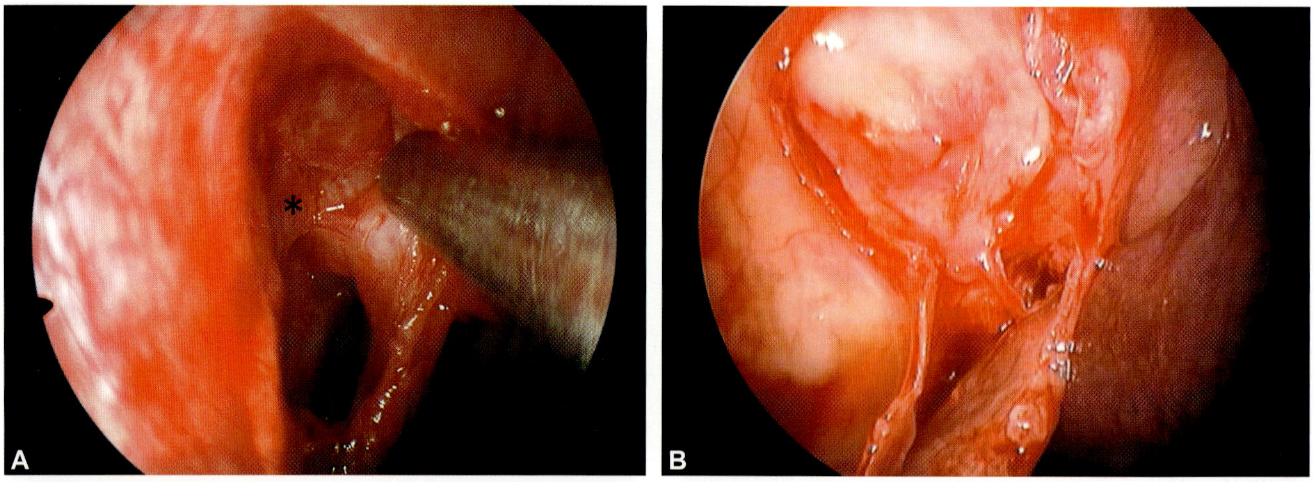

Figs. 18.4A and B: Crista ethmoidalis—This medial projection of bone (asterisk) identifies the site of the SPA and can be removed with rongeurs to better access the vasculature.

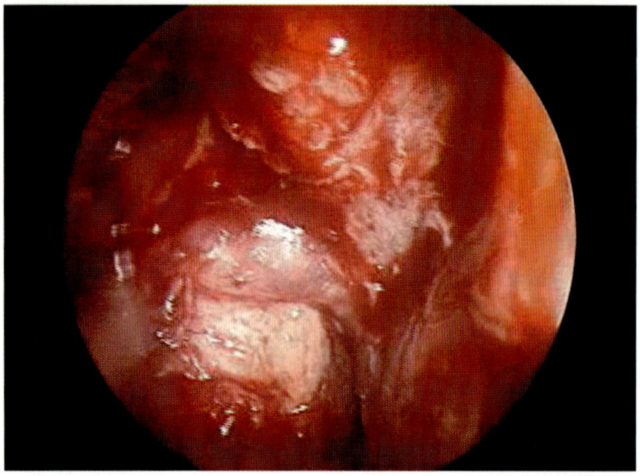

Fig. 18.5: Sphenopalatine artery—The artery is noted to course from lateral to medial in the soft tissue behind the crista ethmoidalis, here it exits the foramen as a single vessel. (Photo courtesy of Bradford Woodworth, MD).

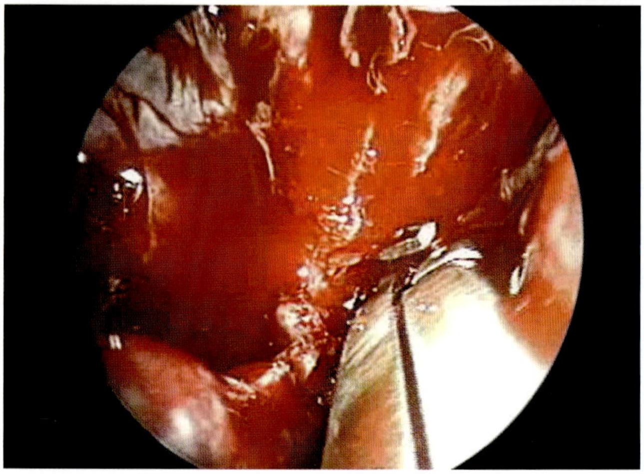

Fig. 18.6: Clipping the artery—Small hemostatic clips are placed, one proximal and one distal to ensure adequacy of ligation. Here, a clip is seen medial to (left of) the applier. (Photo courtesy of Bradford Woodworth, MD).

EXTERNAL LIGATION OF THE ANTERIOR AND POSTERIOR ETHMOID ARTERIES

Basic Concept and Anatomic Considerations

Epistaxis from the anterior and posterior ethmioid arteries is uncommon and is typically seen in patients during or following FESS, or patients who have suffered facial trauma and associated skull base fractures. In the former, if return to the operating room (OR) or theatre is necessary, the initial goal should be to control the bleeding intranasally if possible. In the latter, intranasal approach is not expedient as the dissection has not been previously accomplished.

Both anterior and posterior ethmoid arteries are derived from the internal carotid system and are branches of the ophthalmic artery. The anterior ethmoid artery courses between the superior oblique and medial rectus (Fig. 18.8) to enter the nose through the anterior ethmoid foramen, which typically lies between the second and third ethmoturbinal derivatives (posterior to the ethmoid bulla and either anterior or involved with the basal lamella of the middle turbinate). Once in the nose, the anterior ethmoid artery may lie in a mesentery or remain in the skull base depending on the degree of ethmoid pnuematization and the height of the lateral lamella.[20,21]

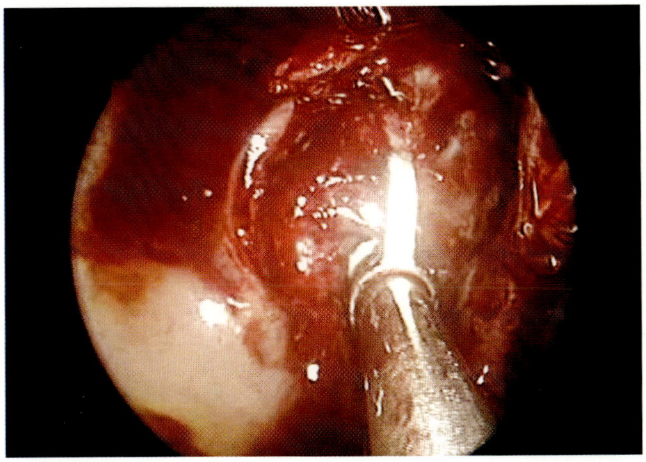

Fig. 18.7: Cauterization of the SPA—Bipolar cautery can be utilized, either in lieu of or in addition to, clip ligation of the artery. (Photo courtesy of Bradford Woodworth, MD).

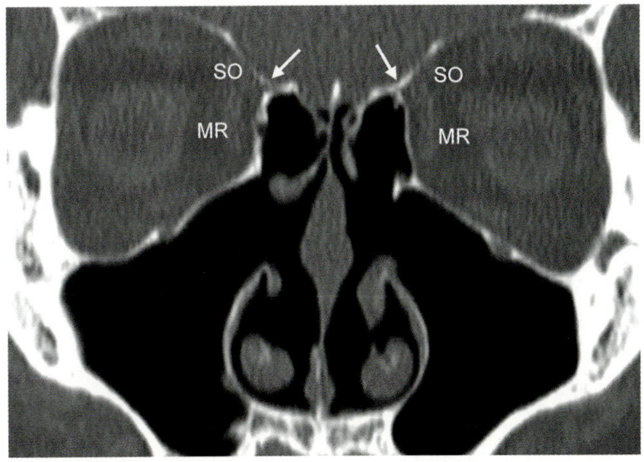

Fig. 18.8: Anterior ethmoid artery—The anterior ethmoid artery (arrows) courses between the superior oblique (SO) and medial rectus (MR) muscles. The projection of bone along the medial orbital wall often appears like a beak and can be used for preoperative identification of the structure.

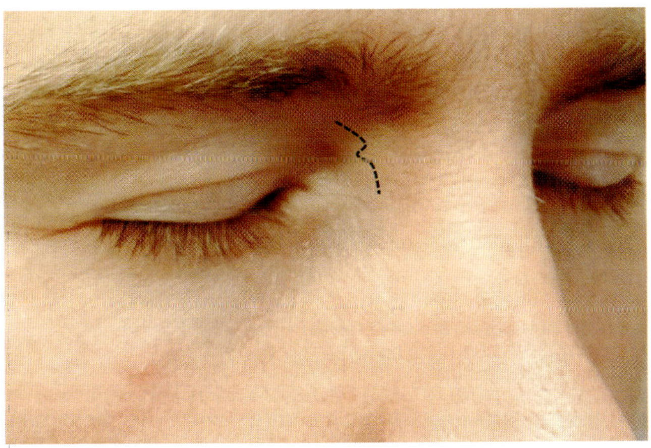

Fig. 18.9: Modified Lynch incision—Use of a pediatric endoscope allows for the utilization of a smaller incision and keeping away from the medial canthus. A broken line can be used to minimize the webbing that may occur with scar contracture.

Externally, the anterior ethmoid artery is approximately 24 mm posterior to the anterior lacrimal crest and lies along the frontoethmoidal suture line. The posterior ethmoid artery is smaller in caliber and less clinically significant. It is found along the roof of the skull base at the junction of the sphenoid and posterior ethmoid sinuses.

Surgical Steps

- A Lynch incision is made with a #15 blade along the superomedial orbital wall in the skin between the medial junction of the upper and lower lids and the nasal dorsum. The incision is curvilinear and is typically about 2.5–3 cm in length. Alternatively, a much smaller incision can be utilized of 1.5–2 cm (Fig. 18.9) when visualization is aided with a 2.7 mm pediatric endoscope.
- Dissection is carried down to the periosteum, which is incised. Often, the distal angular artery or a branch is encountered and requires cauterization.
- Dissection proceeds with a Cottle or Freer elevator in a subperiostal plane. A small malleable retractor to improve exposure during dissection is helpful.
- The anterior lacrimal crest and nasolacrimal sac are identified.
- Release of the medial canthal tendon may be required to aid exposure and allow easier access to the anterior ethmoid and posterior ethmoid arteries. This is usually not necessary when the modified incision is utilized.
- Dissection continues posteriorly along the medial orbital wall along the frontoethmoidal suture line. The anterior ethmoid artery is identified approximately 24 mm posterior to the anterior lacrimal crest. The posterior ethmoid artery is approximately another 12 mm posterior to the anterior ethmoid artery.
- Small hemoclip applier or endoscopic bipolar electrocautery is used to ligate the involved vessel(s).
- The medial canthal tendon is repositioned and secured to the cut end adherent to the periosteum if previously released.
- The wound is closed in layers with reapproximation of the periosteum, dermis, and epidermis. We prefer the use of absorbable suture (6-0 fast-absorbing gut) for the cutaneous closure.

POSTOPERATIVE CONSIDERATIONS

Patients who have been kept in the hospital secondary to significant bleeding may be discharged immediately or watched overnight to confirm resolution of symptoms depending on overall stability. Otherwise, elective procedures for recurrent epistaxis can be treated as any other endoscopic sinus case. Saline irrigations, as in other surgeries, are employed and useful for recovery.

CONCLUSIONS

The vast majority of epistaxis is anterior and is most commonly seen along Little's area. In the rare case of refractory epistaxis of posterior origin, SPA ligation is a highly effective method with minimal morbidity. The majority of posterior nasal bleeds may be treated effectively by this method. The main reason for failure is the lack of control of all the branches of the SPA. There may be up to 3 or more branches, which may exit through separate foramina. Another source of failure may be bleeding from the anterior or posterior ethmoid arteries, which when necessary, may be handled via completely open or endoscopically assisted.

REFERENCES

1. Douglas R, Wormald PJ. Update on epistaxis. Curr Opin Otolaryngol Head Neck Surg. 2007;15(3):180-3. doi: 10.1097/MOO.0b013e32814b06ed [doi].
2. Metson R, Lane R. Internal maxillary artery ligation for epistaxis: An analysis of failures. Laryngoscope. 1988;98(7): 760-4. doi: 10.1288/00005537-198807000-00015 [doi].
3. Snyderman CH, Goldman SA, Carrau RL, et al. Endoscopic sphenopalatine artery ligation is an effective method of treatment for posterior epistaxis. Am J Rhinol. 1999; 13(2): 137-40.
4. Timperley D, Sacks R, Parkinson RJ, et al. Perioperative and intraoperative maneuvers to optimize surgical outcomes in skull base surgery. Otolaryngol Clin North Am. 2010; 43(4):699-730. doi: 10.1016/j.otc.2010.04.002 [doi].
5. Manola M, De Luca E, Moscillo L, et al. Using remifentanil and sufentanil in functional endoscopic sinus surgery to improve surgical conditions. ORL J Otorhinolaryngol Relat Spec. 2005;67(2):83-6. doi: 84576 [pii].
6. Blackwell KE, Ross DA, Kapur P, et al. Propofol for maintenance of general anesthesia: A technique to limit blood loss during endoscopic sinus surgery. Am J Otolaryngol. 1993;14(4):262-6.
7. Chaaban MR, Baroody FM, Gottlieb O, et al. Blood loss during endoscopic sinus surgery with propofol or sevoflurane: A randomized clinical trial. JAMA Otolaryngol Head Neck Surg. 2013;139(5):510-4. doi: 10.1001/jamaoto.2013.2885 [doi].
8. Wormald PJ, van Renen G, Perks J, et al. The effect of the total intravenous anesthesia compared with inhalational anesthesia on the surgical field during endoscopic sinus surgery. Am J Rhinol. 2005;19(5):514-20.
9. Wormald PJ, Athanasiadis T, Rees G, et al. An evaluation of effect of pterygopalatine fossa injection with local anesthetic and adrenalin in the control of nasal bleeding during endoscopic sinus surgery. Am J Rhinol. 2005;19(3):288-92.
10. Douglas R, Wormald PJ. Pterygopalatine fossa infiltration through the greater palatine foramen: Where to bend the needle. Laryngoscope. 2006;116(7):1255-7. doi: 10.1097/01.mlg.0000226005.43817.a2 [doi].
11. Hassmann H. Form, Mabe und Verlaufe der Schä delkanäle. Clinical anatomy of the nose, nasal cavity and paranasal sinuses. In: Lang J. Vol 114. New York: Thieme Medical Publishers; 1989. p. 114.
12. Babin E, Moreau S, de Rugy MG, et al.. Anatomic variations of the arteries of the nasal fossa. Otolaryngol Head Neck Surg. 2003;128(2):236-9. doi: 10.1067/mhn.2003.84 [doi].
13. Schwartzbauer HR, Shete M, Tami TA. Endoscopic anatomy of the sphenopalatine and posterior nasal arteries: Implications for the endoscopic management of epistaxis. Am J Rhinol. 2003;17(1):63-6.
14. Wareing MJ, Padgham ND. Osteologic classification of the sphenopalatine foramen. Laryngoscope. 1998;108(1 Pt 1): 125-7.
15. Simmen DB, Raghavan U, Briner HR, et al. The anatomy of the sphenopalatine artery for the endoscopic sinus surgeon. Am J Rhinol. 2006;20(5):502-5.
16. Kumar S, Shetty A, Rockey J, et al. Contemporary surgical treatment of epistaxis. what is the evidence for sphenopalatine artery ligation? Clin Otolaryngol Allied Sci. 2003;28(4): 360-3. doi: 724 [pii].
17. Leong SC, Roe RJ, Karkanevatos A. No frills management of epistaxis. Emerg Med J. 2005;22(7):470-2. doi: 22/7/470 [pii].
18. Winstead W. Sphenopalatine artery ligation: An alternative to internal maxillary artery ligation for intractable posterior epistaxis. Laryngoscope. 1996;106(5 Pt 1):667-9.
19. Pothier DD, Mackeith S, Youngs R. Sphenopalatine artery ligation: Technical note. J Laryngol Otol. 2005;119(10):810-2. doi: 10.1258/002221505774481354 [doi].
20. Floreani SR, Nair SB, Switajewski MC, et al. Endoscopic anterior ethmoidal artery ligation: A cadaver study. Laryngoscope. 2006;116(7):1263-7. doi: 10.1097/01.mlg.0000221967.67003.1d [doi].
21. Lannoy-Penisson L, Schultz P, Riehm S, et al. The anterior ethmoidal artery: Radio-anatomical comparison and its application in endonasal surgery. Acta Otolaryngol. 2007; 127(6):618-22. doi: 778652548 [pii].

Section 4

Management of Nasal Tumors

Chapters

CHAPTER

19 Surgical Care for Sinus and Nasal Papillomas

Mohamad R Chaaban, Bradford A Woodworth

INTRODUCTION

Papillomas are one of the most common benign sinonasal tumors.[1] Hyams[2] classified papillomas into three types according to their histopathological features and their malignant potential. The two most common forms are the fungiform and the schneiderian or inverted types. Inverted papillomas (IP) have characteristic invaginated epithelium that progresses from the outlining Schneiderian respiratory mucosa to the underlying stroma.[2,3] The fungiform subtype usually arises from the septum and has an exophytic growth pattern. Cylindrical cell papillomas originate from the lateral nasal sinus wall similar to IPs and have a mixed pathology of bright pink granular columellar cells with microcysts mixed with inverted epithelium. Although some authors have regarded these papillomas as distinct entities,[4] others have considered them as hybrid lesions.[2,5,6] Since papillomas are treated in identical fashion with surgical excision, this chapter will generally refer to the management of the inverted type by convention.

Most IPs are unilateral; however, bilateral tumors have been reported.[7] A common feature of IPs is skull base erosion, which may be seen in as high as 75% of patients. However, this does not indicate conversion to malignancy as squamous cell carcinoma is only detected in 10% of cases.[8] Intracranial extension with or without dural involvement is also possible with IPs, but is usually only present in recurrent disease or conversion to malignancy.[9-12]

The exact etiology of IPs is still widely unknown; however, roles for allergy, chronic sinusitis, viral infections, and inflammation have been suggested.[13-15] Stepwise staging for IP grades range from I to IV with I and II representing benign IP, III representing dysplastic IP, and IV representing carcinoma. Viruses as well as genetic disturbances may be related to progression to carcinoma.[16,17] Epstein-Barr virus[18,19] and human papilloma virus (HPV)[20,21] have been linked to IPs with some evidence suggesting HPV is the cause of malignant transformation.[22-24] The HPV subtypes 6, 11, and 16 have been linked to an increased risk of malignant conversion and higher recurrence rate.[25] The overall incidence of malignant transformation is between 5% and 15%.[26]

The clinical manifestations of this tumor are similar to any space occupying lesions of the nose. Typically, an IP presents with unilateral nasal obstruction,[27-29] bleeding,[30] or sinusitis[14]; however, the tumor has to reach a particular size to have these symptoms present. Early tumors usually are asymptomatic and then tend to erode adjacent structures and create symptoms of benign disease.[31,32] Headache and nasal obstruction are the most common presenting symptoms when an IP originates in the sphenoid sinus, whereas facial or dental pain and epistaxis represent common symptoms with conversion to carcinoma.[33] Facial asymmetry and visible tumor in both the nasal and oral cavity may be seen in advanced cases.[34] Tumors involving the ethmoid cavity may present with orbital involvement with signs of proptosis,[35] medial canthal mass, periorbital swelling,[36] blurred vision, epiphora, or diplopia.[36]

On physical examination, IPs are typically unilateral intranasal masses arising from the lateral nasal wall. They involve the maxillary and ethmoid sinuses in 50–80%[37] of cases, but rarely arise within the frontal and sphenoid sinuses (5%).[38]

CLINICAL MANAGEMENT

The surgical management of choice historically has consisted of a medial maxillectomy utilizing a lateral rhinotomy or midface degloving approach. The open approach may provide an en bloc resection. However, this can also be accomplished with endoscopic removal in certain cases as well. Importantly, the premise of an en bloc

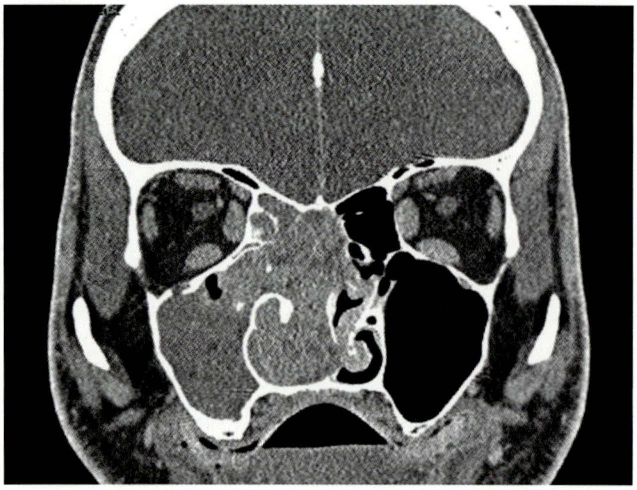

Fig. 19.1: Coronal CT scan shows a right maxillary sinus inverted papilloma with extension to the intranasal cavity.

resection of the entire tumor has been called into question as resection of the tumor pedicle with frozen section control yields low recurrence rates.[34] The possibility of an open approach when planning endoscopic resection should be discussed with the patient since some limitations for endoscopic removal may be present depending on the location, available equipment, and surgeon expertise. The likelihood of a dacryocystorhinostomy should be discussed with the patient preoperatively as well. CT imaging is necessary for evaluation of tumor extension, bony erosion, and computer-assisted surgical navigation (Fig. 19.1). Findings on CT imaging are variable with the typical finding a unilateral opacified sinus.[39-41] The presence of focal hyperostosis or osteitis often predicts with high accuracy the site of origin.[41-43] Calcifications are not always present, but can be seen in various patterns such as punctate, nodular, linear, as well as circular patterns.[44] CT scans have been shown to have a sensitivity of 69% and a specificity of 20%.[45]

Magnetic resonance imaging (MRI) should be obtained for larger tumors and when skull base or orbital erosion is identified. MRI is also helpful to distinguish between retained secretions and tumor particularly on T2 weighted images. The tumor also enhances on T1 with contrast and can differentiate it from enhancement of the mucosa lining with central retained secretions. The appearance of the convoluted cerebriform pattern is a reliable MR feature and can be distinctive in 80% of cases.[46] Features associated with recurrence or malignant transformation include high grade dysplasia, increased mitotic activity, epithelial hyperplasia, and bony invasion.[47-50]

Early detection and locally aggressive surgical management is recommended because of the potential for malignant transformation.[51,52] Medical management has a limited role, but some studies have reported use of antiviral treatment (e.g., interferon and cidofovir) for multiple recurrences and advanced disease involving the orbit and/or the skull base.[52] Chemotherapy[53] and/or radiotherapy are used for advanced malignancies.[54] Radiotherapy may be recommended for aggressive/dysplastic tumors[11] or for poor surgical candidates.[55] It is reasonable to leave benign disease where there is a significant chance of morbidity (e.g., optic nerve) and closely monitor for malignant conversion over time. Endoscopically, IP may look like a polyp with a narrow or broad stalk, but is generally firmer in consistency and is red to pale pink in color. They tend to bleed more than polyps during surgery.[6,56]

STAGING

The most commonly used staging system developed by Krouse[7] divides lesions into T1–T4. T4 lesions extend beyond the paranasal sinuses with either orbital or intracranial extension or are associated with malignancy. Another more recent classification by Cannady et al.[57] that classified these tumors according to their extension into A, B, and C with the highest recurrence rate in group C (extrasinus extension).

SURGICAL OUTCOMES

There has been considerable shift toward endoscopic resections of IPs regardless of their extent. Technological advancements with angled endoscopes, angled drills, as well as surgical navigation have provided better visibility as well as a panoramic view of the mass for thorough evaluation. Surgical goals are primarily complete removal with minimal morbidity. A critical element is the removal of all disease as well as drilling the underlying bone[58], but the extent of disease should dictate the surgical approach. Endoscopic removal has been associated with shorter hospital stays,[59,60] equivalent blood loss,[59-61] as well as less morbidity than open resection.[59,61] Intraoperative findings, and most specifically, the site of attachment of the tumor usually determines whether or not an open approach is needed.[62] A systematic review of 1,060 patients by Busquets and Hwang[63] identified a lower recurrence rate when endoscopic resection was employed when compared with external approaches. In a large retrospective study[34] on 114 patients with inverted papilloma over a 15-year period, the recurrence rate was reported at 15% with a mean disease-free follow up of 40 months. However, primary endoscopic or endoscopically assisted resection of tumors was associated with only a 9% recurrence rate suggesting that total resection during the initial surgery is the best chance for success.

SURGICAL TECHNIQUES

Step 1

The nose is decongested with a topical decongestant. The inferior turbinate mucosa as well as the lateral nasal wall is infiltrated with 1% lidocaine with 1/100,000 epinephrine.

Step 2

If a diagnosis of inverted IP has not been made on previous biopsy, intraoperative biopsy is sent to pathology to rule out carcinoma. Depending on the extent of intranasal extension, the tumor is debulked using a tissue shaver or coblation (Coblator®, ArthroCare ENT, Austin, TX) taking care to meticulously identify areas of attachment (Fig. 19.2).[64-67]

Step 3

The sinuses are opened to an extent that allows complete isolation of the tumor. For tumors involving the medial maxillary wall, a maxillary antrostomy is performed to identify the inferior and medial orbital wall. If the ethmoid skull base, medial orbital wall, frontal sinus, or sphenoid sinus walls are involved, a full endoscopic sinus surgery is generally performed on the affected side.

Step 4

For maxillary inverted IP, a subtotal inferior turbinectomy is performed just posterior to the nasolacrimal duct and Hasner's valve (Fig. 19.3). The posterior stump of the inferior turbinate is cauterized.

Step 5

A medially based nasal floor mucosal flap is elevated and placed medially to cover exposed bone at completion of the case (Fig. 19.4).

Step 6

The medial maxillary wall is removed by penetrating the wall and making anterior, inferior, and posterior cuts with tru-cut forceps and backbiting forceps (Fig. 19.5). If the tumor pedicle is located on the medial maxillary wall, then mucosal frozen sections are taken around the boundaries following removal of the wall. If the tumor is located within the maxillary sinus, the endoscopic medial maxillectomy provides the exposure. Proceed with removal of the tumor, take ½ cm mucosal margins and cauterize and drill the underlying maxillary bone in the area of the original pedicle.

Step 7

Anterior maxillary wall and anterolateral wall locations can be accessed with a transseptal approach if necessary. Further removal of the nasolacrimal duct and creation of a dacryocystorhinostomy can create additional exposure or resected in the case of tumor involvement (Figs. 19.6A and B).

Step 8

The medially based mucosal flap is positioned over the inferior maxillary ridge to help prevent crusting and improve healing postoperatively (Fig. 19.7).[68-70]

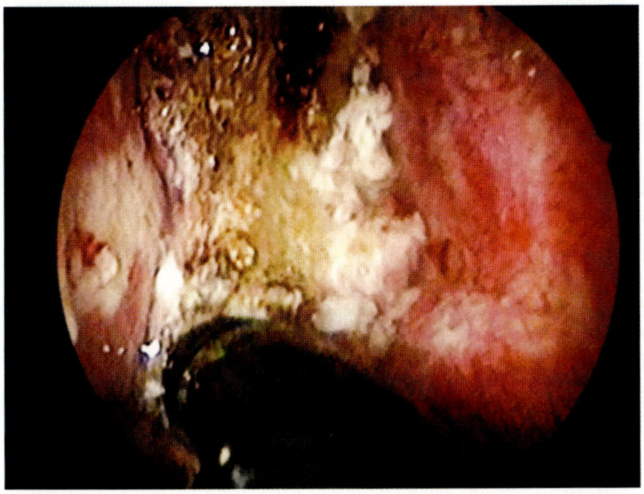

Fig. 19.2: Inverted papilloma filling the right nasal cavity is debulked using radiofrequency coblation to the middle meatus to allow working space.

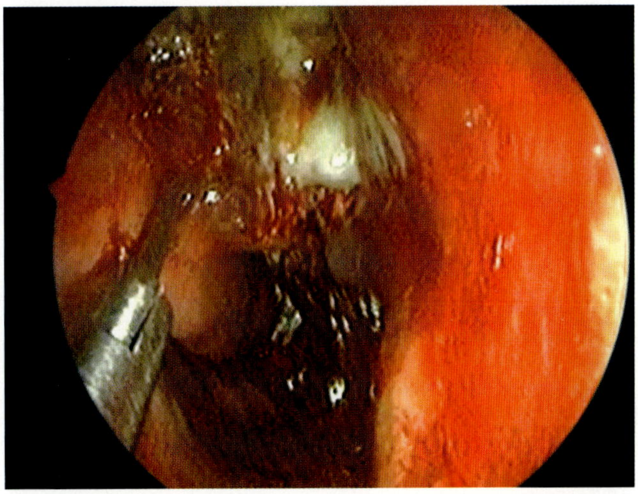

Fig. 19.3: The inferior turbinate is initially removed posterior to Hasner's valve in the inferior meatus.

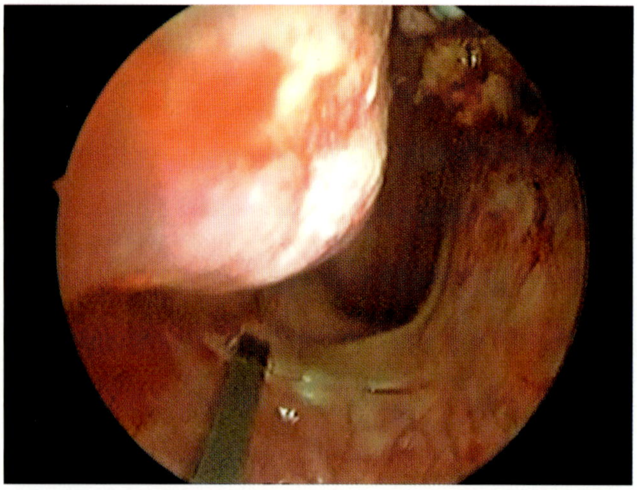

Fig. 19.4: A medially based mucosal nasal floor flap is created with a curved beaver blade.

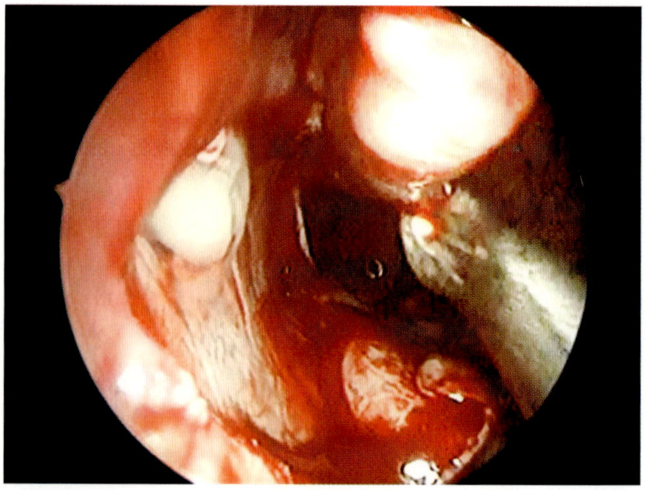

Fig. 19.5: The mucosal flap is positioned medially in the nasal cavity and the medial maxillary wall has been punctured with release of trapped purulent secretions.

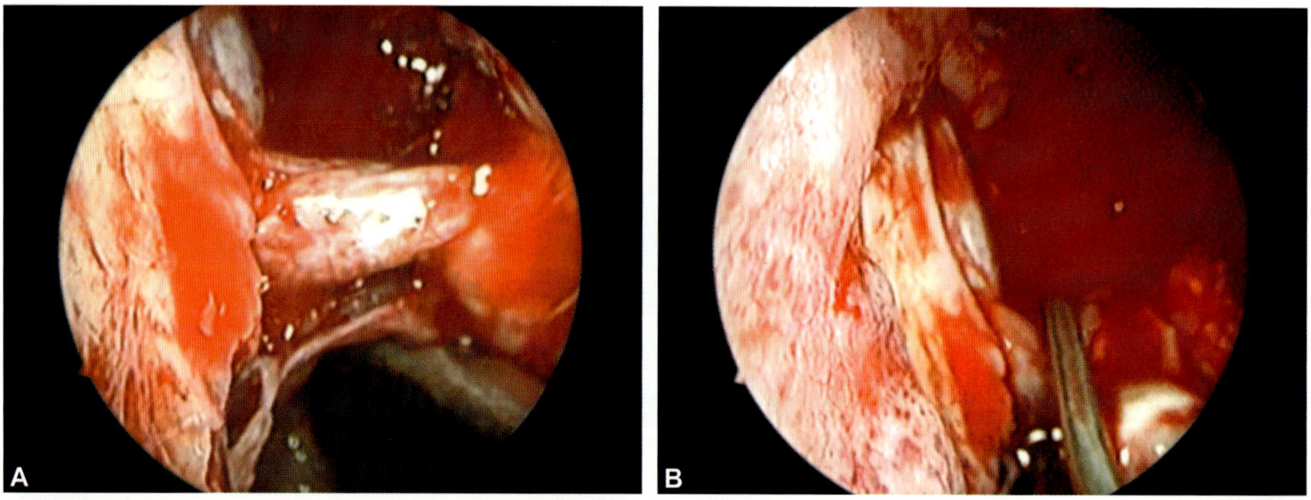

Figs. 19.6A and B: The tumor was noted to involve the lacrimal area so the bone was removed around the nasolacrimal duct (A) and incised with the turbinate scissors (B).

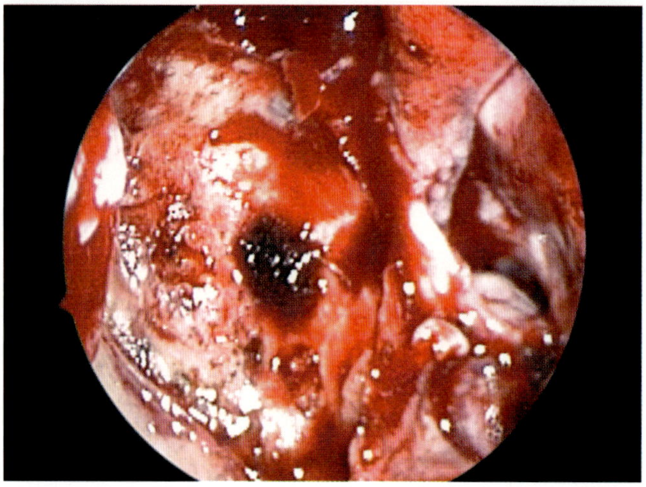

Fig. 19.7: Following removal of the attachment, the underlying mucosa is removed and the bone is drilled to prevent recurrence. Margins around the borders of the medial maxillary wall and posterior maxillary wall pedicle have been cleared by frozen section and the mucosal floor flap placed over the exposed bone of the inferior maxillary ridge.

REFERENCES

1. Buchwald C, Nielsen LH, Nielsen PL, et al. Inverted papilloma: a follow-up study including primarily unacknowledged cases. Am J Otolaryngol. 1989;10(4):273-81.
2. Hyams VJ. Papillomas of the nasal cavity and paranasal sinuses. A clinicopathological study of 315 cases. Ann Otol Rhinol Laryngol. 1971;80(2):192-206.
3. Figuerola E, Liern M, Sanchez Palomero JM, et al. Naso-sinusal inverted papilloma. Acta Otorrinolaringol Esp. 1990; 41(1):35-8.
4. Michaels L. Benign mucosal tumors of the nose and paranasal sinuses. Semin Diagn Pathol. 1996;13(2):113-7.
5. Eggers G, Eggers H, Sander N, et al. Histological features and malignant transformation of inverted papilloma. Eur Arch Otorhinolaryngol. 2005;262(4):263-8.
6. Kaufman MR, Brandwein MS, Lawson W. Sinonasal papillomas: clinicopathologic review of 40 patients with inverted and oncocytic schneiderian papillomas. Laryngoscope. 2002;112(8 Pt 1):1372-7.
7. Krouse JH. Endoscopic treatment of inverted papilloma: safety and efficacy. Am J Otolaryngol. 2001;22(2):87-99.
8. Som PM, Lawson W, Lidov MW. Simulated aggressive skull base erosion in response to benign sinonasal disease. Radiology. 1991;180(3):755-9.
9. Damborenea Tajada J, Campos del Alamo MA, Gil Paraiso P, et al. Endocranial invasion of inverted papilloma. An Otorrinolaringol Ibero Am. 1999;26(1):75-81.
10. Vural E, Suen JY, Hanna E. Intracranial extension of inverted papilloma: An unusual and potentially fatal complication. Head Neck. 1999;21(8):703-6.
11. Bajaj MS, Pushker N. Inverted papilloma invading the orbit. Orbit. 2002;21(2):155-9.
12. Miller PJ, Jacobs J, Roland JT Jr., et al. Intracranial inverting papilloma. Head Neck. 1996;18(5):450-3; discussion 454.
13. Barbieri PG, Tomenzoli D, Morassi L, et al. Sino-nasal inverted papillomas and occupational etiology. Giornale italiano di medicina del lavoro ed ergonomia. 2005;27(4): 422-6.
14. Orlandi RR, Rubin A, Terrell JE, et al. Sinus inflammation associated with contralateral inverted papilloma. Am J Rhinol. 2002;16(2):91-5.
15. Watson MS, Cutting GR, Desnick RJ, et al. Cystic fibrosis population carrier screening: 2004 revision of American College of Medical Genetics mutation panel. Genet Med. 2004;6(5):387-91.
16. Kim JY, Yoon JK, Citardi MJ, et al. The prevalence of human papilloma virus infection in sinonasal inverted papilloma specimens classified by histological grade. Am J Rhinol. 2007; 21(6):664-9.
17. Lawson W, Schlecht NF, Brandwein-Gensler M. The role of the human papillomavirus in the pathogenesis of Schneiderian inverted papillomas: an analytic overview of the evidence. Head Neck Pathol. 2008;2(2):49-59.
18. Gaffey MJ, Frierson HF, Weiss LM, et al. Human papillomavirus and Epstein-Barr virus in sinonasal Schneiderian papillomas. An in situ hybridization and polymerase chain reaction study. Am J Clin Pathol. 1996;106(4):475-82.
19. Macdonald MR, Le KT, Freeman J, et al. A majority of inverted sinonasal papillomas carries Epstein-Barr virus genomes. Cancer. 1995;75(9):2307-12.
20. Syrjanen KJ, Pyrhonen S. Immunoperoxidase demonstration of human papilloma virus (HPV) in dysplastic lesions of the uterine cervix. Arch Gynecol. 1982;233(1):53-61.
21. Weber RS, Shillitoe EJ, Robbins KT, et al. Prevalence of human papillomavirus in inverted nasal papillomas. Arch Otolaryngol Head Neck Surg. 1988;114(1):23-6.
22. Katori H, Tsukuda M. Staging of surgical approach of sinonasal inverted papilloma. Auris Nasus Larynx. 2005; 32(3):257-63.
23. Shen J, Tate JE, Crum CP, et al. Prevalence of human papillomaviruses (HPV) in benign and malignant tumors of the upper respiratory tract. Mod Pathol. 1996;9(1):15-20.
24. Trujillo JM, Wu TC, Mounts P. Characterization of human papillomavirus type 57b: transforming activity and comparative sequence analysis as probes for biological determinants associated with high-risk oncogenic viruses. Virus Genes. 1996;12(2):165-78.
25. Kashima HK, Kessis T, Hruban RH, et al. Human papillomavirus in sinonasal papillomas and squamous cell carcinoma. Laryngoscope. 1992;102(9):973-6.
26. Lesperance MM, Esclamado RM. Squamous cell carcinoma arising in inverted papilloma. Laryngoscope. 1995; 105(2):178-83.
27. Gilain L, Planquart X, Le Lievre G, et al. Inverted papilloma of the nose and paranasal sinuses. Retrospective study of 18 cases. Ann Otolaryngol Chir Cervicofac. 1992;109(8):402-8; discussion 408-409.
28. Luceno V. Naso-sinusal inverse papilloma: a case report. Rev Laryngol Otol Rhinol (Bord). 1999;120(2):103-9.
29. Verhaert E, Ampe W, Depondt M, et al. Medial maxillectomy in transitional papilloma. Acta Otorhinolaryngol Belg. 1992;46(3):273-8.
30. Manasterski J, Leszczynska M. A case of inverted papilloma of the nose and sinuses. Otolaryngol Pol. 2002;56(1):107-9.
31. Moss AL. Inverted papilloma of the nose: an unusual cause of a medial canthal mass. Br J Plast Surg. 1983;36(2):254-7.
32. Zagolski O, Kulisiewicz J, Drazek R. Inverted papilloma of the nose and paranasal sinuses. Otolaryngol Pol. 1999; 53(4):413-5.
33. Cho HJ, Kim JK, Kim K, et al. Endoscopic surgery for inverted papilloma originating from the sphenoid sinus and related clinical characteristics. Acta Otolaryngol. 2008; 128(10):1120-5.
34. Woodworth BA, Bhargave GA, Palmer JN, et al. Clinical outcomes of endoscopic and endoscopic-assisted resection of inverted papillomas: a 15-year experience. Am J Rhinol. 2007;21(5):591-600.
35. Ginsberg J, Polanco GB, Margolin HN, et al. Malignant inverted papilloma characterized by proptosis. Am J Ophthalmol. 1976;82(1):129-35.
36. Karcioglu ZA, Wesley RE, Greenidge KC, et al. Proptosis and pseudocyst formation from inverted papilloma. Ann Ophthalmol. 1982;14(5):443-8.

37. Clarke SR, Amedee RG. Schneiderian papilloma. J La State Med Soc. 1997;149(9):310-5.
38. Phillips PP, Gustafson RO, Facer GW. The clinical behavior of inverting papilloma of the nose and paranasal sinuses: report of 112 cases and review of the literature. Laryngoscope. 1990;100(5):463-9.
39. Unlu HH, Songu M, Ovali GY, et al. Inverted papilloma with new bone formation: report of three cases. Am J Rhinol. 2007;21(5):607-10.
40. Woodruff WW, Vrabec DP. Inverted papilloma of the nasal vault and paranasal sinuses: spectrum of CT findings. AJR Am J Roentgenol. 1994;162(2):419-23.
41. Lawton AW, Karesh JW, Gray WC. Proptosis from maxillary sinus inverted papilloma with malignant transformation. Arch Ophthalmol. 1986;104(6):874-7.
42. Lee DK, Chung SK, Dhong HJ, et al. Focal hyperostosis on CT of sinonasal inverted papilloma as a predictor of tumor origin. AJNR Am J Neuroradiol. 2007;28(4):618-21.
43. Yousuf K, Wright ED. Site of attachment of inverted papilloma predicted by CT findings of osteitis. Am J Rhinol. 2007;21(1):32-6.
44. Lund VJ, Lloyd GA. Radiological changes associated with inverted papilloma of the nose and paranasal sinuses. Br J Radiol. 1984;57(678):455-61.
45. Sukenik MA, Casiano R. Endoscopic medial maxillectomy for inverted papillomas of the paranasal sinuses: value of the intraoperative endoscopic examination. Laryngoscope. 2000;110(1):39-42.
46. Ojiri H, Ujita M, Tada S, et al. Potentially distinctive features of sinonasal inverted papilloma on MR imaging. Am J Roentgenol. 2000;175(2):465-8.
47. Feinmesser R, Gay I, Wiesel JM, et al. Malignant transformation in inverted papilloma. Ann Otol Rhinol Laryngol. 1985;94(1 Pt 1):39-43.
48. Katori H, Nozawa A, Tsukuda M. Histopathological parameters of recurrence and malignant transformation in sinonasal inverted papilloma. Acta Otolaryngol. 2006;126(2):214-8.
49. Woodson GE, Robbins KT, Michaels L. Inverted papilloma. Considerations in treatment. Arch Otolaryngol. 1985;111(12):806-11.
50. Kerschner JE, Futran ND, Chaney V. Inverted papilloma associated with squamous cell carcinoma and adenocarcinoma: case report and review of the literature. Am J Otolaryngol. 1996;17(4):257-9.
51. Lavertu P, Roberts JK, Kraus DH, et al. Squamous cell carcinoma of the paranasal sinuses: the Cleveland Clinic experience 1977–1986. Laryngoscope. 1989;99(11):1130-6.
52. Petersen BL, Buchwald C, Gerstoft J, et al. An aggressive and invasive growth of juvenile papillomas involving the total respiratory tract. J Laryngol Otol. 1998;112(11):1101-4.
53. Nwaorgu OG, Onakoya PA. Inverted papilloma of the nose and paranasal sinuses: a fifteen-year review. African J Med Med Sci. 2002;31(3):191-4.
54. Bernat Gili A, Morais Perez D, Dalmau Galofre J, et al. Malignant rhinosinusal inverted papilloma with orbital involvement. An Otorrinolaringol Ibero Am. 1998;25(4):399-406.
55. Levendag PC, Annyas AA, Escajadillo JR, et al. Radiotherapy for inverted papilloma: a case report. Radiother Oncol. 1984;2(1):13-7.
56. Batsakis JG, Suarez P. Schneiderian papillomas and carcinomas: a review. Adv Anat Pathol. 2001;8(2):53-64.
57. Cannady SB, Batra PS, Sautter NB, et al. New staging system for sinonasal inverted papilloma in the endoscopic era. Laryngoscope. 2007;117(7):1283-7.
58. Minovi A, Kollert M, Draf W et al. Inverted papilloma: feasibility of endonasal surgery and long-term results of 87 cases. Rhinology. 2006;44(3):205-10.
59. Kim YM, Kim HS, Park JY, et al. External vs endoscopic approach for inverted papilloma of the sino-nasal cavities: a retrospective study of 136 cases. Acta Otolaryngol. 2008;128(8):909-14.
60. Sautter NB, Cannady SB, Citardi MJ, et al. Comparison of open versus endoscopic resection of inverted papilloma. Am J Rhinol. 2007;21(3):320-3.
61. Reh DD, Lane AP. The role of endoscopic sinus surgery in the management of sinonasal inverted papilloma. Curr Opin Otolaryngol Head Neck Surg. 2009;17(1):6-10.
62. Wolfe SG, Schlosser RJ, Bolger WE, et al. Endoscopic and endoscope-assisted resections of inverted sinonasal papillomas. Otolaryngol Head Neck Surg. 2004;131(3):174-9.
63. Busquets JM, Hwang PH. Endoscopic resection of sinonasal inverted papilloma: a meta-analysis. Otolaryngol Head Neck Surg. 2006;134(3):476-82.
64. Kostrzewa JP, Sunde J, Riley KO, et al. Radiofrequency coblation decreases blood loss during endoscopic sinonasal and skull base tumor removal. ORL J Otorhinolaryngol Relat Spec. 19 2010;72(1):38-43.
65. Smith N, Riley KO, Woodworth BA. Endoscopic Coblator-assisted management of encephaloceles. Laryngoscope. 2010;120:(12):2535-9.
66. Virgin FW, Bleier BS, Woodworth BA. Evolving materials and techniques for endoscopic sinus surgery. Otolaryngol Clin North Am. 2010;43(3):653-72, xi.
67. Joshi H, Woodworth BA, Carney AS. Coblation for epistaxis management in patients with hereditary haemorrhagic telangiectasia: a multicentre case series. J Laryngol Otol. 2011;125(11):1176-80.
68. Schlosser RJ, Woodworth BA, Gillespie MB, Day TA. Endoscopic resection of sinonasal hemangiomas and hemangiopericytomas. ORL J Otorhinolaryngol Relat Spec. 2006;68(2):69-72.
69. Woodworth BA, Parker RO, Schlosser RJ. Modified endoscopic medial maxillectomy for chronic maxillary sinusitis. Am J Rhinol. 2006;20(3):317-9.
70. Virgin FW, Rowe SM, Wade MB, et al. Extensive surgical and comprehensive postoperative medical management for cystic fibrosis chronic rhinosinusitis. Am J Rhinol Allergy. 2012;26(1):70-5.

CHAPTER

20

Benign Osseous Tumors of the Nose and Sinuses

Spencer C Payne

BACKGROUND

Osteomas

Osteomas are the most common benign tumor of the paranasal sinuses[1] with an increasingly reported incidence of about 3%.[2] Traditionally, the frontal sinus has been considered the major site of involvement[2] but recent studies indicate that the ethmoid may have surpassed this.[3] It is uncertain but potential that this shift is due to an increasing rate of computed tomography scans performed for a variety of reasons resulting in incidental discovery instead of direct symptomaticity. There appears to be a male preponderance with a ratio of 1.5–3:1 and diagnosis is often in the third to fourth decades of life.[4]

There are three main histologic subtypes of osteoma. The ivory type (Fig. 20.1) is composed of dense cortical bone with minimal fibrous component or haversian canals. The trabecular (spongiosum or mature) subtype (Fig. 20.2), however, also contains cancellous bone and comprises these components. A third, mixed type, has both sets of features.

Studies have indicated a slow rate of growth for most osteomas between 0.44 and 6.0 mm/year[5] but accelerated regrowth after removal has been documented.[6] Malignant transformation has not been observed.

Fibrous Dysplasia

Fibrous dysplasia (FD) is an idiopathic bone disorder in which normal bone is replaced by immature woven bone and fibrous tissue (Fig. 20.3). It has monostotic and polyostotic forms, the latter of which is associated with McCune-Albright syndrome. FD of the facial skeleton can involve any of the bones but more commonly involves the frontal, maxilla, and mandible. It is usually asymptomatic but can be painful and/or cause swelling and disfigurement.[7] Typical radiographic features show a ground glass appearance of the bone.

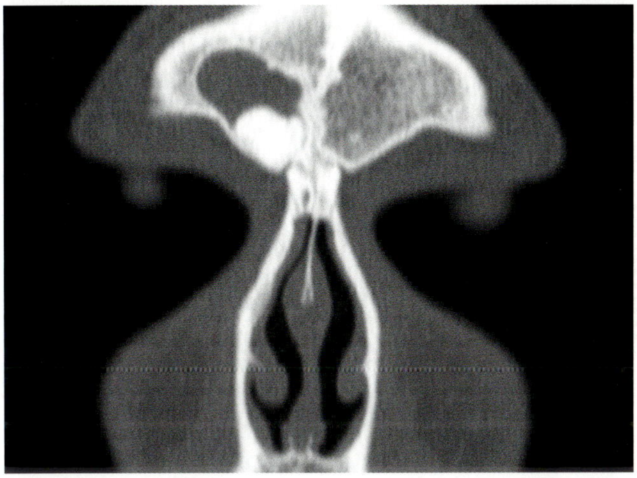

Fig. 20.1: Ivory osteoma—Here, an aplastic left frontal sinus is seen along with a completely opacified right frontal with an inferomedial dense "cue-ball" like osteoma.

SURGICAL REMOVAL

Indications

In the case of osteomas, Smith and Calcaterra[8] originally recommended surgery if the lesion occupied more than 50% of the frontal sinus. Additionally, they and others also advocate for removal in the setting of:

- Rapid growth of the tumor
- Persistent symptoms
- Postobstructive sinus disease
- Bone erosion or facial deformity
- Presence of complications (mucocele, abscess, intracranial extension).

A review by Georglas et al.[9] found that the majority of patients with osteoma presented with headache ranging from 52% to 100% of the cases. This mirror's the author's experience where osteomas are generally found during the workup for a headache. The reader is cautioned however about pursuing surgery in the patient with

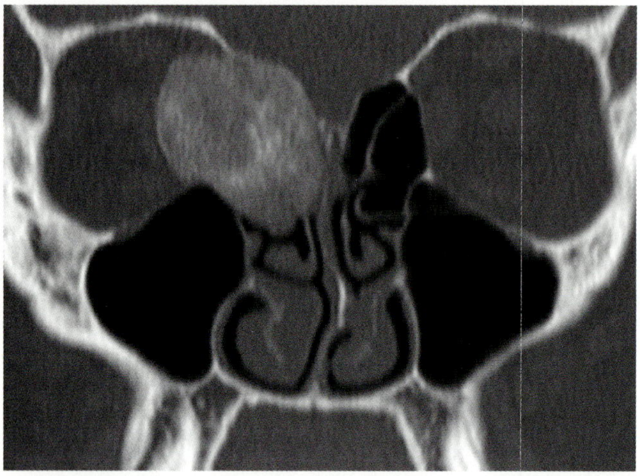

Fig. 20.2: Trabecular osteoma—Expansive osteoma of the ethmoid cavity shows a less dense matrix consistent with a trabecular or cancellous osteoma. Expansion into the orbit resulted in proptosis for this patient.

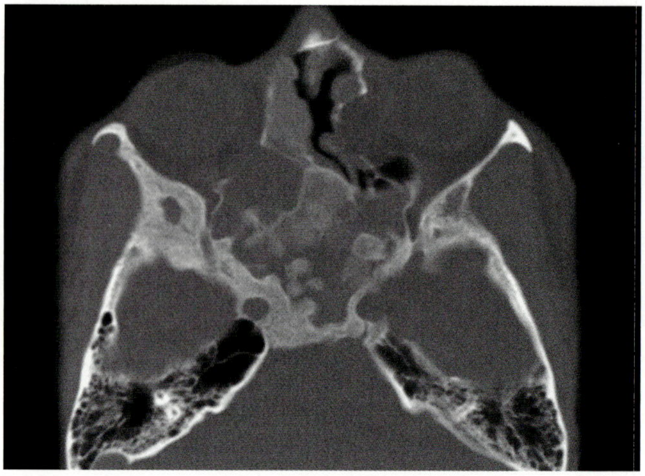

Fig. 20.3: Fibrous dysplasia—Irregular density of the sphenoid and ethmoid sinuses is seen with a ground glass appearance of the more dense bone. MRI evaluation is usually not helpful and often results in a very heterogenous, insidious appearing lesion.

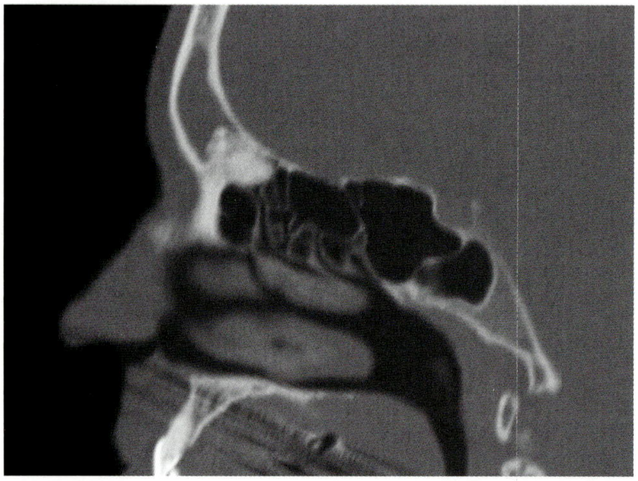

Fig. 20.4: Mixed osteoma—An obstructing frontoethmoidal osteoma of mixed type seen in a patient with a primary complaint of headache.

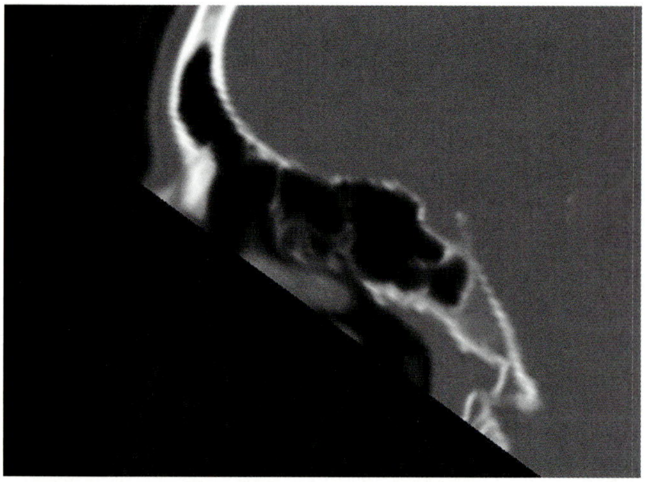

Fig. 20.5: Postoperative CT scan of patient in Figure 20.4—One year later patient had return of headache. CT evaluation revealed no evidence of recurrence.

headache without an extensive evaluation involving assistance from neurological colleagues. Ooi et al.[10] in a recent publication regarding an alternative approach to these lesions stipulate that even in patients with persistent pain observation and multidisciplinary pain clinic consultation should be pursued before resection is considered. Figures 20.4 and 20.5 show the before and after CT scans in a patient whose headaches returned 1 year after osteoma resection despite no recurrence of the lesion. Otherwise it is our policy, in agreement with Ooi et al.[10] that asymptomatic patients can be followed over time with serial CT scans to determine if any growth of the lesion may occur.

Contraindications

Over time, as surgeons have developed experience and techniques such as the Draf III have been refined, the contraindications for endoscopic removal of osteomas have evolved. A review by Chiu et al. in 2005[11] categorized osteomas based on a grading system that further connoted surgical approaches (Table 20.1). Based on this grading scale, they recommended that endoscopic approaches could be utilized for Grade I and II but that an osteoplastic flap was required to properly address Grades III and IV. Seiberling et al.[12] however were able to manage several Grade III and IV tumors endoscopically

Table 20.1: Grading of frontal osteomas according to Chiu et al.[11]

Grades	Characteristics
I	Origin of the osteoma posterior and inferior in the frontal recess; localization of the osteoma medial to a virtual sagittal plane passing through the orbital lamina; anteroposterior (AP) diameter of the tumor is less than 75% of the AP diameter of the frontal sinus
II	As grade I; AP diameter of the tumor greater than 75% of the AP diameter of the frontal recess
III	Origin of the osteoma anterior and/or superior in the frontal sinus and/or osteoma extending lateral to a virtual sagittal plane passing through the orbital lamina
IV	Osteoma fills the entire frontal sinus

through a Draf III approach with only two of them requiring an adjunctive external approach. These authors did note that when the osteoma attached to the skull base that 5–10% of the tumor was left behind to prevent major complications that would not be justified given the natural history of the osteomas.

Surgeons must police themselves and their own abilities before embarking on surgical removal of osteomas. As a result, the relative contraindications for endoscopic removal depending on comfort and skill level are:

- Attachment to posterior table[13]
- Attachment to superior portion of frontal sinus[11,14]
- Less than 1 cm frontal sinus diameter[9,13,15,16]
- Complete obstruction of frontal recess[14]
- Orbital extension[15,16]
- Intracranial extension (though likely absolute for most surgeons)[13,15,16]

Absolute contraindications as suggested by Georglas et al.[9] include:

- Attachment to or erosion of anterior table of frontal sinus
- Extension anterior to nasolacrimal duct.

Surgical Options

A variety of instruments exist to facilitate removal of benign osseous lesions. The most commonly employed are endoscopic drills and burs for which recent advances allow for rotational speeds around 60,000 rpms. When angulated drilling is required however, angular forces and technology typically limits removal to 12,000 rpms. When Gross et al.[17] described the endoscopic-modified Lothrop procedure (EMLP) angulated burs were utilized after first identifying at least one frontal sinus outflow tract. Recently, a group out of Australia published their refinements of the "outside-in" EMLP, which allows for the entire procedure to be completed with mostly straight diamond burs and 0 degree optic scopes.[18] Once an EMLP has been completed, the reach of the surgeon is limited by several factors including the shape and dimension of other instruments as well as visualization.[19] Becker notes that upon completion of a Draf III the average visualized reach in the frontal sinus is ~29.5 mm superior and ~15 mm lateral to the frontal sinus opening that would have been achieved with only a Draf IIA.

Alternative bone removal tools have also been employed. Ehieli et al.[20] recently reported on the use of an ultrasonic bone aspirator to remove a frontal osteoma. They touted its increased safety profile and reduced likelihood of injuring soft tissue compared with a high-speed burr. In our experience, however, this is not always the case and similar care must be employed when utilizing this equipment. An additional advantage may be an augmented ability to control bleeding, which is notably increased during removal of the more trabecular osteomas. The use of piezoelectric devices has also been described.[21] Through the vibrations created by passing an electrical current through ceramic material, these devices can remove bone while sparing soft tissue. The authors note that while the decreased bulk of the device improved maneuverability, bone removal was slower than with standard drills.

As indicated by the above, endoscopic procedures may require adjunctive approaches. The most common is a brow or glabellar rhytid[22] based trephination. When used in concert with pediatric scopes, these approaches can be accomplished with small, less than 10 mm transgressions through the anterior table.

Glabellar Rhytid-Modified Frontal Trephination

- Identify and inject a prominent ipsilateral glabellar rhytid.
- Incision is made with a 15 blade through skin and subcutaneous tissue.
- Blunt dissection with bipolar cautery is continued through the muscle to avoid injury to the supratrochlear neurovascular bundle.

- Incision is carried down to periosteum, which is then incised vertically.
- A 4 or 5 mm diamond burr is then used to access the frontal sinus drilling just above the orbital rim.
- Upon access to the sinus, the opening can be widened with either the drill or the Kerrison rongeurs.
- Pediatric scopes and smaller burs are then employed during removal of the disease.
- At the conclusion of the procedure, a layered repair is completed with periosteum, muscle, and skin closed separately.

Patient Example

A 34-year-old woman, the CT scan for whom is seen in Figure 20.2, presented with a right frontal headache of 1-year duration and mild proptosis without diplopia. Surgical management was deferred by the patient until all medical causes of headache were ruled out and follow up CT scan 1 year later revealed no change in the size of the lesion, but persistent frontal sinus opacification. As her pain was isolated to the right frontal region and she did not wish to risk intracranial or orbital injury, the decision was made to remove only as much of the osteoma as was required to guarantee frontal sinus drainage.

A standard endoscopic approach was performed with removal of the uncinate process and opening of the maxillary sinus. This nicely revealed the ethmoid bulla (Fig. 20.6), which was confirmed by preoperative imaging to be completely opacified by osteoma. Removal of the osteoma began with simple curetting (Fig. 20.7) as the cancellous nature of the osteoma was amenable to rapid bulk reduction in this manner. A drill was brought in to use and using concepts from primary FESS, an inferior approach to the sphenoid was utilized (Fig. 20.8). Upon opening the sphenoid (Fig. 20.9), additional resection was performed superiorly and laterally until running into several high volume intralesional vessels which required monopolar cautery for control. As the preoperative plan was for incomplete resection, we then proceeded with frontal exploration.

The anterior face of the agger nasi was opened using Kerrison rongeurs providing a good view of the roof of the agger (Fig. 20.10). Intraoperative navigation was utilized to confirm a site for entry through the roof the agger, which was then punctured with a curette (Fig. 20.11) and expanded with a curved mushroom punch (Fig. 20.12). A final view of the ostium (Fig. 20.13) was notable for a 9 mm opening. At last follow up (1-year postoperatively), the patient was noted to have resolution of pain, complete remucosalization of the sinus (Figs. 20.14A and B).

CONCLUSION

Benign osseous lesions of the nose and paranasal sinuses appear to be increasing in incidence, likely owing to the increased number of diagnostic scans revealing them incidentally. Given their slow rate of growth, selected observation remains a conservatively appropriate approach. In the setting of complications or persistent symptoms such as headache for which no other cause is determined on multidisciplinary evaluation, surgery can remove the lesion. Depending on surgeon experience and skill, many lesions, even Grade III and IV, can be removed with

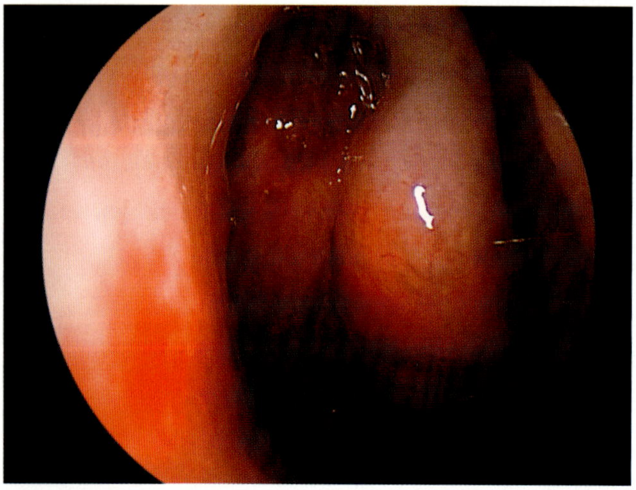

Fig. 20.6: View of ethmoid bulla—Resection of uncinate and maxillary antrostomy have been performed.

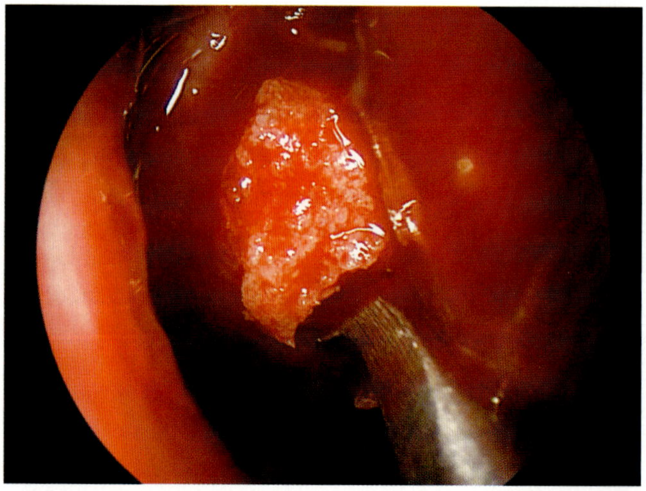

Fig. 20.7: Curettage of osteoma—Initial resection consisted of curettage given the cancellous nature of the lesion allowing for pathologic confirmation.

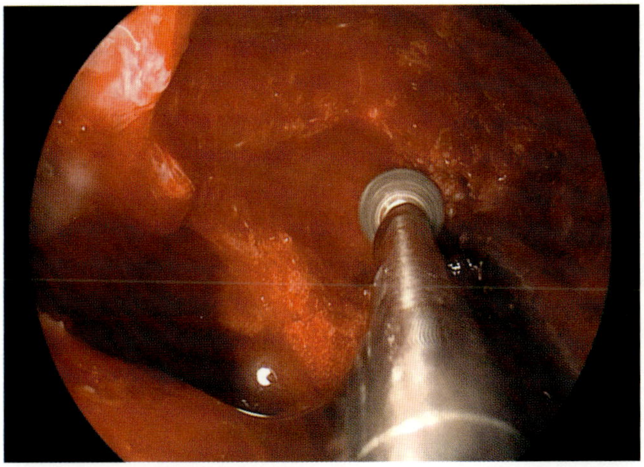

Fig. 20.8: Approach to sphenoid—After initial curettage a high speed drill was used to debulk lesion maintaining an inferior trajectory to the sphenoid.

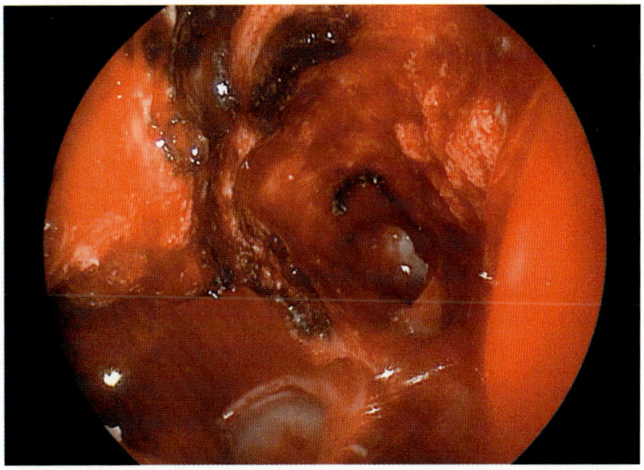

Fig. 20.9: Debulking completed—The opened sphenoid is visible and several areas of cautery are noted which was required to control large intralesional vascular channels.

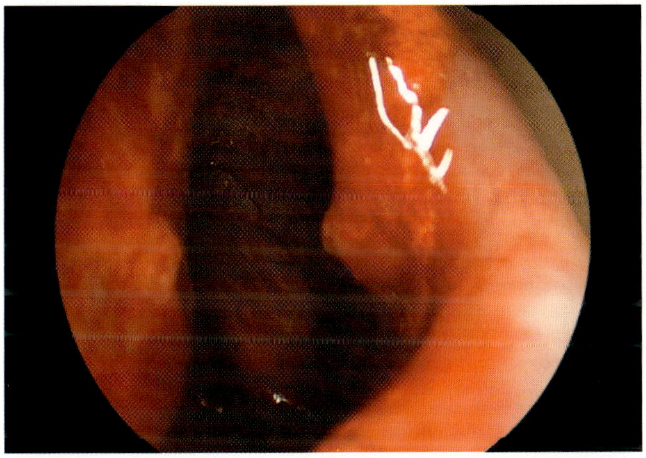

Fig. 20.10: View of agger roof—The anterior face of the agger has been exposed.

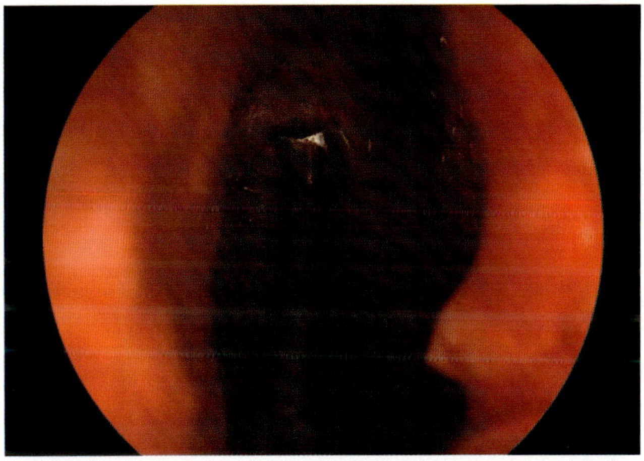

Fig. 20.11: Puncturing agger roof—An angled curette is used to break through the roof into the frontal sinus after confirmation with intraoperative navigation.

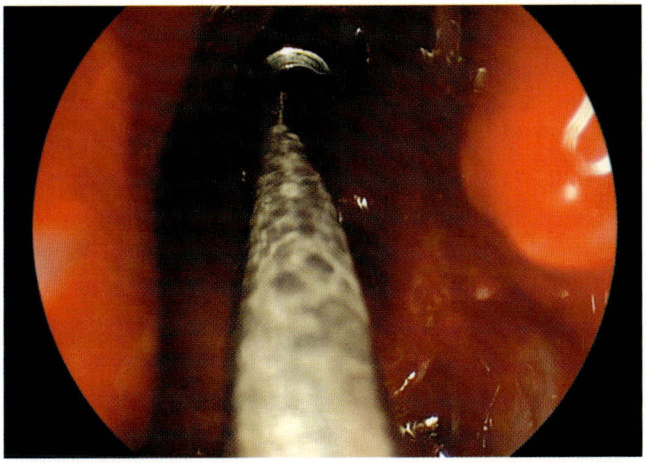

Fig. 20.12: Removal of agger roof—A curved mushroom punch is used to complete the opening to the frontal.

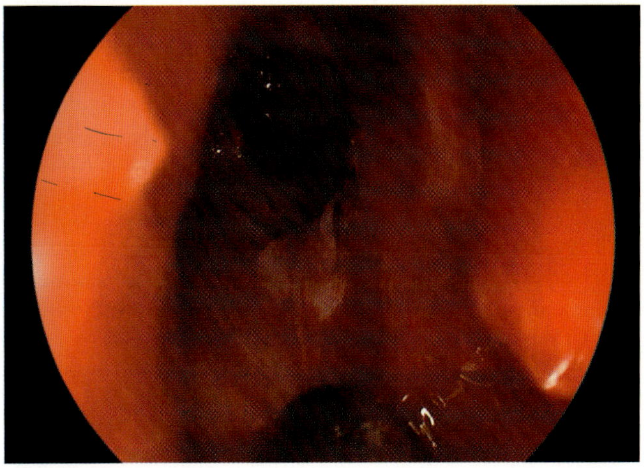

Fig. 20.13: Frontal sinus ostium—A large opening is seen into the frontal sinus, measuring ~9 mm.

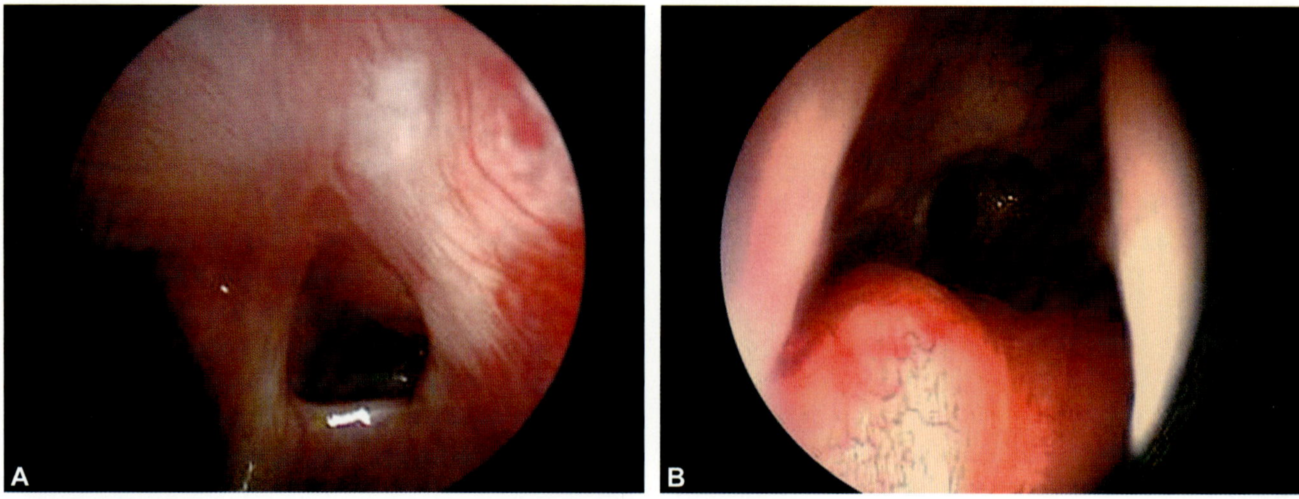

Figs. 20.14A and B: One-year postoperative view—Remucosalization is complete and outflow from the sphenoid (left) and frontal sinus (right) remains patent.

endoscopic or externally assisted endonasal approaches. In the case of complete bone removal circumferentially in the frontal sinus, mucosal grafting may be of benefit.

REFERENCES

1. Broniatowski M. Osteomas of the frontal sinus. Ear Nose Throat J. 1984;63:267-71.
2. Earwalker J. Paranasal sinus osteomas: a review of 46 cases. Skeletal Radiol. 1993;22:417-23.
3. Erdogan N, Demir U, Songu M, et al. A prospective study of paranasal sinus osteomas in 1,889 cases: changing patterns of localization. Laryngoscope. 2009;119:2355-9.
4. Atallah N, Jay M. Osteomas of the paranasal sinus. J Laryngol Otol. 1981;95:291-304.
5. Koivunen P, Löppönen H, Fors AP, et al. The growth rate of osteomas of the paranasal sinuses. Clin Otolaryngol Allied Sci. 1997;22(2):111-4.
6. Gibson T, Walker FM. Large osteoma of the frontal sinus: a method of removal to minimize scarring and prevent deformity. Br J Plast Surg. 1951;4:210-7.
7. Biermann JS. Common benign lesions of bone in children and adolescents. J Pediatr Orthop. 2002;22:268.
8. Smith ME, Calcaterra TC. Frontal sinus osteoma. Ann Otol Rhinol Laryngol. 1989;98:896-900.
9. Georglas C, Goudakos J, Fokkens WJ. Osteoma of the skull base and sinuses. Otolaryngol Clin North Am. 2011;44:875-90.
10. Ooi EH, Glicksman JT, Vescan AD, et al. An alternative management approach to paranasal sinus fibro-osseous lesions. Int Forum Allergy Rhinol. 2011;1:55-63.
11. Chiu A, Schipor I, Cohen N, et al. Surgical decisions in the management of frontal sinus osteomas. Am J Rhinol. 2005;19:191-7.
12. Seiberling K, Floreani S, Robinson S, et al. Endoscopic management of frontal sinus osteomas revisited. Am J Rhinol Allergy. 2009;23:331-6.
13. Castelnuovo P, Valentini V, Giovannetti F, et al. Osteomas of the maxillofacial district: endoscopic surgery versus open surgery. J Craniofac Surg. 2008;19(6):1446-52.
14. Dubin MG, Kuhn FA. Preservation of natural frontal sinus outflow in the management of frontal sinus osteomas. Otolaryngol Head Neck Surg. 2006;134(1):18-24.
15. Schick B, Steigerwald C, el Rahman el Tahan A, et al. The role of endonasal surgery in the management of frontoethmoidal osteomas. Rhinology. 2001;39(2):66-70.
16. Bignami M, Dallan I, Terranova P, et al. Frontal sinus osteomas: the window of endonasal endoscopic approach. Rhinology. 2007;45(4):315-20.
17. Gross WE, Cross CW, Becker D. Modified transnasal endoscopic Lothrop procedure as an alternative to frontal sinus obliteration. Otolaryngol Head Neck Surg. 1995;113:427-34.
18. Chin D, Snidvongs K, Kalish L, et al. The outside-in approach to the modified endoscopic Lothrop procedure. Laryngoscope. 2012;1222:1661-9.
19. Becker SS, Bomeli SR, Gross CW, et al. Limits of endoscopic visualization and instrumentation in the frontal sinus. Otolaryngol Head Neck Surg. 2006;135:917-21.
20. Ehieli E, Chu J, Gordin E, et al. Frontal sinus osteoma removal with the ultrasonic bone aspirator. Laryngoscope. 2012;122;736-7.
21. Gotlib T, Niemczyk K. Transnasal endoscopic piezoelectric-assisted removal of frontal sinus osteoma. Laryngoscope. 2013;123:588-90.
22. Fishero BA, Chen PG, Payne SC. Modified glabellar rhytid incision for frontal sinus trephination. Laryngoscope. In press.

CHAPTER

21 Endoscopic Management of Paranasal Sinus Malignancies

Ameet Singh, Nitin Patel, Arjun Joshi

EPIDEMIOLOGY AND SURVIVAL

Sinonasal malignancies account for less than 3% of neoplasms of the head and neck and occur with a frequency of 0.1 to 0.3 per 100,000 during the first decade of life, with relatively higher rates for Asian and African populations. This frequency rises to seven per 100,0000 by the eighth decade and over 75% of all malignant sinonasal tumors occur in persons older than 50 years.[1,2]

Numerous environmental agents have a causal relationship with sinonasal malignancies. Exposure to wood dust, nickel, chromium, mustard gas, polycyclic hydrocarbons, and aflatoxin has a particular association with squamous cell carcinoma. Furthermore, wood dust and woodworking have been associated with a higher incidence of adenocarcinoma. Tobacco smoke has also been linked with higher incidence of these malignancies.[3] Additionally, human papillomavirus, including subtypes 6, 11, and 18, has been identified in squamous cell carcinoma.[4] A causative association has not been identified however.

Overall, these malignancies occur most commonly in Caucasians, and their incidence in males is twice that of females, likely due to the higher rates of male workers in the occupations listed.[1]

Nasal and paranasal sinus malignancies have shown a 5-year survival rate of 40% according to the Survival, Epidemiology, and End Result database. These data also suggest that the mortality for sinus malignancies has decreased by 11% between 1990 and 2001.[1,5]

HISTOLOGICAL TYPES AND STAGING

Paranasal sinus malignancies are a heterogenous group with significant histologic diversity. Several histological subtypes have been described. Jackson et al.[6] reviewed 115 patients between 1957 and 1974 and reported on the histological distribution. These rates are similar to reviews by Sisson et al.[7] and the Memorial Sloan-Kettering Cancer Center data published in 2007.

The most common sinonasal malignancies are primary epithelial tumors. Of those, the most common lesionsreported are squamous cell carcinomas, followed by adenoid cystic carcinoma (ACC), adenocarcinoma, and mucoepidermoid carcinoma. Less common malignancies include undifferentiated carcinoma, melanoma, olfactory neuroblastoma, and nonepithelial tumors such as sarcomas, lymphoma, and plasmacytomas.[6-8]

Sinonasal Squamous Cell Carcinoma

Squamous cell carcinoma is the most common sinonasal tumor. The majority of these malignancies originate in the maxillary sinus, followed by the nasal cavity, the ethmoid, and rarely, in the sphenoid and frontal sinuses.[2]

Sinonasal ACC

Adenoid cystic carcinoma occurs with a similar frequency as adenocarcinomas but most commonly involves the antrum of the maxillary sinus, followed by the nasal cavity. It is the most frequent salivary type neoplasm in the sinonasal tract. In their ACC series, Lupinetti et al.[9] reported that most patients were Caucasian, nonsmokers and nondrinkers. These tumors are highly neurotropic and frequently associated with bony invasion with skull base involvement and intracranial extension.[2,9]

Sinonasal Adenocarcinoma

Adenocarcinomas make up approximately 4–5% of all sinonasal malignancies. The incidence is less than one case per 100,000 per year, occurring predominantly in men aged 60–65 years. They are more commonly found in the upper nasal cavity and ethmoid sinuses and as mentioned before, have an epidemiologic association with woodworking, furniture making, and leatherwork.[2] Adenocarcinomas tend to be locally aggressive and have a low incidence of distant metastasis.

Sinonasal Mucoepidermoid Carcinoma

Sinonasal mucoepidermoid carcinomas are rare and account for less than 1% of all salivary tumors. The most common site of involvement is the maxillary antrum, followed by the nasal cavity, nasopharynx, and ethmoid sinuses.[2]

Melanoma

Melanoma of the sinuses arises in 1% of cases and may be primary or metastatic. Sinonasal tract melanomas have been reported to occur equally common in men and women, with a higher propensity to affect African Americans. The head and neck represents the most common site of mucosal melanoma. They are most commonly found in the nasal cavity, followed by maxillary sinus, ethmoid sinus and rarely, the frontal sinus.[2,10] Malignant melanomas of the paranasal sinus are usually advanced at the time of diagnosis. In fact, patients often present with regional or distant metastases at the time of initial diagnosis. This often preceded distant metastasis, which is rapidly fatal.[11]

Olfactory Neuroblastoma

Olfactory neuroblastoma or esthesioneuroblastoma arises from the olfactory epithelium and is of neuroendocrine origin. It occurs over a wide age range and generally has a bimodal distribution at ages 10–20 and 50–60 years, with a similar incidence amongst males and females. No hereditary patterns or racial predilections have been described.[2,12]

Sinonasal Undifferentiated Carcinoma

Sinonasal undifferentiated carcinoma (SNUC) is a rare, aggressive malignancy that is thought to be of neuroendocrine origin. It is often advanced when first appreciated on imaging or physical examination. There have been less than 100 reported cases in the literature.[13] There is a male predominance, with a broad range of presentation ranging from the third to the ninth decades. Although there are no known etiologic associations, some cases have been reported to occur following radiation for nasopharyngeal carcinoma.[2,14]

Sarcomas

Sinonasal sarcomas including chondrosarcomas, osteogenic sarcomas, and fibrosarcomas are rare. Overall, they account for 4–10% of all sarcomas, and less than 1% of all head and neck malignancies.[2] Although the metastatic potential and oncological outcome of these sarcomas arising from the sinuses are variable among the different histological types, the local behavior is similar and usually infiltrative.

Lymphoid Tumors

The paranasal sinuses are an uncommon site for primary lymphoid tumors. Most often, these lesions are non-Hodgkin lymphomas, which can be classified into the B and T-NK subtypes according to lymphocytic phenotypes. These subtypes display differences in incidence, epidemiology, and cell type between Asian and Western countries.[2]

Metastatic Tumors

Metastatic lesions to the sinuses occur infrequently and usually present with advanced stage of primary disease. The highest incidence is in the sixth and seventh decades. Metastatic tumors of the sinonasal tract originate from renal carcinoma in more than 50% of cases; however, they may also arise from the breast and lung. Metastases most commonly involve the maxillary, ethmoid, frontal, and sphenoid sinus in descending order.[2]

Staging

The American Joint Committee on Cancer (AJCC) has established staging for nasal cavity and paranasal sinus carcinomas. The TNM classification (Table 21.1) has been designated for staging for cancer of the maxillary sinus, the nasal cavity, and ethmoid sinus.

EVALUATION

History and Physical

Tumors of the sinonasal tract generally appear with symptoms similar to those caused by inflammatory sinus disease. These symptoms include nasal airway obstruction (most common), headache, epistaxis, facial pain,

Table 21.1: AJCC Staging of nasal and paranasal sinus tumors

Stage	*Maxillary*	*Nasal cavity & ethmoid*
T1	Tumor limited to maxillary sinus mucosa with no erosion or destruction of bone	Tumor restricted to any 1 subsite, with or without bony invasion
T2	Tumor causing bone erosion or destruction, including extension into the hard palate and/or middle nasal meatus, except extension to posterior wall of the maxillary sinus and pterygoid plates	Tumor invading 2 subsites* in a single region or extending to involve an adjacent region within the nasoethmoidal complex, with or without bony invasion
T3	Tumor invades any of the following: bone of the posterior wall of the maxillary sinus, subcutaneous tissues, floor or medial wall of the orbit, pterygoid fossa, ethmoid sinuses	Tumor extends to invade the medial wall or floor of the orbit, maxillary sinus, palate, or cribriform plate
T4a	Tumor invades the anterior orbital contents, skin of the cheek, pterygoid plates, infratemporal fossa, cribriform plate, sphenoid or frontal sinuses	Tumor invades any of the following: anterior orbital contents, skin of the nose or cheek, minimal extension to the anterior cranial fossa, pterygoid plates, sphenoid or frontal sinuses
T4b	Tumor invades any of the following: orbital apex, dura, brain, middle cranial fossa, cranial nerves other than maxillary division of trigeminal nerve (V2), nasopharynx, or clivus	Tumor invades any of the following: orbital apex, dura, brain, middle cranial fossa, cranial nerves other than maxillary division of trigeminal nerve (V2), nasopharynx, or clivus

*Regions and Subsites–Nasal Cavity: Septum, Floor, Lateral Wall, Vestibule; Maxillary Sinus; Ethmoid: Left, Right

hyposmia, and nasal discharge. However, until the tumor has grown to infiltrate cranial nerve foramina, displace facial/orbital bones, or sufficiently enlarged to obstruct a sinus ostium, patients are frequently asymptomatic, resulting in a delay in diagnosis. Findings suggestive of malignancy include mass effect on the orbit (proptosis, diplopia, blurry vision), oral cavity (palatal mass, loose dentition), or cranial nerve deficits including cranial nerves II, III, IV, V1, V2, and VII.

Nasal Endoscopy and Biopsy

Nasal endoscopy is important to establish a working diagnosis of a paranasal sinus malignancy. Tumors within the sinonasal cavity are ideally sampled endoscopically prior to treatment planning. Palpation of the tumor may provide useful clinical information such as vascularity and points of attachment. Imaging (computed tomography [CT], magnetic resonance imaging [MRI], and angiography) may be considered before biopsy. Biopsy may be performed in most patients in the office under local anesthesia. Bleeding may be controlled with cautery, hemostatic materials, and/or packing. Highly vascular or deeply seated tumors may be better suited for biopsy in the operating room. Specimens are usually sent in formalin and fresh media, especially if cytology is desired.

Computed Tomography

Computed tomography is the imaging choice for all paranasal sinus malignancies. CT is critical for demonstrating the extent of the lesion, bony erosion (lamina papyracea, skull base), and intracranial extension. The use of contrast provides information about tumor vascularity and proximity of the malignancy to the carotid artery.

Magnetic Resonance Imaging

Magnetic resonance imaging is desirable to define soft tissue extent of disease. In particular, MRI is able to differentiate between tissue density and retained secretions. Furthermore, MRI provides detail on orbital and brain involvement as well as perineural spread. It also has less artifact in the setting of dental fillings and does not involve exposure to radiation.

Angiography

Angiography is helpful to determine the involvement of the paranasal sinus neoplasm with the internal carotid system. In vascular tumors, angiography is essential to determine the tumor extent and anatomy of feeding vessels and as an approach for embolization.

Positron Emission Tomography

Positron emission tomography (PET) is an important modality for evaluation of metastatic disease. The presence of distant disease may alter the treatment strategy from curative to a palliative surgical resection. Alternatively, a CT of neck, chest, abdomen, and pelvis with contrast may be used to accurately stage the patient and evaluate for metastasis.

OPEN MANAGEMENT OF PARANASAL MALIGNANCIES

The majority of patients with sinonasal malignancies have advanced (T3-T4) disease at the time of diagnosis. The standard approach for a majority of patients has been multimodality treatment, usually accomplished with surgical resection followed by radiotherapy for locally advanced disease.

The gold standard for advanced paranasal malignancies has been the anterior craniofacial approach first described by Ketcham in 1963.[15] Classic open procedures for management of sinonasal tumors will be briefly reviewed. External ethmoidectomy, which is the most limited operation, is appropriate for the removal of small tumors in the ethmoidal region through an incision in the lateral wall of the nose. An inferior medial maxillectomy can be performed through a lateral rhinotomy or sublabial approach for resection of tumors involving the medial wall of the antrum and the inferior turbinate and involves margins laterally to infraorbital foramen, inferiorly to floor of nose, superiorly to lacrimal fossa and posteriorly to dorsal end of inferior turbinate.

A medial maxillectomy may be used for larger malignancies involving the lateral nasal wall without extension into the orbit, anterior cranial fossa or alveolus. An extended lateral rhinotomy incision is used to remove lateral nasal wall, including all turbinate issue and the ethmoid and maxillary sinuses. A radical maxillectomy is performed using a Weber-Ferguson incision and removes the maxilla with the nasal bone, ethmoid sinuses, and in some cases, the pterygoid plates. This procedure may be performed with or without orbital exenteration depending on evidence of orbital invasion.

Craniofacial resection is the gold standard open approach for advanced sinonasal malignancies, including those involving the anterior skull base. It represents an advantage in surgical removal, allowing clearance of disease along the cribriform plate, and better access to the anterior skull base. The approach is generally performed with the neurosurgery team and involves a combination of coronal and anterior or lateral facial incisions.

In an international collaboration of 17 institutions, the 5-year overall, disease-specific and recurrence-free survival rates ranged from 45% to 53% for patients treated with craniofacial resection. Surgical margins, histological findings, and intracranial extent were independent predictors of survival.[16] In another report, additional factors with a significant impact on survival were identified, including deep involvement of the orbit, lateral wall of sphenoid sinus, brain, and postoperative recurrence.[17] The very nature of the craniofacial resection implies a complication rate that ranges from approximately 26% to 49%.[18]

Nonoperative Management (Radiation and Chemotherapy)

Primary radiotherapy is not typically employed for the treatment of sinonasal malignancy due to the proximity of critical vital structures (brain, optic nerve, etc.). Adverse effects of primary radiotherapy include cataracts, optic neuritis, osteoradionecrosis, conjunctivitis, and cerebritis with encephalomalacia. For unresectable lesions in with poor surgical candidates, radiation therapy alone appears to be a viable option but is often palliative rather than curative.

Adjuvant radiotherapy may be employed for advanced local disease in order to improve local control. Chemotherapy can be used as a radiation sensitizer. The addition of radiation therapy postoperatively has been demonstrated to improve local recurrence rates and is commonly used in the treatment of sinonasal cancer.[19] There have been several reports in the literature demonstrating increased survival and overall improvement in stage III/IV disease with the addition of chemotherapy to surgery and radiation.

In 2007, Guntinas-Lichius et al.[20] reported an overall increased 5-year disease-free survival rate for patients who received radical surgery followed by postoperative radiation versus patients who received nonsurgical therapy in their cohort of 229 patients. Furthermore, Dulguerov et al.[1] made a similar conclusion with 220 patients in their data on outcome analysis. In 2009, Mendenhall et al.[21] reported the results of 109 patients with sinonasal malignancies. This group also concluded that the local control and cause-specific survival is better after surgery and radiation compared with definitive radiation therapy.[21]

However, with regard to comparing the outcome results of these treatment modalities, there may be a selection bias as it can be assumed that the patients selected for nonsurgical therapy were more likely to have unresectable disease. Jansen et al.[22] analyzed this bias and identified parameters associated with selection of radiotherapy alone, all of which were related to feasibility of successful surgical removal. The parameters for selection of radiotherapy alone included age over 65 years, clinical T4 stage, and radiographic evidence of skin, nasopharynx, palate, and/or skull base invasion.[22]

The role of chemotherapy for the treatment of tumors of the sinonasal tract as a single agent has traditionally

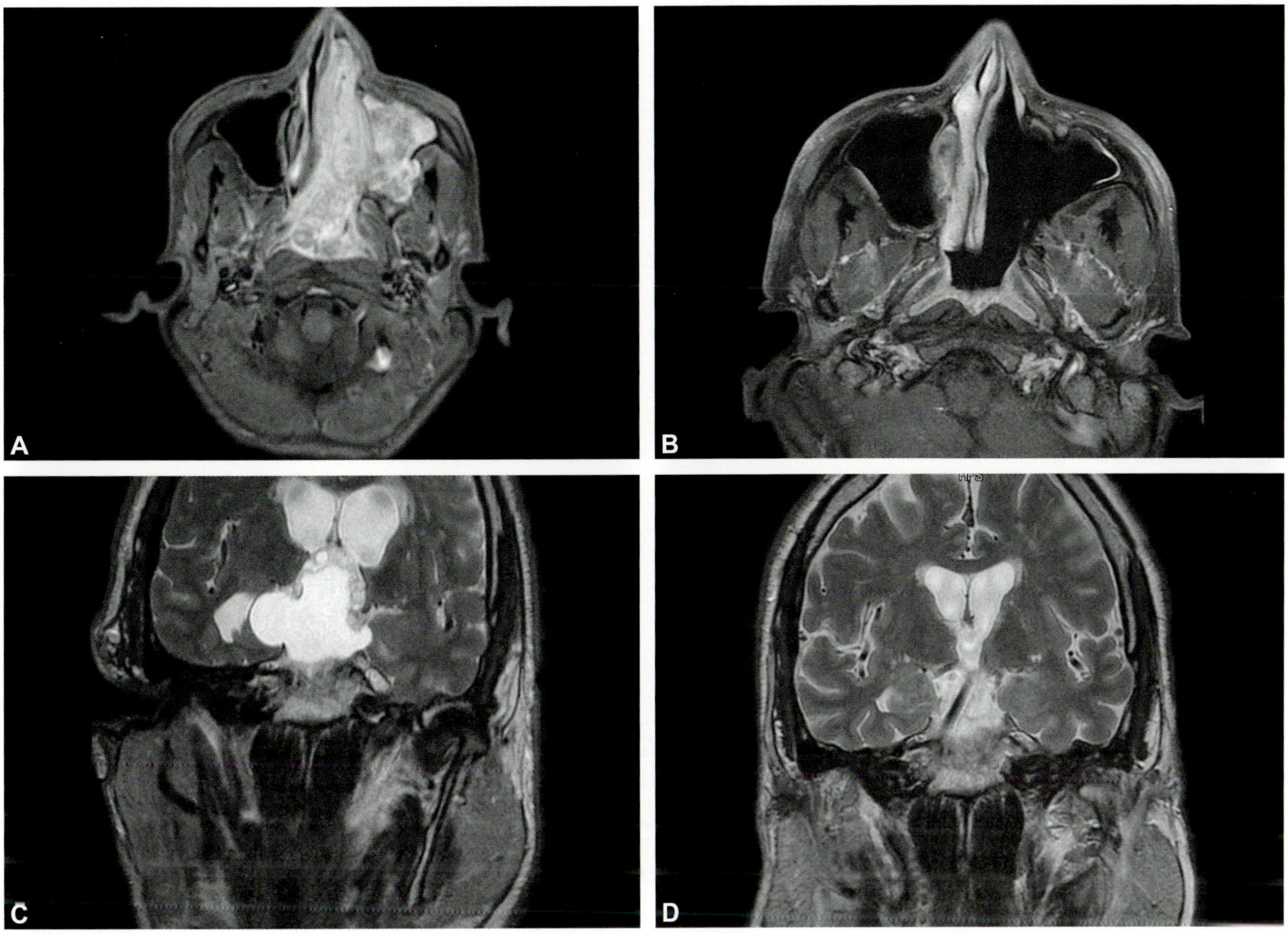

Figs. 21.1A to D: (A) Large juvenile nasal angiofibroma involving the nasal cavity, nasopharynx, pterygopalatine, and infratemporal fossae. (B) Two-year postoperative imaging after successful endoscopic resection of the large juvenile nasal angiofibroma. (C) Extensive solid and cystic craniopharyngioma involving the Circle of Willis. (D) Two-year postoperative imaging after endoscopic resection of the extensive craniopharyngioma.

been thought to be palliative, using its cytoreductive effect to relieve pain and obstruction or debulk a massive lesion. There has generally been a low level of interest for its use as a primary treatment of advanced sinonasal malignancy.

In summary, the current status of conventional treatment for malignant sinonasal tumors is radical surgical excision followed by adjuvant radiation therapy is preferred, whereas radiation therapy alone or combined with chemotherapy is used for patients who are not ideal surgical candidates.

ENDOSCOPIC MANAGEMENT OF SINONASAL MALIGNANCIES

The advancement in instrumentation, techniques, and surgical experience has allowed for the endoscopic management of increasingly complex sinonasal pathology. Over the past few decades, endoscopic surgeons have successfully managed benign extracranial (e.g., inverted papilloma, juvenile nasal angiofibromas) as well as intracranial (e.g., pituitary adenomas) tumors[23,24] (Figs. 21.1A to D). Encouraged by the benefits of endoscopic techniques (panoramic visualization, magnification, ability to look around corners, functional preservation of critical or uninvolved structures, and excellent cosmesis), experienced surgeons have begun to treat selected sinonasal malignancies endoscopically.

Initially, surgeons were appropriately cautious about managing sinonasal malignancies endoscopically. The gold standard for advanced paranasal sinus malignancies has been the anterior craniofacial resection with postoperative radiotherapy.[15] In the early stages of development, the inability to perform en-bloc resection, potential difficulty in obtaining negative margins, lack of refined instrumentation, and techniques (especially for reliable skull base reconstruction) limited the role of endoscopic surgery in sinonasal malignancies.

There were several criticisms made against the use of endoscopic surgery for advanced sinonasal malignancies. One of them was the inability of endoscopic techniques to achieve an en-bloc resection in order to achieve optimal disease-free survival. However, it is not clear that an en-bloc resection is necessary to ensure negative margins. In a paper on anterior craniofacial resection of paranasal sinus malignancies, McCutcheon et al.[25] reported that "Given the anatomic limitations of this region, however, the oncologic ideal of a wide, en bloc resection was rarely achieved..." Other authors have also suggested that since the majority of sinonasal tumors originate in the inherently unstable ethmoidal complex, piecemeal resection via any approach (open or endoscopic) is unavoidable.[19,26] Furthermore, additional data suggest that piecemeal resection of laryngeal or skin malignancies does not compromise oncologically sound outcomes.[27,28]

Achieving negative margins in paranasal sinus malignancies is a critical independent predictor of survival.[16] The perceived difficulty in obtaining negative margins via endoscopic surgery has not been demonstrated in practice and the literature. Experienced rhinologic surgeons have attained negative margins with endoscopic approaches as readily as transcranial approaches, assuming there was no significant disease extending laterally above the orbits and no orbital exenteration was required.[26,29,30] Likewise, despite aggressive attempts to achieve negative margins through craniofacial or transfacial approaches, recurrences rates approach 50%, indicating that this goal may be impracticable in a subset of patients regardless of the approach.[31] Therefore, a less morbid and minimally invasive approach may be preferable. Finally, palliative debulking for advanced sinonasal malignancies is better tolerated using an endonasal endoscopic approach.[32]

Oncological Paradigm for Endoscopic Surgery

The oncological paradigm for sinonasal malignancies via the endoscopic approach remains unchanged. Complete tumor extirpation with negative margins remains the primary objective for the surgical management of these tumors. Obtaining negative margins are critical since they have been shown to be an independent predictor of survival. Although minimizing morbidity and decreasing the adverse impact on the patient's quality of life is important, no effort must be spared to remove all macroscopically involved tissue (e.g., dura, periorbita). Preserving vision and neurologic function while at the same time maintaining a normal physical appearance for the patient is an important goal.

Previous contraindications (bony erosion of skull base, lamina papyracea, and nasal floor, involvement of brain parenchyma or orbit, extension into the pterygopalatine and infratemporal fossa, and involvement of the frontal sinus or lacrimal pathway) to endoscopic resection of sinonasal malignancies have been overturned with advancements in instrumentation, techniques and experience. More contemporary contraindications for the endoscopic approaches for sinonasal malignancies include extensive brain parenchyma involvement, extension of intracranial disease lateral to the mid-pupillary line, extensive palatal/skin involvement, and/or extensive circumferential involvement of the carotid arteries[2] (Figs. 21.2A to D).

Instrumentation for Endoscopic Surgery

Advancement in instrumentation has enabled endoscopic surgeons to address increasing complex sinonasal malignancies. A high definition endoscopic (1,080 p) camera with display and a variety of straight and angled telescopes (0°, 30°, and 45°) are requisite for any endoscopic approach. High-definition imaging provides subtle visual clues that enhance a surgeon's ability to resect sinonasal malignancies.

Straight and angled endoscopic instruments (cutting instruments, endoscopic scissors) as well as fine dissectors in good working condition are essential for tumor mobilization, and resection. Powered instrumentation including shavers and high-speed drills is necessary for soft tissue and bone removal. High-speed drills must be capable of handling a variety of cutting, diamond, and rough diamond burrs for safe and effective removal of bone.

An ultrasonic aspirator based on piezoelectric technology (Sonopet Ultrasonic Aspirator, Stryker Corp., Kalamazoo, MI, USA) for both bone and soft tissue removal may be used for endoscopic surgery for endonasal malignancies. It has proved especially useful around critical neurovascular structures, and can be safely utilized to skeletonize the carotid artery and/or optic nerve. Another recently introduced device (NICO Myriad, NICO Corp., USA) that acts as a "micro-microdebrider" provides variable suction, and side-cutting capabilities to aid in intracranial endoscopic tumor resection.

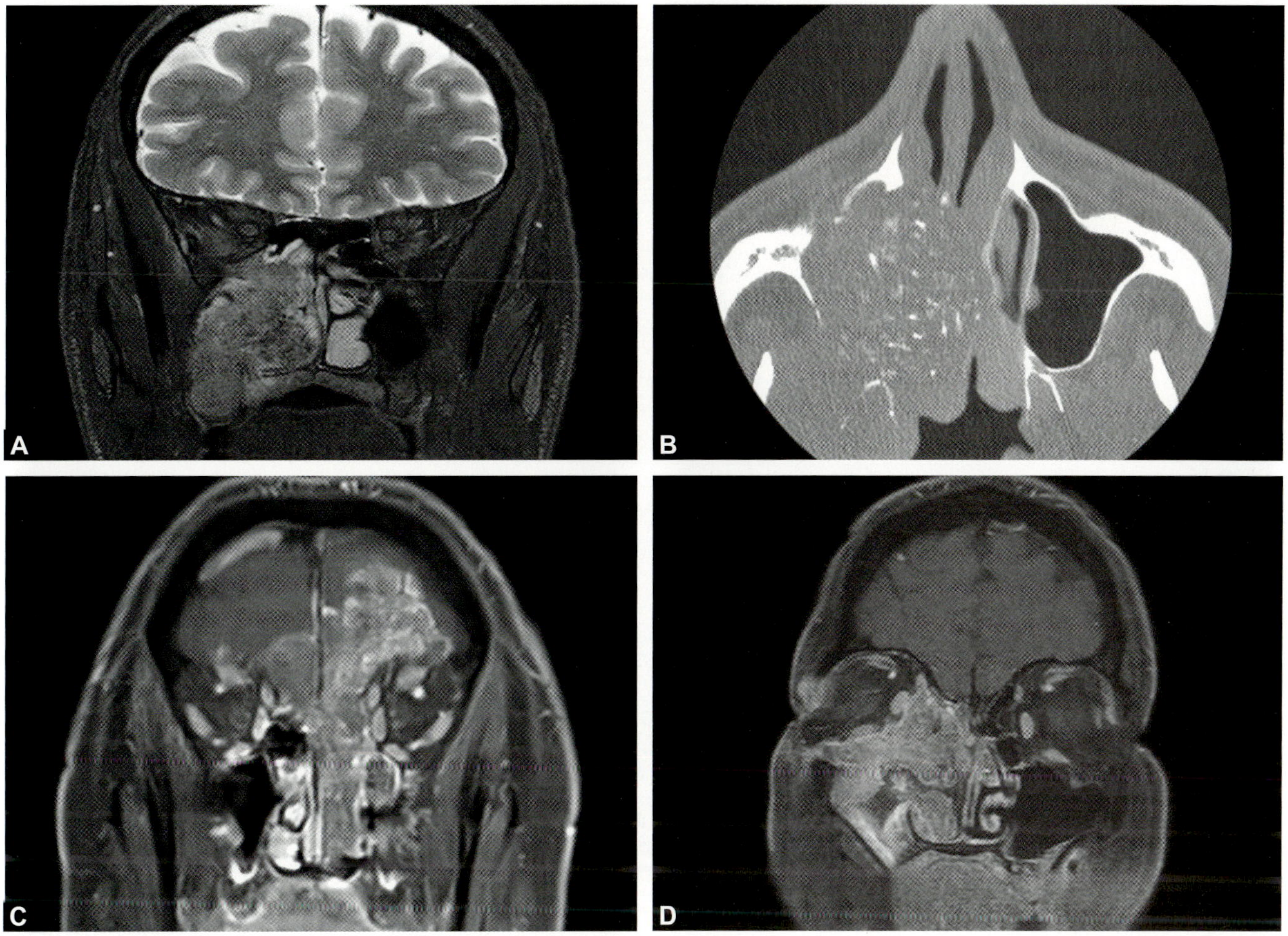

Figs. 21.2A to D: (A and B) Large adenoid cystic carcinoma with palatal and anterior maxillary wall erosion not amenable to pure endoscopic resection. (C) Large neuroendocrine carcinoma with extensive far lateral intracranial extension not currently advisable for pure endoscopic resection. (D) Large paranasal malignancy with frank orbital invasion.

A computer-assisted surgical navigation system (such as Medtronic, Stryker, or Brain Lab) is routinely used on all cases. Triplanar imaging can help the surgeon preoperatively and intraoperatively to create a three-dimensional representation of the tumor, and its proximity to critical neurovascular structures. In cases of extensive tumor, the tip of a shaver, drill, or ultrasonic aspirator may be registered to allow for continuous navigation.

A number of bipolar cautery devices (Take-Apart Bipolar, Landolt Cautery, Wormald Bipolar Forceps) are available for hemostasis during endoscopic surgery for sinonasal malignancies. The use of bipolar cautery, which has minimal spread of heat, is used to control bleeding especially when in close proximity to the skull base and orbit.

Finally, a variety of hemostatic materials (Surgiflo or Floseal, Bone wax, Thrombin, Surgicel) are essential for every case. A 8–10 Fr Foley catheter (with the tip cut off) is routinely available to tamponade any catastrophic arterial bleeding. This is especially true for cases where the ethmoidal or sphenopalatine vessels are buried in the tumor or there is concern for encasement or erosion of a parent vessel (carotid, vertebral, basilar).

Operative Techniques for Tumor Excision

Specific resection techniques for sinonasal malignancies have been described with the goal of accomplishing complete tumor resection with negative margins. A combination of the outside-in technique (dissecting around the tumor in a submucoperiosteal plane), and inside-out technique (resecting the central tumor prior to the periphery) are usually employed for tumor resection.[33] Nicolai et al.[29] reporting on one of the largest international experiences with endoscopic resection of sinonasal

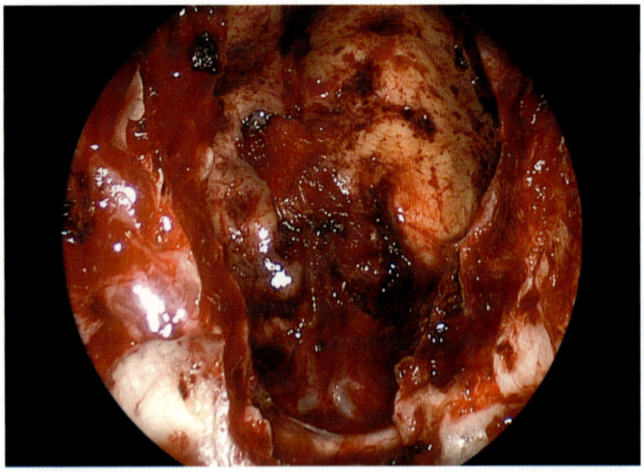

Fig. 21.3: Intraoperative endoscopic anterior craniofacial resection for esthesioneuroblastoma.

malignancy is a proponent of central debulking followed by "centripetal" dissection of the tumor beginning with peripheral mucosal incisions far from the tumor to guarantee negative margins. Meticulous accounting of tumor attachments must be performed to accomplish complete tumor extirpation with negative margins. Intraoperative frozen sections are extensively utilized during the surgery to ensure a three-dimensional resection with negative margins.

Specific combinations of endoscopic surgical techniques described can be utilized for tumor extirpation. Extended maxillary sinusotomies and medial maxillectomy can be used for sinonasal tumors of the maxillary sinuses. Endoscopic approaches to the pterygopalatine and infratemporal fossa are also available for tumors extending to the far lateral infraorbital skull base.[34] Select sinonasal malignancies involving or invading the orbit may benefit from orbital decompression with removal of the lamina papyracea or endoscopic power-assisted orbital exenteration.[26] Extended frontal sinusotomies or frontal drill out procedures (Draf I, IIa, IIb, III) are often necessary for tumors involving the frontoethmoidal and frontal region or to prevent iatrogenic frontal sinusitis after skull base reconstruction.[35] Multidisciplinary endoscopic approaches with neurosurgical colleagues for malignancies involving the anterior skull-base (cribriform, ethmoidal, sella, suprasellar) or posterior skull-base (clival) are often necessary for complete removal of sinonasal malignancies (Fig. 21.3). Several modifications are available to approach sinonasal malignancies. These include the Denker's modification for far-lateral access to the maxillary sinus, infratemporal fossa,[36] staggered septal perforations,[37] anterior maxillary ports, and posterior/superior septectomies.

Skull Base Reconstruction

Skull base reconstruction for cerebrospinal fluid (CSF) leak repair is necessary for patients undergoing dural resection for paranasal sinus malignancies. A multilayered closure of the skull base is critical for successful closure of CSF leaks.[38] Small defects with a low-flow leak may be closed with a small amount of Gelfoam or autologous fat, followed by a rigid buttress (e.g., quadrangular cartilage, vomer, porous polyethylene plate plate), and overlayed with a tissue sealant (Tisseel, Baxter Inc. or Duraseal, Confluent Surgical Inc). Larger defects require an inlay fascial graft (fascia lata, rectus abdominis) or acellular dermal allograft (Alloderm, Lifecell Corporation), a rigid buttress, and a tissue sealant. Multiple techniques that include gasket seal,[39] bilayer button,[40] and modified one-piece gasket seal[41] have been described in the literature (Figs. 21.4A and B). Secondary closure with vascularized reconstruction is often utilized for large defects to significantly reduce postoperative CSF leaks.[42] The easily harvested vascularized nasoseptal flap[43] is often not available for skull base reconstruction in patients with paranasal sinus malignancies. Other vascularized flaps (endoscopic-assisted pericranial flap, tunneled temporoparietal fascia flap) have shown to be equally successful in reducing postoperative CSF leaks.[44] Lumbar drainage is used in cases of a high volume preoperative CSF leak, extended skull base defects, large body habitus, concern regarding the closure, or for a small persistent leak after skull base reconstruction.

Postoperative Care

Postoperative care for patients is tailored based on the approach, dural involvement, reconstructive strategy, and lumbar drain utilization. Patients undergoing extracranial resection of tumor are observed overnight and discharged the following day. Patients with dural or intracranial dissection with utilization of a lumbar drain are monitored in the intensive care unit with frequent neurological checks, lumbar drain monitoring, and close observation for CSF leaks. A postoperative head CT may be obtained for any clinical concern for intracranial bleeding or pneumocephalus. Lumbar drainage is usually utilized for 3–5 days. Broad spectrum antibiotics (vancomycin or first generation cephalosporin) are utilized.

The type of reconstruction and packing dictates postoperative management. Usually sinonasal debridement is initiated approximately 1 week after surgery. In most cases, an absorbable biofragmentable foam (Nasopore,

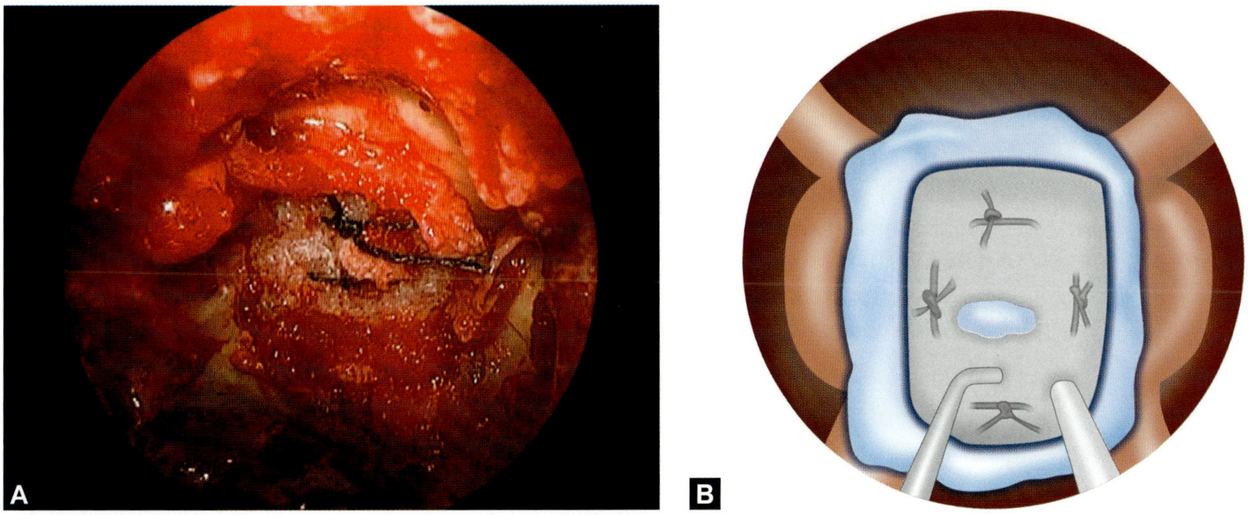

Figs. 21.4A and B: (A) One piece modified "gasket seal" technique for extended skull base reconstruction. (B) Artist's rendition of a one piece modified "gasket seal".

Stryker) is used for packing, which fragments during the postoperative period, and can be easily suctioned during sinonasal debridement. Copious saline irrigation, sometimes with topical antibiotics and steroid are utilized to clear hemostatic agents, packing, blood, crusting, and secretions. Patients are instructed to refrain for nose blowing and avoid strenuous activity for 10–14 days. A small subset of patients suffers from long-term crusting because of the persistent mucociliary dysfunction.

Postoperative Surveillance

The purpose of postoperative surveillance is to detect locoregional recurrence with the hope of prompt treatment salvage. Choosing the method of surveillance is highly dependent on tumor histology, biology, patterns of tumor spread (bone or nerve), location of tumor, and reconstruction strategy.

Endoscopic examination is the mainstay of surveillance and should be performed based on the type of pathology, margin status, and location of tumor. Our routine protocol is to examine the patient every 6 weeks for the first 3 months, and every 3 months for the next 3 years thereafter. After 3 years, the patient can be seen on a biannual basis for follow-up. At 5 years post-treatment, surveillance should proceed annually to monitor for other primary tumors—especially in cases where adjuvant radiation therapy was administered.

The length of follow-up required to deem a patient "cured" is highly variable and depends on the histology and growth pattern of the tumor. For example, patients with slow growing tumors such as ACC, should be followed for longer intervals beyond 5 years before suggesting that a "cure" has been accomplished.

Computed tomography is helpful for patients where the original pathology involved deep bony structures (such as the pterygoid plates, anterior or middle fossa floor). However, it is not necessary for a routine surveillance paradigm.

Magnetic resonance imaging is useful for evaluation of mesenchymal structures, such as nerves, vasculature, and whole organs (e.g., brain, eyes). MRI surveillance is usually reserved for tumors with a propensity for perineural invasion (e.g., ACC, esthesioneuroblastoma) or for surgical cases where a reconstructive graft was introduced into the surgical field. In these patients, MRI is critical for surveillance since any recurrence may be hidden under a reconstructive graft and not visible during nasal endoscopy.

Positron emission tomography imaging with CT overlay has gained tremendous popularity over the past 10 years primarily for pretreatment staging and posttreatment restaging purposes. The resolution of PET/CT has been demonstrated to be 1 cm, which may not be directly applicable to sinonasal malignancies, as recurrences may not be detected as readily. In addition, PET/CT has other limitations, as it measures metabolic activity and may not always directly correlate with tumor recurrence. Based on the resolution and propensity for generating false positive results, PET imaging is employed strictly for initial staging purposes. Restaging is typically performed with conventional MRI or CT scans. For biopsy proven recurrences, PET/CT may be performed for staging prior to treatment.

OUTCOMES FOR ENDOSCOPIC MANAGEMENT OF SINONASAL MALIGNANCIES

Multiple reports have been published over the past decade examining the role of endoscopic management of sinonasal malignancies. Initial series included small numbers of patients with limited follow-up. There was also a selection bias for early-stage tumors as well as relatively favorable histologic malignancies (e.g., olfactory neuroblastoma). Stammberger et al.[45] reported good outcomes and better functional preservation with endoscopic surgery in a series of 18 patients. Similarly, Carrau et al.[46] reported a disease-free survival of 95% in a series of 20 patients with a 22 month follow-up. The majority of patients in both series were olfactory neuroblastoma, which carry a more favorable prognosis compared with all other paranasal sinus malignancies.

In another small series of early stage tumors with diverse histopathology, Podboj and Smid[47] reported a single tumor recurrence after a median follow-up of 67 months. That same year, Lund et al.[48] reported a 68% disease-free survival in a larger series of 49 patients treated with endoscopic surgery. There was a selection bias for favorable malignant histologies (over 50% were adenocarcinoma or olfactory neuroblastoma), and early-stage tumors (over 75% were staged T1 or T2).[48]

Larger series demonstrating the benefits of endoscopic surgery in paranasal sinus malignancies have been published in the recent literature. In one of largest studies from a European Center, Nicolai et al.[29] reported on 184 patients with sinonasal malignancies, 134 of whom were treated exclusively with endoscopic surgery. Over half of the patients had adenocarcinoma or olfactory neuroblastoma with an even distribution of tumors across all T stages. There was a selection bias for endoscopic surgery for lower T stage tumors. The disease-free survival with a follow-up of 34.1 months was 91.4% for the endoscopic group versus 58.8% for the open craniofacial group. Nearly 50% of the patients underwent some form of adjuvant treatment, which included radiotherapy and/or chemotherapy.[29] In the largest US series, Hanna et al.[30] treated 120 patients, of which 93 were treated with endoscopic surgery alone. The series had a lower proportion of patients with adenocarcinoma (14%) than the European series with equal representation of tumors across all T stages. The 5-year and 10-year disease-free survival was 87% and 80%, respectively.[30]

In a unique paper examining the role of endoscopic surgery for exclusively late stage (T3 and T4) sinonasal tumors, Batra et al.[49] noted a 67.6% disease-free survival at 31.7 months with a projected 60% 5-year disease-free survival. Although it was a small series with limited follow-up, these outcomes were similar for open anterior craniofacial approaches with a similar histologic distribution. The series reported a low complication with good function outcomes.[49]

An evidence-based review for endoscopic versus open craniofacial approaches for paranasal sinus malignancies was recently performed. The authors concluded that endoscopic approaches for esthesioneuroblastoma may provide higher survival rates compared with open approaches (Level 2A evidence). They also found encouraging 2-year survival data for SNUC, and similar rates of long-term survival for sinonasal melanoma with endoscopic approaches (Level 4 evidence). The data for endoscopic approaches for adenocarcinoma and nasopharyngeal carcinoma were lacking (Level 4 evidence).[50] Accrued data for endoscopic resection of SCC mirror the overall survival rate of open anterior craniofacial approaches, albeit the follow-up period at present is limited to less than 4 years.[51]

CONCLUSION

The advancements in endoscopic instrumentation and surgical experience with benign pathology encouraged surgeons to examine the role of endoscopic surgery in sinonasal malignancy. Endoscopic approaches have reduced the morbidity compared with transcranial and transfacial approaches. Although accrued outcome data are promising for utilizing endoscopic surgery for many sinonasal malignancies, long-term follow-up is lacking. It is imperative that the gains in disease-free survival for paranasal sinus malignancies achieved by transfacial and transcranial approaches be maintained. If the intent is curative, endoscopic surgeons should ensure that they are prepared to achieve complete tumor extirpation with negative margins for all patients with paranasal sinus malignancies.

REFERENCES

1. Dulguerov P, Jacobsen MS, Allal AS, et al. Nasal and paranasal sinus carcinoma: are we making progress? A series of 220 patients and a systematic review. Cancer. 2001;92(12): 3012-29.
2. Lund VJ, Stammberger H, Nicolai P, et al. European position paper on endoscopic management of tumours of the nose, paranasal sinuses and skull base. Rhinol Suppl. 2010; (22):1-143.

3. Caplan LS, Hall I, Levine RS, et al. Preventable risk factors for nasal cancer. Ann Epidemiol. 2000;10:186-91.
4. Kashima HK, Kessis T, Hruban RH, et al. Human papillomavirus in sinonasal papillomas and squamous cell carcinoma. Laryngoscope. 1992;102(9):973-6.
5. Davies L, Welch HG. Epidemiology of head and neck cancer in the United States. Otolaryngol Head Neck Surg. 2006; 135:451-7.
6. Jackson RT, Fitz-Hugh GS, Constable WC. Malignant neoplasms of the nasal cavities and paranasal sinuses: (a retrospective study). Laryngoscope. 1977;87:726-36.
7. Sisson GA Sr, Toriumi DM, Atiyah RA. Paranasal sinus malignancy: a comprehensive update. Laryngoscope. 1989; 99(2):143-50.
8. Hoppe BS, Stegman LD, Zelefsky MJ, et al. Treatment of nasal cavity and paranasal sinus cancer with modern radiotherapy techniques in the postoperative setting—the MSKCC experience. Int J Radiat Oncol Biol Phys. 2007; 67:691-702.
9. Lupinetti AD, Roberts DB, Williams MD, et al. Sinonasal adenoid cystic carcinoma: the M.D. Anderson Cancer Center experience. Cancer. 2007;110:2726-31.
10. Thompson LD, Wieneke JA, Miettinen M. Sinonasal tract and nasopharyngeal melanomas: a clinicopathologic study of 115 cases with a proposed staging system. Am J Surg Pathol. 2003;27(5):594-611.
11. Dauer EH, Lewis JE, Rohlinger AL, et al. Sinonasal melanoma: a clinicopathologic review of 61 cases. Otolaryngol Head Neck Surg. 2008;138(3):347-52.
12. Rinaldo A, Ferlito A, Shaha AR, et al. Esthesioneuroblastoma and cervical lymph node metastases: clinical and therapeutic implications. Acta Otolaryngol. 2002;122(2):215-21.
13. Frierson H Jr. Sinonasal undifferentiated carcinoma. In: Barnes L (Ed). Pathology and Genetics of Head and Neck Tumours. Lyon: IARC Press; 2005. p. 19.
14. Cerilli LA, Holst VA, Brandwein MS, et al. Sinonasal undifferentiated carcinoma: immunohistochemical profile and lack of EBV association. Am J Surg Pathol. 2001;25(2): 156-63.
15. Ketcham AS, Wilkins RH, Van Buren JM, et al. A combined intracranial facial approach to the paranasal sinuses. Am J Surg. 1963;106:698-703.
16. Ganly I, Patel SG, Singh B, et al. Craniofacial resection for malignant paranasal sinus tumors: Report of an International Collaborative Study. Head Neck. 2005;27(7):575-84.
17. Suarez C, Llorente JL, Fernandez De Leon R, et al. Prognostic factors in sinonasal tumors involving the anterior skull base. Head Neck. 2004;26:136-44.
18. Suarez C, Ferlito A, Lund VJ, et al. Management of the orbit in malignant sinonasal tumors. Head Neck. 2008;30(2): 242-50.
19. Robbins KT, Ferlito A, Silver, C, et al. Contemporary management of sinonasal cancer. Head Neck. 2011;33(9):1352-65.
20. Guntinas-Lichius O, Kreppel MP, et al. Single modality and multimodality treatment of nasal and paranasal sinuses cancer: a single institution experience of 229 patients. Eur J Surg Oncol. 2007;33:222-8.
21. Mendenhall WM, Amdur RJ, Morris CG, et al. Carcinoma of the nasal cavity and paranasal sinuses. Laryngoscope. 2009;119:899-906.
22. Jansen EPM, Keus RB, Hilgers FJ, et al. Does the combination of radiotherapy and debulking surgery favor survival in paranasal sinus carcinoma? Int J Radiat Oncol Biol Phys. 2000;48:27-35.
23. Singh A, Anand VK, Schwartz TH. Endoscopic approaches to the pterygopalatine fossa and infratemporal fossa. In: Rhinology: Diseases of the Nose, Sinuses, and Skull Base. New York: Thieme Publishers; 2012.
24. Tabaee A, Anand VK, Barrón Y, et al. Endoscopic pituitary surgery: a systematic review and meta-analysis. J Neurosurg. 2009;111(3):545-54.
25. McCutcheon IE, Blacklock JB, Weber RS, et al. Anterior transcranial (craniofacial) resection of tumors of the paranasal sinuses: surgical technique and results. Neurosurgery. 1996;38:471-9; discussion 479-480.
26. Batra PS, Luong A, Kanowitz SJ, et al. Outcomes of minimally invasive endoscopic resection of anterior skull base neoplasms. Laryngoscope. 2010;120:9-16.
27. Steiner W, Vogt P, Ambrosch P, et al. Transoral carbon dioxide laser microsurgery for recurrent glottic carcinoma after radiotherapy. Head Neck. 2004;26:477-84.
28. Vuyk HD, Lohuis PJ. Mohs micrographic surgery for facial skin cancer. Clin Otolaryngol Allied Sci. 2001;26:265-73.
29. Nicolai P, Battaglia P, Bignami M, et al. Endoscopic surgery for malignant tumors of the sinonasal tract and adjacent skull base: a 10-year experience. Am J Rhinol. 2008;22: 308-16.
30. Hanna E, DeMonte F, Ibrahim S, et al. Endoscopic resection of sinonasal cancers with and without craniotomy: oncologic results. Arch Otolaryngol Head Neck Surg. 2009; 135(12):1219-24.
31. Patel SG, Singh B, Polluri A, et al. Craniofacial surgery for malignant skull base tumors: report of an international collaborative study. Cancer. 2003;98:1179-87.
32. Tabaee A, Nyquist GG, Anand VK, et al. Palliative endscopic surgery in advanced sinonasal and anterior skull base neoplasms. Otolaryngol Head Neck Surg. 2010;142(1): 126-8.
33. Batra PS, Lanza DC. Endoscopic power-assisted orbital exenteration. Am J Rhinol. 2005;19(3):297-301.
34. Hofstetter CP, Singh A, Anand VK, et al. The endoscopic, endonasal, transmaxillary transpterygoid approach to the pterygopalatine fossa, infratemporal fossa, petrous apex, and the Meckel cave. J Neurosurg. 2010;113(5):967-74.
35. Chen C, Selva D, Wormald PJ. Endoscopic modified Lothrop procedure: an alter- native for frontal osteoma excision. Rhinology. 2004;42(4):239-43.
36. Prosser JD, Figueroa R, Carrau RL, et al. Quantitative analysis of endoscopic endonasal approaches to the infratemporal fossa. Laryngoscope. 2011;121(8):1601-5.
37. Robinson S, Patel N, Wormald PJ. Endoscopic management of benign tumors extending into the infratemporal fossa: a two-surgeon transnasal approach. Laryngoscope. 2005; 115:1818-22.

38. Tabaee A, Anand VK, Brown SM, et al. Algorithm for reconstruction after endoscopic pituitary and skull base surgery. Laryngoscope. 2007;117(7):1133-7.
39. Leng LZ, Brown S, Anand VK, et al. "Gasket-seal" watertight closure in minimal-access endoscopic cranial base surgery. Neurosurgery. 2008;62(5)(suppl 2):ONSE342-3; discussion ONSE343.
40. Luginbuhl AJ, Campbell PG, Evans J, et al. Endoscopic repair of high-flow cranial base defects using a bilayer button. Laryngoscope. 2010;120(5):876-80.
41. Wessell A, Singh A, Litvack Z. One-piece modified gasket seal technique. J Neurol Surg B Skull Base. 2013;74(5):305-10.
42. McCoul ED, Anand VK, Singh A, et al. Long-term effectiveness of a reconstructive protocol using the nasoseptal flap after endoscopic skull base surgery. World Neurosurg. 2012. pii: S1878-8750 (12):905-9.
43. Hadad G, Bassagasteguy L, Carrau RL, et al. A novel reconstructive technique after endoscopic expanded endonasal approaches: vascular pedicle nasoseptal flap. Laryngoscope. 2006;116:1882-6.
44. Patel MR, Taylor RJ, Hackman TG, et al. Beyond the nasoseptal flap: outcomes and pearls with secondary flaps in endoscopic endonasal skull base reconstruction. Laryngoscope. 2014;124(4):846-52.
45. Stammberger H, Anderhuber W, Walch C, et al. Possibilities and limitations of endoscopic management of nasal and paranasal sinus malignancies. Acta Otorhinolaryngol Belg. 1999;53:199-205.
46. Carrau RL, Kassam AB, Snyderman CH, et al. Endoscopic transnasal anterior skull base resection for the treatment of sinonasal malignancies. Oper Tech Otolaryngol Head Neck Surg. 2006;17:102-10.
47. Podboj J, Smid L. Endoscopic surgery with curative intent for malignant tumors of the nose and paranasal sinuses. Eur J Surg Oncol. 2007;33:1081-6.
48. Lund V, Howard DJ, Wei WI. Endoscopic resection of malignant tumors of the nose and sinuses. Am J Rhinol. 2007;21:89-94.
49. Batra PS, Luong A, Kanowitz SJ, et al. Outcomes of minimally invasive endoscopic resection of anterior skull base neoplasms. Laryngoscope. 2010;120:9-16.
50. Rawal RB, Gore MR, Harvey RJ, et al. Evidence-Based Practice Endoscopic Skull Base Resection for Malignancy. Otolaryngol Clin North Am. 2012;45:1127-42.
51. Harvey RJ, Winder M, Parmar P, et al. Endoscopic skull base surgery for sinonasal malignancy. Otolaryngol Clin North Am. 2011;44(5):1081-140.

Section 5

Endoscopic Skull Base Surgery

Chapters

CHAPTER

22

Advanced Endoscopic Skull Base Anatomy

Aaron P Wessell, Joseph C Watson, Ameet Singh

INTRODUCTION

Endoscopic skull base surgery has emerged as a preferred technique for access to lesions of the midline anterior skull base, representing a unique collaboration between otolaryngologists and neurosurgeons. Advances in endoscopic technology have sparked an evolution in endoscopic pituitary and skull base surgery offering superior visualization, improved patient comfort, and reduced hospital stays.[1] The goal of this chapter is to introduce surgeons to the extra- and intracranial skull base anatomy from a transnasal perspective.

LATERAL NASAL WALL

The paranasal sinuses serve as natural corridors for accessing pathologies of the anterior skull base. Progression from anterior to posterior within the nasal cavity reveals the following structures: the uncinate process, ethmoidal bulla, basal lamellae of the middle, superior, and supreme turbinates, and sphenoid sinus. Constant landmarks include the uncinate process, anterior face of the ethmoidal bulla, basal lamella of the middle turbinate, and the anterior face of the sphenoid sinus (Fig. 22.1). Variable landmarks include the posterior wall of the ethmoid bulla, and lamellae of the superior and supreme turbinates.

The lateral nasal wall possesses three to four mucosalized bony projections, called turbinates (conchae), which include the inferior, middle, superior, and occasionally the supreme turbinates. Each turbinate has an associated meatus, or air-filled space, below, named for the corresponding turbinate positioned above. The turbinates are important anatomical structures within the nasal cavity, serving to warm, humidify, and purify air (Fig. 22.1). The middle turbinate serves as an important anatomical landmark. It is derived from the ethmoturbinal, and consists of an anterior buttress, posterior buttress, horizontal and vertical lamellae. The middle turbinate

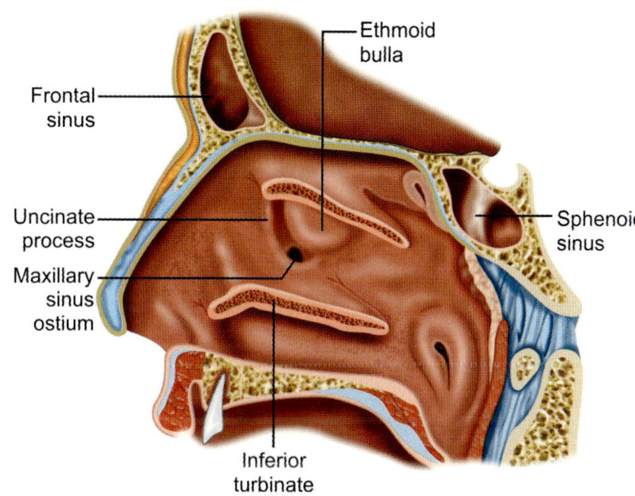

Fig. 22.1: Constant and parallel landmarks of the lateral nasal wall.

attaches to the lateral nasal wall in the agger nasi and posterior ethmoid regions via the anterior buttress and posterior buttress, respectively. It also attaches to the lateral cribriform plate lamella (LCPL), which separates the cribriform plate from the ethmoid roof (Fig. 22.2). The basal lamella (horizontal lamella) serves as the border between the anterior and posterior ethmoid cells. Middle turbinate preservation is preferred except in select cases of malignancy or expanded approaches to the skull base. Preservation of the middle turbinate maintains nasal architecture and provides maximal surface for humidification and filtration of air.

The uncinate process is a crescent bony lamina positioned on the lateral nasal wall, lateral to the middle turbinate, extending from the maxillary sinus ostium (SO), inferiorly, to the frontal recess, superiorly. It serves as the medial wall of the ethmoid infundibulum, a three-dimensional space that drains the maxillary, frontal, and anterior ethmoidal sinuses. Frontal sinus drainage is dependent on the position of the superior attachment of

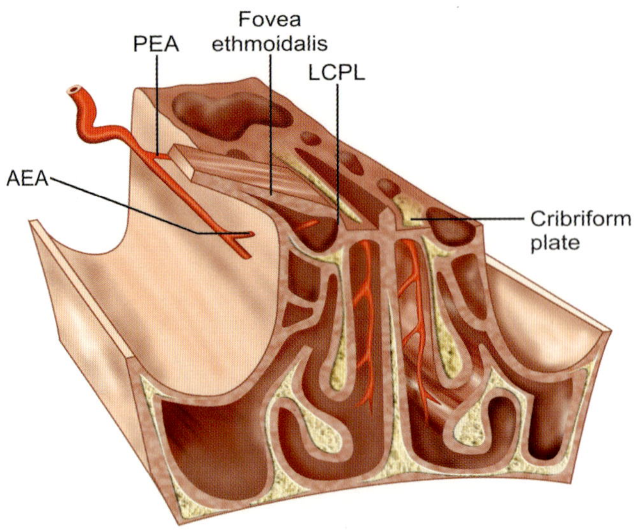

Fig. 22.2: Cribriform plate, lateral cribriform plate lamella, fovea ethmoidalis, and branches of the ophthalmic artery.
(AEA: Anterior ethmoidal artery; LCPL: Lateral cribriform plate lamella; PEA: Posterior ethmodial artery).

the uncinate process. It drains into the middle meatus if the uncinate process attaches to the lamina papyracea, and into the ethmoid infundibulum if it attaches to the skull base or middle turbinate (Fig. 22.2).

The ethmoid bulla resides posterior to the uncinate process and is the largest anterior ethmoid cell. It lies anterior to the basal lamella of the middle turbinate and often extends superiorly to the skull base. Occasionally, the bulla may be connected to the skull base by a vertical lamella, called the bulla lamella (Fig. 22.1). The superior border of the bulla can be formed either by a suprabullar cell or a cleft called the suprabullar recess. Behind the ethmoid bulla is a space, termed the retrobullar recess, which if present often communicates superiorly with the suprabullar recess. The anterior ethmoidal artery (AEA) is usually located within millimeters of the bulla lamella traveling with an upward trajectory as it courses in the lateral to medial direction. The AEA resides at the base of the frontal recess if the bulla lamella is not present (Fig. 22.2).

The osteomeatal complex (OMC) serves as a three-dimensional functional space composed of the uncinate process, ethmoid infundibulum, ethmoid bulla, and middle turbinate. The borders of the OMC are defined by the middle turbinate medially, lamina papyrecea laterally, the frontal recess superiorly, and the maxillary SO inferiorly. Scarring of the OMC must be avoided during endoscopic skull base approaches to eliminate any anatomical or functional obstruction that could potentially lead to chronic rhinosinusitis (Fig. 22.1).

FRONTAL SINUS/RECESS

The frontal recess is a variably sized anatomical space at the level of the frontal SO. Most commonly, it is bound anteriorly by the posterior wall of the agger nasi cell, posteriorly by the anterior wall of the ethmoidal bulla, or suprabullar recess, superiorly by the frontal sinus, medially by the LCPL, and laterally by the lamina papyracea. A conglomeration of accessory cells complicates frontal recess anatomy. These include the four types of frontal cells, and supraorbital cells. The four types of frontal sinus cells (I–IV) are all located superior to the agger nasi cell, the most anterior ethmoidal air cell. A Type I frontal cell is a single cell that lies above the agger nasi cell. Type II cells are multitiered cells that lie above the agger nasi cell and may or may not pneumatize into the frontal sinus. Type III cells are single cells that pneumatize at least 50% into the frontal sinus. Type IV cells are contained entirely within the frontal sinus, with no apparent connection to the frontal recess.[2] Supraorbital ethmoid air cells may also pneumatize into the frontal sinus, displacing the posterior wall of the frontal sinus anteriorly. Frontal recess dissection with a thorough understanding of its anatomical variation is necessary to provide access to pathology of the anterior cranial fossa, which include tumors, mucoceles, and CSF leaks.[3]

ETHMOID BONE/FOVEA ETHMOIDALIS

The ethmoid bone is located at the anterior base of the cranium between the two orbits. The medial component of the ethmoid bone is a cruciate membranous bone composed of the crista galli, cribriform plate, and perpendicular ethmoidal plate. The crista galli is a thick piece of bone, resembling a "cock's comb" in shape, that extends intracranially to attach to the falx cerebri. This dural attachment is often transected during an endoscopic anterior craniofacial resection to remove the crista galli. The cribriform plate possesses numerous perforations through which the olfactory fibers pass to the superior turbinate, nasal septum, and middle turbinate (Fig. 22.2). The perpendicular plate of the ethmoidal bone is oriented perpendicular to the cribriform plate and forms the superior nasal septum which aligns with the quadrangular cartilage anteroinferiorly and the vomer posteroinferiorly. The vomer may be harvested and used as a rigid buttress for skull base reconstruction. Care should be taken to preserve the olfactory fibers of the superior septum while performing a posterior septectomy or harvesting a nasoseptal flap.

The vertical lamella of the middle turbinate separates the anterior skull base into the fovea ethmoidalis laterally and the cribriform plate medially. The fovea ethmoidalis maintains an inferiorly sloping trajectory when advancing in posteromedial direction along the skull base (Fig. 22.2). A thorough understanding of this relationship is crucial to prevent inadvertent violation of the skull base during endoscopic surgery. The orbital plate and the LCPL form the roof of the ethmoid bone. The orbital plate is thicker and oriented horizontally, whereas the LCPL is thinner, ranging from 0.05 to 0.2 mm in thickness, and oriented vertically.[4] The junction of the LCPL and the cribriform plate form the olfactory cleft, where the dura is tightly adherent to bone. The olfactory cleft is classified according to its depth, with greater depths increasing the risk of intracranial complications including CSF leaks. A deep Type III (8–16 mm) olfactory cleft is more likely to be violated than a more shallow Type I (1–3 mm) olfactory cleft.[5]

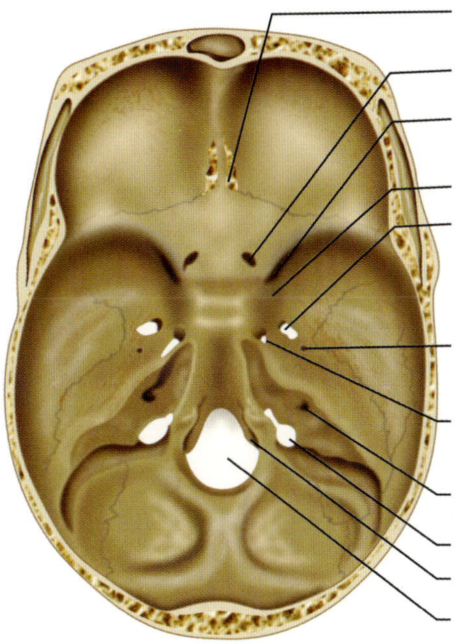

Fig. 22.3: Cranial foramina.

SPHENOID BONE/ SPHENOID SINUS

The sphenoid bone is a butterfly shaped bone that lies in the middle anterior cranial base. It is composed of a central body, a single greater and lesser wing laterally, and pterygoid processes inferiorly. Each pterygoid process gives rise to a medial and lateral pterygoid plate, separated by a pterygoid fossa. The lesser wing of the sphenoid bone and the planum sphenoidale (PS) form the medial anterior cranial fossa, which houses the olfactory tracts and gyrus rectus. The medial portion of the middle cranial base consists of the sphenoid body, tuberculum sella, sella turcica, middle and posterior clinoid processes, and dorsum sellae. The lateral aspect of the middle cranial base is formed by the lesser and greater wings of the sphenoid bone, which contains the temporal lobe (Fig. 22.3).

Several critical neurovascular structures traverse foramina contained within the sphenoid bone. The superior orbital fissure (SOF), positioned between the junction of the lesser and greater wings, transmits cranial nerves III, IV, V-1, and VI, and the sympathetic fibers to the orbit. The optic canals carry the optic nerves, separated from the SOF by a ridge of bone called the optic strut. Other foramina located between the body and greater wing of the sphenoid include the foramen rotundum, pterygoid canal, foramen ovale, and foramen spinosum. The foramen rotundum and pterygoid canal carry the maxillary nerve (V_2) and vidian nerve (VN), respectively, leading into the pterygopalatine fossa (PPF). The foramen ovale is located at the posterior aspect of the lateral pterygoid plate and transmits the mandibular nerve (V_3). The foramen spinosum transmits the middle meningeal artery and is located lateral to foramen lacerum on the infratemporal surface of the greater wing of the sphenoid bone (Fig. 22.3).

Extensive knowledge of sphenoid anatomy is essential to safely and effectively perform transphenoidal surgery, the workhorse approach for endoscopic skull base surgery. The sphenoid sinus is a large paired paranasal sinus located posterior to the ethmoid sinuses. The sphenoid is completely or incompletely divided into various compartments by bony septa. These septations often adjoin the posterior wall of the sinus overlying the carotid artery, with as many as 87% of sphenoid septations inserting at the carotid artery, commonly in the parasellar and paraclival segments.[6] As such, caution should be exercised to ensure atraumatic removal and avoidance of catastrophic vascular injury. In recent studies, as visualized on CT scan and endoscopic dissection, 48–54% of sphenoid sinuses contain one septation, 33–41% contain two septations, and anywhere from 13% to 18% contain three or more septations.[6,7] Only 11% of specimens have an isolated midline septation on endoscopic dissection (Fig. 22.4).[6]

Pneumatization of the sphenoid sinus is highly variable and can extend as far laterally as the sphenoid wings, and inferiorly to the clivus and foramen magnum.[35] Pneumatization occurs in a progressive fashion during

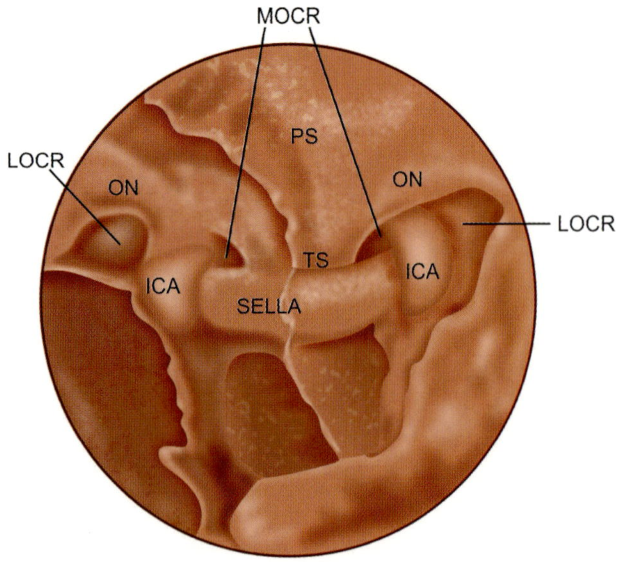

Fig. 22.4: Endoscopic sphenoid sinus anatomy.
(LOCR: Lateral opticocarotid recess; MOCR: Medial opticocarotid recess; ON: Optic nerve; ICA: Internal carotid artery; TS: Tuberculum sella; PS: Planum sphenoidale).

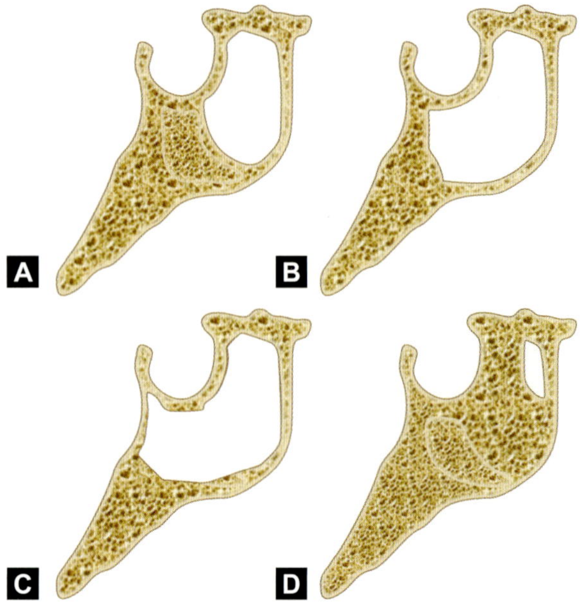

Figs. 22.5A to D: Sphenoid sinus pneumatization.
(A: Presellar; B: Sellar; C: Postsellar; D: Conchal).

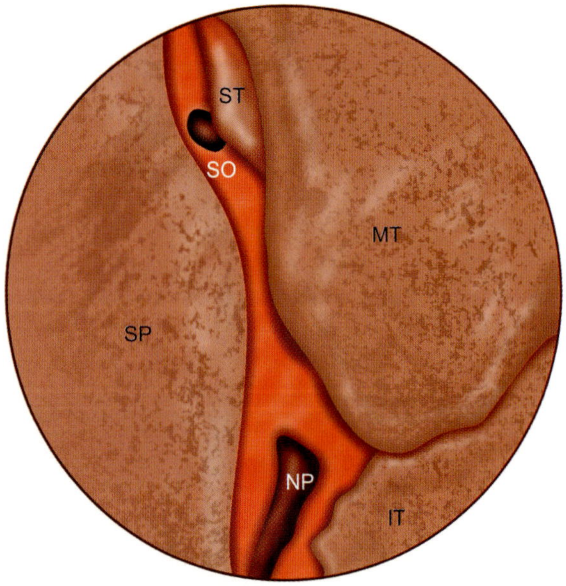

Fig. 22.6: Natural sphenoid ostium.
(SO: Sphenoid ostium; ST: Superior turbinate; MT: Middle turbinate; NP: Nasopharynx; IT: Inferior turbinate; SP: Septum).

childhood. Therefore, incomplete or partial pneumatization is far more common in the pediatric population. The historically accepted classification scheme for sphenoid sinus pneumatization patterns includes three types, sellar (80%), presellar (17%), and conchal (3%),[8] as originally proposed by Hammer and Radberg (Figs. 22.5A to D).[9] Preoperative imaging is crucial to evaluating such variations in sphenoid sinus anatomy in order to ensure safe entry into the sinus and access to the target lesions.

The sphenoid SO is located approximately half way up the anterior wall of the sphenoid sinus, positioned 21.21 ± 6.02 mm superolateral to the posterior choana and 4.85 cm ± 2.89 mm lateral of midline.[10] The postero-inferior end of the superior turbinate is a useful reference point for localizing the SO. The SO resides approximately 10.6 ± 3.0 mm above the posterior inferior border of the superior turbinate, draining medial to the turbinate in 83% of cases.[11] The SO can be visualized with gentle lateralization of the superior turbinate in the sphenoethmoid recess, enclosed by the septum medially, superior turbinate laterally, cribiform plate superiorly, and the nasal floor inferiorly. The sphenoid sinus can also be accessed past the posterior ethmoidal cells through the medial-inferior triangle of the sphenoid face. This approach avoids risk to the optic nerve and carotid artery in the superior-lateral triangle. The sphenoid sinus can also be accessed through a transpterygoid approach (Fig. 22.6).[12]

The Onodi (sphenoethmoid) cells are posterior ethmoid air cells that pneumatize posterior, lateral, and superior to the sphenoid face. The Onodi cell is of practical importance given its intimate relationship with the surrounding optic nerves, carotid arteries, sphenoid sinus and sella, and should be recognized on preoperative imaging. Complete removal of the Onodi cells may be

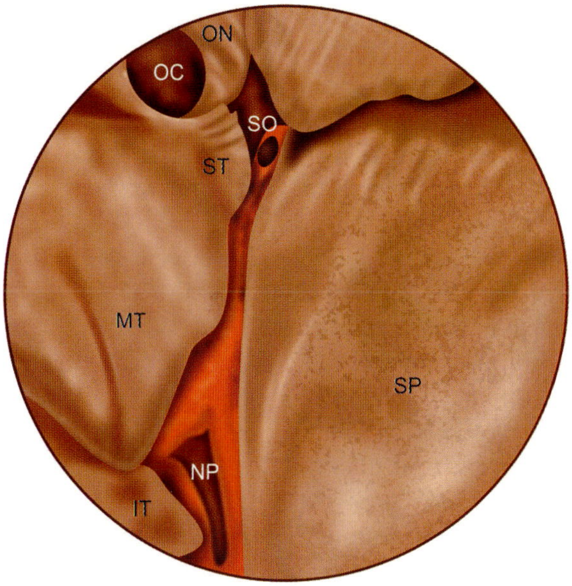

Fig. 22.7: Onodi cell.
(OC: Onodi cell; ON: Optic nerve; SO: Sphenoid ostium; IT: Inferior turbinate; MT: Middle turbinate; ST: Superior turbinate; NP: Nasopharynx; SP: Septum).

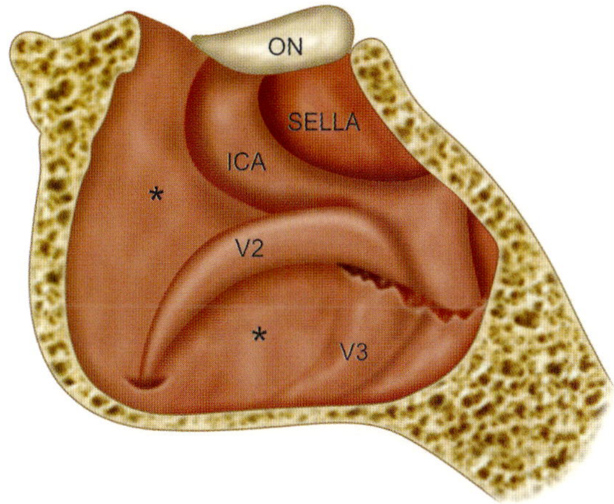

Fig. 22.8: Lateral sphenoid sinus wall.
(*depressions; V3: Mandibular nerve; V2: Maxillary nerve).

required to achieve adequate visualization of tumors in the sellar and parasellar regions. Historically, the Onodi cell has been described according to CT imaging with a reported prevalence ranging from 1.3 to 8%.[13-15] Anatomical studies have reported a prevalence of Onodi cells ranging from 1 to 39%.[14,16-20] However, more recent radiographic studies have demonstrated Onodi cells in as many as 65.3% of patients, present both unilaterally and bilaterally.[21] A greater prevalence of Onodi cell pneumatization has been described among those from East Asia (Fig. 22.7).[22]

The sella lies within the midline posterior wall of the sphenoid sinus, superior to the intra-sphenoidal clivus, separated by the sellar-clival junction. Superior and anterior to the sella lies the PS, separated from the sella by a thick bony ridge, termed the tuberculum sellae (TS), which corresponds to the chiasmatic sulcus intracranially (Fig. 22.4). The lateral wall of the sphenoid sinus involves four bony prominences and three depressions. The bony prominences from superior to inferior include the prominences of the optic nerve, parasellar ICA, maxillary (V2), and mandibular (V3) divisions of trigeminal nerve. The three bony depressions include the lateral opticocarotid recess (LOCR), the depression between cavernous sinus apex and V2, and the depression between V2 and V3 (Fig. 22.8). The LOCR is delineated superolaterally by the optic nerve and inferomedially by the parasellar ICA. The floor of the optic canal forms the LOCR superiorly, the SOF inferiorly, and the lateral border of the carotid prominence medially.[23] It corresponds to the optic strut and anterior clinoid processes intracranially. This bone that forms the LOCR can be thin or absent altogether, producing a dehiscence of the ICA.[24] The oculomotor nerve may also be found inferiorly within this recess (Fig. 22.4). The next recess is a triangular region with the base located at the parasellar carotid and apex corresponding to the SOF. The third recess, between V2 and V3, represents an embryologic fusion plane of the basisphenoid called Sternberg's canal. Lateral sphenoid sinus encephaloceles and CSF leaks can be found within this recess secondary to dehiscence.[8,24] Another recess, termed the medial opticocarotid recess (MOCR), is located at the intersection of the optic canal, carotid canal, sella and anterior cranial base, and corresponds to the medial clinoid intracranially. The MOCR has been described as an important "keyhole" landmark in skull base surgery. With its position at the medial aspect of the ICA sulcus, the MOCR offers an entry point for access to surrounding structures, while providing a safe border for prevention of injury to the adjacent paraclinoid ICA (Fig. 22.8).[23]

SELLAR/SUPRASELLAR ANATOMY

The pituitary gland is located in the center of the cranial base, supported by a bony saddle, called the sella turcica (i.e., "Turkish saddle"). The diaphragma sellae forms a dural roof of the sella turcica, which covers the pituitary gland.[23] The sella turcica is surrounded by a number of neurovascular structures including the optic nerves, optic

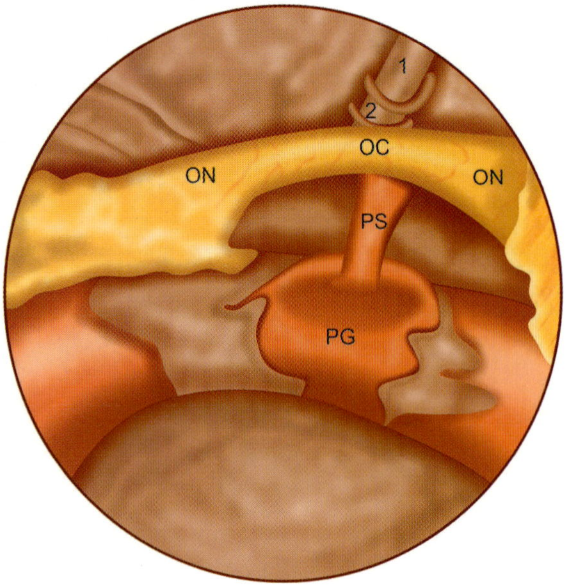

Fig. 22.9: Sellar anatomy.
(PG: Pituitary gland; PS: Pituitary stalk; OC: Optic chiasm; ON: Optic nerve; 1 and 2: Anterior cerebral circulation).

chiasm and anterior circulation superiorly; the cavernous sinuses, internal carotid arteries, and multiple cranial nerves laterally; and the brainstem and posterior circulation posteriorly. Because of the high density of neurovascular structures located superiorly, laterally, and posteriorly in relation to the pituitary gland, anterior approaches have become the preferred approach to the sellar region (Fig. 22.9).

The cavernous sinuses reside along the lateral aspect of the sphenoid sinus, sella and pituitary gland, spanning from the SOF, anteriorly, to the petrous apex, posteriorly. The medial walls of the cavernous sinus abut the lateral wall of the pituitary gland, often separated by a single layer of dura, thus allowing sellar tumors to extend laterally into the cavernous sinus. The internal carotid artery lies medially within the cavernous sinus. The carotid artery enters the cavernous sinus after leaving the foramen lacerum and turning abruptly forward, traversing the sinus in a horizontal direction before passing upward along the lateral aspect of the anterior clinoid process. The intracavernous carotid artery is fixed at multiple points, which include bony rings of the anterior and middle clinoid processes and carotid sulcus. The intracavernous carotid artery provides blood supply to sellar contents via the meningohypophyseal trunk (Fig. 22.10).[25]

Venous channels running along the border of the diaphragma sellae and pituitary gland connect the bilateral cavernous sinuses. These intercavernous sinuses are located anterior, posterior, and inferior to the pituitary gland. If the anterior and posterior intercavernous sinuses connect, the entire venous channel is called the circular sinus. The largest, constant, intercavernous sinus is the posterior basilar sinus located behind the dorsum sellae and upper clivus. The anterior intercavernous sinus is often larger than the posterior basilar sinus and can occasionally occupy the entire anterior sellar wall. This can result in intraoperative bleeding during a transsphenoidal procedure, which can be controlled with compression of the venous channel and packing with, or application of, hemostatic agents. Multiple other combinations of intercavernous sinuses may occur.[25,26]

Many nerves reside within the cavernous sinus including, superiorly to inferiorly, the oculomotor (CN III), trochlear (IV), ophthalmic (V_1), and abducens (VI) nerves. Cranial nerves III, IV, and V_1 lie between two dural leaves of the lateral sinus wall. CN III enters the cavernous sinus anterior and lateral to the dorsum sellae, and lies slightly anteromedial to CN IV. V_1 enters the sinus inferiorly and traverses upward to exit through the SOF. CN VI penetrates the cavernous sinus at the posteroinferior border running medial and parallel to the ophthalmic nerve. CN VI is bordered medially by the lateral wall of the intracavernous carotid (Fig. 22.11).[27] The ascending postganglionic sympathetic fibers to the eye, including Muller's muscles, enter the cavernous sinus with the carotid artery, follow the abucens nerve to the SOF and then follow V_1 to the orbit.

The optic nerves pass through the suprasellar region and anterior incisural space. The anterior incisural space spans from the anterior border of the brainstem upward around the optic chiasm to the midline position of the subcallosal space.[28] The optic nerves exit the optic canals medial to the anterior clinoid processes and travel in a posterior, medial, and superior trajectory towards the optic chiasm. The optic tracts leave the chiasm and traverse posteriorly and laterally around the cerebral peduncles to enter the midline incisural space (Fig. 22.12). The optic chiasm is positioned inferior to the junction of the anterior wall and floor of the third ventricle. Structures situated superior to the optic chiasm include the anterior cerebral and anterior communicating arteries, lamina terminalis, and third ventricle. Laterally to the optic chiasm lie the internal carotid arteries, posteriorly lies the infundibulum, whereas the diaphragma sellae and pituitary gland are seated beneath the optic chiasm. The infundibular recess lies at the base of the pituitary stalk behind the chiasm (Fig. 22.13).[29]

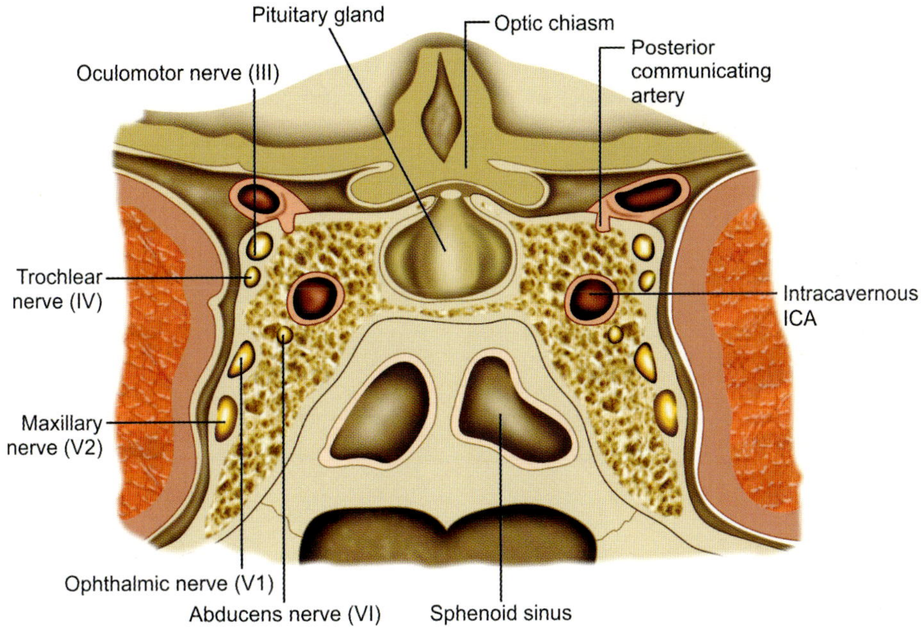

Fig. 22.10: Coronal section of cavernous sinus.

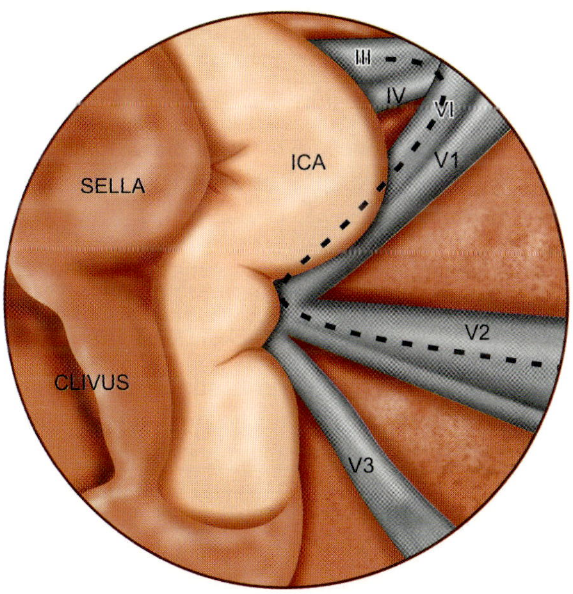

Fig. 22.11: Cavernous sinus neural anatomy. Cavallo's triangles. Cranial nerves are labeled (III, IV, V1, V2, V3) ICA: Internal carotid artery; CL: Clivus.

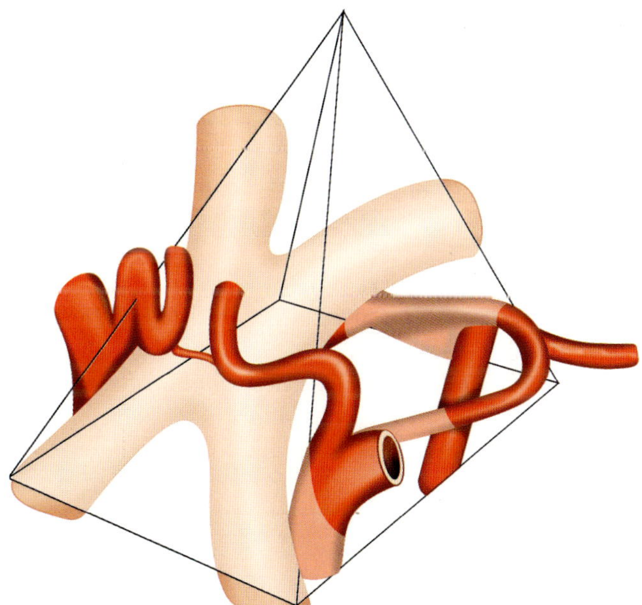

Fig. 22.12: Perneczky's pyramid. *Adapted* from Ref. 36.

CLIVAL/BASILAR REGION

The clivus is positioned at the center of the skull base and is formed by the posterior portion of the sphenoid body (basisphenoid) and occipital bone (basiocciput). It can be divided into thirds, comprised of intrasphenoidal (upper one-third) and extrasphenoidal (lower two-thirds) components. The upper third of the clivus is formed by the basisphenoid and dorsum sellae, the middle third by the portion of the basiocciput above the petroclival fissures, and the lower third by the lower part of the basiocciput. The tectorial membrane overlies the clival dura in the basioccipital portion of the clivus. The largest intercavernous sinus, the basilar sinus, passes from the dorsum sellae to the lower clivus connecting the posterior aspect of both cavernous sinuses.[26] Exposure through the inner dural layer and arachnoid reveals critical neurovascular structures such as the vertebral arteries, basilar

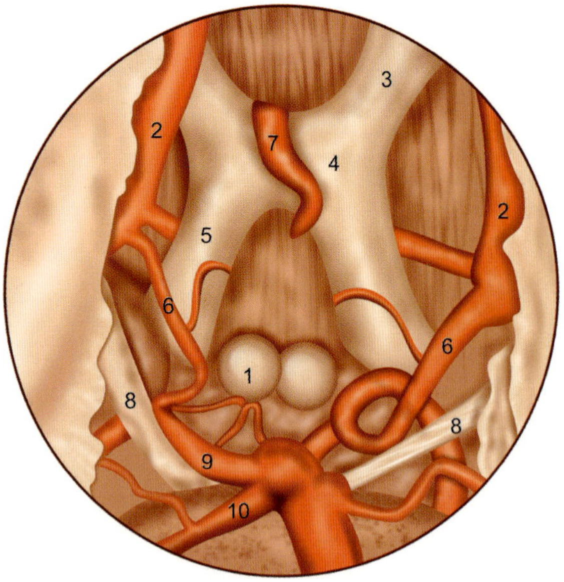

Fig. 22.13: Suprasellar anatomy.
(1: Mammillary body; 2: Internal carotid artery; 3: Optic nerve; 4: Optic chiasm; 5: Optic tract; 6: Posterior communicating artery; 7: Pituitary stalk; 8: Oculomotor nerve; 9: Posterior cerebral artery; 10: Superior cerebellar artery).

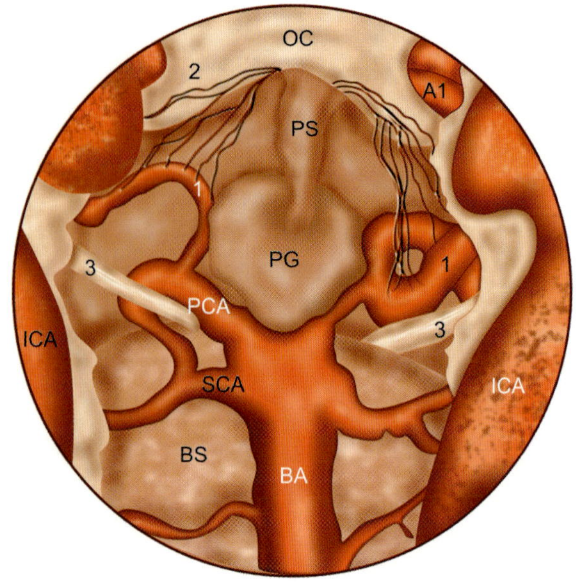

Fig. 22.14: Clival anatomy.
(PG: Pituitary gland; PS: Pituitary stalk; OC: Optic chiasm; ON: Optic nerve; PCA: Posterior cerebral artery; SCA: Superior cerebellar artery; BA: Basilar artery; BS: Brainstem; ICA: Internal carotid artery; 1: Posterior communicating artery; 2: Optic tract; 3: Oculomotor nerve; A1: Anterior cerebral artery, first division).

artery, and its branches (superior cerebellar arteries, anterior inferior cerebellar arteries) posterior cerebral arteries, the brainstem and cranial nerves III, IV, V, and VI (Fig. 22.14).

The oculomotor nerve (CN III) arises from the medial side of the cerebral peduncle, in the interpeduncular cistern, and courses between the superior cerebellar and posterior cerebral arteries. The oculomotor nerve travels in the lateral wall of the interpeduncular cistern, enters the roof of the cavernous sinus and traverses downward in the superior and lateral corner of the cavernous sinus. The trochlear nerve (CN IV) has a particularly long intracranial course, arising below the inferior colliculi and advancing around the dorsal midbrain, coursing under the tentorial edge, and piercing the roof of the cavernous sinus near the anterior tentorial attachment. The trigeminal nerve (CN V) arises from the midpons and divides into its three main branches, ophthalmic (V1), maxillary (V2), and mandibular (V3), at the anterior margin of the trigeminal ganglion. The ophthalmic division (V1) travels in the anteroinferior portion of the cavernous sinus. The medial aspect of the maxillary nerve (V2) flanks the sphenoid sinus as it courses inferior to the cavernous sinus, producing a prominence in the lateral wall of the sphenoid sinus. The abducens nerve (VI) originates near the lower margin of the pons and can pass either above or below the anteroinferior cerebellar artery. CN VI passes through the prepontine cistern and pierces the dura of the clivus at Dorello's canal to enter the posterior aspect of the cavernous sinus near the superior border of the petrous apex (Fig. 22.15).[26]

VASCULAR ANATOMY SELLAR/SUPRASELLAR REGION

The meningohypophyseal trunk, the largest branch of the intracavernous carotid artery, provides the majority of the bloody supply to the sellar region. The meningohypophyseal artery exits the intracavernous carotid artery at the level of the dorsum sellae and gives rise to the inferior hypophyseal artery. The inferior hypophyseal artery travels medially, where it anastomoses with its counterpart from the contralateral side, and provides circulation to the posterior pituitary and dura of the sellar floor (Fig. 22.16).

The perforating branches of the internal carotid artery also supply the optic nerve, chiasm, optic tract, infundibulum, and floor of the third ventricle. The superior hypophyseal artery originates from the supraclinoid portion of the carotid artery, and travels medially beneath the floor of the third ventricle, where it connects with its counterpart from the opposite side to form a vascular ring around the infundibulum (Fig. 22.16). The first branch of the internal carotid artery is the ophthalmic

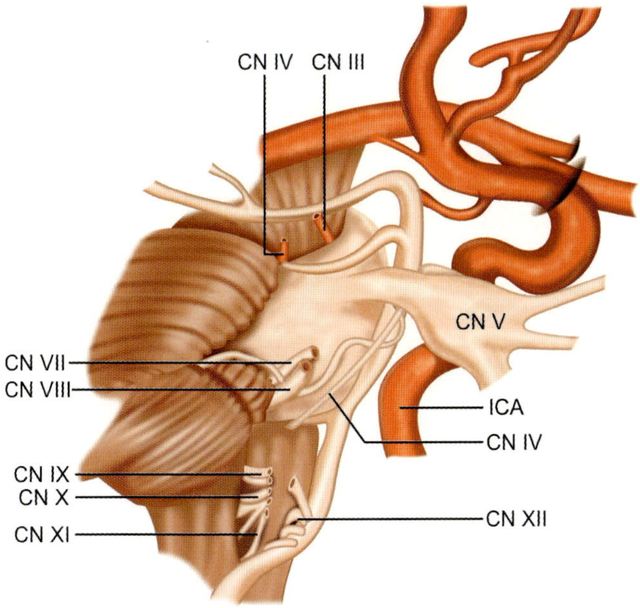

Fig. 22.15: Cranial nerves.
(CN III: Oculomotor nerve; CN IV: Trochlear nerve; CN V: Trigeminal nerve; CN VI: Abducens nerve; CN VII: Facial nerve; CN VIII: Vestibulocochlear nerve; CN IX: Glossopharyngeal nerve; CN X: Vagus nerve; CN XI: Accessory nerve; CN XII: Hypoglossal nerve; ICA: Internal carotid artery).

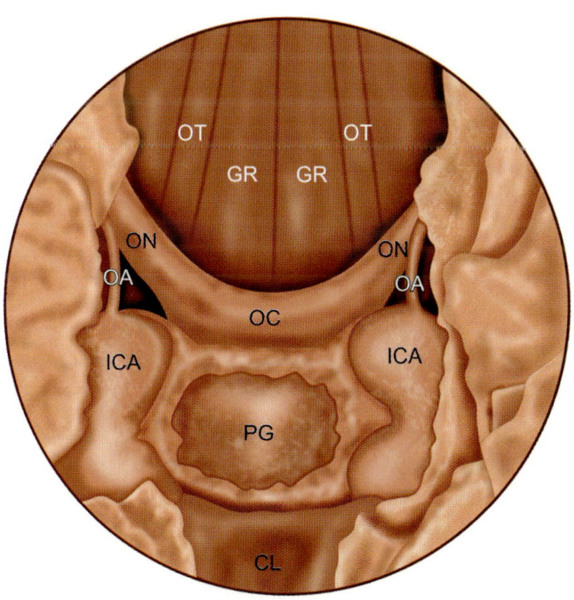

Fig. 22.17: Anterior cranial fossa.
(OA: Ophthalmic artery; OC: Optic chiasm; ON: Optic nerve; OT: Olfactory tract; GR: Gyrus rectus).

artery, which enters the optic canal just below the optic nerve. It most commonly arises from the supraclinoid portion of the carotid artery, but can also arise from the intracavernous carotid[30] and, rarely, from the middle meningeal artery (Fig. 22.17).[31]

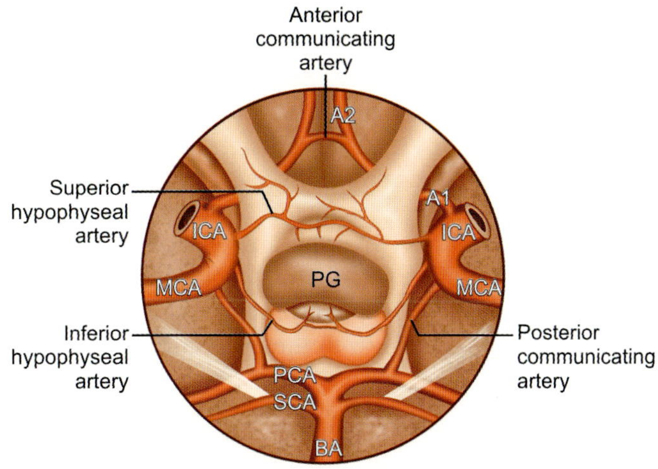

Fig. 22.16: Sellar/suprasellar vascular anatomy.
(PCA: Posterior cerebral artery; SCA: Superior cerebellar artery; BA: Basilar artery; MCA: Middle cerebral artery).

The suprasellar area harbors the circle of Willis. The anterior circle of Willis (the anterior cerebral and anterior communicating arteries) borders the anterior wall of the third ventricle. The anterior cerebral artery arises from the internal carotid artery and passes anteromedially above the optic nerve and chiasm, where it typically anastomoses with the contralateral artery at the interhemispheric fissure.[24] The convergence of the bilateral A1 segments typically occurs above the optic chiasm, forming the anterior communicating artery (ACom). Perforating branches arise from the anterior cerebral and anterior communicating arteries that supply the third ventricle, hypothalamus, fornix, and the anterior part of the basal ganglia and internal capsule (the recurrent artery of Heubner) (Fig. 22.16).[25]

The posterior communicating artery arises from the posterior wall of the internal carotid and travels posteromedially inferior to the optic tracts and floor of the third ventricle to join the posterior cerebral artery (Fig. 22.16). Branches from the posterior communicating artery provide blood supply to the optic chiasm, thalamus, hypothalamus, and internal capsule. The anterior choroidal artery originates from the internal carotid artery, posteriorly, above the origin of the posterior communicating artery. The anterior choroidal artery travels in close proximity to the inferior surface of the optic tract as it progresses posteriorly between the uncus and cerebral peduncle to ultimately supply the optic tract, globus pallidus, genu of the internal capsule, posterior part of the third ventricle, and ultimately the lateral choroid plexus. The venous channels within the suprasellar region are not typically transgressed during surgical exposure and are therefore less of a concern for intraoperative bleeding. Tributaries of the basal vein of Rosenthal drain this region, traveling between the midbrain and temporal lobes feeding into the internal cerebral vein complex at the vein of Galen. The internal cerebral veins often travel in the roof of the third ventricle where they join caudally near the pineal body to form the great vein Galen, as mentioned. Fortunately, the internal cerebral veins are rarely involved with surprasellar pathology, but great care must be exercised if preoperative imaging suggests any close anatomical relation with these structures.

PTERYGOPALATINE FOSSA

The PPF is an inverted pyramidal space, which serves as a portal for a number of endoscopic approaches to the anterolateral skull base.[32-34] This pyramidal region is formed by the pterygoid posteriorly, the maxilla anterolaterally, the perpendicular plate of the palatine bone medially, and the body of the sphenoid superiorly. The PPF communicates with the infratemporal fossa (ITF) laterally via the pterygomaxillary fissure. This region is of particular importance given its intimate relationship with many critical structures, including branches of the internal maxillary artery (IMA), the VN, maxillary nerve, and pterygopalatine ganglion. The PPF can be divided into two compartments, with its anterior compartment containing fat and blood vessels and its posterior compartment containing neural components (Fig. 22.18).

The pterygopalatine branches of the IMA include the posterior superior alveolar artery, infraorbital artery, descending palatine artery, pharyngeal artery, artery of the pterygoid canal, and sphenopalatine artery. The sphenopalatine artery branches carry blood to several vascularized pedicled flaps utilized for endoscopic skull base reconstruction. Specifically, the posterior lateral nasal artery supplies the nasal turbinates and the posterior septal artery, with its anastomoses with the ethmoidal arteries, supplies the posterior nasal septum. The pterygoid venous plexus, which is positioned between the masticator, temporal, and the internal and external pterygoid muscles, provides venous drainage from this region (Fig. 22.18).

The pterygopalatine (sphenopalatine) ganglion, residing in the PPF, is one of four parasympathetic ganglia in the head and neck. The nerves associated with the ganglion include the VN, pharyngeal nerve, descending palatine nerves, nasopalatine nerves, and the posterior superior nasal nerve. The VN carries preganglionic parasympathetic fibers from the greater petrosal nerve and postganglionic sympathetic fibers from the deep petrosal

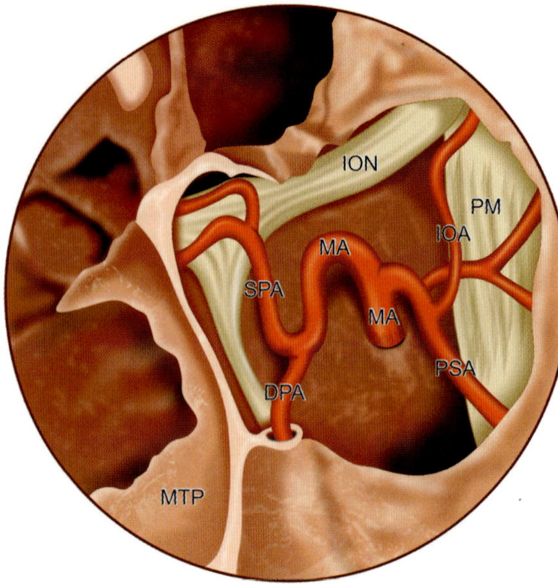

Fig. 22.18: Neurovascular pterygopalatine anatomy.
(ION: Infraorbital nerve, IOA: Infraorbital artery; PSA: Posterior superior alveolar artery; MA: Maxillary artery; SPA: Sphenopalatine artery; DPA: Descending palatine artery; MTP: Medial pterygoid plate).

nerve. The VN travels through the vidian canal and its parasympathetic fibers then synapse on the pterygopalatine ganglion. The parasympathetic branches then distribute to the nose, palate and lacrimal gland through the foramina in the PPF. The VN serves as a valuable surgical landmark for localizing the petrous ICA during supra- and infrapetrous transpterygoid approaches (Fig. 22.19). The maxillary nerve (V2) enters the PPF through the foramen rotundum, distributes its branches, and then continues as the infraorbital nerve through the infraorbital canal, which separates the PPF from the ITF laterally. Primary lesions of the PPF are rare. However, this region may contain metastatic disease or serve as a conduit for local extension of sinonasal or pharyngeal lesions into the ITF, petrous apex, orbital apex, or middle cranial fossa (MCF). There are eight different foramina that transmit various neurovascular structures through the PPF. The infraorbital nerve, zygomatic nerve, infraorbital vessels, and ophthalmic vein pass through the inferior orbital fissure anteriorly to communicate with the orbit. Medially, the sphenopalatine foramen carries the sphenopalatine artery into the nasal cavity, and laterally, the maxillary vessels pass through the pterygomaxillary fissure to communicate with the ITF. Inferiorly, the greater and lesser palatine canals transmit the greater and lesser palatine nerves and vessels, which supply the palate. Three of the eight foramina reside posteriorly within the PPF, including the foramen rotundum, the vidian (pterygoid)

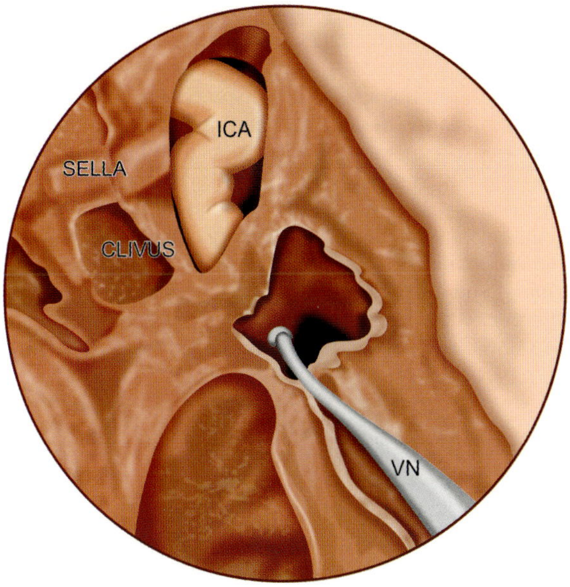

Fig. 22.19: Vidian nerve.

canal, and the pharyngeal (palatovaginal) canal. The foramen rotundum transmits V2, while the vidian canal, located 7–10 mm inferomedial to foramen rotundum, carries the VN to the pterygopalatine (sphenopalatine) ganglion. Branches of the IMA supply the nasopharynx as they pass through the pharyngeal canal located at the lateral part of the posterior choanae.[33]

REFERENCES

1. Lee SC, Senior BA. Endoscopic skull base surgery. Clin Exp Otorhinolaryngol. 2008;1(2):53-62.
2. DelGaudio JM, Hudgins PA, Venkatraman G, et al. Multiplanar computed tomographic analysis of frontal recess cells: effect on frontal isthmus size and frontal sinusitis. Arch Otolaryngol Head Neck Surg. 2005;131(3):230-5.
3. Kuhn F. Lateral nasal wall and sinus surgical anatomy: contemporary understanding. In: Maintenance Manual for Lifelong Learning. New York: Thieme; 2001.
4. Wormold PJ. Anatomy of the frontal recess and frontal sinus. In: Wormold PJ, (Eds). Endoscopic Sinus Surgery. 2nd ed. New York: Thieme; 2005. pp. 54-69.
5. Keros P. Uber die praktische Bedeutung der Niveauunterschiede de lamina cribrosa des Ethmoids. In: Laryngol Rhinol Otol (Stuttgart). 1965;41:808-13.
6. Fernandez-Miranda JC, Prevedello DM, Madhok R, et al. Sphenoid septations and their relationship with internal carotid arteries: anatomical and radiological study. Laryngoscope 2009;119(10).
7. Poirier J, Duggal N, Lee D, et al. Sphenoid sinus septations: Unpredictable anatomic landmarks in endoscopic pituitary surgery. J Otolaryngol Head Neck Surg. 2011;40(6):489-92.
8. Singh A, Roth J, Anand VK, et al. Anatomy of the pituitary gland and parasellar areas. In: Schwartz TH, Anand VK (Eds). Endoscopic Pituitary Surgery—A Comprehensive Guide. New York: Thieme; 2011.
9. Hammer G, Radberg C. The sphenoidal sinus: an anatomical and roentgenologic study with reference to transsphenoid hypophysectomy. Acta Radiol. 1961;56:401-22.
10. Gupta T, Aggarwal A, Sahni D. Anatomical landmarks for locating the sphenoid sinus ostium during endoscopic endonasal approach: a cadaveric study. Surg Radiol Anat. 2013;35(2):137-42.
11. Kim HU, Kim SS, Kang SS, et al. Surgical anatomy of the natural ostium of the sphenoid sinus. Laryngoscope. 2001; 111(9):1599-602.
12. Bolger WE, Keyes AS, Lanza DC. Use of the superior meatus and superior turbinate in the endoscopic approach to the sphenoid sinus. Otolaryngol Head Neck Surg. 1999;120: 308-13.
13. Bansberg SF, Harner SG, Forbes G. Relationship of the optic nerve to the paranasal sinuses as shown by computed tomography. Otolaryngol Head Neck Surg. 1987;96:331-5.
14. Driben JS, Bolger WE, Robles HA, et al. The reliability of computerized tomographic detection of the Onodi (Sphenoethmoid) cell. Am J Rhinol. 1998;12(2):105-11.
15. Kosling S, Wagner F, Schulz HG, et al. Knocherne variationen im koronaren nasennebenhohlen-CT. Fortschr Rontgenstr. 1993;159:506-10.
16. Dixon FW. A comparative study of the sphenoid sinus (A study of 1600 skulls). Ann Otol Rhinol Laryngol. 1937;46: 687-98.
17. Lang J. Uber die Cellulae ethmoidales posteriores und ihre Beziehungen zum Canalis opticus. HNO. 1988;36:49-53.
18. Mellinger WI. The optic nerves and their relations in the sphenoidal region. Tr Pacific Coast Oto-Ophth Soc. 1937; 22:85-94.
19. Van Alyea OE. Ethmoid labyrinth: anatomic study, with consideration of the clinical significance of its structural characteristics. Arch Otolaryngol. 1939;29:881-902.
20. Van Alyea OE. Sphenoid sinus: anatomic study, with consideration of the clinical significance of the structural characteristics of the sphenoid sinus. Arch Otolaryngol. 1941;34:225-53.
21. Tomovic S, Esmaeili A, Chan NJ, et al. High-resolution computed tomography analysis of the prevalence of onodi cells. Laryngoscope. 2012;122(7):1470-3.
22. Yuntao L, Jun P, Songtao Q, et al. Pneumatization of the sphenoid sinus in Chinese: the differences from Caucasian and its application in the extended transsphenoidal approach. J Anat. 2011;219:132-42.
23. Labib MA, Prevedello DM, Fernandez-Miranda JC, et al. The medial opticocarotid recess: an anatomic study of an endoscopic "key landmark" for the ventral cranial base. Neurosurgery. 2013;72(1 suppl operative):66-76;discussion 76.
24. Barañano CF, Curé J, Palmer JN, et al. Sternberg's canal: fact or fiction? Am J Rhinol Allergy. 2009;23(2):167-71.
25. Rhoton AL Jr. The sellar region. Neurosurgery. 2002;51 (4 suppl):S335-74.

26. Rhoton AL. The anterior and middle cranial fossa. Neurosurgery. 2002;51(suppl 1):273-302.
27. Joo W, Yoshioka F, Funaki T, et al. Microsurgical anatomy of the abducens nerve. Clin Anat. 2012;25(8):1030-42.
28. Ono M, Ono M, Rhoton AL Jr., et al. Microsurgical anatomy of the region of the tentorial incisura. J Neurosurg. 1984; 60(2):365-99.
29. Rhoton AL. The Orbit and Sellar Region: Microsurgical Anatomy and Operative Approaches. New York: Thieme; 1996.
30. Huynh-Le P, Natori Y, Sasaki T. Surgical anatomy of the ophthalmic artery: its origin and proximal course. Neurosurgery. 2005;57(4 suppl):236-41, discussion 236-41.
31. Liu Q, Rhoton AL Jr. Middle meningeal origin of the ophthalmic artery. Neurosurgery. 2001;49(2):401-6, discussion 406-7.
32. Alfieri A, Jho HD, Schettino R, et al. Endoscopic endonasal approach to the pterygopalatine fossa: anatomic study. Neurosurgery. 2003;42(2):374-78, discussion 378-80.
33. Hofstetter CP, Singh A, Anand VK, et al. The endoscopic, endonasal, transmaxillary transpterygoid approach to the pterygopalatine fossa, infratemporal fossa, petrous apex, and the meckel cave. J Neurosurg. 2010;113(5):967-74.
34. Kassam AB, Vescan AD, Carrau RL, et al. Expanded endonasal approach: vidian canal as a landmark to the petrous internal carotid artery. J Neurosurg. 2008;108(1):177-83.
35. Wang J, Bidari S, Inoue K, et al. Extensions of the sphenoid sinus: a new classification. Neurosurgery. 2010;66(4):797-816.
36. Perneczky A, Tschabitscher M, Resch KDM. Endoscopic Anatomy for Neurosurgery. Stutgart, NY: George Thieme; 1993.

CHAPTER

23

Management of CSF Rhinorrhea

Mohamad R Chaaban, Bradford A Woodworth

ETIOLOGY

Cerebrospinal fluid (CSF) leaks are classified according to etiology into either secondary to trauma, spontaneous, neoplasm, or congenital. When considering surgical repair of defects in the skull base, there are several factors that need to be addressed. These include the presence or absence of an encephalocele or intracranial hypertension as well as the site and size of the defect. The management of CSF leaks depends on the etiology with the success rate over 90% in multiple studies with the minimally invasive transnasal endoscopic technique.[1-3]

Trauma

Traumatic CSF leaks are caused by either blunt or penetrating trauma with patients either presenting early with active leak or late with meningitis, delayed leak or encephaloceles. Conservative treatment is usually adequate for traumatic leaks; however, there has been reported a 29% incidence of meningitis in patients that were not surgically managed.[4]

Neoplasm

CSF leaks due to a neoplasm occur as a result of erosion of the tumor into the skull base of the anterior or middle cranial fossa or as a result of resection of the tumor. Removal of these tumors can be performed endoscopically in select cases or through an open approach and requires an adequate, water tight seal between the sinonasal and intracranial cavities. Endoscopic reconstruction consists of multilayer repairs. While a variety of tissues may be utilized, a vascularized nasoseptal flap has been demonstrated to improve the rate of CSF leak recurrences. Endoscopic-assisted craniofacial resection or traditional craniofacial resection are most commonly repaired with a pericranial flap or combination of pericranial and a nasoseptal flap if available.[5]

Congenital

Congenital encephaloceles are historically divided into sincipital and basal encephaloceles.[6] Basal encephaloceles are intranasal and further divided into transethmoidal, sphenoethmoidal, sphenomaxillary, spheno-orbital, transsphenoidal, as well as transtemporal.[7] The most common ones encountered arise from the cribriform plate.[6] Transethmoidal encephaloceles typically originate from the foramen cecum with a deviated crista galli and variable extension into the cribriform or ethmoidal roof. These encephaloceles are likely caused by the failure of closure of the fonticulus frontalis.[6] Another type of ethmoidal encephalocele exists with a normal foramen cecum. Patients typically have a low lying skull base with a funnel-shaped defect. Transsphenoidal congenital encephaloceles are either intrasphenoidal or true transsphenoidal[8] with the latter presenting as a mass that protrudes into the nose or nasopharynx and is usually associated with coexisting facial, optic as well as central nervous system (CNS) abnormalities.[9] CSF leaks originating in the lateral recess of the sphenoid sinus have been described as a congenital origin from a persistent embryonic canal called a lateral craniopharyngeal canal (Sternberg's canal)[10]; however, the location of this canal as originally described in the literature is medial to the foramen rotundum, which does not explain the existence of sphenoid sinus CSF leaks that occur lateral to the maxillary nerve.[11,12] CSF leaks from the sphenoid lateral recess are thus always acquired and most commonly spontaneous.

Spontaneous

As opposed to the excellent repair rates seen with other causes of CSF leaks, the success rates for spontaneous CSF leak have varied in the literature between 25% and 87%.[13] These patients may present with or had a history of signs and symptoms of elevated intracranial hypertension as part of the syndrome of idiopathic intracranial hypertension (IIH) with pulsatile tinnitus, headache, as well as visual disturbances.[14-18] In a 5-year prospective evaluation of endoscopic spontaneous CSF leak repair, the majority of patients (45 out of 48) had radiologic and clinical symptoms associated with elevated intracranial pressure (ICP).[19] Radiologically, these patients have partial or total empty sella reported in up to 85%.[19,20] In addition, other features of elevated ICP may be seen including arachnoid pits, encephaloceles, dilated Meckel's caves, and dural ectasias.[18] Similarly, clinical as well as demographic similarities have been found between patients with IIH, formerly known as pseudotumor cerebri, and patients with spontaneous CSF leaks. Patients with spontaneous CSF leaks are commonly obese middle-aged females and tend to have an average body mass index of 36.[21-28] The most common areas for spontaneous CSF leaks to occur include the lateral recess of sphenoid, frontal sinus as well as the cribriform plate of ethmoid.[16] Patients with IIH typically present with pulsatile tinnitus, balance problems, headache as well as visual disturbances. The exact pathophysiology is still unknown regarding the occurrence of spontaneous CSF leaks. The role of obesity suggests increased intra-abdominal and thoracic pressure causes decreased venous return and cerebral venous outflow thereby preventing CSF absorption. In support of this theory, the incidence of raised intra-abdominal and ICP was much higher in morbidly obese patients compared with controls in one study.[29] Regardless of the reason for CSF pressure elevation, the constant pulsatile forces on the skull base leads to erosion at sites of inherent weakness.

DIAGNOSIS

There are a variety of methods to diagnose a CSF leak. Currently, the most commonly accepted test is evaluation of nasal fluid for beta-2 transferrin as there is a low false positive and false negative rate.[30] For localization, imaging in the form of CT and CT cisternography can be utilized. CT scan provides bony detail of the cranial base that can also be used for computer-assisted intraoperative surgical navigation (Fig. 23.1). The primary drawback of CT is the lack of differentiation between CSF/encephalocele formation and other soft tissue opacification. Additionally, the site of dehiscence may not necessarily indicate the site of active leakage as some defects may be present without active CSF leak. Indeed, spontaneous CSF leaks are commonly associated with multiple areas of attenuated bone. To resolve this problem, injecting intrathecal contrast in CT cisternography may be utilized to localize active leakage. It is quite useful for sphenoid sinus leaks since it acts as a reservoir; however, this may miss intermittent CSF leaks, particularly in sites other than the sphenoid. This test has a sensitivity between 48% and 96%.[30] An advantage of MRI over CT scan is the ability to distinguish between CSF and other opacified soft tissue through the use of fast spin echo with fat suppression and image reversal.[31] MRI has a sensitivity of 85–92% and specificity of up to 100% for localizing CSF leaks[30,32] This imaging modality provides detailed brain imaging revealing encephaloceles, tumor, and signs of elevated ICP such as empty sella, dural ectasia, and optic nerve findings (e.g., dilated optic nerve sheath, vertical tortuosity, and scleral blunting). MRI should be viewed as complementary to CT as it does not provide detailed bony anatomy. The radionuclide cisternogram involves injection of a radioactive marker intrathecally with placement of intranasal pledgets. Although this technique has been used to detect intermittent leaks, the test is not recommended because of unacceptable false positive rates.[19,30] Finally, the injection of intrathecal fluorescein with endoscopic examination is very useful for detecting active leakage at the time of surgery, especially for spontaneous CSF leaks (high rates of multiple leaks) and comminuted fractures of the skull base. Fluorescein is not FDA approved because of reports of neurotoxicity and seizures that have occurred when administered at high concentrations and rapid infusions. Diluting 0.1 mL of 10% Fluorescein in 10 mL of patient's CSF and injecting it slowly over a 10–15 min appears to be safe with minimal

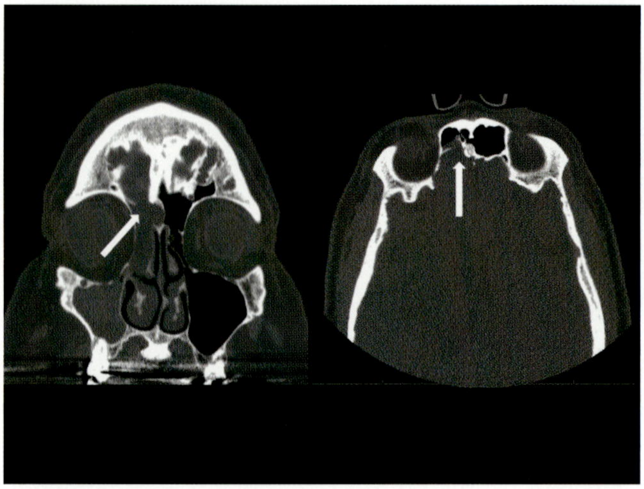

Fig. 23.1: Coronal (right) and axial (left) CT scans of a patient with a right frontal sinus posterior (arrows) table defect with encephalocele.

complications in nearly 20 years of use.[19] Intrathecal fluorescein is more helpful in patients who already have their skull base skeletonized. While it aids in localization, the green staining of CSF also assists with ensuring a watertight seal following repair.

MANAGEMENT OF CSF LEAKS

Skull base defect reconstructive techniques can vary depending on the site, etiology, and preference of the surgeon. There are a number of repair materials available including dural substitutes (e.g., xenografts, cadaveric dermis), structural support materials (e.g., bone, cartilage, synthetics), and mucosal grafts or flaps. Structural support grafts do not appear to be necessary, but are utilized commonly for spontaneous leaks associated with intracranial hypertension for the theoretical value. Vascularized nasoseptal flaps or other vascularized local flaps are also preferred for larger defects.[33] The general surgical technique requires removing several millimeters of the mucosa surrounding the defect since the sinus mucosal gland secretions may lead to mucoceles or lifting the graft off the surgical site. Stripping the mucosa can lead to osteoneogenesis and aid in future structural support for the defect. For spontaneous CSF leaks with documented elevated ICP postoperatively above 15 cm H_2O, medical treatment with acetazolamide is recommended.[34] Acetazolamide is a carbonic anhydrase inhibitor that decreases CSF production up to 48% and may decrease the recurrence of CSF leak.[34] For multiple defects, significantly elevated ICP (>30 cm H_2O), or for those who failed medical management with acetazolamide, neurosurgical evaluation is recommended for ventriculoperitoneal (VP) shunt insertion. VP shunts consist of a shunt valve as well as ventricular and peritoneal catheters. Complications from permanent diversion of CSF include infection, obstruction, malfunction, and over- or underdrainage. For this reason, VP shunts should be carefully selected for patients with high pressure who recur or those with significantly high pressure and/or multiple defects. Careful postoperative management of these spontaneous CSF leaks with pressure measurements assists with the detection of individuals who may require shunting.

Surgical Technique for Repair of CSF Leaks

Step 1

Application of a topical decongestant as well as injecting the septum with local anesthesia (1% lidocaine with 1/100,000 epinephrine) in preparation for harvesting a septal flap.

Step 2

Depending upon the location of the encephalocele and the exposure, an endoscopic sinus surgery including sphenoidotomy, ethmoidectomy, maxillary antrostomy, and frontal sinusotomy are performed for exposure. If the exposure is limited by an encephalocele, then meticulous reduction with an endoscopic bipolar or radiofrequency coblation (Coblator®, ArthroCare ENT, Austin, TX) will provide the necessary operative visualization (Figs. 23.2 and 23.3).[24,35] It is important that the encephalocele is not reduced in a narrow field.

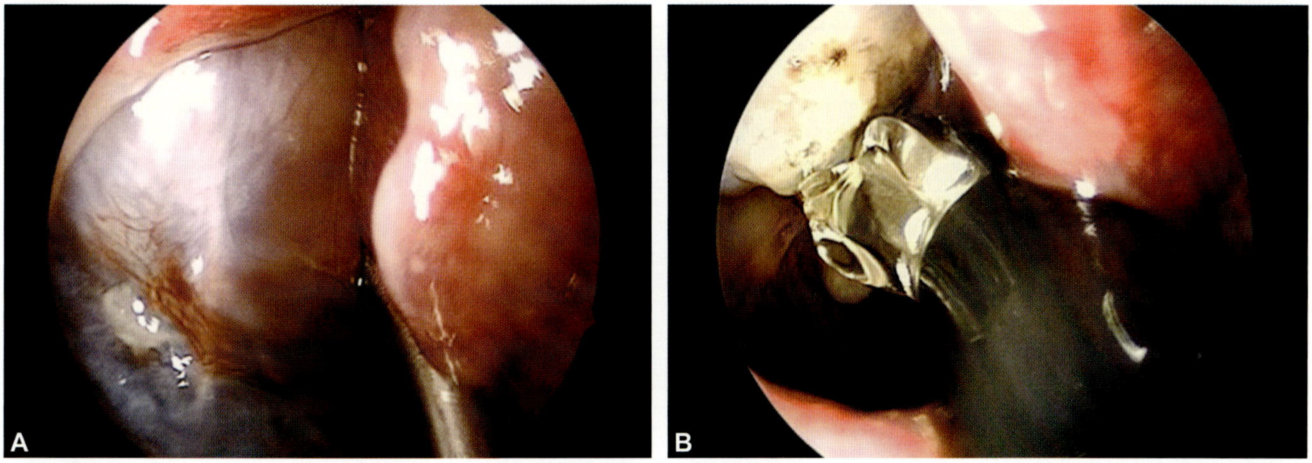

Figs. 23.2A and B: An encephalocele is identified emanating from the right frontal sinus within the middle meatus (A). After opening the maxillary and other surrounding sinuses, the encephalocele is meticulously ablated and reduced with complete hemostasis using the Coblator® (ArthroCare ENT, Austin, TX) (B).

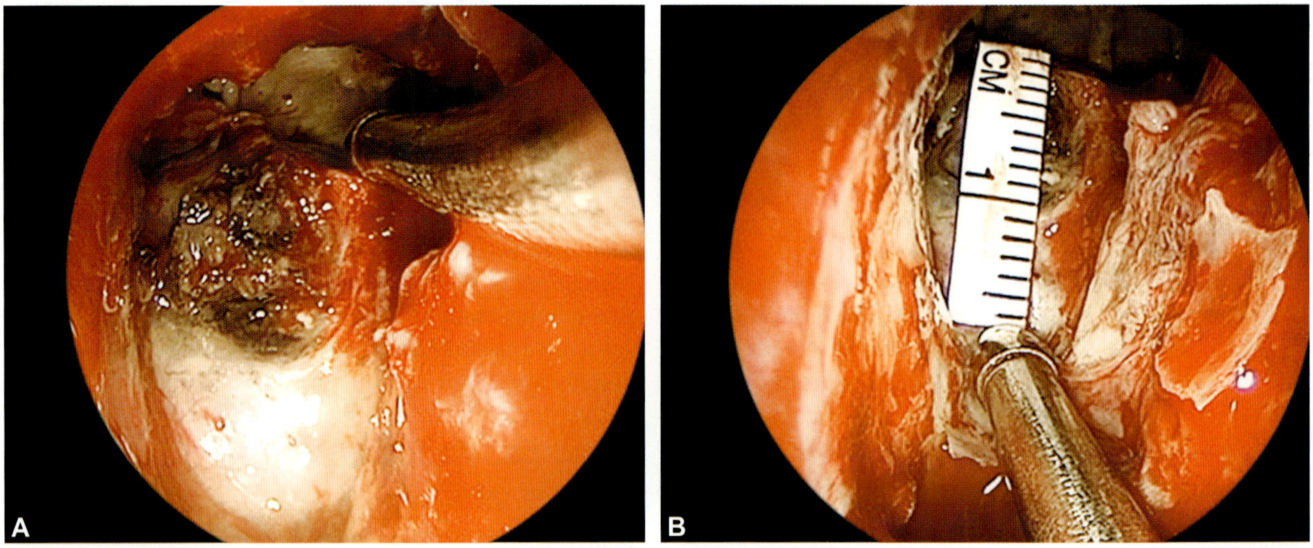

Figs. 23.3A and B: The encephalocele has been completely removed and the frontal sinus opened (A). The cranial base defect is measured with a ruler endoscopically to judge graft size (B).

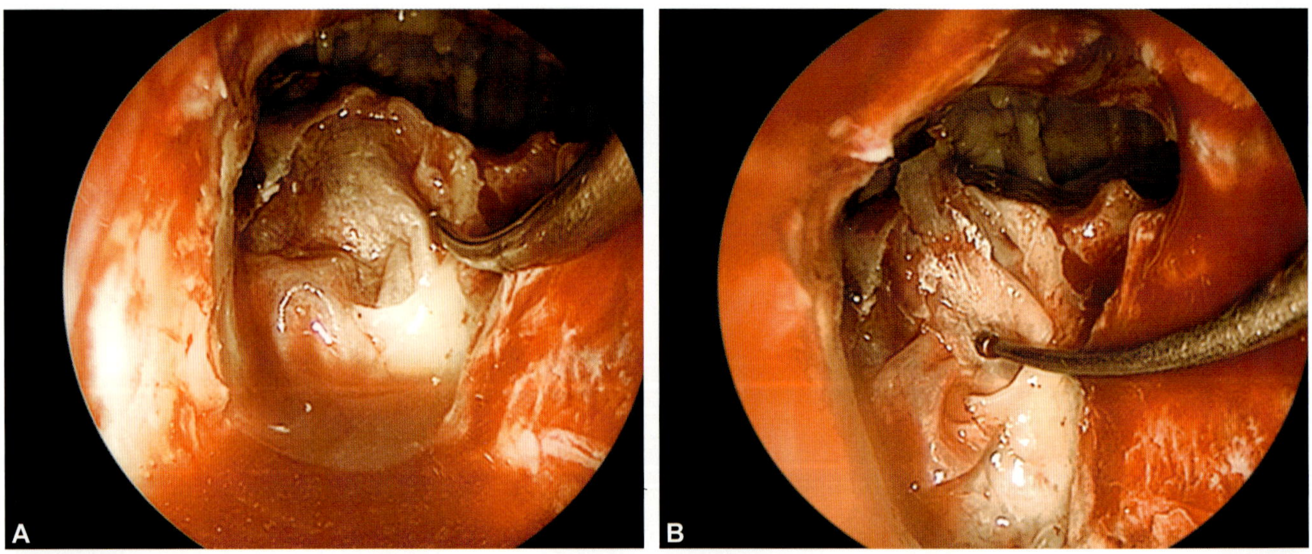

Figs. 23.4A and B: A multilayer reconstruction is performed using porcine small intestine submucosal xenograft (Biodesign®, Cook Medical, Bloomington, IN) (A). An underlay bone graft is also positioned in the epidural space (B).

Step 3

The sinus mucosa surrounding the defect is coagulated and meticulous hemostasis is maintained.

Step 4

A multilayer reconstruction is used for reconstruction for defects larger than several mm (Figs. 23.4A and B). An underlay graft with fascia, cadaveric dermis, or xenograft is placed in an epidural fashion. A bone graft is also placed in the epidural space if intracranial hypertension is suspected. Overlay grafts with fascia, mucosa, or vascularized pedicled local flaps (e.g., nasoseptal flap) are positioned and fixated with fibrin glue (Evicel®, Somerville, NJ) (Figs. 23.5 and 23.6).

Step 5

Support packing with gelfoam or other absorbable packing and removable cotton spacer in a nonlatex gloved finger counteracts coughing or other val salva upon extubation and postoperatively during the first week of graft healing.

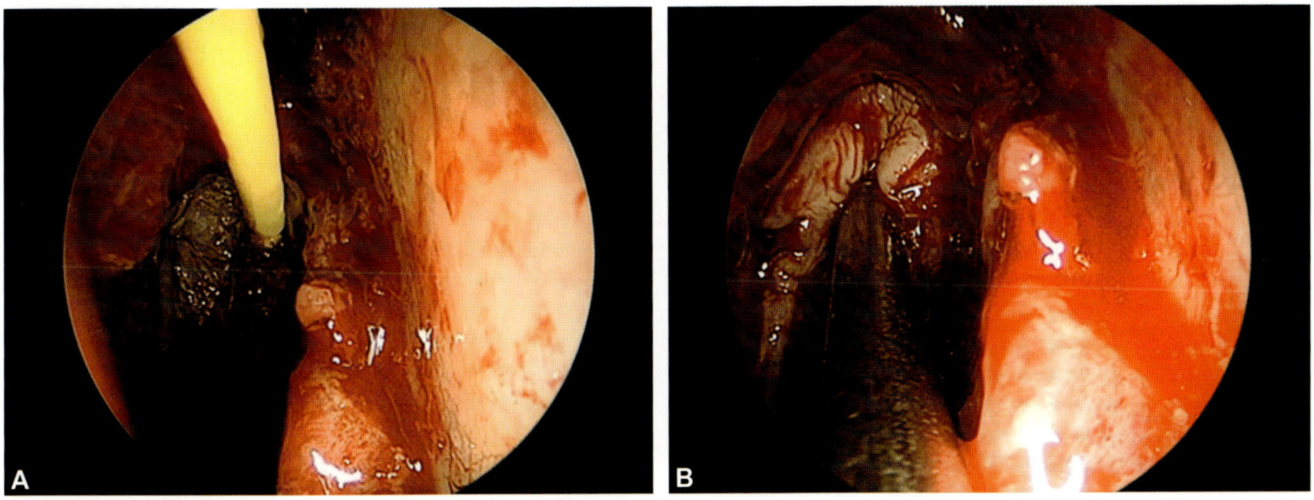

Figs. 23.5A and B: Fibrin glue (Evicel®, Somerville, NJ) helps keep the graft in place (A). A nasoseptal flap is placed over the defect and into the frontal sinus (B).

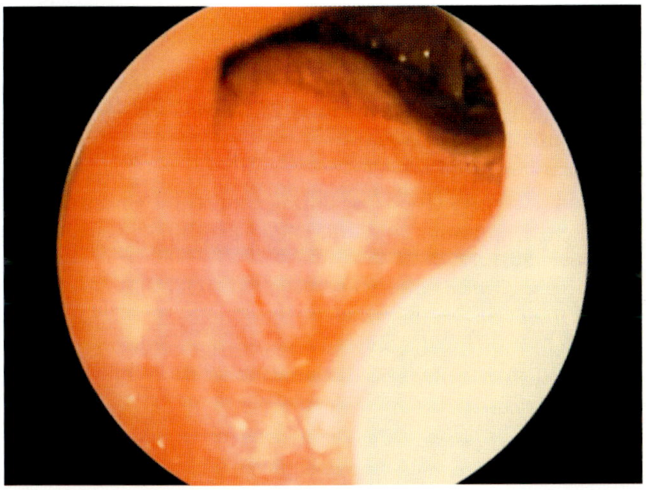

Fig. 23.6: Transnasal 70° endoscopic view of the nasoseptal flap covering the right posterior table defect at 6 months. It is important to avoid collateral damage during and following the repair by meticulous postoperative management to keep the sinuses patent.

REFERENCES

1. Banks CA, Palmer JN, Chiu AG, et al. Endoscopic closure of CSF rhinorrhea: 193 cases over 21 years. Otolaryngol Head Neck Surg. 2009;140(6):826-33.
2. Mattox DE, Kennedy DW. Endoscopic management of cerebrospinal fluid leaks and cephaloceles. Laryngoscope. 1990;100(8):857-62.
3. Schick B, Ibing R, Brors D, et al. Long-term study of endonasal duraplasty and review of the literature. Ann Otol Rhinol Laryngol. 2001;110(2):142-7.
4. Bernal-Sprekelsen M, Bleda-Vazquez C, et al. Ascending meningitis secondary to traumatic cerebrospinal fluid leaks. Am J Rhinol. 2000;14(4):257-9.
5. Chaaban MR, Chaudhry A, Riley KO, et al. Simultaneous pericranial and nasoseptal flap reconstruction of anterior skull base defects following endoscopic-assisted craniofacial resection. Laryngoscope. 2013;123:2383-6.
6. Woodworth BA, Schlosser RJ, Faust RA, et al. Evolutions in the management of congenital intranasal skull base defects. Arch Otolaryngol Head Neck Surg. 2004;130(11):1283-8.
7. David DJ. Cephaloceles: classification, pathology, and management—a review. J Craniofac Surg. 1993;4(4):192-202.
8. Woodworth BA, Neal JG, Schlosser RJ. Sphenoid sinus cerebrospinal fluid leaks. Op Tech Otolaryngol. 2006;17:37-42.
9. Moore MH, Lodge ML, David DJ. Basal encephalocoele: imaging and exposing the hernia. Br J Plast Surg. 1993;46(6):497-502.
10. Castelnuovo P, Dallan I, Pistochini A, et al. Endonasal endoscopic repair of Sternberg's canal cerebrospinal fluid leaks. Laryngoscope. 2007;117(2):345-9.
11. Mirza S, Thaper A, McClelland L, et al. Sinonasal cerebrospinal fluid leaks: management of 97 patients over 10 years. Laryngoscope. 2005;115(10):1774-7.
12. Zuckerman J, Stankiewicz JA, Chow JM. Long-term outcomes of endoscopic repair of cerebrospinal fluid leaks and meningoencephaloceles. Am J Rhinol. 2005;19(6):582-7.
13. Hubbard JL, McDonald TJ, Pearson BW, et al. Spontaneous cerebrospinal fluid rhinorrhea: evolving concepts in diagnosis and surgical management based on the Mayo Clinic experience from 1970 through 1981. Neurosurgery. 1985;16(3):314-21.
14. Illing E, Chaaban MR, Riley KO, et al. Porcine small intestine submucosal graft for endoscopic skull base reconstruction. Int Forum Aller Rhinol. 2013;3:928-32.
15. Chaaban MR, Illing E, Riley KO, et al. Acetazolamide for high intracranial pressure cerebrospinal fluid leaks. Int Forum Allergy Rhinol. 2013;3:718-21.
16. Chaaban MR, Illing E, Riley KO, et al. Spontaneous cerebrospinal fluid leak repair: A five-year prospective evaluation. Laryngoscope. 2013;105:70-5.

17. Jones V, Virgin F, Riley K, Woodworth BA. Changing paradigms in frontal sinus cerebrospinal fluid leak repair. Int Forum Allergy Rhinol. 2012;2:227-32.
18. Woodworth BA, Palmer JN. Spontaneous cerebrospinal fluid leaks. Curr Opin Otolaryngol Head Neck Surg. 2009; 17(1):59-65.
19. Woodworth BA, Prince A, Chiu AG, et al. Spontaneous CSF leaks: A paradigm for definitive repair and management of intracranial hypertension. Otolaryngol Head Neck Surg. 2008;138(6):715-20.
20. Schlosser RJ, Bolger WE. Spontaneous nasal cerebrospinal fluid leaks and empty sella syndrome: a clinical association. Am J Rhinol. 2003;17(2):91-6.
21. Radhakrishnan K, Thacker AK, Bohlaga NH, et al. Epidemiology of idiopathic intracranial hypertension: a prospective and case-control study. J Neurol Sci. 1993; 116(1):18-28.
22. Woodworth BA, Schlosser RJ, Palmer JN. Endoscopic repair of frontal sinus cerebrospinal fluid leaks. J Laryngol Otol. 2005;119(9):709-13.
23. Purkey MT, Woodworth BA, Hahn S, et al. Endoscopic repair of supraorbital ethmoid cerebrospinal fluid leaks. ORL J Otorhinolaryngol Relat Spec. 2009;71(2):93-8.
24. Smith N, Riley KO, Woodworth BA. Endoscopic Coblator-assisted management of encephaloceles. Laryngoscope. 2010;120:(12):2535-9.
25. Hatch NU, Riley KO, Woodworth BA. Endoscopic removal of a bullet penetrating the middle cranial fossa. Skull Base Rep 2011;1(1):47-50.
26. Schuster D, Riley KO, Cure JK, et al. Endoscopic resection of intracranial dermoid cysts. J Laryngol Otol. 2011;125(4): 423-7.
27. Virgin F, Baranano CF, Riley K, et al. Frontal sinus skull base defect repair using the pedicled nasoseptal flap. Otolaryngol Head Neck Surg. 2011;145:338-40.
28. Chaaban MR, Woodworth BA. Complications of skull base reconstruction. Adv Otorhinolaryngol. 2013;74:148-62.
29. Bloomfield GL, Ridings PC, Blocher CR, et al. A proposed relationship between increased intra-abdominal, intrathoracic, and intracranial pressure. Crit Care Med. 1997; 25(3):496-503.
30. Schlosser RJ, Bolger WE. Nasal cerebrospinal fluid leaks: critical review and surgical considerations. Laryngoscope. 2004;114(2):255-65.
31. Eljamel MS. Fractures of the middle third of the face and cerebrospinal fluid rhinorrhoea. Br J Neurosurg. 1994;8(3): 289-93.
32. Woodworth BA, Schlosser RJ. Repair of anterior skull base defects and CSF Leaks. Op Tech Otolaryngol. 2006;18: 111-6.
33. Hadad G, Bassagasteguy L, Carrau RL, et al. A novel reconstructive technique after endoscopic expanded endonasal approaches: vascular pedicle nasoseptal flap. Laryngoscope. 2006;116(10):1882-6.
34. Chaaban MR, Illing E, Riley KO, et al. Acetazolamide for high intracranial pressure CSF leaks. Int Forum Aller Rhinol. 2013;3:718-21.
35. Kostrzewa JP, Sunde J, Riley KO, et al. Radiofrequency coblation decreases blood loss during endoscopic sinonasal and skull base tumor removal. ORL J Otorhinolaryngol Relat Spec. 2010;72(1):38-43.

CHAPTER

24

Sellar and Parasellar Approaches

Spencer C Payne, Robert G Louis, John A Jane

BACKGROUND

Sellar Pathology

Pituitary tumors represent 10–15% of all primary brain tumors and as many as 20% of surgically resected brain tumors.[1] These tumors are traditionally categorized in two dichotomous manners based on size and functionality with fairly high association between them. Patients presenting with clinical symptoms due a hypersecretory tumor (e.g., Cushings, acromegaly, or prolactinoma) are classified as functional. Typically, these lesions are often also microadenomas (defined as less than 1.0 cm) as the patients present with symptoms before the tumor has significantly grown in size. Conversely, patients with nonfunctioning tumors typically do not present until the tumors have grown in size resulting in mass-effect, typically the homonymous hemianopsia of optic chiasm compression. Often, these exceed 1 cm in size and are categorized as macroadenomas. While the functioning and nonfunctioning tumors tend to also segregate into micro- and macroadenomas, respectively this overlap is not always "respected" and delays in diagnosis or those diagnosed incidentally may result in cross-over. Of the nonfunctioning macroadenomas, up to 10% may present with pituitary apoplexy, having bled into themselves. These tumors are not only usually larger upon diagnosis with extrasellar extension, but are typically associated with sphenoid mucosal edema, resulting in a more challenging approach and resection.

Preoperative Imaging

While computed tomography is the gold-standard for evaluation of the nose and paranasal sinuses for most endoscopic sinonasal surgery, magnetic resonance imaging with contrast is the modality of choice for pituitary tumors. Smaller tumors often appear isointense on T1 and T2 weighted series. Contrasted series usually reveal a relative hypointensity of the lesion and can be important in determining the approach and explorations when tumors are small. Macroadenomas appear slightly differently, often with mixed appearance on T1 and T2 that is relatively isointense with variable enhancement on contrasted series. Despite gross alteration in the size and shape of the sella, the pituitary infundibulum can usually be identified and traced to a small rim of enhancement indicating the location of residual, normal gland. For the surgeon desiring anatomical detail of the sphenoid or posterior ethmoid sinuses for operative planning, T2 and/or contrasted series are often adequate for demonstrating the thin mucosal layers overling bony septations similar to the standard CT scan. That being said, in revision cases, or massive extrasellar tumors where the usual sinonasal architecture has been dramatically altered, additional CT evaluation is both warranted and recommended.

Preoperative Lab Evaluation

Typically, these tests are arranged and managed by endocrinologists who must remain pivotal members of the team, but the surgeon should be cognizant of the significant physiologic derangements which can be present before embarking on the surgical management of these tumors. Prolactinomas represent approximately 40% of all pituitary adenomas[2] and are the only functional adenomas for which medical therapy is the primary modality of treatment. As such, the evaluation of prolactin levels after radiographic diagnosis of a sellar lesion is essential. It is not uncommon to find mildly elevated prolactin levels in patient with macroadenomas because of an anti-inhibitory effect resulting from stalk compression. Consequently, levels lower than 200 ng/mL may be consistent with other macroadenomas, pregnancy, or other physiologic causes. Determination of adrenal corticotrophic hormone (ACTH) production and/or cortisol levels are also important, not only in the setting of Cushing's disease, but also to evaluate for potential hypocortisolism, which can have significant detrimental effects if supplementation and stress dosing are not provided in the perioperative setting.

Surgical Approaches

The goals of pituitary surgery are (1) the normalization of excess hormone secretion, (2) alleviation of any mass effect, and (3) preservation of normal pituitary function. The sublabial transseptal microscopic approach has been the traditional method for accessing the sella for years. Modifications of this technique have included a transnasal transseptal which suffers from a narrowed approach and risk of alar avulsion. The advantage however was the decreased pain and healing time compared with the sublabial approach. The technique has been further modified to include the use of endoscopes, but overtime even this has progressed to the endonasal transsphenoidal approach as described below. Two recent series have indicated that when direct comparison is made between surgeons experienced in microscopic and endoscopic approaches the success rates are comparable for both functional (e.g., acromegaly[3]) and nonfunctional tumors[4] indicating that in terms of the goals noted above, the approaches are equivalent. The advantage of the endoscopic approach however, is the improved visualization that comes from superior illumination and views afforded by angled endoscopes, albeit this may be more important for macro-versus microadenomas. Further, studies have indicated that the endoscopic approach typically results in decreased operating time, fewer rhinologic complications, less pain, and shorter postoperative stays[5] all of which are important secondary outcomes to the rhinologist and skull base surgeon.

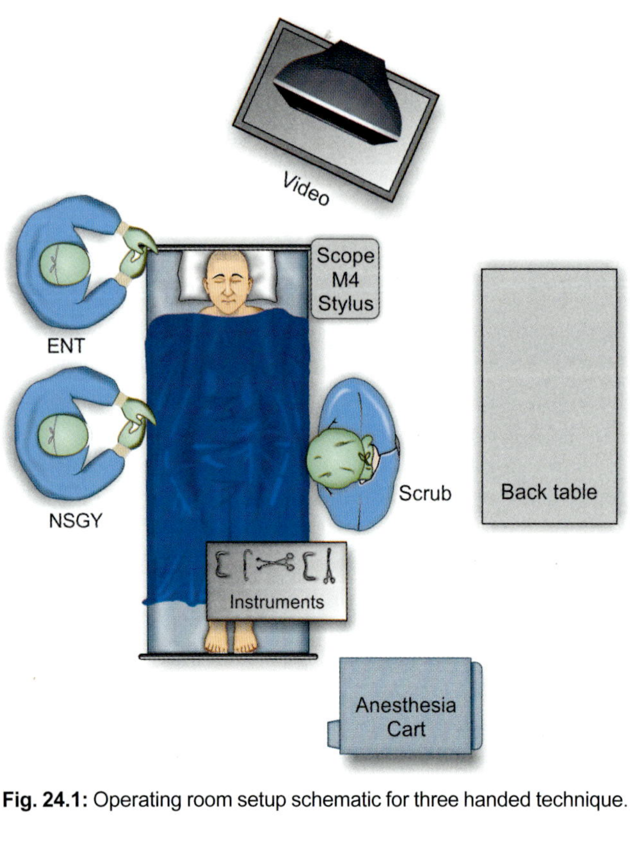

Fig. 24.1: Operating room setup schematic for three handed technique.

O.R. SETUP AND PATIENT POSITIONING

The operating table is turned at least 180° away from the anesthesia cart to provide sufficient room for the surgeon and the equipment (Figs. 24.1 and 24.2). The right-handed surgeon will find it easiest to be on the patient's right side with the scrub and back table across the patient on their left side. The video cart should be positioned at around the 1 or 2 o'clock position to facilitate an ergonomic view. The IGS tower, if being used, can be positioned either to the left of the video tower. Appropriate reversal of this setup can be utilized for the left handed surgeon.

Before draping, any anesthetic monitoring cables are elevated off the floor and secured to the bed to minimize discomfort and optimize the operative area for standing or sitting. Once draped, the various cables (light, endoscope, and powered instrumentation) and suction tubes are secured to the bed. This prevents movement during the case which can often limit the maneuverability of the surgeon's hand as the cables can be weighty.

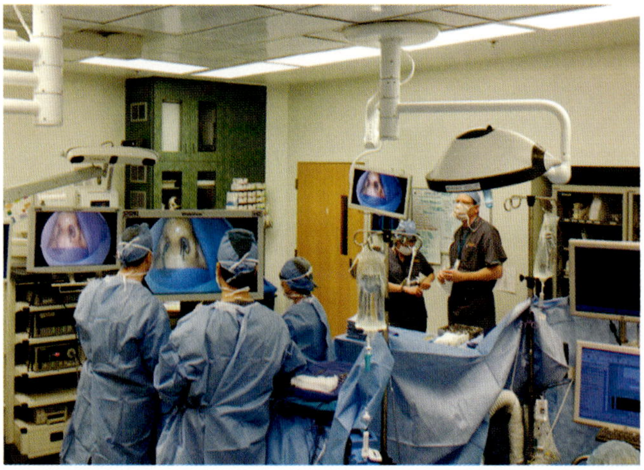

Fig. 24.2: OR layout demonstrating location of endoscopy tower and surgical navigation and location of personnel.

As was noted in Chapter 6, positioning of the patient can greatly improve visualization of the sinuses by decreasing blood loss.[6] Either the head of bed can be elevated or the patient is placed in a reverse trendelenburg position of about 20°–30° in order to reduce central venous pressure and subsequent venous and capillary bleeding. Alternatively, a beach chair positioning can be utilized.

PATIENT PREPARATION

Nasal Preparation

Preparation of the nose begins in the preoperative suite with three applications, separated by 5–10 min, of oxymetazoline sprays. In the operating room, once general anesthesia has been induced and monitoring established, preparation of the patient can begin. The room is setup as noted above and any stereotactic registration is performed. The eyes, which have usually been taped by the anesthesiology team, can be left as such. Unlike in standard sinus surgery where the eyes are typically left uncovered beyond this, we generally prefer to protect the eyes with adhesive foam goggles. These are slightly modified by tearing up the middle to extend the nasal opening but leaving them connected along the superior edge. The medial/nasal edges are splayed, applied to the cheeks lateral to the nasolabial folds, and then further rotated superolaterally before affixing the lateral aspects to the lateral orbital rims. This helps (1) prevent any inadvertent nasal collapse possibly induced by the goggles as well as (2) splay the nostrils into a more open stance to facilitate the passage of instruments during surgery.

While the nose is likely colonized with any number of normal flora, attempts should be made to reduce the bacterial load of the skin and vestibule to prevent any introduction of any "less benign" bacterial into the intracranial space. The nostrils are cleaned with betadine solution and 2–3 oxymetazoline soaked ½ by 3" pledgets are then placed bilaterally between the turbinates and the septum under direct inspection. There is debate regarding the appropriate vasoconstrictor in sinus surgery.[7] The safest overall is oxymetazoline, which is why we generally use it preferentially. Phenylephrine should be avoided because of its increased side effect profile. Topical epinephrine, used 1:1,000 to 1:5,000 can be employed for better hemostasis but the surgeon is cautioned to avoid in patients with cardiac history and to employ mechanisms and/or protocols to guarantee against accidental injection (such as coloring with fluorescein). The nose, cheeks, upper lip, and nasal edges of the eye goggles are then painted with betadine. There should be no issue with betadine accidentally getting into the eyes, but betadine scrub should be avoided, as this will be a significant ocular irritant. The face is then toweled off with three towels such that a triangular opening is left exposing the nasal tip and nostrils.

Further draping is dictated by any plans for adjunctive procedures such as abdominal fat graft or fascia lata graft harvesting. Our preference is to always plan for a possible abdominal fat graft harvest, preparing the abdomen with betadine paint and toweled out, covering with an iodinated adhesive drape, and marking the area with a clip so it can be palpated below the drapes if access is needed later.

Effective Nasal Cleaning and Suctioning

After sufficient time has elapsed, usually upon completion of equipment set-up and a time-out where the surgical plan and patient specific concerns are discussed amongst members of the operative suite team, the nose should be suctioned and the procedures commenced. As simple an act as nasal suctioning can play a large role in minimizing trauma to the nose. At this early point and throughout the case, care should be taken to enter the nose carefully without applying any suction and proceed first to the nasopharynx, which often serves as the reservoir for saliva, mucus and blood. Suction is then applied and blood is cleared from the nose from posterior to anterior. In this manner, the oftentimes sharp edge of the suction is less likely to cause inadvertent trauma. It is also important to not dwell on cut surfaces throughout the case but focus only on removing blood pools and not areas where coagulation has already occurred. Failure to do so may disrupt the clots and reinitiate bleeding. Instead warm saline irrigation (104°F) can be a miraculous adjunct for the surgeon to deal with areas of persistent oozing.

Nasal Inspection

After nasal preparation is complete, the nose is inspected and the need for a septoplasty is further assessed. For optimal surgery, and adequate degree of freedom for the surgical instruments, it is important to identify any anatomical limitations at this point. Pay close attention to whether superior dorsal deflection, often at the superior most portion of the bone-cartilaginous junction of the septum, prevents access to or visualization of the middle turbinate (Fig. 24.3). If necessary, an endoscopic septoplasty can be performed (*see* Chapter 13). Often correction of isolated inferior septal spurs is not necessary, but

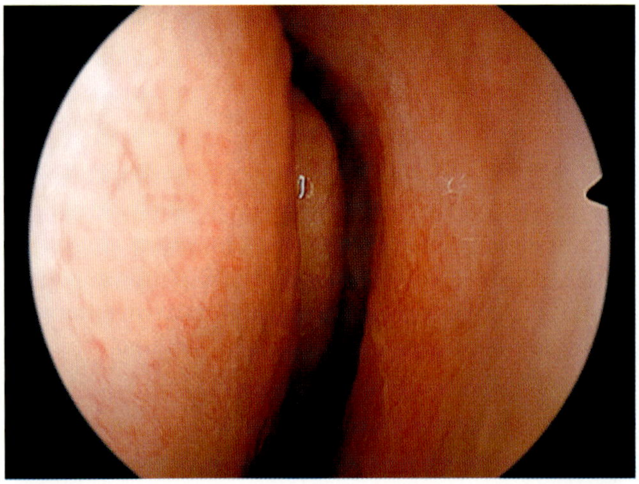

Fig. 24.3: Superior dorsal deflection of the septum narrows the operative corridor between the septum and middle turbinate and may require septoplasty to correct and avoid significant mucosal disruption during surgery.

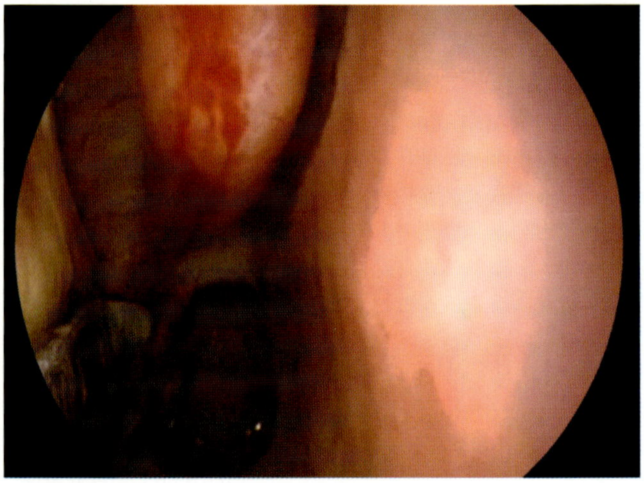

Fig. 24.4: Lateralizing the inferior turbinate.

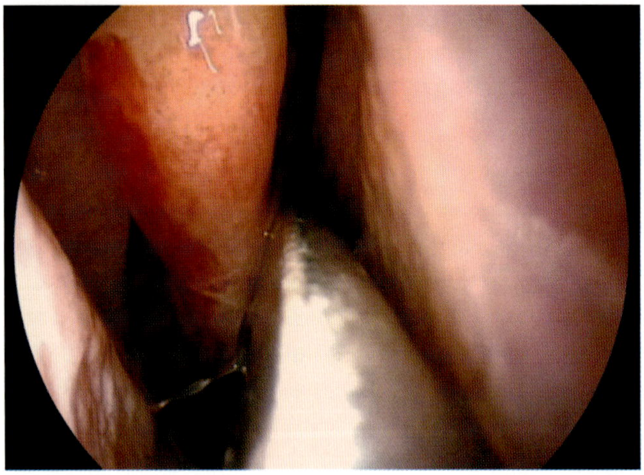

Fig. 24.5: Lateralizing the middle turbinate—It is important to start low on the middle turbinate and remain at a 30° trajectory.

the surgeon should recognize that their presence may tend to inadvertently drive the approach more superiorly and employ efforts to correct this.

OPERATIVE APPROACH

Nasal Injection

After draping the nose is injected with a focus on the middle turbinate in three locations (*see* Fig. 9.2): (1) over the axilla at the junction of the turbinate and the lateral wall with more lateral positioning to help guide any bleeding from the injection site away from the middle meatus, (2) inferolaterally on the head of the middle turbinate, and (3) posteriorly along the inferior aspect of the turbinate. The vestibular vibrissae can then be trimmed, but discussion with the neurosurgical colleagues regarding this should take place. There is some disagreement on whether cut remnants of these left the nose may pose a risk for later contamination of the intradural space. As such, we generally avoid it unless adjunctive measures for the approach (septal or sinus manipulation) are required.

Turbinate Lateralization and Sphenoidotomy

Steps

1. The inferior turbinate is first in- and then out-fractured using a Freer or Cottle elevator. We find it often easier to start the outfracturing more posteriorly and work anteriorly (Fig. 24.4). Care should be taken to use the convex aspect of the elevator as the point of contact with the turbinate and not the tip. This is true for the next step as well.
2. Staying low, on a 30° trajectory to the sphenoid ostium, the lower aspect of the middle turbinate is lateralized and the endoscope advanced to permit visualization of the tip of the elevator at all times (Fig. 24.5). It is a common mistake to assume that the trajectory should be higher than along the lower aspect of the middle turbinate. Care should be taken to avoid approaching the superior aspect or axilla of the middle turbinate as this will quickly bring you to, and possibly through, the posterior cribriform plate.
3. Identify the superior turbinate and superior meatus. Upon doing so, the elevator can be rotated such that

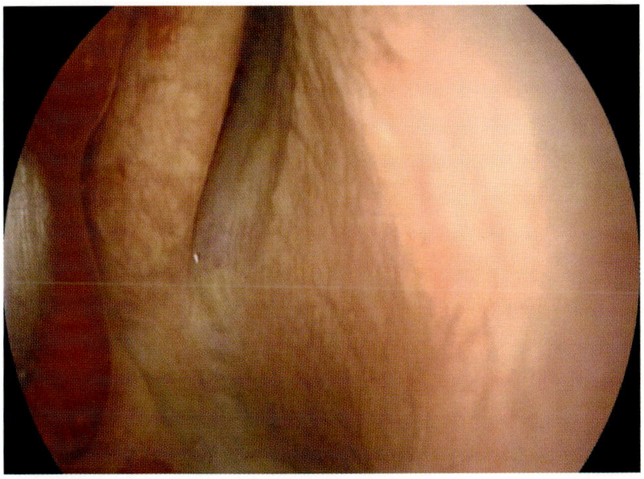

Fig. 24.6: Laterlization of the middle turbinate tail—With full lateralization the superior turbinate can be seen as well as, often times, the sphenoid os as seen just medial to the superior turbinate.

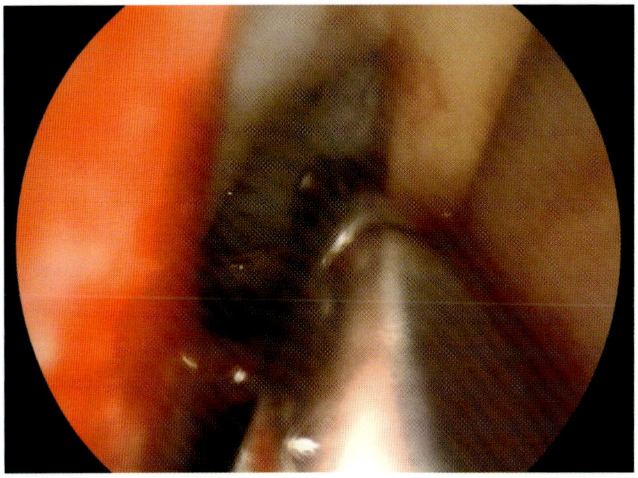

Fig. 24.7: Resection of superior turbinate—Using straight biting forcpes, the inferior portion of the turbinate is incised.

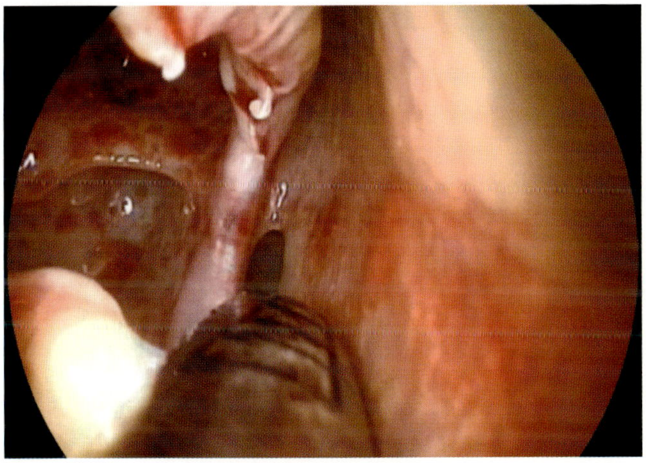

Fig. 24.8: Posterior ethmoids—An "inside-out" posterior ethmoidectomy has been completed with the superior turbinate removed and the anterior wall of the sphenoid visible.

the concave surface is then facing laterally. The tip of the instrument can then be slipped into the inferior portion of the superior meatus such that the elevator "hugs" the basal lamella of the middle turbinate. Firm, steady pressure on this inferoposterior aspect of the turbinate will result in a final "give" and lateralization of the turbinate (Fig. 24.6).

Alternatively, the middle turbinate, as advocated by other authors, can be resected. We have not found this to be necessary in the majority of cases with the exception of very narrow nasal cavities and/or some pediatric patients. If pursued, resection of the turbinate can be performed with straight or curved turbinate scissors aimed inferiorly. The incision should be initiated just superior to the bulbous head and care taken to not cut too close to the axilla. Failure to do so can result in postoperative lateralization of the turbinate remnant with subsequent scarring and iatrogenic frontal sinus disease. The incision continues posteriorly and inferiorly effectively separating and removing the sagittal component of the turbinate from the coronal and axial portions.

4. The inferior portion of the superior turbinate is then resected. A thru-cutting forcep is opened laterally and serial cuts are made advancing posteriorly with each cut until the face of the sphenoid is removed (Fig. 24.7).
5. A 4 mm standard microdebrider is then used to remove the remainder of this tissue clean the edges of the original incision. We prefer at this point to fully open up what is usually a single dominant posterior ethmoid cell (Fig. 24.8). Doing so establishes the lamina and provides for maximal exposure for any lateral parasellar lesions and further prevents postoperative ethmoid mucocele formation.
6. The sphenoid ostium is palpated, if not already palpable, and opened laterally with the sharp end of the Cottle elevator.
7. 2-mm Kerrison rongeurs can then be inserted and used to expand the opening laterally and superiorly. If the bone of the sphenoid face is rather thick and unable to be fractured as noted in Step 2, the Kerrison itself can be used initially. Inserting it upside-down will align the 45° tip perfectly with the orientation of the sphenoid ostium. Once through the ostium with the tip, it can be rotated to face superolaterally and the ostium expanded as noted.

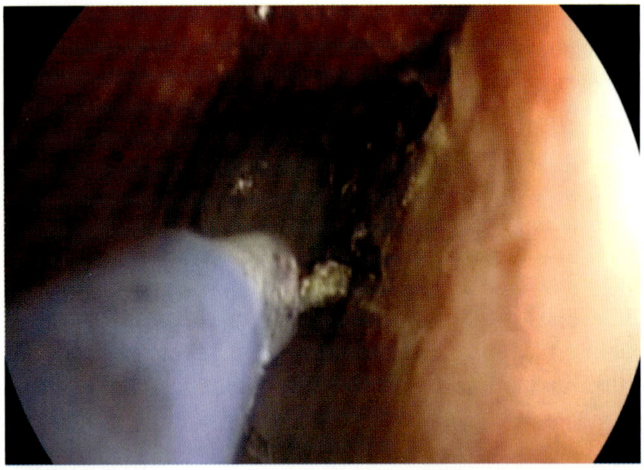

Fig. 24.9: Septal mucosal cuts—An insulated monopolar needle bovie with a specifically bent tip completes the inferior limb of the mucosal incision for the septectomy.

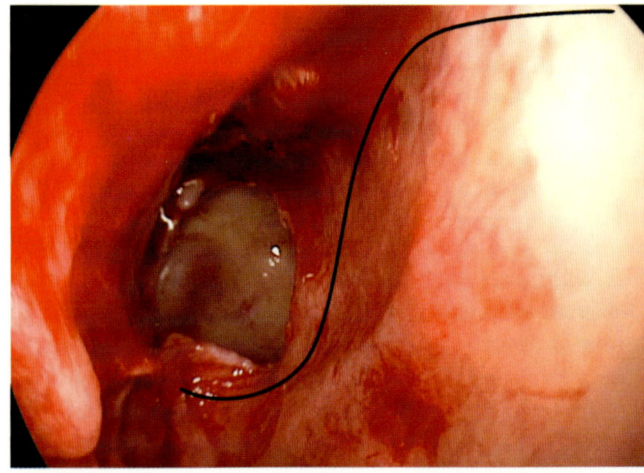

Fig. 24.10: Incision for rescue flap—The posterior septum is visible with an S-shaped incision planned for a rescue flap. Black line marks the incision.

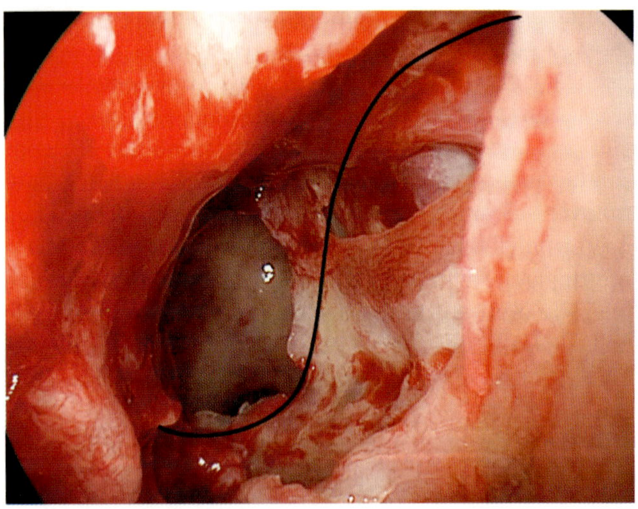

Fig. 24.11: Rescue flap—The incisions have been made and the mucosal flap has been elevated inferiorly.

8. The opening is cleaned with the microdebrider and further work with up-biting thru-cutting forceps expands the opening to the lamina and skull base.

Extension of Sphenoid Opening

Steps

9. Mucosal removal for septectomy: An extended insulated needle tip bovie is used to incise a rectangular shaped area of mucosa on the posterior septum. We find it easiest to accomplish this when the tip of the needle is reshaped twice with two 45° bends such that it cuts perpendicular to its long axis. The inferior portion of the incision is made first, starting at the inferior aspect of the sphenoid ostium, carrying this medially onto the septum and anteriorly to the original extent of the superior turbinate (note: this can be extended anteriorly as necessary for access, but this landmark serves as a good starting place). The superior incision is created approximately at the level at which the superior turbinate was resected and brought anterior as well (Fig. 24.9). A vertical incision dropped at the anterior extent of the horizontal incisions is then made. The mucosa is elevated off the septum posteriorly and removed with microdebrider. The prior incisions establish a level below which lies the posterior nasoseptal artery and we prefer to preserve this mucosa both to avoid iatrogenic vascular injury, which may result in immediate or postoperative hemorrhage, as well as preserve the pedicle in the event a septal flap is needed.

Alternate Rescue Flap Technique

10. In situations where there is a good possibility that a nasoseptal flap (NSF) (*see* Chapter 30) may be needed for reconstructive purposes, but its use not guaranteed, an alternative "rescue flap" incision can be used. Instead of making the cuts as noted above a single S-shaped incision is made which parallels the superior cut of a NSF (Figs. 24.10 and 24.11). Still using a needle point monopolar cautery as noted above an incision is started at the inferior aspect of the sphenoid ostium and is brought medially and on to the septum. The incision is the curved superiorly,

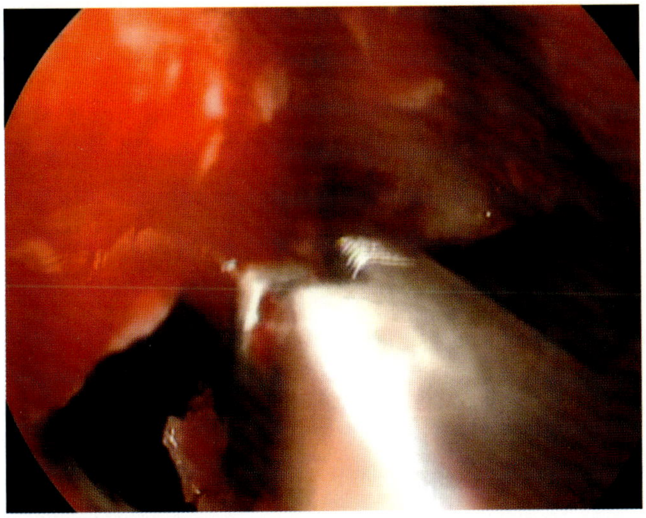

Fig. 24.12: PPE resection—Thru-cutting forceps separate the PPE from skull base to prevent inadvertent transmission of force and subsequent CSF leak.

in an S-shape and turned anteriorly at the level of the cut portion of the superior turbinate (approximately 1.5 cm from nasal vault). The incision is carried anteriorly to about mid- middle turbinate. The flap is then elevated inferiorly.

11. Elevation of mucosa off the sphenoid rostrum: The sharp end of a Cottle elevator is then used to elevate the mucosa from superior to inferior. Applying gentle force at the anterior extent of removed-mucosa area first with progressively inferior dissection as the elevation advances posteriorly will provide for a quick elevation while minimizing potential laceration/tearing. We usually switch to a small 7- or 8-frasier suction to complete the elevation along the rostrum after initial mucosal dissection as this facilitates visualization while the mucosa and bone bleed during elevation. This is done in a medial-lateral-medial sweeping fashion.
12. Inferior bone removal: A down-biting Kerrison is then brought in and the sphenoid ostium extended inferiorly. We prefer to start the removal lateral with a slight counterclockwise rotation (clockwise if on the left side) of the Kerrison rongeur. Paired with medial placement of the endoscope this greatly facilitates visualization and preservation of the mucosal flap. The dissection continues as inferior as is necessary such that a straight suction can be placed inferior to the pituitary sella. Bone is removed as medial as possible, usually to where the septum transitions to the intersinus septum.
13. Steps 1–11 are then repeated on the contralateral side.

Completion of Posterior Septectomy and Sphenoid Clearing

Steps

14. A Cottle elevator is then used to create a vertical fracture of the perpendicular plate of the ethmoid (PPE), often just anterior to the prior mucosal elevation and this is extended superiorly and inferiorly. Occasionally, the PPE is thickened and may require drilling to initiate a separation from the anterior septal components.
15. A thru-cutting forceps, or straight turbinate scissor, is then used to cut the superior attachment of the PPE posteriorly as far as possible (Fig. 24.12), but at least to the extent where the cribriform/ethmoid roof transitions to the sphenoid bone and its rather thick planum sphenoidale. Doing so will minimize accidental skull base fracture and subsequent cerebrospinal fluid (CSF) leak during bone removal.
16. A large pituitary forceps can then be used to grasp the bony septum and sphenoid keel and with a quick rocking mechanism can be removed fairly easily, often without the need for further drilling.
17. The intersinus septum is then removed from anterior to posterior and taken to the face of the sella. Care must be taken for septa that extend laterally within the sinus as these usually attach to bone anchored over the paraclival carotid and/or syphon. If bone removal is needed to access the sellar or parasellar areas it should only be done with drilling or thru-cutting instruments or rongeurs as grasping and twisting could result in inadvertent injury and rupture of the internal carotid artery (ICA). The completed opening is seen in Figure 24.13.

Transgressing the Sella—Optional

18. Sellar bone can then be removed as desired. For a right handed surgeon, this is often best started at the inferior, patient's left side of the sella. The bone may be quite thin in this area if a macroadenoma is the underlying pathology, and bone removal may be easily started with the sharp end of a small Cottle elevator (alternatively, a pie knife or disk elevator may also be of use). Otherwise, gentle circular drilling can thin the bone in this area enough that overlying bone can be flaked away.
19. The remainder of the bone is removed with Kerrison rongeurs. To maximize tumor access, we remove the entire bone off the sella with the lateral extent of the dissection determined by visualization of the medial

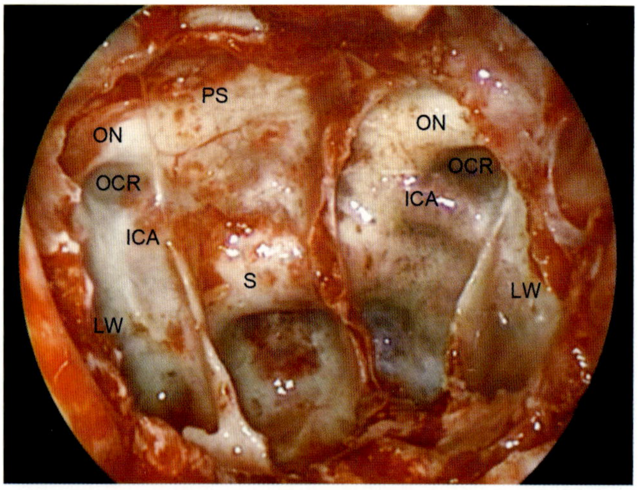

Fig. 24.13: Completed opening—The sphenoid has been opened widely such that lateral walls (LW) and the planum sphenoidale (PS) are clearly in view with the sella (S) centrally. The lateral optico-carotid recesses are also clearly seen (OCR) with optic nerve (ON) and internal carotid artery (ICA) abutting them.

aspect of the cavernous sinus, which can often be noted as a transition to a more blue appearing area of dura. Accidental injury to the cavernous or the paired superior and inferior intercavernous sinuses can often be easily managed with either bipolar cautery or a thrombin/collagen matrix (such as FloSeal® or Surgiflo®).

The bone removal can continue depending on the extent of the underlying pathology with care taken in the area lateral to the sella as the optic nerve and ICA can be found in these areas and iatrogenic injury may be difficult to avoid. Dural incision at our institution is usually reserved for the neurosurgical team and beyond the scope of this text. It is however, at this point that we move from a two to three-handed technique, keeping the endoscope in the patient's right nares such that instruments can be passed below it as well as contralaterally.

Pearls

- The inferior extent of the approach is defined by the inferior extent of the pathology. For simple pituitary adenomas, bone of the sphenoid face is removed until a suction can be passed easily below the sella or extent of the tumor. In some cases it may require complete removal of the bone as well as drilling of the floor and clivus. Otherwise complete removal of the pathology will be difficult.
- The lateral extent of the sphenoidotomy is also defined by the lateral extent of the tumor. Removal of the entire sphenoid face to the orbital lamina bilaterally, afforded by opening the posterior ethmoids after superior turbinate resection, ensures both visualization and access to the lateral extent of the sphenoid. For lesions that extend lateral to the lateral wall of the sphenoid, a total ethmoidectomy with middle turbinate removal may be necessary to fully access the lesion.
- The superior opening should be high enough that the planum can be visualized with the scope just outside the sphenoid sinus. This "maximal" exposure is often tempered by a desire to preserve olfaction and aggressive removal of superior turbinate and septum all the way to skull base should be avoided. Extension of only the posterior portion of the septectomy and posterior most portions of the superior turbinate will result in some olfactory epithelial loss, but this is usually not noticeable by the patient.

Conclusion of the Operation

Before final reconstruction of the sella, the nose is copiously irrigated with warm sterile saline to encourage hemostasis and remove debris. Reconstruction then ensues as described in Chapter 30. Following this the middle turbinates are returned to a more natural position by gently medializing them. If significant mucosal trauma has occurred during the approach or tumor resection, absorbable materials can be placed throughout the nose as necessary such as Nasopore® or Gelfilm®. For substantial injury, we will place 0.020" thick silastic sheeting, secured in place with a nylon suture to the columella, which is removed after the second postoperative week.

POSTOPERATIVE COURSE

Nasal Care

Saline irrigations and sprays serve as a major adjunct to the patient's postoperative care. Unless an intraoperative CSF leak is encountered, saline irrigations are started on the first postoperative day (POD). We generally recommend rinsing with two bottles, three times daily using standard commercially available bottles and salt-packets with distilled water. Additionally, saline nasal spray is helpfully applied throughout the day on an hourly basis. Should an intraoperative CSF leak have occurred, we wait until the POD#3 to begin rinses, but saline sprays are initiated immediately. At any point, should there be a concern for a postoperative leak, all saline sprays and irrigations are held for 24 h until the source of salty drainage can be further elucidated.

Complications

CSF Rhinorrhea

Postoperative CSF leak rates are variable across series but our overall incidence is around 2%. Confirmation of CSF rhinorrhea is includes discontinuation of nasal saline as noted above and laboratory analysis of nasal fluid for Beta-2 (Tau) transferrin is recommended. Depending on the institution this lab may or may not be available immediately and management should not be delayed if obvious drainage on tilt procedure with head hanging forward is present. While lumbar drainage can be considered, it is our experience that the efficacy is inconsistent. Surgical reexploration and repair should be performed with techniques utilized from Chapter 30.

Epistaxis

Management of the patient with epistaxis can be difficult. Often this is minor capillary or venous oozing and can be controlled with topical decongestants (e.g., oxymetazoline) and/or warm saline irrigations. Of greatest concern is bleeding from the ICA, which can be catastrophic, or the cavernous sinus. Fortunately, it is our experience that this is extremely rare, but evaluation should be geared toward ruling this out, especially in the setting of high volume, intermittent bleeding. In this setting, CT angiogram should be attempted and, if the etiology remains uncertain, formal angiogram with or without embolization of nasal feeder vessels can be attempted. Operative control of epistaxis may also be warranted and bleeding from the posterior nose can be controlled often with bipolar cautery, especially if resulting from injury to the posterior septal artery. Additional management of epistaxis is discussed in Chapter 18. Otherwise, directed packing with absorbable materials is usually sufficient.

Hyposmia

One would assume that loss of smell would be significant in patients undergoing a transsphenoidal approach to the skull base considering the tissue removal, which often occurs to access the pathology. Hart et al.[8] and Sowerby et al.[9] both found however that mean smell scores returned to normal by the third postoperative month, even when middle turbinectomy was performed.[9] This mirrors our experience as most patients do not note or complain of olfactory loss. The team from the University of Western Ontario, however, reported a 100% olfactory disturbance.[10] All of their patients in their series, though, had undergone NSF reconstruction and a follow-up study by the same group[11] indicated that NSF portended a worse smell outcome than without (90% mild or moderate hyposmia vs. 40% mild hyposmia when not used). Patient counseling and postoperative care should be able to prepare and minimize complaints in this regard. Further, NSF reconstruction should be reserved for more significant leaks. In the event of postoperative edema, rhinitis, or sinusitis, topical nasal steroid, potentially administered in a Mygind's or head-hanging-back position should be considered.

CONCLUSION

A growing body of literature supports the endoscopic approach for the management of sellar/parasellar lesions as having equivalent if not superior outcomes as more traditional, microscopic approaches. Proper evaluation of the patient preoperatively with radiographic and laboratory diagnostics can ensure a well planned procedure with minimal surprises. While serious postoperative complications associated with the endoscopic approach are rare, their anticipation can guide discussions with the patient regarding their postoperative course and expectations. Hyposmia can likely be detected in a significant number of patients but this is likely not subjectively bothersome in the absence of NSF reconstruction.

REFERENCES

1. Jane Jr JA, Sulton LD, Laws Jr ER. Surgery for primary brain tumors at United States academic training centers: results from the Residency Review Committee for neurological surgery. J Neurosurg. 2005;103:789.
2. Vance ML, Thorner MO. Prolactinomas. Endocrinol Metab Clin North Am. 1987;16(3):731-53.
3. Starke RM, Raper DMS, Payne SC, et al. Endoscopic vs. microsurgical transsphenoidal surgery for acromegaly: Outcomes in a concurrent series of patients using modern criteria for remission. J Clin Endocrinol Metab. 2013;98: 3190-8.
4. Dallapiazza R1, Bond AE, Grober Y, et al. Retrospective analysis of a concurrent series of microscopic versus endoscopic transsphenoidal surgeries for Knosp Grades 0-2

nonfunctioning pituitary macroadenomas at a single institution. J Neurosurg. 2014 Jul 4:1-7.

5. Rotenberg B, Tam S, Ryu WH, et al. Microscopic versus endoscopic pituitary surgery: a systematic review. Laryngoscope. 2010;120(7):1292-7.
6. Timperley D, Harvey RJ. Perioperative and intraoperative techniques to improve surgical outcomes in skull base surgery. Otolaryngol Clin North Am. 2010;43:699-730.
7. Higgins TS, Hwang PH, Kingdom TT, et al. Systematic review of topical vasoconstrictors in endoscopic sinus surgery. Laryngoscope. 2011;121:422-32.
8. Hart CK, Theodosopoulos PV, Zimmer LA. Olfactory changes after endoscopic pituitary tumor resection. Otolaryngol Head Neck Surg. 2010;142(1):95-7.
9. Sowerby LJ, Gross M, Broad R, et al. Olfactory and sinonasal outcomes in endoscopic transsphenoidal skull-base surgery. Int Forum Allergy Rhinol. 2013;3(3):217-20.
10. Rotenberg BW, Saunders S, Duggal N. Olfactory outcomes after endoscopic transsphenoidal pituitary surgery. Laryngoscope. 2011;121(8):1611-3.
11. Tam S, Duggal N, Rotenberg BW. Olfactory outcomes following endoscopic pituitary surgery with or without septal flap reconstruction: a randomized controlled trial. Int Forum Allergy Rhinol. 2013;3(1):62-5.

CHAPTER 25

Endoscopic Endonasal Anterior Cranial Fossa Approaches

Anand V Germanwala, Tarik Ibrahim, Ameet Singh

INTRODUCTION

Endoscopic endonasal techniques in the midsagittal plane to approach the anterior cranial fossa can be subdivided into transtubercular, transplanar, transcribriform, and transfrontal modules. These modules represent the anterior continuum of the skull base extending from the sella (Figs. 25.1A and B). A variety of pathologies can be successfully treated, including frontal sinus disease, benign or malignant sinonasal tumors, intracranial neoplasms, cerebrospinal fluid leaks, encephaloceles, and other masses. Extensive study of preoperative imaging, including thin section computed tomography (CT) and magnetic resonance imaging (MRI) must be performed to assess the lesion and surrounding anatomy to determine if the endonasal corridor provides the best surgical treatment option for the patient. Additional approaches, including eyebrow and frontosphenotemporal craniotomy, should be considered for anterior skull base lesions encasing or extending lateral to the internal carotid artery, or extending far lateral to the midline of the orbit.[1] In addition, anterior skull base malignancies with skin or orbital involvement are better addressed using purely open or a combination of open and endoscopic techniques.[2] Image guidance is a useful intraoperative adjunct and can enhance safety during extensive skull base procedures. For intra-arachnoidal cases, continuous neurophysiological monitoring can be utilized to provide additional information during surgery.

EXTRACRANIAL SURGICAL APPROACH

The patient is placed supine on the operating table, and the head is placed above the heart and turned slightly to the right. For intra-arachnoidal cases or complex extra-arachnoidal/extradural cases, the head is often immobilized in Mayfield pins to aid in accurate image guidance/navigation. A greater amount of neck extension is advantageous for transcribriform/transethmoidal and

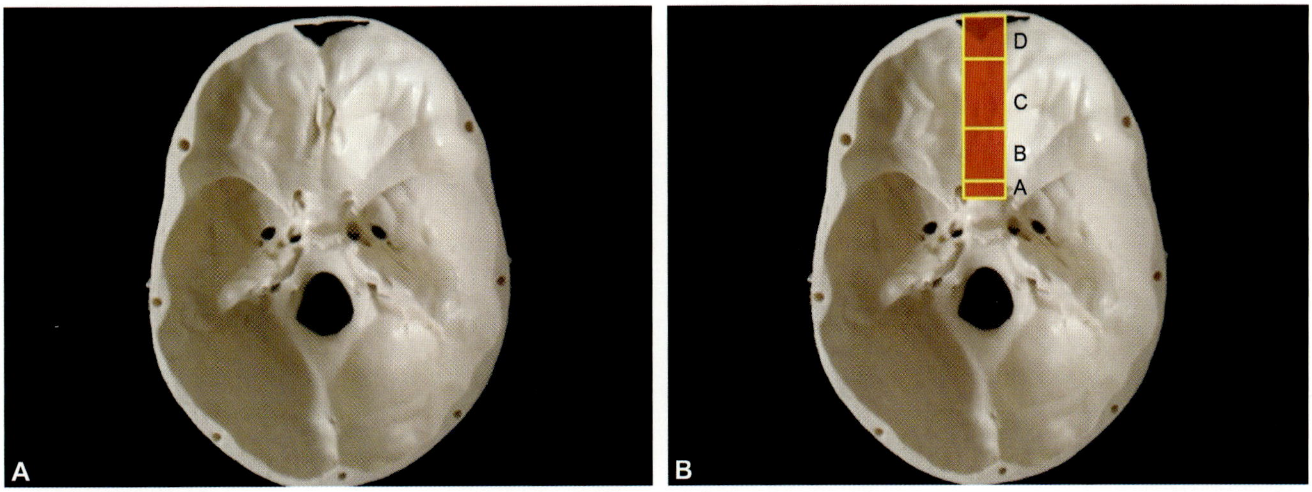

Figs. 25.1A and B: (A) Axial view of the anterior skull base with (B) identification of the different anterior skull base endoscopic endonasal modules.
(A: Transtubercular; B: Transplanar; C: Transcribriform; D: Transfrontal).

transfrontal approaches. Limited use of a single dose of prophylactic IV antibiotic may be sufficient for pathologies with limited intracranial involvement. However, broad spectrum antibiotics are typically recommended for extensive extracranial and most intracranial pathologies.[3] Baseline neurophysiological monitoring is confirmed after patient positioning for intra-arachnoidal cases. The nasal cavity is decongested with vasoconstricting agents such as topical adrenaline (1:1,000) or 4% cocaine. The inferior turbinates are gently out-fractured to widen the nasal corridor and nasal valve. This maneuver increases the physical space necessary for instrumentation but also increases the amount of light in the nasal cavity and paranasal sinuses. Bilateral sphenopalatine foramina are infiltrated with local anesthesia (e.g., 1% lidocaine with 1:100,000 epinephrine) to vasoconstrict the branches of the sphenopalatine artery to reduce intra-operative bleeding. Additional injections are performed along the nasal floor, middle turbinates, and superior posterior septum. If a large high flow CSF leak is anticipated, a pedicled vascularized flap (e.g., nasoseptal flap) is usually harvested during the initial approach and vasoconstriction of the ipsilateral sphenopalatine foramen is avoided. Alternatively, the pedicle to the nasoseptal flap may be preserved and a vascularized flap may be harvested if necessary. A septoplasty may be performed to widen the nasal corridor, and/or harvest vomeric bone for rigid skull base reconstruction as necessary. A partial or complete middle turbinate resection may also be performed to further widen the nasal airway as deemed necessary for the surgical approach.

The details of the extracranial approach are dictated by the size, location, and type of pathology. Transtubercular and transplanum approaches require a posterior septectomy to aid in a bi-nostril three- or four-handed technique. Usually, the endoscope is placed on the right, elevating the vestibule superiorly in order to increase space for other instruments.

Unilateral or bilateral posterior ethmoidectomies help provide panoramic views of the skull base as well as allow the endoscope to "park" away from other surgical instruments during the bi-nostril approach. Onodi cells (posterior, lateral, and superior pneumatization of ethmoid cells) must be identified preoperatively and opened to provide adequate visualization of the entire sphenoid sinus. Partial superior and/or middle turbinate resections are sometimes necessary for adequate exposure. However, all attempts should be made to preserve these structures to maintain sinonasal function (humidification, filtration).[4] Extensive bilateral sphenoidotomies along with removal of the sphenoid rostrum and sphenoid roof/floor must be performed to allow unfettered access to the sella and suprasellar, planum, and clival regions. Vertical, horizontal, and/or oblique bony septations are removed and smoothened carefully, especially those attached to the internal carotid artery. This is important to prevent any inadvertent catastrophic vascular injuries.

Transcribriform and transfrontal approaches typically require a combination of unilateral or bilateral maxillary sinusotomies, complete ethmoidectomies, and wide sphenoidotomies. The fovea ethmoidalis is often completely skeletonized from the posterior frontal recess to the planum sphenoidale, and from lamina papyracea to lamina papyracea. A superior and posterior septectomy is often necessary for a bi-nostril approach to larger sinonasal or intradural lesions. Although complete unilateral or bilateral middle turbinate removal is sometimes necessary for exposure, every attempt must be to preserve normal sinonasal anatomy.[4] Lesions that extend anterior to the anterior ethmoidal arteries usually require a modified Lothrop for complete exposure of the sloping frontoethmoidal skull base.[5] This is necessary not only for unhindered access to the frontal sinus but also to prevent iatrogenic frontal sinusitis after skull base reconstruction.

TRANSTUBERCULAR APPROACHES

Transtubercular approaches require removal of the tuberculum, the portion of skull base bone in between the chiasmatic sulcus that separates the sella from the planum (Figs. 25.2A and B).[6] This approach exposes the superior intercavernous sinus, which must be meticulously cauterized, and permits entry into the suprasellar space/cistern after dural opening. The anterior/superior extent of the diaphragma sella attaches to the undersurface of the dura in this region. Therefore, a transtubercular dural opening will result in entering the diaphragma/subarachnoid space with CSF egress, and plans for dural reconstruction must be anticipated from the beginning. Once CSF is encountered, adequate brain relaxation can be achieved within several seconds. Similar to microsurgical principles, central debulking of tumors with circumferential sharp dissection can be performed using ultrasonic aspirators with endonasal attachments, endonasal skull-base dissectors, and shafted microinstruments.

Prior to surgical intervention, imaging must be studied to identify the location of the optic chiasm (prefixed vs. postfixed), infundibulum, carotid arteries, anterior

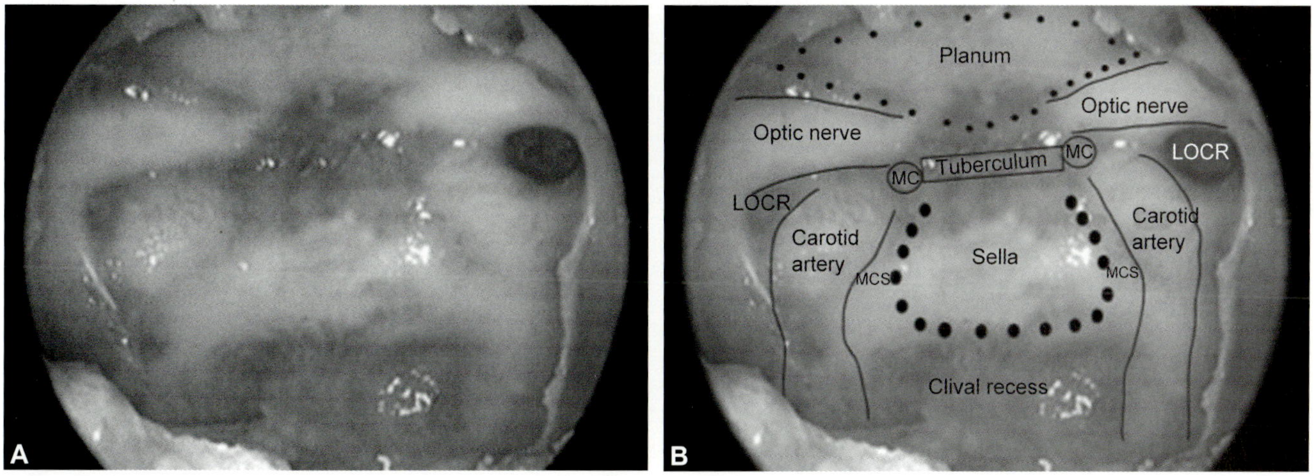

Figs. 25.2A and B: Endoscopic endonasal view of the sella, tuberculum, and planum following sphenoidotomies and ethmoidectomies.[7] (LOCR: Lateral opticocarotid recess; MC: Medial clinoid; MCS: Medial cavernous sinus).

cerebral arteries, and surgical lesion.[8] Care must be taken during bony removal to identify the carotid protuberances and location of the optic nerves. Continuous irrigation can mitigate heat generation and dispersal from drilling and prevent thermal injury to the nearby optic nerves. It is important to recognize the limitations with this approach. Lesions that extend lateral to the optic nerve cannot be safely removed through an endonasal corridor without significant risk to the optic nerve. Additional surgical options, including eyebrow or frontosphenotemporal craniotomy, should be considered. The endoscopic endonasal transtubercular module can be combined with transsellar approaches for infundibular tumors, tuberculum meningiomas, craniopharyngiomas, large pituitary adenomas, and other large sellar masses, limited to the midline, that extend into the suprasellar space and require additional exposure (Figs. 25.3A and B). The initial dural opening commonly is in the midline, and often is merely an anterior extension from a sellar dural opening with cauterization of the intervening superior intercavernous sinus. Dural openings are typically expanded laterally after exploration and identification of the nearby neurovascular structures.

TRANSPLANAR APPROACHES

The planum extends anteriorly from the tuberculum to the posterior aspect of the crista galli. Transplanar approaches are merely an anterior extension of the transtubercular module and require additional bone removal of the sphenoid roof. The planum bone is thinned with a diamond bit drill, and the bone resection classically occurs in an anterior to posterior direction with rongeurs. For planar dural-based masses, such as meningiomas, the endoscopic endonasal transplanar approach allows for interruption of tumor blood supply by cauterizing the dura prior to its opening. In addition, branches of the anterior and posterior ethmoidal arteries are disrupted prior to tumor removal. These techniques usually lead to a lower rate of blood loss during tumor resection. Intradurally, this module permits further anterior exposure of the subfrontal lobes. This additional exposure provides a better angle for exploration of additional suprasellar structures, including the infundibular recess and third ventricle, with little to no brain retraction. This module is often combined with transsellar and transtubercular approaches and allows the surgical team visualization of the superior aspect of sellar masses with suprasellar extension (Figs. 25.4A and B). Close inspection of the preoperative MRI/CT must be performed to assess the proximity of the anterior cerebral arteries. For lesions that extend lateral to the meridian of the orbit, additional surgical options, including craniotomy, should be considered.

TRANSCRIBRIFORM/ TRANSETHMOIDAL APPROACHES

The cribriform plate of the ethmoid bone and fovea ethmoidalis (ethmoidal roof) extend from the posterior wall of the frontal sinus to the anterior edge of the planum. The vertical lamella of the middle turbinate divides the cribriform plate (medially) from the fovea ethmoidalis (laterally). Numerous small perforations in the cribriform bone permit passage of olfactory filaments that connect to the olfactory bulbs and provide the sense of smell.[9]

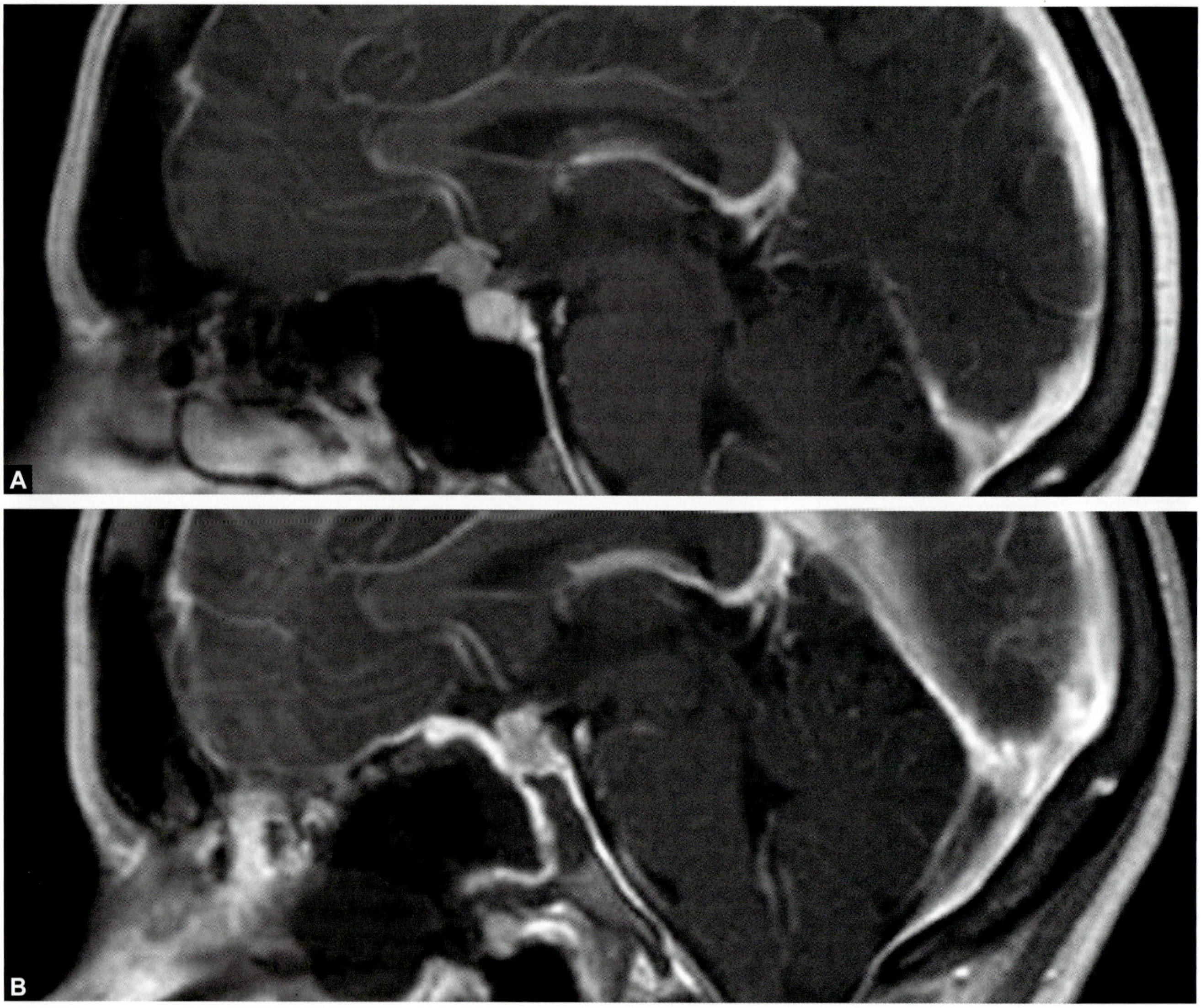

Figs. 25.3A and B: (A) Preoperative midsagittal contrasted MRI revealing a growing tubercular mass. Note the location of the anterior cerebral arteries. (B) Postoperative midsagittal contrasted MRI revealing gross total resection of confirmed meningioma and dural reconstruction with a pedicled vascularized nasoseptal flap.

Thus, a unilateral approach may preserve olfaction. Anatomically, the cribriform plate ultimately ends in the crista galli, a thick ridge of bone that provides dural attachment for the falx cerebri. This dural attachment is often transected during certain transcribriform approaches to intracranial pathologies.

The approach to resect transcribriform/transethmoidal pathology is often modified on the size, precise location, and type of tumor.[10] A small cribriform cerebrospinal fluid leak can be addressed with a simple unilateral transnasal approach which requires minimal work in the paranasal sinuses. In contrast, a large olfactory groove meningioma requires extensive paranasal sinus dissection which often includes bilateral maxillary antrostomies, frontoethmoidectomies, sphenoidotomies, and often frontal sinusotomies. Bilateral partial or complete middle turbinectomies with complete skeletonization of the fovea ethmoidalis must be completed prior to bony anterior skull base removal. Closure for CSF leaks and encephaloceles requires complete exenteration of the ethmoidal septations, identification of the leak, denuding of surround mucosa, followed by multilayered closure. Small CSF leaks may be closed with onlay mucoperichondrial grafts, whereas larger leaks usually require a combination of underlay/onlay grafts and/or vascularized flaps. Benign or malignant sinonasal tumors require

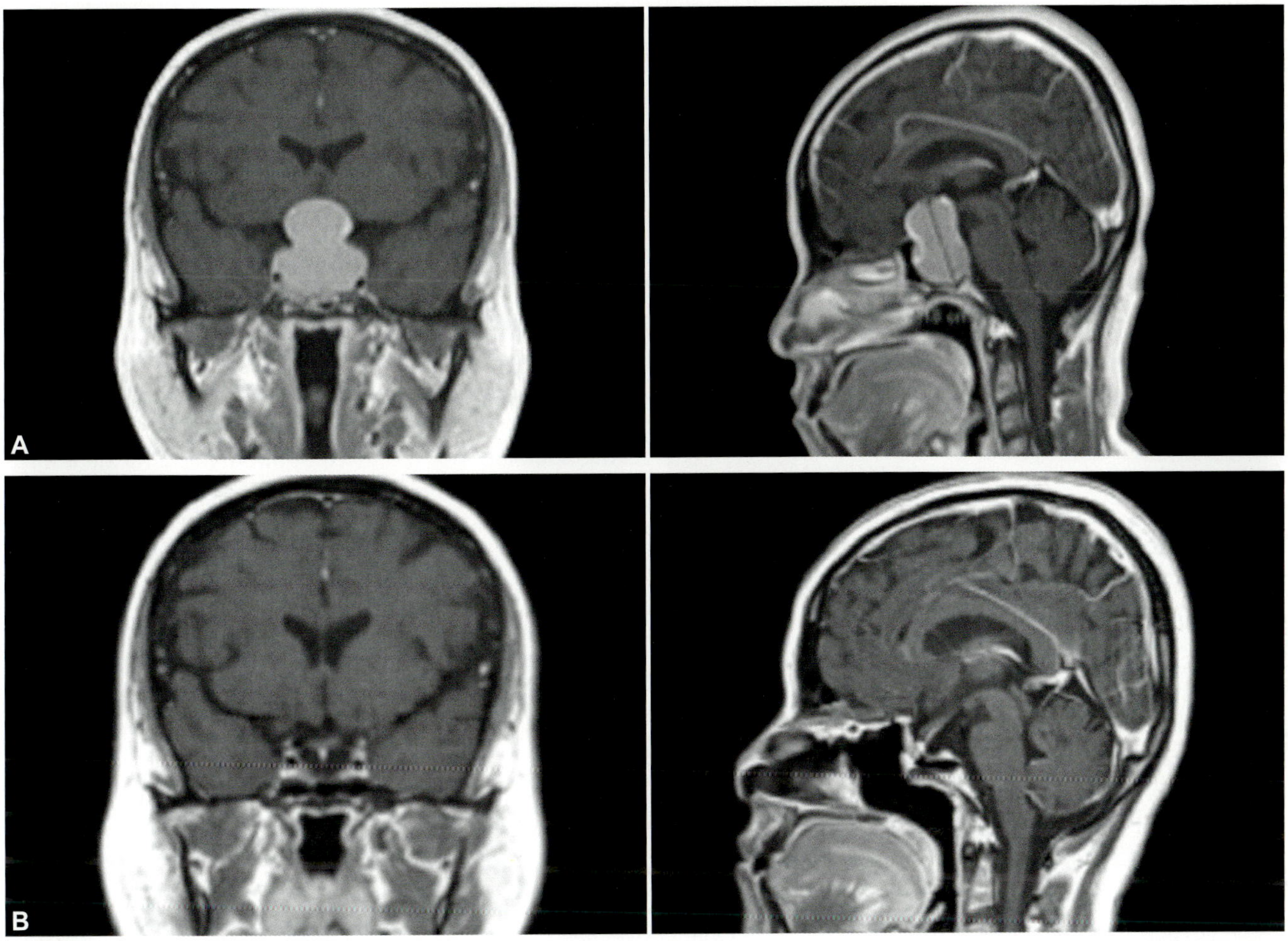

Figs. 25.4A and B: (A) Preoperative coronal and sagittal contrasted MRI revealing large pituitary tumor with suprasellar extension and chiasmatic compression. A combined transsellar, transtubercular, and posterior transplanar approach was performed given the large suprasellar extension. (B) Postoperative coronal and sagittal contrasted MRI revealing gross total resection, decompression of the chiasm, and pedicled vascularized nasoseptal flap.

careful review of all preoperative imaging since these tumors have often destroyed a significant portion of the normal ethmoidal anatomy. Intracranial tumors (e.g., olfactory groove meningiomas) require significant extracranial and intracranial work.

Preoperative and intraoperative attention must be paid to the location of the anterior and posterior ethmoidal arteries, both branches of the ophthalmic artery. The anterior ethmoidal artery, the larger of the two, courses in the anterior ethmoidal sulcus and enters the olfactory fossa after it exits the orbit. It provides the majority of blood supply to the anterior ethmoidal sinuses, and, to a lesser extent, the frontal sinus. Meticulous ligation (bipolar cautery or hemoclips) of this vessel must be performed to avoid the development of a retroorbital hematoma from retraction of a proximal bleeding stump into the orbit. The posterior ethmoidal artery, usually found approximately 13 mm posterior to the anterior ethmoidal artery, primarily supplies the superior nasal septum, and posterior ethmoidal sinuses and must also be properly identified and ligated.[9,11] Ligation of the ethmoidal arteries is imperative to prevent significant intraoperative bleeding and decrease blood supply to surgical field and intracranial tumor.

Visualization of the cribriform/ethmoidal region from an endonasal vantage following ethmoidectomies usually requires the use of angled endoscopes (30°, 45°, and 70°). Dissecting instruments and drills are usually placed above the endoscope to maintain visualization. The variations in bone thickness must be kept in mind to avoid inadvertent injury to the underlying dura. High-speed drilling with a coarse diamond bit is classically performed by drilling horizontal osteotomies immediately posterior to the posterior wall of the frontal sinus and at the junction of

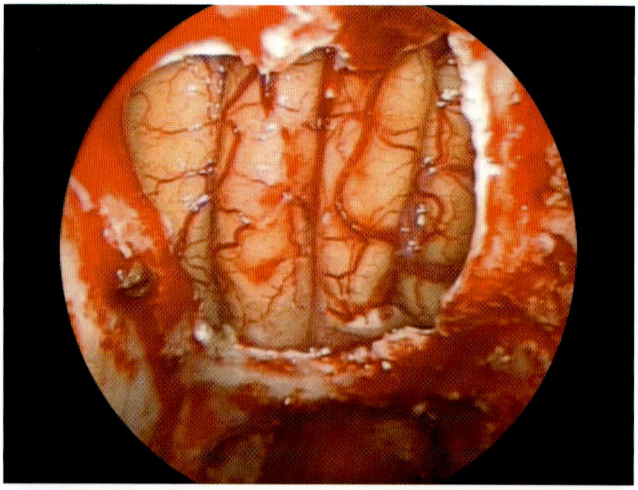

Fig. 25.5: Intraoperative endoscopic endonasal transcribriform approach showing dural and midline falx resection and exposure of the subfrontal lobes bilaterally after resection of a sinonasal undifferentiated carcinoma. Dural reconstruction in this case was with a pedicled endoscopic pericranial flap.[14]

the cribriform and planum. These osteotomies are then followed by drilling along the lateral aspect of the cribriform parallel to the superomedial aspect of the orbit. The lamina papyracea can be removed if needed. Careful rongeuring in an anterior to posterior direction permits exposure of the dura, which is limited laterally by the presence of the orbits. The crista galli is often egg-shelled and then fractured. Given the presence of the olfactory filaments, small CSF leaks are likely to be encountered. Dural openings are classically performed on each side in trap-door fashion and flapped against the midline falx attachment. This attachment is then cut sharply in an anterior to posterior fashion. Such an approach should allow visualization of the olfactory bulbs and subfrontal lobes of the brain (Fig. 25.5).

TRANSFRONTAL APPROACHES

Transfrontal approaches provide access to pathology involving the floor and posterior wall of the frontal sinus. These approaches require a modular dissection through the frontoethmoidal cells and frontal recess based on the type, size, and location of the pathology. The dissection is largely performed in the frontal recess, defined anteriorly by the frontal beak, posteriorly by the sloping skull base, medially by the vertical lamellae of the middle turbinate, and laterally by the orbit. The complexity of dissecting in the frontal recess arises from the variability of the type and position of cells inhabiting this recess which include agger nasi cells, frontal cells (Types I–IV), suprabullar cells, supraorbital cells, and interfrontal sinus septal cells.[12] Different pathologies require a variable amount of dissection in the frontal recess to achieve the desired access and exposure.

Frontal sinus and frontal recess pathology such as erosive mucoceles, CSF leaks, encephaloceles, and osteomas may be addressed with a combination of extended frontal sinus techniques. These techniques include the Draf "extended drainage" procedures originally described for addressing inflammatory chronic sinusitis.[13] A Draf I approach (complete frontoethmoidectomy) may be used to address small ethmoidal tumors, and CSF leaks and/or encephaloceles of the fovea ethmoidalis. Draf IIa approaches (frontal sinus floor removal between the lamina papyracea and middle turbinate) and Draf IIb (frontal sinus floor removal between the lamina papyracea and nasal septum) can be used to access unilateral pathology of the frontal recess such as larger frontoethmoidal tumors, or small intradural tumors (e.g., olfactory groove meningiomas), as well as larger CSF leaks and/or encephaloceles. Draf III approaches (modified Lothrop) are the most extensive of the transfrontal approaches that allow unfettered access to frontal sinus tumors, encephaloceles, and anterior intradural pathology. This approach creates a single, common frontal outflow tract by removing the superior septum, intersinus septum, and frontal sinus floors bilaterally. A modified Lothrop approach is usually employed for lesions anterior or extending anterior to the anterior ethmoidal artery.[5] This approach is used not only for adequate access to remove skull base pathology located anterior to the anterior ethmoidal artery but also ensure that the frontal sinus is unobstructed after skull base reconstruction (Fig. 25.6).

SKULL BASE RECONSTRUCTION

Dural reconstruction for anterior skull base approaches is often performed with multilayered closure followed with pedicled vascularized tissue. Vascularized reconstruction for most transtubercular and transplanum approaches can be achieved with robust nasoseptal flaps. Even the vast majority of transcribriform and/or transethmoidal defects may be reconstructed with either nasoseptal or middle turbinate flaps. The flap pedicle is often placed along the lamina papyracea to ensure adequate length for even the most anterior defects. Alternatively, avascular grafts, bipedicled nasoseptal flaps (Janus flap), or pedicled vascularized endoscopic pericranial flaps

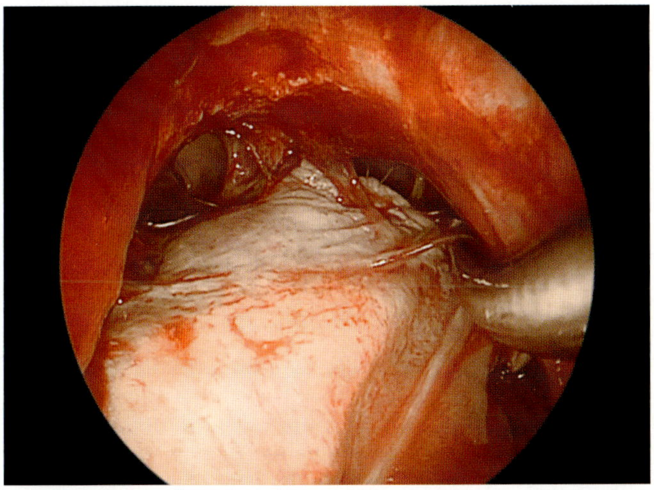

Fig. 25.6: Intraoperative endoscopic modified Lothrop approach during endoscopic transcribriform/transethmoidal skull base approach to an olfactory groove meningioma. Dural reconstruction was performed with a modified "gasket-seal" and vascularized nasoseptal flap.

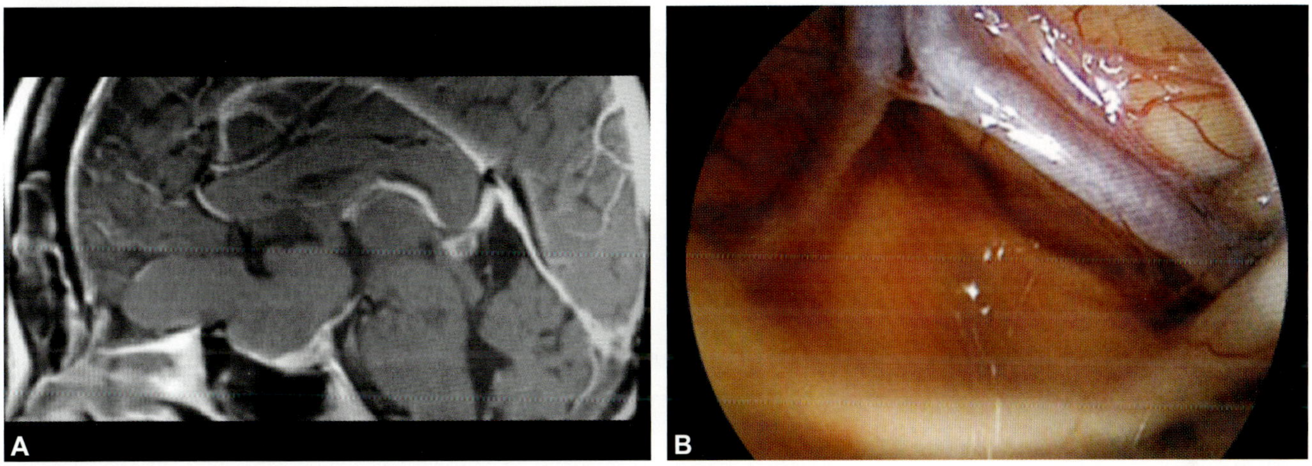

Figs. 25.7A and B: (A) Preoperative midsagittal contrasted MRI revealing a large anterior skull base mass with mass effect on the optic apparatus, subfrontal lobes, and anterior cerebral arteries. A combined transsellar, transtubercular, transplanar, and transcribriform approach was performed for wide fenestration of loculated contents after initial results revealed a skull base cyst. (B) Exploration following evacuation of cyst contents revealed good visualization of the anterior cerebral artery complex.

can be used for extensive skull base reconstruction.[14,15] Although vascularized pedicled flaps have revolutionized the reconstruction of endoscopic skull base defects, the importance of multilayered reconstruction cannot be over emphasized. Multilayered reconstruction techniques such as the "gasket seal" closure, "bilayer button" closure, or "Alloderm sling" prior to secondary vascularized closure are critical to avoiding postoperative CSF leaks and preventing inadvertent intracranial injury during flap take-down for redo surgery.[16-19]

CONCLUSION

Endoscopic endonasal approaches to the anterior skull base are categorized into these four modules that merely represent an extension of each other. The location of the lesion and surgical goals dictate the approach, and these modules can be combined in order to provide the optimal surgical exposure (Figs. 25.7A and B). Surrounding anatomy must always be kept in mind to minimize complications.[20] Limitations do exist for the endonasal corridor, and additional surgical options must be kept in mind. However, with strong multidisciplinary teams, great success can be achieved after careful and thoughtful analysis of preoperative imaging.

ACKNOWLEDGMENT

We would like to recognize and thank Dr. Murugappan Ramanathan, Jr. and Dr. Adam M. Zanation for images from our mutual surgical cases.

REFERENCES

1. Solares CA, Ong YK, Synderman CH. Transnsal endoscopic skull base surgery: what are the limits? Curr Opin Otolaryngol Head Neck Surg. 2010;18(1):1-7.
2. Eloy JA, Vivero RJ, Hoang K, et al. Comparison of transnasal endoscopic and open craniofacial resection for malignant tumors of the anterior skull base. Laryngoscope. 2009;119(5):834-40.
3. Brown SM, Anand VK, Tabaee A, et al. Role of perioperative antibiotics in endoscopic skull base surgery. Laryngoscope. 2007;117:1528-32.
4. Nyquist GG, Anand VK, Brown S, et al. Middle turbinate preservation in endoscopic transsphenoidal surgery of the anterior skull base. Skull Base. 2010;20(5):343-7.
5. Seiberling K, Wormald, PJ. Frontal sinus management in skull base surgery. In: Transnasal Endoscopic Skull Base and Brain Surgery. New York: Thieme; 2012:115-20.
6. de Notaris M, Solari D, Cavallo LM, et al. The "suprasellar notch," or the tuberculum sellae as seen from below: definition, features, and clinical implications from an endoscopic endonasal perspective. J Neurosurg. 2012;116(3):622-9.
7. Germanwala AV, Zanation AM. Endoscopic endonasal approach for clipping of ruptured and unruptured paraclinoid cerebral aneurysms: case report. Neurosurgery. 2011; 68(1 Suppl Operative):234-9; discussion 240.
8. Gulsen S, Dinc AH, Unai M, et al. Characterization of the anatomic location of the pituitary stalk and its relationship to the dorsum sellae, tuberculum sellae and chiasmatic cistern. J Korean Neurosurg Soc. 2010;47(3):169-73.
9. Singh A, Wessell A. Surgical anatomy and physiology for the skull base surgeon. Oper Tech Otolaryngol-Head Neck Surg. 2011;22(3):183-252.
10. Anand VK, Kacker A, Siebert MJ, et al. Endoscopic endonasal transethmoidal transcribriform, transfovea ethmoidalis appraoch to the anterior cranial fossa and skull base. Neurosurgery. 2010;66(5):883-9.
11. Abuzayed B, Tanriover N, Gazioglu N, et al. Endoscopic endonasal anatomy and approaches to the anterior skull base: a neurosurgeon's viewpoint. J Craniofac Surg. 2010; 21(2):529-37.
12. Kuhn F. Lateral nasal wall and sinus surgical anatomy: Contemporary understanding. In: Maintenance manual for lifelong learning. New York: Thieme; 2001.
13. Draf W. Endonasal frontal sinus drainage type I-III according to Draf. In: The Frontal Sinus. Berlin: Springer-Verlag; 2005, pp. 219-32.
14. Patel MR, Shah RN, Snyderman CH, et al. Pericranial flap for endoscopic anterior skull-base reconstruction: clinical outcomes and radioanatomic analysis of preoperative planning. Neurosurgery. 2010; 66(3):506-12; discussion 512.
15. Anand VK, Singh A, Schwartz TH. Janus flap: bilateral nasoseptal flaps for anterior skull base reconstruction. Otolaryngology-Head Neck Surg. 2010;142(3):327-31.
16. Germani RM, Vivero R, Herzallah IR, et al. Endoscopic reconstruction of large anterior skull base defects using acellular dermal allograft. Am J Rhinol. 2007;21(5):615-8.
17. Luginbuhl AJ, Campbell PG, Evans J, et al. Endoscopic repair of high-flow cranial base defects using bilayer button. Laryngoscope. 2010;120(5):876-80.
18. Leng LZ, Brown SM, Anand VK, Schwartz TH. "Gasket seal" water tight closure in minimal-access endoscopic cranial base surgery. Neurosurgery. 2008;62(5 Suppl 2):ONSE342-3.
19. Hadad G, Bassagasteguy L, Carrau RL, et al. A novel reconstructive technique after endoscopic exapnded endonasal approach: vascular pedicle nasoseptal flap. Laryngoscope. 2006;116(10):1882-6.
20. Singh A, Germanwala A. Management of post-operative complications of skull base surgery. Oper Tech Otolaryngol: Head Neck Surg. 2011;22 (3):237-45.

CHAPTER 26

Endoscopic Clival Approaches

Ameet Singh, Alan Siu, Zachary N Litvack

INTRODUCTION

Surgery for pathology of the clivus has traditionally been performed through transfacial and/or (combined) transcranial corridors, resulting in significant morbidity to patients. These approaches were necessary to obtain adequate exposure for tumor removal without jeopardizing adjacent vital neurovascular structures. Over the past two decades, advancements in endoscopic sinus surgery, the keyhole concept in neurosurgery, and development of advanced instrumentation and visualization, we have collectively witnessed a leap forward in the surgical management of lesions of the skull base. The incorporation of the endoscope into neurosurgery has especially benefited the minimally invasive surgical treatment of clival pathology. We aim to discuss diagnostic evaluation, surgical anatomy, and describe in detail the operative technique and advantages of endoscopic approaches to lesions of the clivus.

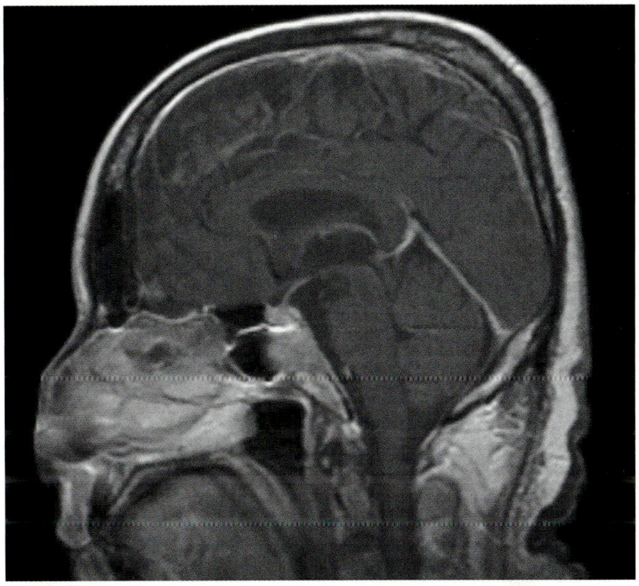

Fig. 26.1: Ideal midline tumor (chordoma) for endoscopic skull base approach to the clivus.

INTEGRATION OF THE ENDOSCOPE FOR CLIVAL APPROACHES

Advantages

The introduction of the endoscope in treating clival pathologies evolved largely in an effort to develop less-invasive techniques that minimize brain retraction/exposure injury and improve cosmesis. These less-invasive techniques have steadily decreased complications and improved outcomes over the past decade. The advent of enhanced optics through technological improvements in image magnification and illumination has resulted in an advantage of the endoscope as a mainstay of minimally invasive skull base surgery.[1-3] The endoscope carries several advantages as the principal visualization tool when compared with the operating microscope,[4,5] primarily in maintaining illumination (without tissue desiccation), improving resolution, and the ability to offer angled views without the need to increase exposure.[6,7]

Surgery with an endoscope displays the greatest advantage when operating through a narrow external corridor in an attempt to preserve anatomy, as is the case when approaching the upper clivus anteriorly through a transsphenoidal corridor, or mid and lower-clivus through an transnasal corridor.[8] The endoscopic endonasal approach offers a direct route to the clivus with little-to-no neurovascular manipulation. The most amenable pathologies for an endoscopic approach are the small midline lesions with limited lateral extension (Fig. 26.1). Additionally, angled lenses can be used to easily expand viewing angles to gain a panoramic appreciation for the resection cavity and its adjacent structures without needing additional osteotomies to increase the line of sight. In comparison, a transcranial approach to this same region would be considerably more invasive, requiring greater bone removal and neurovascular retraction. For a direct anterior approach (i.e., transoral), the soft palate may need to be split, thus avoiding potentially complex wound healing scenarios, oropharyngeal dysphagia and velopharyngeal insufficiency.

Disadvantages

A steep learning curve has been recognized when transitioning to a purely endoscopic approach.[9,10] The most touted difficulties in adopting the endoscope are unfamiliarity with the new instruments, loss of stereoscopic vision, and developing the muscle memory necessary to operate in a narrow field without feedback from direct three-dimensional visualization.[11,12] These differences can result in disorientation and compromise appreciation for the regional anatomy.

The optimal clival lesion for complete resection is one that is midline with minimal lateral extension. Conversely, extensive lateral involvement rostral and dorsal to the paraclival segment of the carotid or extensive dorsal extension to involve the vertebrobasilar circulation and surrounding cranial nerves can be difficult to safely access and manipulate through the deep narrow operative corridor. Bleeding from the intercavernous sinus and ventral occipital dural plexus can prove challenging to control, and can easily cloud the endoscopic view in inexperienced hands. Thus, it is critical for the endoscopic surgeon to fully appreciate the regional anatomy and anticipate such issues.

Judicious selection of the approach must take into consideration the underlying pathology and the overall goals of the surgery, whether it is to biopsy, marsupialize, debulk, or achieve a gross total resection. A transcranial approach may be a favorable alternative to direct endonasal approach, but we still advocate an endoscopic assisted approach to "look around corners" and minimize the surgical exposure.

SURGICAL ANATOMY

Clival/Basilar Region

The clivus is formed by the posterior midline portion of the sphenoid body (basisphenoid) and occipital bone (basiocciput). It is divided into the intrasphenoidal (upper one-third) and extrasphenoidal (lower two-thirds) clivus. The upper third is formed by the dorsum sellae and basisphenoid, the middle third by the portion of the basiocciput above the petroclival fissures, and the lower third is formed by the lower part of the basiocciput. The tectorial membrane lies dorsal to the clival dura (but is effectively fused to it) in the lower two-thirds of the clivus. The intracranial surface of the upper two-thirds of the clivus is concave and faces the pons. The basilar plexus, the largest and most prominent of the intercavernous sinus, lies between two layers of dura and extends from the dorsum sellae to the lower clivus.

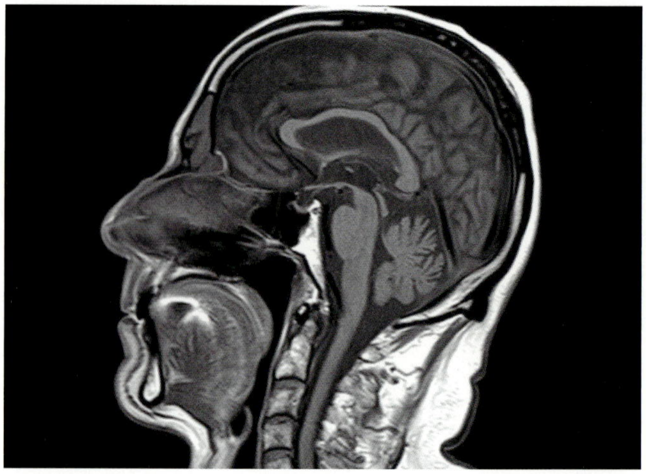

Fig. 26.2: Sagittal image demonstrating the "intrasphenoidal" upper one-third of the clivus, and the inferior one-third of the clivus contained within the posterior nasopharynx.

Seen from the ventral-caudal (i.e., endonasal) side, the upper third of the clivus is entirely contained within (and accessible through) the sphenoid sinus. The middle third is typically "infrasphenoidal" and reached through taking down the mucosa of the choanae, drilling of the vomer, and below the floor of the sphenoid. The inferior third is contained entirely within the posterior nasopharynx, and access therein (via an endonasal route) may be limited by the hard palate (Fig. 26.2).

Sphenoid Sinus

The sphenoid sinus is the gateway to the large majority of endoscopic approaches to the clivus and some petroclival pathology. An intimate knowledge of its anatomy is imperative for any endoscopic skull base surgeon.

The sphenoid sinus ostium, frequently utilized to access the sinus, is located approximately 1.5 cm superior to the posterior choanae on the anterior sphenoid sinus wall. It is elliptical in shape and found at the junction of the inferior and middle thirds of the superior turbinate. It is visualized in the sphenoethmoidal recess enclosed by the septum medially, superior turbinate laterally, cribriform plate superiorly, and the nasal floor inferiorly

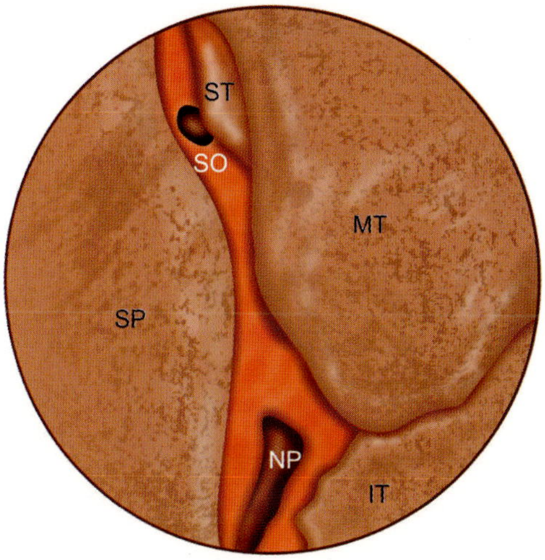

Fig. 26.3: Natural sphenoid ostium.
(SO: Sphenoid ostium; ST: Superior turbinate; MT: Middle turbinate; NP: Nasopharynx; IT: Inferior turbinate; SP: Septum).

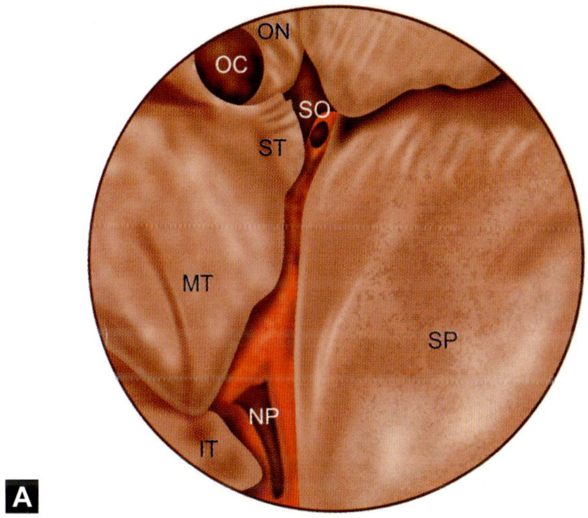

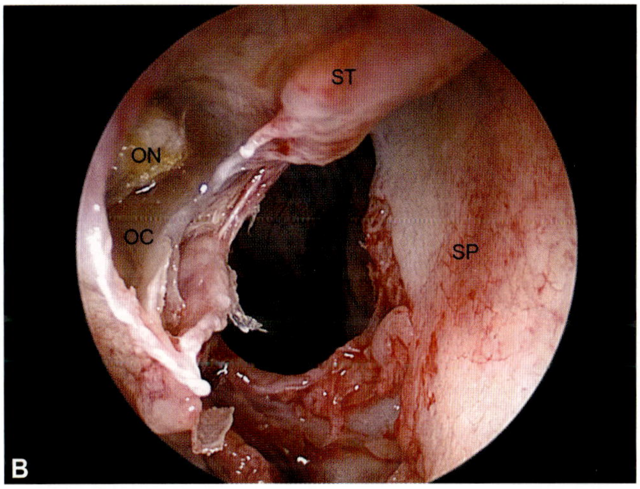

Figs. 26.4A and B: (A and B) Onodi cell.
(OC: Onodi cell; ON: Optic nerve; SO: Sphenoid ostium; IT: Inferior turbinate; MT: Middle turbinate; ST: Superior turbinate; NP: Nasopharynx; SP: Septum).

(Fig. 26.3). The sphenoid sinus may also be entered past the posterior ethmoid cells through the medial-inferior triangle of the sphenoid face. This avoids any risk to the optic nerve and carotid artery located in the superior-lateral triangle. It may also be accessed through a transpterygoid approach, lateral to the middle turbinate. However, this approach is more frequently utilized to reach lateral sphenoid pathology in the region of Sternberg's Canal, but may be useful for approaches to the petroclival junction.[13]

The Onodi (sphenoethmoidal) cell is a posterior ethmoidal cell, which pneumatizes posterior, lateral, and superior to the sphenoid face. It is present in 7–25% of Caucasian patients, and nearly 50% of patients from the Far East.[6] It may often encompass the optic nerve and/or internal carotid artery (ICA) making them vulnerable to injury if not recognized preoperatively (Figs. 26.4A and B).

The body of the sinus is a large paired paranasal sinus located posterior to the ethmoid sinuses. It is divided by complete and incomplete bony septations that occur in various orientations (vertical, horizontal, and oblique). These septations often localize to the carotid artery, underscoring the importance of atraumatic dissection to avoid a catastrophic vascular injury. A recent study of sphenoid sinuses demonstrated that 85% had at least one septation, and 41% had at least two septations inserted into the internal carotid arteries on computed tomography. The same study found that in cadavers, 89%

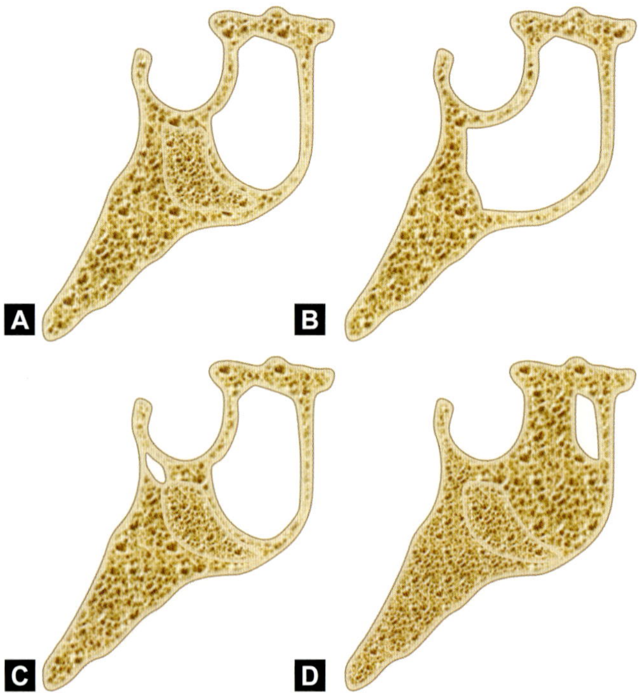

Figs. 26.5A to D: Sphenoid sinus pneumatization. (A: Presellar; B: Sellar; C: Postsellar; D: Conchal).

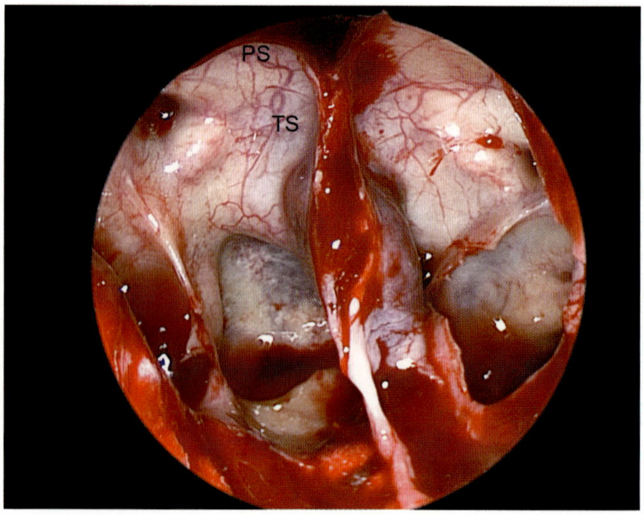

Fig. 26.6: The midline posterior sphenoid sinus wall with the tuberculum sella (TS) separating the sella from the planum sphenoidale (PS).

of sinuses had one septation, and 48% had two septations inserting into the carotid artery. Only 13% of specimens had a isolated midline septation.[14]

Pneumatization of the sphenoid sinus is highly variable and can extend as far as the clivus and foramen magnum inferiorly, and the sphenoid wings laterally. Three major pneumatization patterns for sphenoid sinus include the sellar (80%), presellar (17%), and conchal (3%) configurations.[15] A sellar sphenoid is pneumatized anterior and inferior to the sellar prominence; a presellar configuration is pneumatized only anterior to the sella, and a conchal sphenoid sinus has minimal to absent pneumatization. A conchal configuration poses an especially challenging situation during transclival approaches since the surgeon has to rely heavily on image guidance to identify critical structures (e.g., internal carotid arteries). An additional pneumatization pattern that occurs infrequently is called the postsellar or retrosellar configuration where the sella appears as a prominence along the sphenoid planum rather than the posterior wall of the sphenoid sinus (Figs. 26.5A to D).

Posterior Sphenoid Wall

A thorough knowledge of endoscopic sphenoid anatomy is critical for performing transsphenoidal transclival surgery, the workhorse approach. The midline posterior wall of the sphenoid sinus reveals the sella, inferior to which lies the intrasphenoidal clivus separated by the sellar–clival junction. Rostral to the sella lies the planum sphenoidale (PS), which is separated from the sella by the tuberculum sella (TS), which corresponds to the chiasmatic sulcus intracranially (Fig. 26.6).

Lateral Sphenoid Wall

The lateral wall of the sphenoid sinus reveals four prominences and three depressions. The four prominences from superior to inferior include the bony prominences of the optic nerve, the parasellar ICA, the maxillary (V2), and mandibular (V3) divisions of the trigeminal nerve. The three bony depressions include the lateral opticocarotid recess (LOCR), the depression between the cavernous sinus apex and V2, and the depression between V2 and V3. The LOCR is bound by the optic nerve superolaterally, and parasellar ICA inferomedially. It corresponds to the base of the optic strut intracranially. The oculomotor nerve (CN III) may also be found inferiorly in this recess. The medial opticocarotid recess, located at the medial intersection of the optic canal, and carotid protuberance, corresponds to lateral tubercular crest (and not as often thought the middle clinoid) intracranially.[16] Finally, the region between V2 and V3 represents an embryologic fusion plane of the basi-sphenoid called Sternberg's canal. Lateral sphenoid sinus encephaloceles from the middle cranial fossa may be found in this region secondary to a dehiscence (Fig. 26.7).

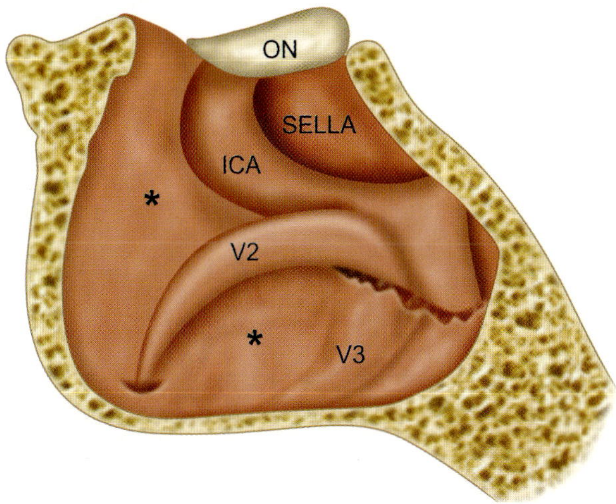

Fig. 26.7: Lateral sphenoid sinus wall.
(*depressions; V3: Mandibular nerve; V2: Maxillary nerve).

THE ENDOSCOPIC APPROACH TO THE CLIVUS

The Operative Team

We routinely utilize a multidisciplinary team approach that includes neurosurgery, otolaryngology, neurophysiology, and neuroanesthesiology—regardless of whether the lesion is purely intranasal, transclival, or intradural. This allows the team to build their comfort level with working together, learn relevant paranasal and neuroanatomy from each other, and refine technique for challenging cases. Ideally, each member has additional specialized training in both endoscopic and open skull base surgery.

Perioperative Physical Examination

A thorough neurologic exam with special consideration to all the cranial nerves is necessary prior to operative intervention (i.e., VI, IX, X, XI, XII). A visual field examination and/or ophthalmology consult is important especially if the orbit or optic nerve is involved. Endoscopic examination of the sinonasal cavity is recommended to document anatomic variations such as septal spurs or deviations, turbinate hypertrophy, septal mucosa integrity, as well as any extension of clival pathology into the sinonasal cavity. For lesions that do extend into the sinonasal cavity, preoperative biopsy provides additional information for operative planning and goals of surgery (debulking vs. gross total resection).

Preoperative Imaging

Preoperative imaging studies include a neuronavigation-specific maxillofacial computed tomograph (CT) or computed tomographic angiogram (CTA) head and an magnetic resonance image (MRI) of the brain with and without contrast. CT allows for the assessment of bony architecture including paranasal anatomic variants, extent of sphenoid sinus pneumatization, intersinus septations in proximity to the carotid arteries, presence of skull base erosion, integrity of the lamina papyracea, and location of the internal carotid arteries, optic nerves and cavernous sinuses (Fig. 26.8A). We find CT angiography extremely helpful for simultaneous visualization of bony and vascular structures. This is particularly important when tumor involvement with the carotid artery, vertebrobasilar system or dural sinuses is noted. The intercarotid distance at the paraclival segments (best seen on axial or coronal reconstructions) and thickness of clivus (best seen on sagittal reconstructions) are important indicators influencing preoperative planning (Fig. 26.8B). MRI is important for delineating soft tissue architecture, in particular, differentiating between tumor or inflammatory lesions (sarcoid, rheumatoid) which often involve the clivus. High resolution T2 sequences (CISS, BFFE, or similar) are often helpful in determining whether the dura has been violated, and if so, whether there is a an arachnoid plane (visualized as a cuff of CSF) between the lesion and the vertebrobasilar circulation and/or brainstem itself (Figs. 26.8C and D).

Neurophysiologic Monitoring

Neurophysiological monitoring with somatosensory evoked potentials is recommended for all cases involving the paraclival carotid or extending transclival intradural. Additional monitoring of motor activity, with the option of stimulated electromyography (EMG), depends on the location and extent of the lesion. CN VI may be monitored with EMG electrodes in the lateral rectus muscle (placed through the lateral canthus), CN IX may be monitored with EMG electrodes sutured into the soft palate, CN X may be monitored with EMG electrodes in a specialized endotracheal tube, and CN XII may be monitored with electrodes in the tongue.

Lumbar Subarachnoid Drain

We do not routinely place a drain for every case. However, placement of a preoperative lumbar drain is considered (on a case-by-case basis) if a large dural defect with a high flow cerebrospinal fluid leak is anticipated.

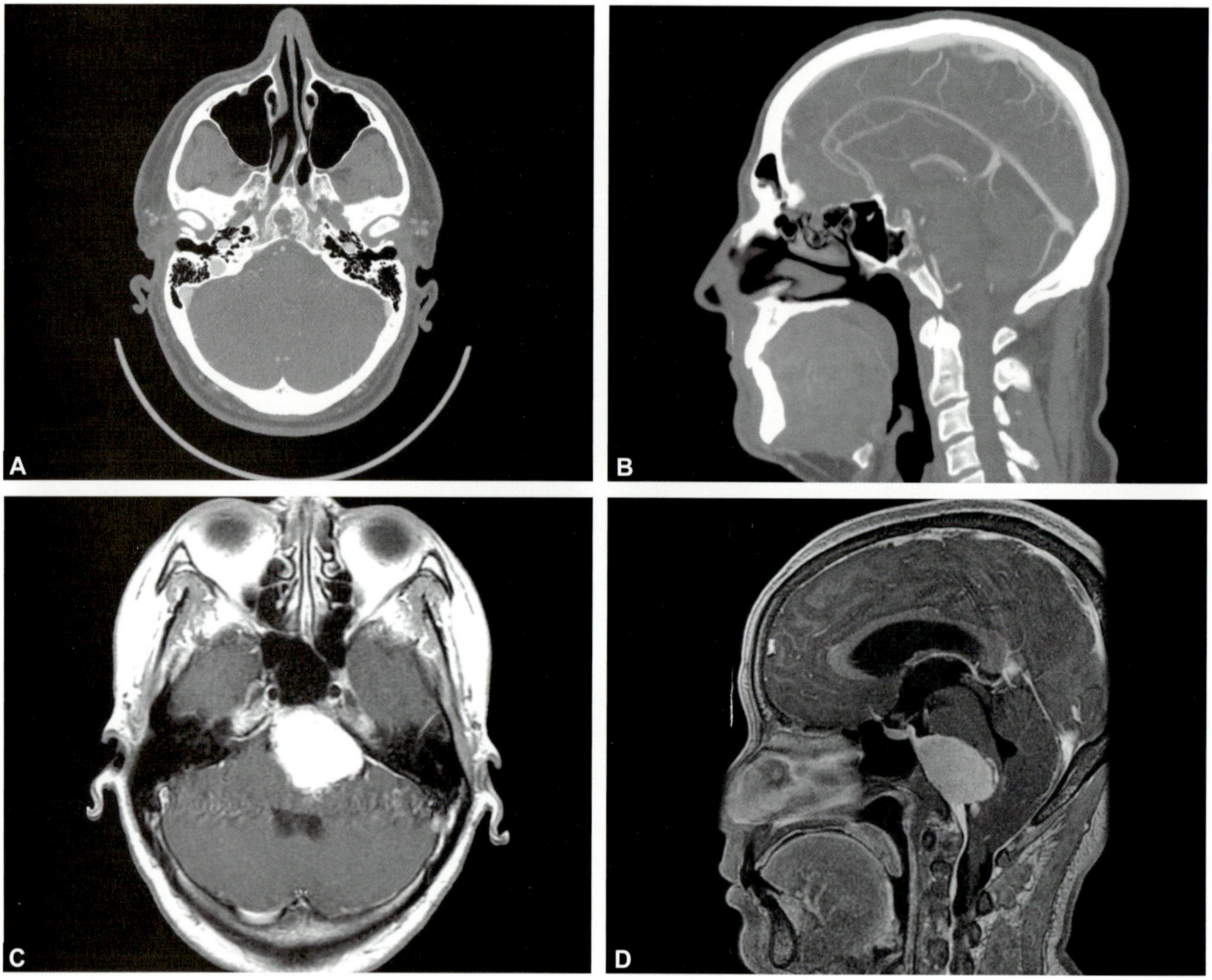

Figs. 26.8A to D: CT, CT angiogram, and MRI images of a large extra- and intradural chordoma.

Equipment

Endoscopic approaches to the clivus require specialized instrumentation beyond the standard set of sinus instruments and/or standard micro-neurosurgical instruments. We strongly recommend investing in a high-definition (1,080 p) camera and tower, and a variety of straight and angled telescopes (0°, 30°, and 45°). Some advocate the use of long telescopes (30 cm) during the three-handed/two surgeon portions of the case, though we find that a standard 18 cm length is sufficient and does not lead to excessive crowding at the nares.

A computer-assisted surgical navigation system (such as Medtronic, Stryker, or Brain Lab) is routinely utilized on all cases. In cases of extensive tumor, or tumor encased in clival bone, we register the tip of a drill or ultrasonic aspirator (see below) to the system to allow continuous navigation while working.

High-speed drills with MIS attachments, capable of handling a variety of cutting, diamond, and rough diamond burrs are important for safe and efficient removal of clival bone. More recently, we have switched over to utilizing an ultrasonic aspirator based on an piezoelectric motor (Sonopet Ultrasonic Aspirator, Stryker Corp., Kalamazoo, MI, USA) for both bone and soft tissue removal. It has proved especially useful around critical neurovascular structures, and can be safely utilized to skeletonize the carotid artery and/or optic nerve (Fig. 26.9).

Specialized nonbayonetted straight and angled long endoscopic instruments are essential for tumor mobilization and resection. These instruments are available from a variety of manufacturers (Karl Storz, Aesculap, Mizuho),

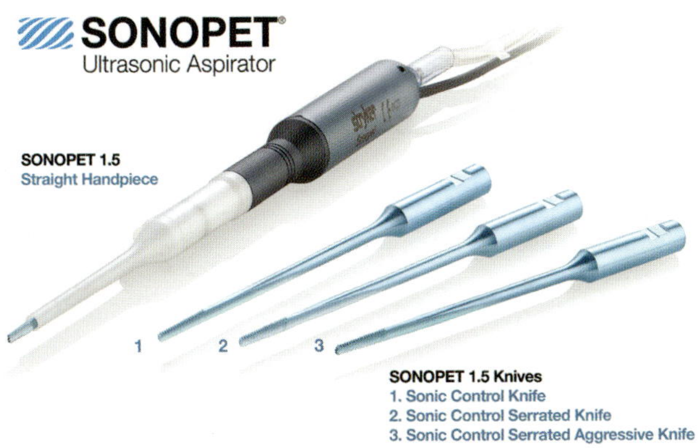

Fig. 26.9: Ultrasonic aspirator based on a piezoelectric motor.

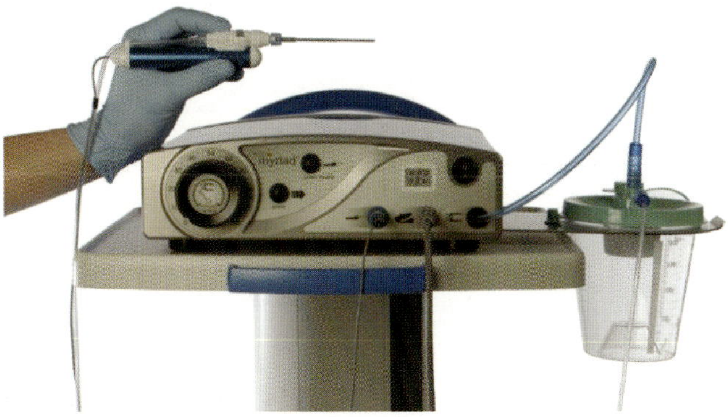

Fig. 26.10: Nonheating generating, oscillating, cutting, and tissue removal. "microdebrider" used for endoscopic and open neurosurgical procedures.

but share common designs revolving around a tubular shaft with movement on either end, rather than a typical "scissor" formation seen in most micro-neurosurgical instruments. We routinely utilize a recently introduced device (NICO Myriad, NICO Corp., USA), which acts as a "micro-microdebrider" similar to arthroscopic shavers and powered sinus debriders, providing variable suction and side cutting capabilities. This has significantly improved endoscopic tumor resection (Fig. 26.10).

Finally, a variety of hemostatic materials (Surgiflo or Floseal, bone wax, thrombin, Surgicel) are important to set up and have available at the beginning of every case. If there is concern for encasement or erosion of a parent vessel (carotid, vertebral, basilar), we routinely have an 8–10 Fr Foley catheter (with the tip cutoff) on the field to place intranasally to tamponade catastrophic arterial bleeding.

Operative Approach

The patient is intubated orotracheally and preoperative antibiotics are given within one hour of incision. Although studies suggest that a weight appropriate does of cefazolin is adequate for antibiotic coverage, other authors have suggested broader antibiotic coverage for expanded intradural skull base surgery.[17] For cases in which dural transgression is planned, we routinely use a third generation cephalosporin with good CSF penetration (ceftriaxone) and vancomycin for the perioperative antibiotics.

The endotracheal tube is usually taped to the left lower corner of the mouth (for the right-handed surgeon) and 4% cocaine-soaked cottonoids are placed in the nasal cavity for decongestion and vasoconstriction of the sinonasal mucosa. Corticosteroids may be given at the discretion of the surgeon, but we advocate not routinely utilizing preoperative steroids, which allows for immediate postoperative day morning cortisol testing to ensure integrity of the anterior pituitary for upper clival lesions.

The patient is positioned in a "beach-chair" position, with the bed reflexed such that the torso is elevated 15°–20°, and the legs are dropped to decrease tension on the lumbar plexus. The head may be placed in pin-fixation (for optical tracking navigation), or on a cerebellar headrest (for active IR or electromagnetic tracking). The head is typically flexed an additional 15°–30° depending on the target—upper clival lesions require less flexion, and lower clival lesions are better approached with the patient hyper flexed at the neck. The head is also anterolisthesed relative to the shoulders to raise the face off the chest, allowing better access for the surgeons (Fig. 26.11). Preoperative imaging is thoroughly reviewed and image guidance registration and verification is performed. The face is prepped in standard fashion with chlorhexidine (taking care to keep it away from mucosa) or chloroxylenol-based solution. If a high flow cerebrospinal fluid leak is anticipated, the abdomen or thigh is prepped to harvest a fat and/or rectus sheath fascia graft for a multilayered reconstruction.

Nasal Portion

Nasal endoscopy is initiated and the septum, middle turbinates, inferior turbinates, nasal floor, sphenoethmoidal

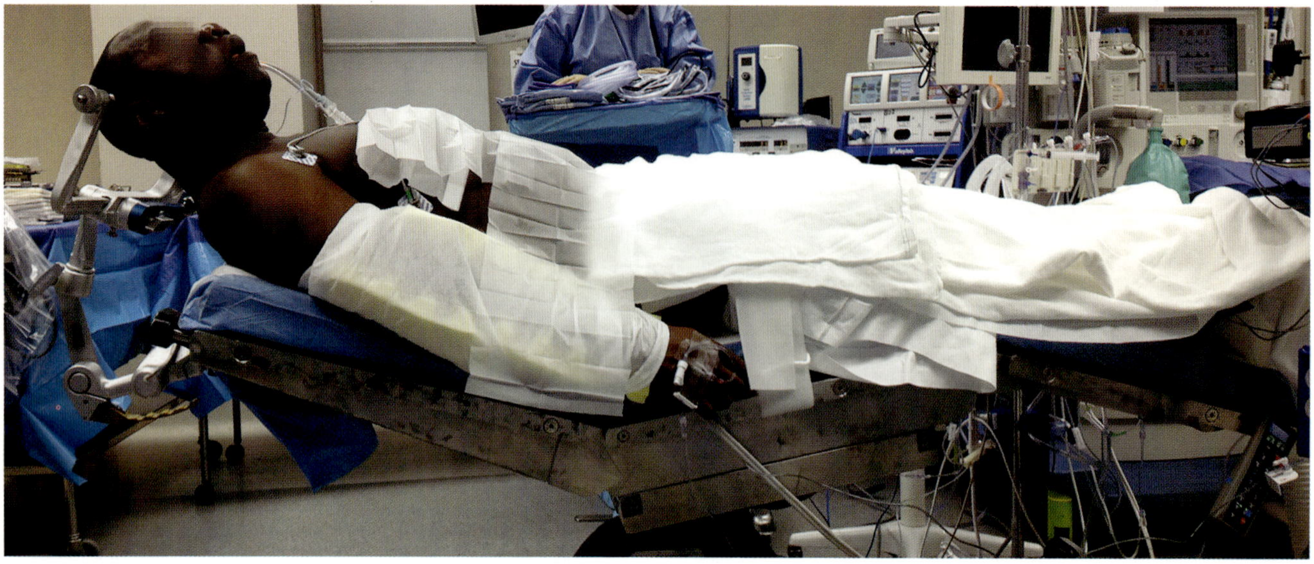

Fig. 26.11: Patient "beach-chair" positioning for endoscopic skull base approach to the clivus.

recesses, and septal mucosa are examined. The vertical lamella of the middle turbinates, the superior turbinates, superior septum, nasal floor, and columella are injected with a local anesthetic (e.g., 1% lidocaine with 1:100,000 epinephrine) to provide vasoconstriction of the nasal mucosa during the endoscopic approach to the clivus. Injection of local anesthesia directly near the pedicle is avoided to prevent arterial vasospasm, especially if harvesting a nasoseptal flap for secondary skull base reconstruction.

If a large dural defect with a high-flow cerebrospinal fluid is anticipated, a vascularized nasoseptal flap for secondary skull base closure is harvested prior to the bulk of the approach. The pedicle of the nasoseptal flap as originally described[18] is supplied by the posterior septal branch of the sphenopalatine artery (Fig. 26.12). The cuts to design the pedicle are made first by incising the arch of the columellar mucosa from midline laterally to approximately 2/3 the circumference of the arch, with a Colorado tip bovie at low power (10–15 Watts). We find it easiest to do with an angled Colorado needle tip. A second incision for the pedicle is made from the medial side of the sphenoid ostium across the rostrum toward its junction with the perpendicular plate of the ethmoid. The superior incision is made 1 cm inferior to the cribriform region in order to preserve the olfactory fibers to the nasal septum. It is important to use the lowest power setting on the Bovie (or a cold knife) to prevent thermal injury to the olfactory nerves. The inferior incision may be made along the premaxillary crest or laterally along the nasal floor if additional flap width is desired. Again, care should be taken so as to not cause a thermal injury to the palatine nerve. The anterior incision may be performed all the way to include the columellar skin if necessary. The flap is then harvested with a combination of sharp or blunt elevators. Typically, the flap is placed in the nasopharynx, however, for extensive transclival approaches, a large maxillary antrostomy is performed so that the flap may be safely stored in the ipsilateral maxillary sinus. This requires releasing the sphenopalatine artery from its foramen in order to provide a sufficient arc of rotation to place the flap in the maxillary sinus. If the clival lesion extends to involve the nasal septum and/or pedicles, alternative vascularized flaps may be harvested. These

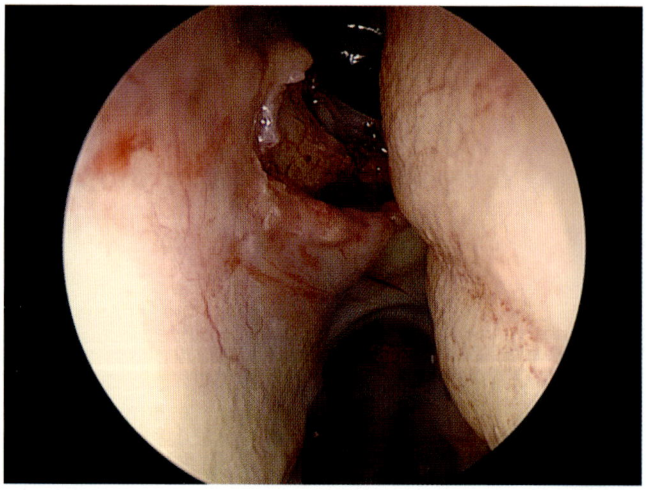

Fig. 26.12: Pedicle of a left nasoseptal flap vascularized by posterior septal artery, a branch of the sphenopalatine artery.

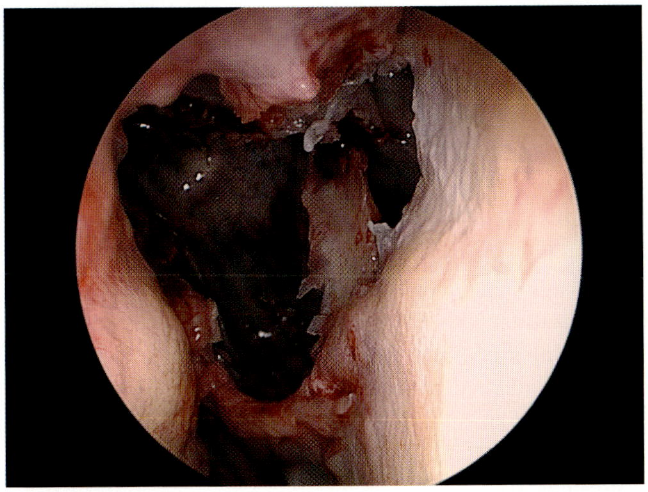

Fig. 26.13: A posterior septectomy and wide bilateral sphenoidotomy allowing for a bi-nostril approach to the intrasphenoidal clivus.

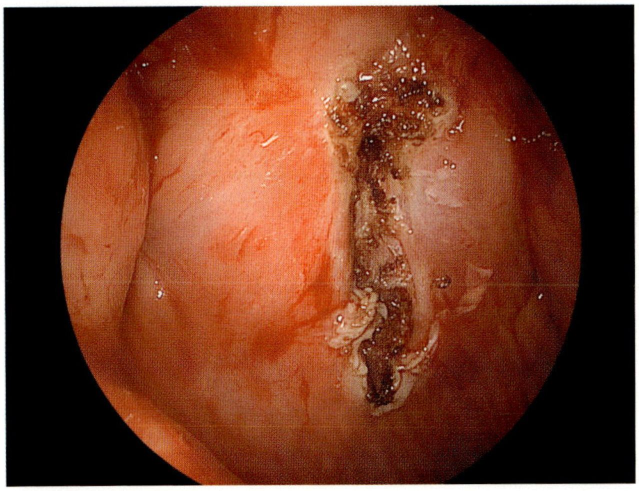

Fig. 26.14: Vertical nasopharyngeal incision to approach an extra-sphenoidal clival lesion.

include the inferior turbinate flap, middle turbinate flap, lateral nasal wall flap, palatal flap, or endoscopic pericranial flap. Discussion of these flaps is covered elsewhere and is beyond the scope of this chapter.[19]

The inferior turbinates are lateralized with a Boise or Freer elevator to provide greater room for maneuvering. The middle turbinates and superior turbinates are also gently lateralized to improve visualization of the sphenoid ethmoidal recesses and sphenoid ostia. Although, middle turbinate preservation is preferred, partial or complete resection may be performed to improve access to the clivus. Care must be taken to ensure that the natural frontal sinus ostia is not obstructed during complete middle turbinate resection. In patients with a congenitally narrow aperture, resection of a single middle turbinate may be necessary to provide room to "park" the telescope while the other surgeon works in a bi-nostril fashion. Similarly, a septoplasty may be performed if septal deviations or spurs prevent adequate visualization or passing of instruments to the clivus. If a flap is harvested, it is important to keep the contralateral septal mucosa intact to prevent ischemia and septal perforations. Meticulous hemostasis during the sinonasal approach is important not only to prevent postoperative epistaxis but also maintain a dry field during the endoscopic approach. Bleeding from the sinonasal cavity during the clival approach may frequently soil the endoscope and make tumor removal infinitely more tedious. Control of bleeding from branches of the sphenopalatine artery, anterior and posterior ethmoidal arteries must be performed during the approach.

A transsphenoidal approach is necessary for the vast majority of endoscopic approaches to the clivus. The natural sphenoid ostia are identified and enlarged using circular "mushroom" punches or Kerrison rongeurs. A posterior septectomy is performed to enable a bi-nostril approach to the clivus (Fig. 26.13). Wide removal of the anterior sphenoid face superiorly, laterally, and inferiorly is performed with a variety of instruments, which include Kerrison rongeurs. Care should be taken to avoid injury to the posterior ethmoidal arteries that course at the junction of the PS and fovea ethmoidalis. Once the anterior face of the sphenoid sinus is addressed, extensive removal of the sphenoid floor is carried out. As previously noted, in cases where anatomy is distorted due to presellar or conchal aeration of the sinus or tumor, the drill or bone-cutting ultrasonic aspirator may be registered to the navigation system to allow safe and efficient removal of the floor of the sphenoid. The distance between the paraclival internal carotid arteries dictates the width of the endoscopic approach to the clivus. Frequent image guided verification of anatomical landmarks and careful micro-Doppler examination of the paraclival carotid arteries is recommended during removal of the sphenoid floor and clivus. For approaches to the middle and inferior third of the clivus, a single midline vertical incision in the mucosa of the nasopharynx/pharynx be made. This incision is typically not necessary, as the mucosa of the choanae and posterior nasopharynx may be mobilized and deflected inferiorly (Fig. 26.14).

Resection of Clival Lesions

Once the initial exposure is complete, it is useful to begin to work as a two-surgeon, three to four handed team. The

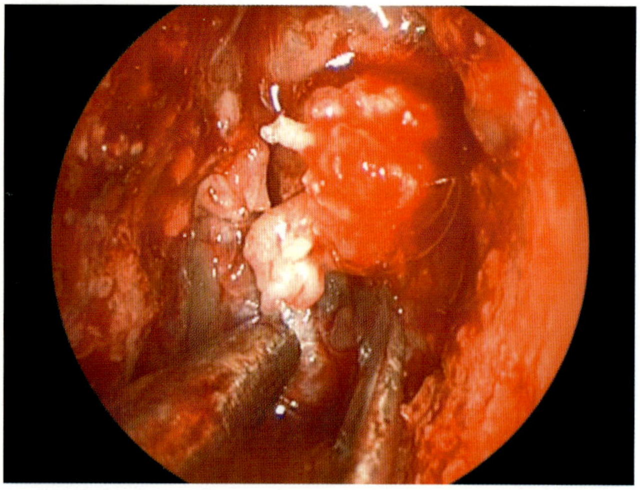

Fig. 26.15: Endoscopic microneurosurgical dissection of an extra- and intradural chordoma with Fukushima suctions, and blunt dissectors.

cosurgeon or first assist will stand shoulder to shoulder (on the left of the primary surgeon) and drive the endoscope. Alternatively, a pneumatic or robotic endoscope holder may be employed. For the majority of the case, the endoscope will be in the patient's right nostril, balanced against the ventral tip of the columella, while the primary surgeon will place a left-handed instrument (usually a suction) below the telescope in the same nostril. This leaves the (right-handed) surgeon complete freedom in the left nostril to use the primary dissecting/cutting instrument with their dominant hand.

Dissection often begins with a blunt or ball-tipped dissector (similar to a lumbar nerve hook, or a Janetta or Fukushima ball-tip) to bluntly define the edge of the lesion and separate it from surrounding structures (Fig. 26.15). For most clival lesions, if possible it is critical, as early as possible, to define and protect the adventitia of the carotid artery. For extensive lesions, after confirmation with image guidance, internal debulking is started, working primarily in the midline. Depending on the texture of lesion, this may be simple suction and curettage, or require more aggressive instrumentation such as a microdebrider or ultrasonic aspirator. The general modus operandi is to create a "safe-zone" midline and ventral, and then working with ring curettes, hooks, and ball-tipped dissectors, collapse and deliver the tumor into this safe zone. More fibrotic and adherent masses do not take well to this technique, and sharp dissection with micro scissor may be required. Extreme caution should be taken while performing sharp dissection off midline—the carotid is often more medial than the surgeon realizes. Frequent confirmation with microdoppler and navigation is advised—especially early in one's experience. Once the bulk of the tumor is removed, and the surgeon has taken advantage of the safe-zone created by the mass of the tumor, the remainder is taken off its adhesions to surrounding structures.

Quite often, the full thickness of the dura is not involved. If it is partially involved, for most pathologies it is advisable to leave an intact dura after curettage of the periosteal dura. Not only does this significantly decrease the complexity of the case in terms of avoiding reconstruction, but dura serves as a hearty natural barrier to the extension of sinonasal and osseous tumors into the central nervous system. Once the curettage and debridement is complete, there may be vigorous venous bleeding from the occipital plexus. This may be staunched with either fibrin epoxy (Tisseel, Baxter, USA or Evicel, Johnson and Johnson, USA) or powdered thrombin-foam complexes (FloSeal, Baxter, USA or SurgiFlo, Johnson and Johnson, USA).

Removal of lesions that extend more laterally to involve the petro-clival junction (or arise therein, such as cholesterol granuloma) or the retrocarotid space is facilitated by working with a "side-looking" 30° scope. A common fallacy, early in endoscopic skull base surgery is to assume that if you can see it, you can reach it. This is not at all true when working with angled scopes, which require angled suctions, angled dissectors, and often extension of the exposure through Bolger's box or transpterygoid to allow the surgeon to reach what he/she can visualize. This is where frequently working together as a team produces rewards, as the neurosurgeon may convey these needs or the otorhinolaryngologist may anticipate these needs before they arise, and adjust the exposure accordingly.

Reconstruction of Clival Defects

Extradural clival defects after biopsy or removal of extracranial lesions do not require any significant reconstruction. If no dura is exposed after completion of the resection, bony edges, and spurs are smoothed out using diamond or rough-diamond burrs on a high speed drill. This includes clival bone, intersinus sphenoid septations, and edges of the sphenoid face. The heat generated by drilling with a diamond friction bit improves bony hemostasis and decortication encourages rapid mucosalization in the postoperative period. Large venous channels within the clivus (which frequently communicate with the occipital plexus) may be packed with paraffin bone wax or hemostatic foams.

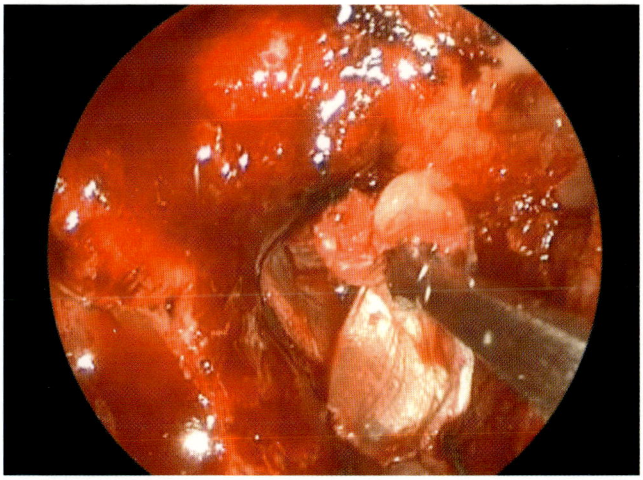

Fig. 26.16: Multilayered endoscopic skull base reconstruction of a high flow cerebrospinal fluid leak with fascia lata after chordoma resection.

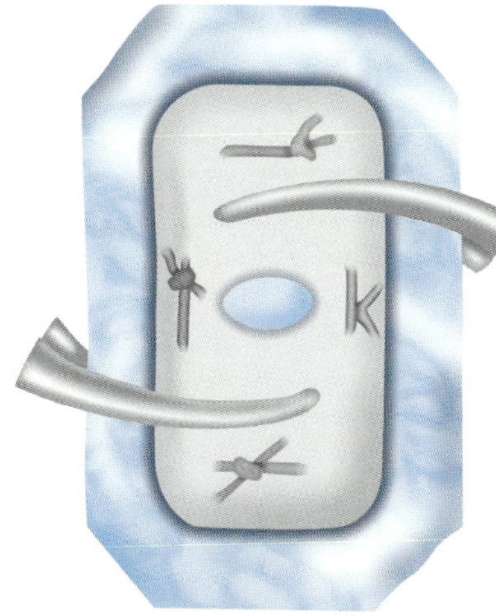

Fig. 26.17: Modified gasket seal for closure of high flow cerebrospinal fluid leaks using a one-piece construct of fascia lata and a rigid polyethylene buttress.

If the dura is exposed but not entered after resection, it may be left alone or covered with a free mucosa grafts after the surrounding bony edges are smoothened. Internal carotid artery adventitial exposure is typically covered with a mucosal or vascularized pedicled flap. The type of pathology may influence this decision. Free grafts are often held in place with fibrin epoxy or a hydrogel (Duraseal, Covidien, USA).

Reconstruction after intradural tumor resection requires a multilayered reconstructive strategy. Clival defects are usually large dural defects with a high flow cerebrospinal fluid leak. The resection cavity may be packed with fat to obliterate the dead space and prevent pooling of cerebrospinal fluid. A multilayered closure using either fascia, dural substitute, or Alloderm is used to close the high flow cerebrospinal fluid defect (Fig. 26.16). A variety of techniques have been used and reported in the literature which include the gasket seal, bilayer button and Alloderm reconstruction. The gasket seal and variations thereof[20] are dependent on a bony defect which sometimes may not be available after extensive endoscopic clival surgery. When possible, we prefer to use a modified gasket seal consisting of autologous rectus sheath fascia, Porex™ plate without extensive fat grafting as described by Wessel et al.[20] (Fig. 26.17). Secondary closure of the clival defect with a vascularized pedicle flap (e.g., nasoseptal flap) is now routine since their use has resulted in a significant decrease in postoperative cerebrospinal fluid leaks. A vascularized flap must be large enough to cover all bony edges of the defect without any tension. It also must placed flush with the bone from its pedicle to most distal point (Fig. 26.18). The flap is covered with a tissue sealant (e.g., fibrin glue or hydrogel) and buttressed with nasal packing (Fig. 26.19). Our preferred packing is a bio-fragmentable foam (Nasopore; Stryker, Kalamazoo, USA), which fragments in the postoperative period and may be easily suctioned and removed during endoscopic postoperative debridement (Fig. 26.19). Mucosal hemostasis may be achieved with monopolar and/or bipolar cautery as well as various hemostatic agents. Packing may be used to tamponade any minor bleeding. We often place a nasal splint on the side of harvesting the nasoseptal flap to encourage mucosalization and decrease synechiae formation. We do not routinely place non-absorbable anterior packs, or utilize Foley catheters to buttress the flap as these may cause necrosis and pressure ulceration.

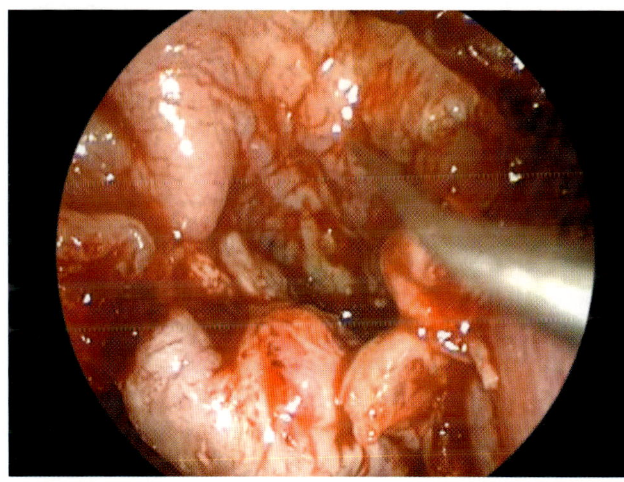

Fig. 26.18: Vascularized nasoseptal flap placed over the primary multilayered reconstruction to ensure a water-tight closure.

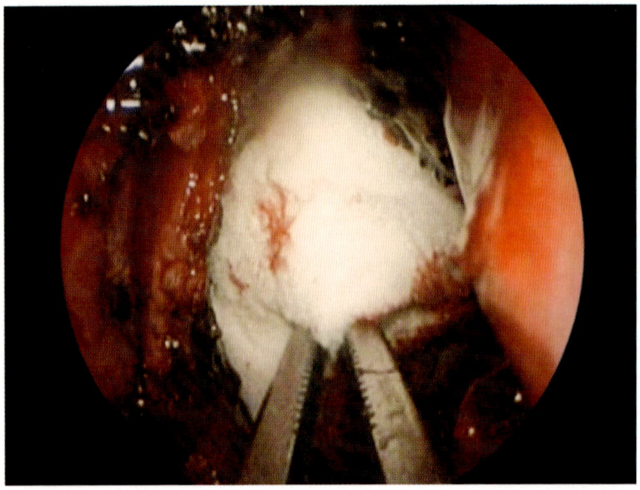

Fig. 26.19: Reinforced multilayered skull base reconstruction with a biofragmentable foam.

CONCLUSION

Endoscopic approaches to the clivus have resulted in a significant decrease in morbidity for patients with clival pathology. Improvements in visualization, availability of specialized instrumentation, and widening clinical experience have made endoscopic approaches the preferred technique for resection of clival lesions. Introduction of various multilayered reconstruction techniques, and vascularized pedicled flaps have significantly reduced postoperative cerebrospinal fluid leaks, the "Achilles heel" for extended endoscopic skull base surgery.

REFERENCES

1. Siomin V, Constantini S. Basic principles and equipment in neuroendoscopy. Neurosurg Clin N Am. 2004;15(1):19-31.
2. Prevedello DM, Doglietto F, Jane JA Jr., et al. History of endoscopic skull base surgery: its evolution and current reality. J Neurosurg. 2007;107(1):206-13.
3. Li KW, Nelson C, Suk I, et al. Neuroendoscopy: past, present, and future. Neurosurg Focus. 2005;19(6):E1.
4. Spencer WR, Das K, Nwagu C, et al. Approaches to the sellar and parasellar region: anatomic comparison of the microscope versus endoscope. Laryngoscope. 1999;109(5):791-4.
5. Catapano D, Sloffer CA, Frank G, et al. Comparison between the microscope and endoscope in the direct endonasal extended transsphenoidal approach: anatomical study. J Neurosurg. 2006;104(3):419-25.
6. Perneczky A, Fries G. Endoscope-assisted brain surgery: part 1—evolution, basic concept, and current technique. Neurosurgery. 1998;42(2):219-24; discussion 224-15.
7. Fries G, Perneczky A. Endoscope-assisted brain surgery: part 2—analysis of 380 procedures. Neurosurgery. 1998;42(2):226-31; discussion 231-22.
8. Schwartz TH, Fraser JF, Brown S, et al. Endoscopic cranial base surgery: classification of operative approaches. Neurosurgery. 2008;62(5):991-1002; discussion 1002-5.
9. O'Malley BW, Jr., Grady MS, Gabel BC, et al. Comparison of endoscopic and microscopic removal of pituitary adenomas: single-surgeon experience and the learning curve. Neurosurg Focus. 2008;25(6):E10.
10. Snyderman CH, Fernandez-Miranda J, Gardner PA. Training in neurorhinology: the impact of case volume on the learning curve. Otolaryngol Clin North Am. 2011;44(5):1223-8.
11. Yang I, Wang MB, Bergsneider M. Making the transition from microsurgery to endoscopic trans-sphenoidal pituitary neurosurgery. Neurosurg Clin N Am. 2010;21(4):643-51, vi.
12. Singh A, Saraiya R. Three-dimensional endoscopy in sinus surgery. Curr Opin Otolaryngol Head Neck Surg. 2013;21(1):3-10.
13. Bolger WE, Keyes AS, Lanza DC. Use of the superior meatus and superior turbinate in the endoscopic approach to the sphenoid sinus. Otolaryngol Head Neck Surg. 1999; 120(3):308-13.
14. Fernandez-Miranda JC, Prevedello DM, Madhok R, et al. Sphenoid septations and their relationship with internal carotid arteries: anatomical and radiological study. Laryngoscope. 2009;119(10):1893-6.
15. Singh A, Roth J, Anand VK, et al. Anatomy of the Pituitary Gland and Parasellar Region in: Endoscopic Pituitary Surgery. New York: Thieme; 2011.
16. Kassam A, Snyderman CH, Mintz A, et al. Expanded endonasal approach: the rostrocaudal axis. Part II. Posterior clinoids to the foramen magnum. Neurosurg Focus. 2005; 19(1):E4.
17. Brown SM, Anand VK, Tabaee A, et al. Role of perioperative antibiotics in endoscopic skull base surgery. Laryngoscope. 2007;117(9):1528-32.
18. Hadad G, Bassagasteguy L, Carrau RL, et al. A novel reconstructive technique after endoscopic expanded endonasal approaches: vascular pedicle nasoseptal flap. Laryngoscope. 2006;116(10):1882-6.
19. Nyquist GG, Anand VK, Singh A, et al. Janus flap: bilateral nasoseptal flaps for anterior skull base reconstruction. Otolaryngol Head Neck Surg. 2010;142(3):327-31.
20. Wessell A, Singh A, Litvack Z. One-piece modified gasket seal technique. J Neurol Surg Part B. 2013;74(5):305-10.

CHAPTER

27

Endoscopic Transodontoid Approach

James D Phillips, Bradford A Woodworth

INTRODUCTION

Anterior surgical access to the craniovertebral junction and the rostral cervical spine had been attempted as early as 1935.[1] Subsequent advancements in surgical technique yielded the transoral approach, which became the gold standard for operative exposure.[2] Using microscopic assistance, a number of pathologies were addressed in this manner: basilar invagination, congenital anomaly (often associated with Chiari malformation), rheumatoid arthritis with resultant compression or pannus formation, odontoid fractures, and neoplasms. However, the transpalatal technique was accompanied by the morbidity associated with division of the soft palate, including edema, airway obstruction, alterations in swallow mechanism requiring nasogastric tube placement, or voice changes from velopalatal insufficiency.[3,4] Considering that pathology may require both extradural and intradural exposure, there is a risk for bacterial seeding of the meninges from saliva in the oropharynx. Additionally, use of the operative microscope requires line-of-sight visualization and thus certain anatomical limitations are imposed. Particularly in instances of progressive basilar invagination or when more extensive dissection of the foramen magnum is required, the hard palate can begin to obstruct the surgeon's view.[5,6]

In light of these concerns and limitations, and with the burgeoning applications of transnasal endoscopic approaches to the skull base, an alternative to the transoral approach was developed. Early cadaveric studies explored and confirmed the feasibility of a transnasal endoscopic approach to the dens.[7,8] In 2005, Kassam et al.[9] published a case report utilizing transnasal techniques in a 73-year-old female with a pannus from rheumatoid arthritis causing compression at the atlantoaxial joint. Using rigid endoscopes, an endoscopic drill, and an ultrasonic aspirator, the odontoid process was resected in conjunction with a posterior spinal fusion of the occiput to the C3 vertebra. At a month follow-up, the patient had regained complete strength in her extremities.

APPLICATIONS

Although the endoscopic endonasal transodontoid approach is a useful technique for exposing the anterior craniovertebral junction, the clinical situations in which this type of access is required are relatively rare. The most common disease entity reported in the literature for which it has been applied is odontoid pannus formation from rheumatoid arthritis.[10,11] The integrity of the anterior C1 arch may be maintained during removal, which obviates the need for posterior fixation and the resultant impairment of rotational movement.[10] Neoplasms that affect the craniovertebral junction, though exceedingly rare, are also candidates for resection or biopsy using the transnasal corridor. Lesions include primary soft tissue sarcomas or meningioma, but metastases from distant sites such as the breast or the prostate may also present in this location.[11]

In pediatric patients, the transodontoid approach is suitable for a number of congenitally derived malformations. Basilar invagination from upward migration of the odontoid process is accessible for decompression with this technique (Figs. 27.1A and B).[12,13] Spinal abnormalities may be addressed in the setting of a type 1 Arnold-Chiari malformation, traditionally a diagnostic and therapeutic dilemma.[14,15] Down syndrome patients who manifest with atlantoaxial instability may be decompressed when posterior spinal fixation has failed.[16]

The transodontoid surgical approach allows enough exposure to adequately reconstruct the posterior cranial fossa to prevent postoperative cerebrospinal fluid (CSF) leak. This may be accomplished in a layered fashion to ensure the integrity of the repair.[17-22] Larger defects may require use of a pedicled vascularized nasoseptal flap.[23,24]

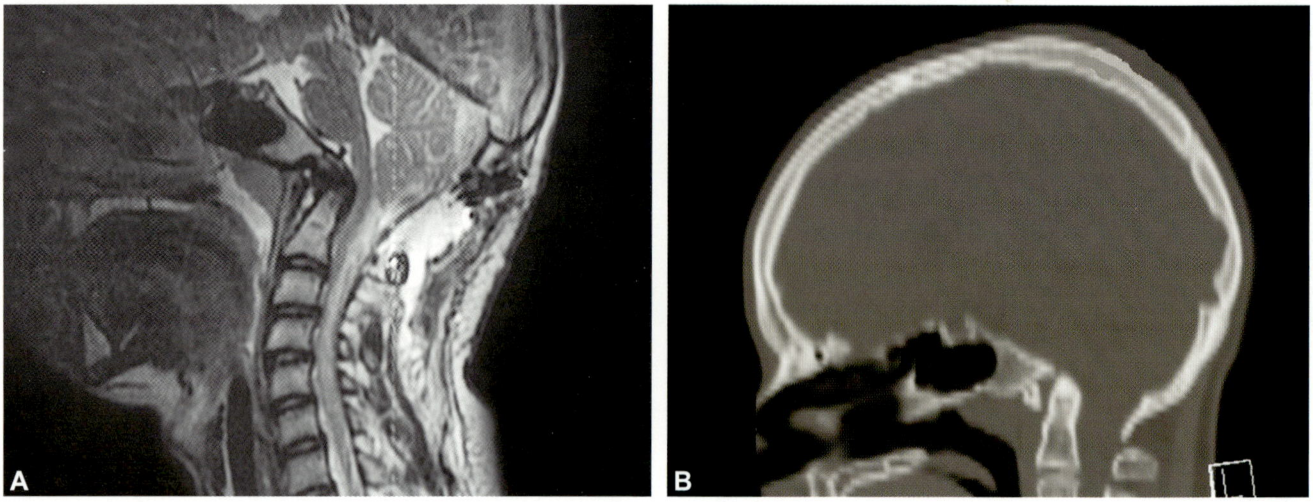

Figs. 27.1A and B: (A) A sagittally oriented T2 weighted magnetic resonance image showing basilar invagination as a result of a bony malformation of the skull base. Note the compressed brainstem. (B) The same patient imaged with computed tomography in a sagittal plane. The bony anatomy of the dens and skull base is better delineated.

LIMITATIONS

Endonasal transodontoid surgery has a number of restrictive anatomic limitations that must be considered preoperatively. Inferiorly, the plane of the approach is determined by the bony skeleton of the nose and palate. An imaginary landmark termed the nasopalatine line connects the most anterior tip of the bony pyramid of the nose to the most posterior aspect of the hard palate and defines the inferior extent of dissection.[11,25] Inferior access may be influenced by cervical mobility and the degree of basilar invagination, but de Almeida et al.[11] found that the mean intersection of the nasopalatine line and the spinal column was 8.9 mm above the base of C2 commonly enabling full exposure of the base of the odontoid process. Neurovascular structures, including the carotid artery and vidian nerves, represent the lateral limits of the transodontoid surgery.

Concerns regarding the endonasal approach include the unnecessary exposure of vital structures such as the carotid arteries and the vidian nerves (although not always necessary), the increased distance between the surgical orifice and the spine, and the inconvenience of coordinating two surgeons (neurosurgeon and rhinologist).[9] Pillai et al.[26] performed a cadaveric study suggesting that the same principles of endoscopic assistance and image guidance may be applied to a transoral approach with adequate visualization of the craniovertebral junction in a comparable fashion to the operating microscope. Another cadaveric study examined the relative strengths and weaknesses of the transoral and transnasal exposures along the length of the most rostral aspects of the spine and suggested that both may be used on a single case in a complimentary fashion.[27] Technical advancements, such as robotic surgery, are under continuing investigation.

TECHNIQUE

Although surgical techniques may vary, it is important to respect a number of set principles to the transodontoid approach that should be consistent across operators. Acquiring CT scans for image-guided systems are crucial adjuncts for intraoperative computer-assisted navigation. Magnetic resonance imaging (MRI) is also useful if the surgeon would like to fuse computed tomography (CT) and MRI for image guidance.

After the induction of general anesthesia and an orally placed endotracheal tube, the patient is placed in Mayfield pins in a neutral position. The sinus navigation system is calibrated, and topical decongestant medication is placed in the nares.

Exposure may be obtained by proceeding directly to wide sphenoidotomies (Fig. 27.2), although some individuals may have enough operative room with lateralization of the inferior turbinates. Structures may be removed depending on the working space necessary for three or four-handed technique; err on the side of preservation of normal anatomy when possible. The posterior aspect of the nasal septum may be removed for greater access. Once this exposure is granted, the wide field allows for the safe identification of the carotid arteries, vidian nerve

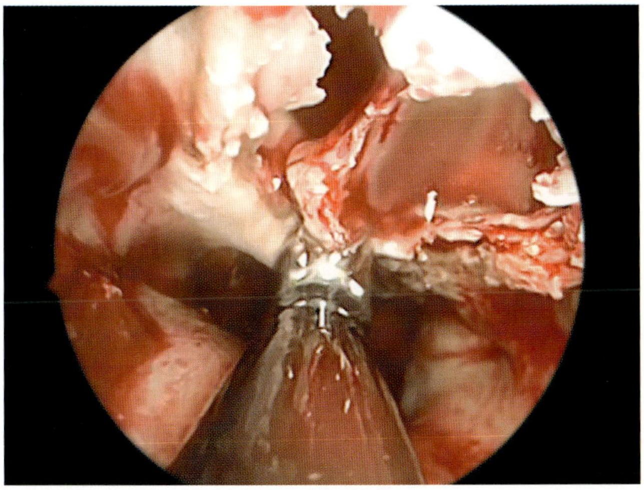

Fig. 27.2: Bilateral wide sphenoidotomies with posterior septectomy provides working space and visualization of relative landmarks.

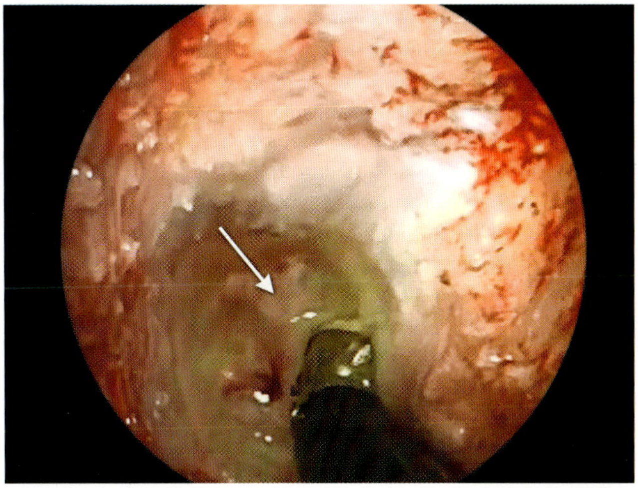

Fig. 27.3: Dissection proceeds from the sphenoid floor and along the clivus. Radiofrequency coblation is a useful method by which to incise and remove the soft tissue of the nasopharynx in a relatively bloodless manner. A superior incision along the base of the sphenoid sinus and superior clivus can be combined with posterolateral nasopharyngeal incisions (medial to the Eustachian tubes) to create an inferiorly based flap or, as in this case, the tissue ablated taking care to limit removal to above the closure of the palate. The anterior aspect of the dens is visualized (arrow).

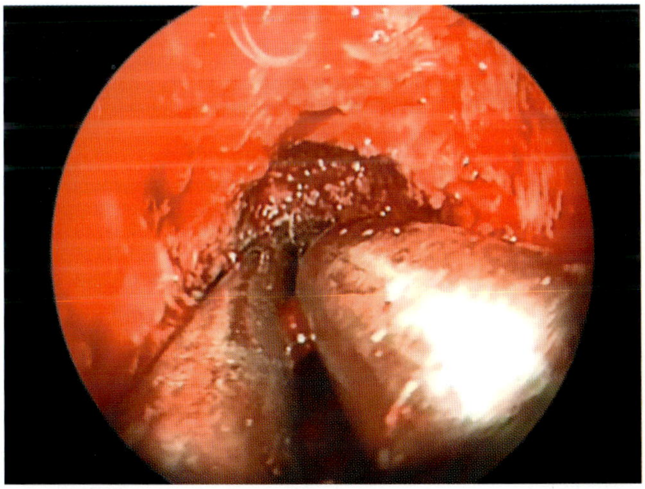

Fig. 27.4: The three-handed technique is demonstrated, allowing for instrumentation while simultaneously resecting the odontoid process. The center of the dens is cored out with the drill.

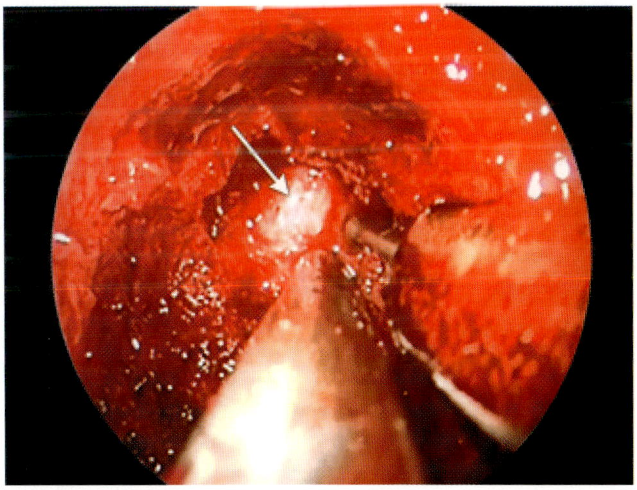

Fig. 27.5: The posterior cranial fossa dura is exposed (arrow) and the edges of the dens are thinned with the drill.

and pterygoid plates if necessary. Caudally, the field may extend between the mucosa of the eustachian tubes.

The mucosa of the nasopharynx may be elevated from the underlying basipharyngeal fascia, creating an inferiorly based mucosal flap or removed entirely taking care to stay superior to palatal closure to avoid velo-pharyngeal insufficiency. Next, the basipharyngeal fascia is removed, exposing the bony sphenoid floor and ventral clivus. Radiofrequency coblation is useful for removing the fascia and exposing bone (Fig. 27.3).[23,24,28-33] The occipital condyles, the C1 and C2 vertebrae including the dens, and the foramen magnum can be exposed with this technique. Once the odontoid process is encountered, the bone is removed with endoscopic drills and Kerrison punches (Figs. 27.4 to 27.6). The entire procedure is extradural so no grafting is necessary unless a CSF leak

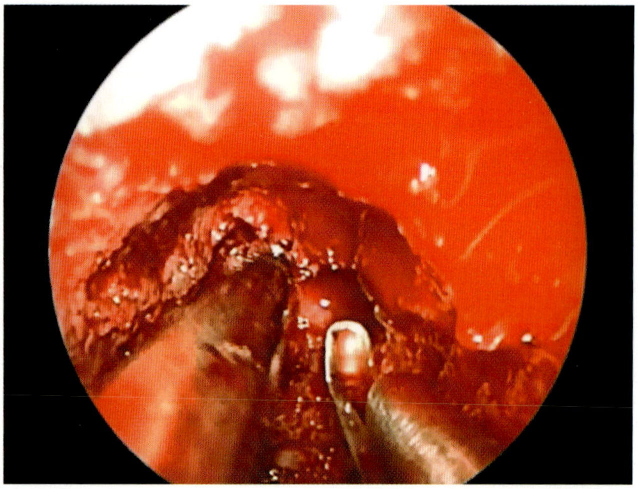

Fig. 27.6: The remnants of the odontoid process are removed with Kerrison punches.

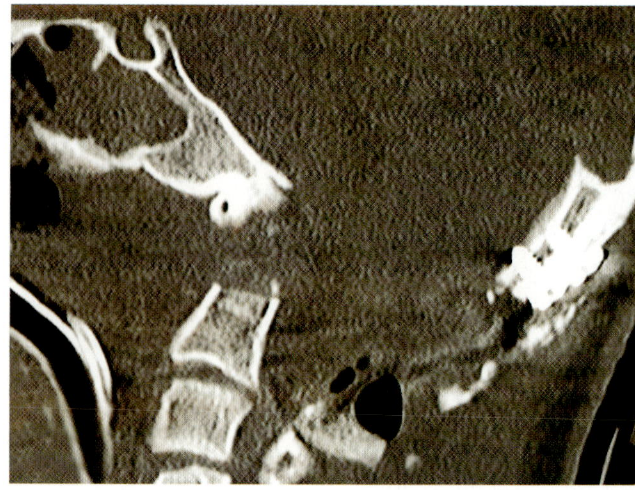

Fig. 27.7: Intraoperative CT scan reveals the odontoid process has been removed and the brainstem completely decompressed.

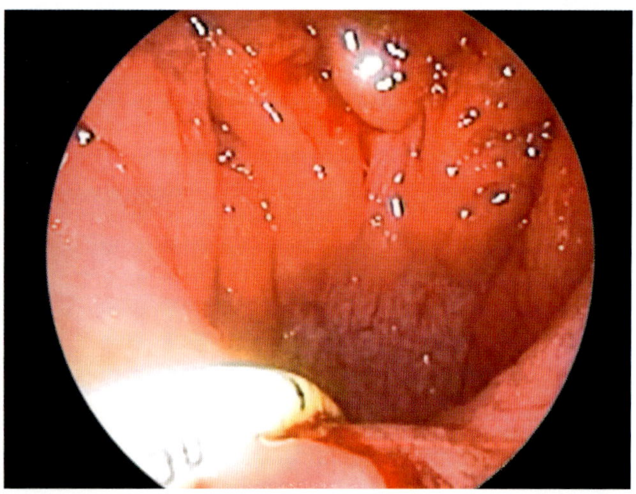

Fig. 27.8: At 6 weeks postoperatively, the transnasal endoscopic view demonstrates a well-healed nasopharynx. There is a nasogastric feeding tube due to incomplete recovery of his lower cranial nerve dysfunction at that point. The patient had a full recovery with no velopharyngeal insufficiency once lower cranial nerve function returned.

is created. Intraoperative CT scans may be helpful to ensure completeness of resection prior to extubation (Fig. 27.7).[34,35] Postoperatively, the nasopharynx is completely healed at 6 weeks (Fig. 27.8).

CONCLUSION

The endoscopic endonasal transodontoid approach to the skull base is a useful and potentially powerful tool in the armamentarium of the skull base surgeon. The relative and absolute indications for the approach continue to be delineated, and will take time to define due to relative paucity of disease processes. Advancements in instrumentation and visualization, such as robotic surgery, will continue to facilitate broadening applications of endoscopic techniques.

REFERENCES

1. Greenberg AD, Scoville WB, Davey LM. Transoral decompression of atlanto-axial dislocation due to odontoid hypoplasia. Report of two cases. J Neurosurg. 1968;28(3):266-9.
2. Merwin GE, Post JC, Sypert GW. Transoral approach to the upper cervical spine. Laryngoscope. 1991;101(7 Pt 1):780-4.
3. Jones DC, Hayter JP, Vaughan ED, et al. Oropharyngeal morbidity following transoral approaches to the upper cervical spine. Int J Oral Maxillofac Surg. 1998;27(4):295-8.
4. Daniels SK, Mahoney MC, Lyons GD. Persistent dysphagia and dysphonia following cervical spine surgery. Ear Nose Throat J. 1998;77(6):470, 473-5.
5. Frempong-Boadu AK, Faunce WA, Fessler RG. Endoscopically assisted transoral-transpharyngeal approach to the craniovertebral junction. Neurosurgery. 2002;51(5 Suppl):S60-6.
6. Welch WC, Kassam A. Endoscopically assisted transoral-transpharyngeal approach to the craniovertebral junction. Neurosurgery. 2003;52(6):1511-2.
7. Alfieri A, Jho HD, Tschabitscher M. Endoscopic endonasal approach to the ventral cranio-cervical junction: anatomical study. Acta Neurochir (Wien). 2002;144(3):219-25.
8. Messina A, Bruno MC, Decq P, et al. Pure endoscopic endonasal odontoidectomy: anatomical study. Neurosurg Rev. 2007;30(3):189-94.
9. Kassam A, Thomas AJ, Snyderman C, et al. Fully endoscopic expanded endonasal approach treating skull base lesions in pediatric patients. J Neurosurg. 2007;106(2 Suppl):75-86.

10. Iacoangeli M, Gladi M, Alvaro L, et al. Endoscopic endonasal odontoidectomy with anterior C1 arch preservation in elderly patients affected by rheumatoid arthritis. Spine J. 2013;13:542-8.
11. de Almeida JR, Zanation AM, Snyderman CH, et al. Defining the nasopalatine line: the limit for endonasal surgery of the spine. Laryngoscope. 2009;119(2):239-44.
12. Yu Y, Wang X, Zhang X, et al. Endoscopic transnasal odontoidectomy to treat basilar invagination with congenital osseous malformations. Eur Spine J. 2012;22:1127-36.
13. Patel AJ, Boatey J, Muns J, et al. Endoscopic endonasal odontoidectomy in a child with chronic type 3 atlantoaxial rotatory fixation: case report and literature review. Childs Nerv Syst. 2012;28(11):1971-5.
14. Scholtes F, Signorelli F, McLaughlin N, et al. Endoscopic endonasal resection of the odontoid process as a standalone decompressive procedure for basilar invagination in Chiari type I malformation. Minim Invasive Neurosurg. 2011;54(4):179-82.
15. Grammatica A, Bonali M, Ruscitti F, et al. Transnasal endoscopic removal of malformation of the odontoid process in a patient with type I Arnold-Chiari malformation: a case report. Acta Otorhinolaryngol Ital. 2011;31(4):248-52.
16. Magrini S, Pasquini E, Mazzatenta D, et al. Endoscopic endonasal odontoidectomy in a patient affected by Down syndrome: technical case report. Neurosurgery. 2008;63(2): E373-4.
17. Illing E, Chaaban MR, Riley KO, et al. Porcine small intestine submucosal graft for endoscopic skull base reconstruction. Int Forum Allergy Rhinol. 2013;3:928-32.
18. Chaaban MR, Illing E, Riley KO, et al. Spontaneous cerebrospinal fluid leak repair: a five-year prospective evaluation. Laryngoscope. 2014;124(1):70-5.
19. Chaaban MR, Illing E, Riley KO, Woodworth BA. Acetazolamide for high intracranial pressure cerebrospinal fluid leaks. Int Forum Allergy Rhinol. 2013;3(9):718-21.
20. Jones V, Virgin F, Riley K, et al. Changing paradigms in frontal sinus cerebrospinal fluid leak repair. Int Forum Allergy Rhinol. 2012;2(3):227-32.
21. Chaaban MR, Conger B, Riley KO, et al. Transnasal endoscopic repair of posterior table fractures. Otolaryngol Head Neck Surg. 2012;147(6):1142-7.
22. Alexander NS, Chaaban MR, Riley KO, et al. Treatment strategies for lateral sphenoid sinus recess cerebrospinal fluid leaks. Arch Otolaryngol Head Neck Surg. 2012;138(5): 471-8.
23. Chaaban MR, Chaudhry A, Riley KO, et al. Simultaneous pericranial and nasoseptal flap reconstruction of anterior skull base defects following endoscopic-assisted craniofacial resection. Laryngoscope. 2013; 123:2383-6.
24. Virgin F, Baranano CF, Riley K, et al. Frontal sinus skull base defect repair using the pedicled nasoseptal flap. Otolaryngol Head Neck Surg. 2011;145(2):338-40.
25. Lega BC, Kramer DR, Newman JG, et al. Morphometric measurements of the anterior skull base for endoscopic transoral and transnasal approaches. Skull Base. 2011;21(1): 65-70.
26. Pillai P, Baig MN, Karas CS, et al. Endoscopic image-guided transoral approach to the craniovertebral junction: an anatomic study comparing surgical exposure and surgical freedom obtained with the endoscope and the operating microscope. Neurosurgery. 2009;64(5 Suppl 2):437-42; discussion 442-4.
27. Seker A, Inoue K, Osawa S, et al. Comparison of endoscopic transnasal and transoral approaches to the craniovertebral junction. World Neurosurg. 2010;74(6):583-602.
28. Schuster D, Riley KO, Cure JK, et al. Endoscopic resection of intracranial dermoid cysts. J Laryngol Otol. 2011;125(4): 423-7.
29. Joshi H, Woodworth BA, Carney AS. Coblation for epistaxis management in patients with hereditary haemorrhagic telangiectasia: a multicentre case series. J Laryngol Otol. 2011;125(11):1176-80.
30. Blount A, Riley KO, Woodworth BA. Juvenile nasopharyngeal angiofibroma. Otolaryngol Clin North Am. 2011;44(4): 989-1004.
31. Virgin FW, Bleier BS, Woodworth BA. Evolving materials and techniques for endoscopic sinus surgery. Otolaryngol Clin North Am. 2010;43(3):653-72.
32. Smith N, Riley KO, Woodworth BA. Endoscopic Coblator-assisted management of encephaloceles. Laryngoscope. 2010;120(12):2535-9.
33. Kostrzewa JP, Sunde J, Riley KO, et al. Radiofrequency coblation decreases blood loss during endoscopic sinonasal and skull base tumor removal. ORL J Otorhinolaryngol Relat Spec. 2010;72(1):38-43.
34. Woodworth BA, Chiu AG, Cohen NA, et al. Real-time computed tomography image update for endoscopic skull base surgery. J Laryngol Otol. 2008;122(4):361-5.
35. Chennupati SK, Woodworth BA, Palmer JN, et al. Intraoperative IGS/CT updates for complex endoscopic frontal sinus surgery. ORL J Otorhinolaryngol Relat Spec. 2008; 70(4):268-70.

CHAPTER 28

Endoscopic Approaches to the Pterygopalatine and Infratemporal Fossa

James D Phillips, Bradford A Woodworth

BACKGROUND OF SURGICAL INTERVENTION AT THE ANTERIOR LATERAL SKULL BASE

Because of the deep anatomic location and neurovascular structures, traditional open surgical access to lateral skull base lesions has a high chance of morbidity for patients. These lesions extend lateral to the plane of the medial maxillary wall (including the maxillary antrum, the pterygopalatine fossa (PPF) and pterygoid plates, the infratemporal fossa (ITF), and the lateral third of the clivus to the petroclival junction),[1] and were historically considered inoperable. In the 1980s, Fisch et al.[2,3] challenged this notion and developed open techniques to approach the lateral skull base. Later surgeons expanded upon these techniques in an attempt to streamline the approach with additional maneuvers such as orbitozygomatic osteotomies[4] and small temporal craniectomies or craniotomies.[5]

As transnasal endoscopic sinus surgery broadened in scope and popularity, surgeons explored this approach to the lateral skull base in search of better visualization while avoiding external scars or bony deformities.[6,7] Maneuvers such as the contralateral transseptal approach,[8] extended maxillotomy, and/or partial resection of the pyriform aperture[1] were developed to augment the ability of rigid telescopes to visualize lateral areas normally limited by the bony anatomy of the nasal skeleton. This improved access for three or four-handed techniques between two surgeons to optimize the dissection.

PERTINENT ANATOMY AND TYPICAL LESIONS

Posterior to the maxillary sinus, below the middle cranial fossa, and medial to the mandible, the pterygopalatine and ITF represent complex anatomy with major neurovascular conduits from the cranium to the face and the distal body. The ITF contains the parapharyngeal and masticator spaces.[9] Traditionally, the stylopharyngeal aponeurosis has separated the parapharyngeal space into pre- and poststyloid units, with the prestyloid compartment containing primarily the fat between the medial pterygoid and tensor veli palatini muscles and the poststyloid containing more neurovascular structures. These include the internal carotid artery (ICA), the internal jugular vein, and cranial nerves IX–XII. The masticator space contains the muscles of mastication as well as palatal musculature, the tensor veli palatini and the levator veli palatini. The internal maxillary artery (IMA), third branch of the trigeminal nerve (V3), and the eustachian tube also pass through this space.

The PPF is generally described as an inverted pyramidal space defined by the pterygoid plates posteriorly, the ascending process of the palatine bone anteromedially, and the posterior wall of the maxillary sinus antrum anterolaterally.[10] The pterygomaxillary fissure lies laterally and connects the PPF to the ITF. Its neurovascular contents include the continuation of the IMA and its terminal branches, the second branch of the trigeminal nerve (V2), and the sphenopalatine ganglion. Primary tumors of the PPF are primarily vascular (juvenile nasopharyngeal angiofibromas) or neurogenic (e.g., Schwannoma) in origin. However, the PPF must be transversed to gain access to the pterygoid recess of the sphenoid sinus where spontaneous encephaloceles are common (Figs. 28.1A and B) and for exposure of the foramen rotundum or foramen ovale.[11]

The ITF may contain the breadth of skull base lesions. These include benign lesions of intracranial origin such as meningiomas, schwannomas, and craniopharyngiomas as well as those of extracranial origin such as angiofibromas, inverted papillomas, and cholesteatomas.[12-15] Additional considerations are masses of primary basicranial origin such as encephaloceles with or without concomitant

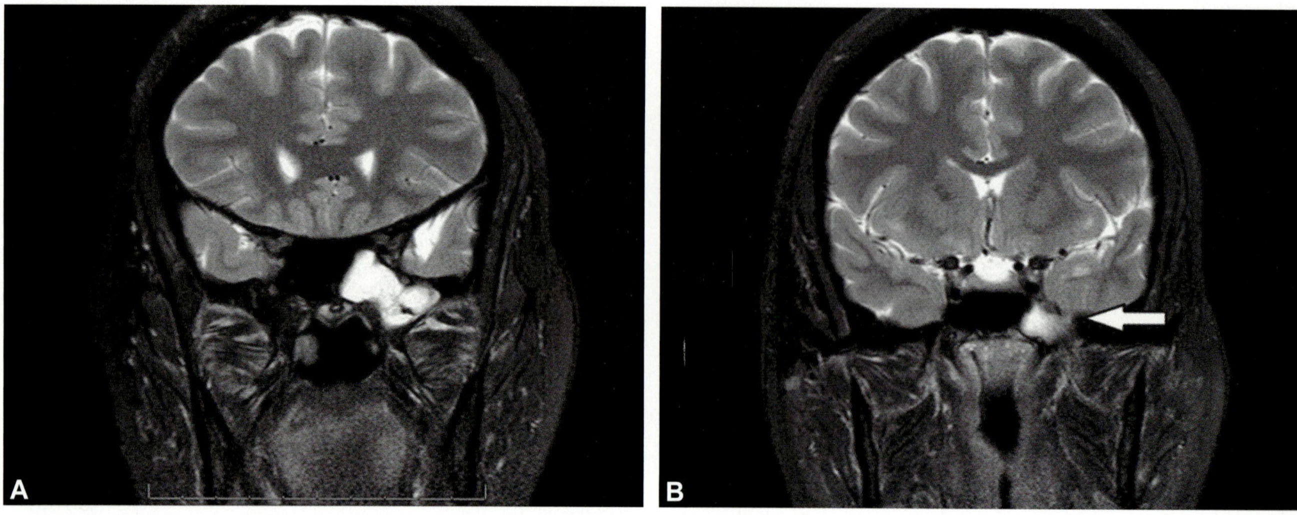

Figs. 28.1A and B: Coronal sections of a T2 weighted MRI shows CSF density in the left sphenoid sinus (left) then an encephalocele arising from the temporal lobe (right—arrow) that is herniating into the lateral pterygoid recess.

cerebrospinal fluid (CSF) leaks, fibrous dysplasia, dermoids, and chordomas.[16-21] Malignant lesions may also present at the lateral skull base. These include malignancies of salivary gland origin, lymphomas, undifferentiated carcinoma, esthesioneuroblastoma, and distant metastases from the lung, breast, or prostate.[22,23] Radiographic evaluation with computed tomography, magnetic resonance imaging (MRI), and angiography (select cases) are invaluable for determining likely pathology and operative planning.

SURGICAL TECHNIQUES

Step 1

Preoperative considerations include orotracheal intubation, nasal decongestion, and possible lumbar puncture ± lumbar drain–either for determination of intracranial pressure or the injection of fluorescein for the localization of CSF leaks.[16,24] Angiography with embolization may be necessary for juvenile nasopharyngeal angiofibromas or other extremely vascular lesions.[15] The implementation of radiographic intraoperative navigation is paramount and well supported by the literature for advanced endonasal skull base procedures.[25-27] The patient is positioned supine on the surgical table and may be placed in slight reverse-Trendelenburg to assist with intraoperative bleeding.

Step 2

Using rigid 0° and angled endoscopes, the surgeon performs a standard functional endoscopic sinus surgery including a wide maxillary antrostomy to the posterior wall, complete ethmoidectomy, sphenoidotomy, and skeletonization of the skull base.

Step 3

With the posterior wall of the maxillary sinus exposed, the mucosa is elevated. The sphenopalatine neurovascular bundle may be identified and dissected in a medial to lateral direction.

Step 4

The bone of the posterior wall of the maxillary sinus is removed with an endoscopic drill, Kerrison punches, and curettes (Figs. 28.2 and 28.3). Switching to angled endoscopy (30° or 45°) is recommended if not using a transseptal approach.

Step 5

The pterygopalatine fascia is incised (Fig. 28.4) and blunt dissection is carefully performed through the adipose tissue of this space until the IMA and neural structures are defined (Fig. 28.5).

Step 6

Posterior to the vascular branches of the IMA, the neural structures of the vidian and infraorbital nerves as well as the sphenopalatine ganglion are preserved (Fig. 28.5). The infraorbital nerve may be followed from its branch point from V2 at the foramen rotundum coursing towards the infraorbital fissure and pterygomaxillary fissure, defining the border between the PPF and the ITF.

Step 7

Dissection at this point is dictated by the ultimate area of concern. The IMA is ligated as necessary for exposure (Fig. 28.6). The anterior aspect of the pterygoid plates may be identified and resected to enter into the lateral

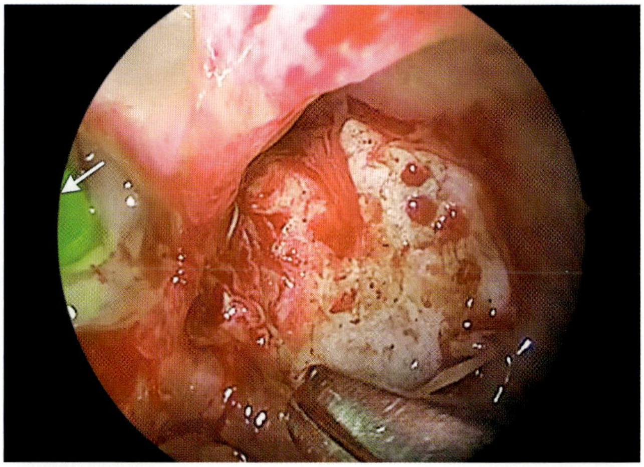

Fig. 28.2: Visualization of the posterior maxillary wall after wide left maxillary antrostomy and sphenoidotomy with a 30° endoscope. The posterior maxillary mucosa is removed. Green fluorescein staining of the cerebrospinal fluid from intrathecal injection is noted emanating from the sphenoid sinus (arrow).

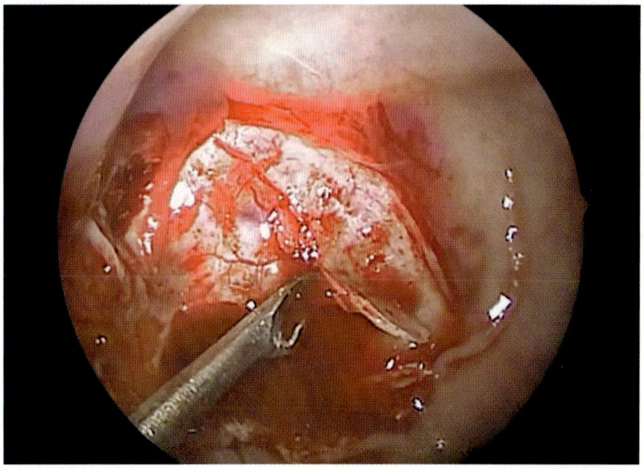

Fig. 28.3: The posterior wall of the maxillary sinus is rarefied with an endoscopic diamond bur drill followed by removal with a curette.

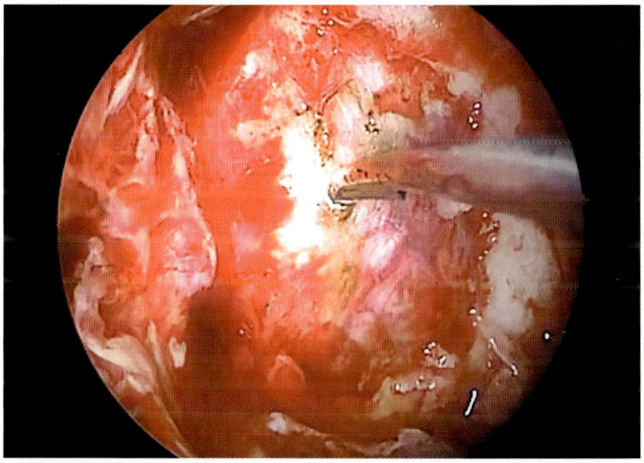

Fig. 28.4: After the bone is removed, the pterygopalatine fascia is incised with a sickle knife.

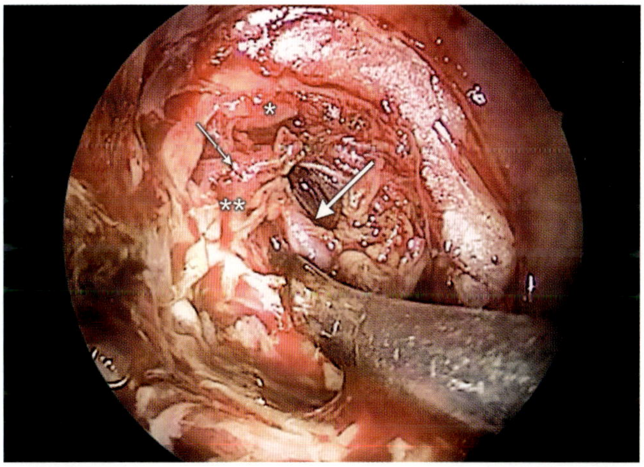

Fig. 28.5: The adipose tissue of the pterygopalatine fossa is bluntly dissected away to expose the neurovascular structures (large arrow, internal maxillary artery; small arrow, pterygopalatine ganglion with branches to infraorbital nerve* and descending palatine nerve**).

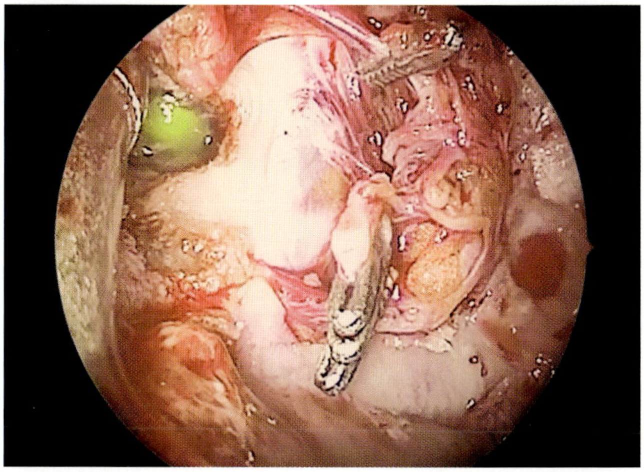

Fig. 28.6: The internal maxillary artery is clipped and divided.

sphenoid recess (Figs. 28.7 and 28.8). Alternatively, the lateral pterygoid plate may be separated from its muscular attachments to expose the ITF.

ADDITIONAL CONSIDERATIONS

High Flow Vascular Injury

One of the most feared complications of this approach is injury to the ICA, which can lead to rapid exsanguination or cerebral ischemia for the patient. Though occurring infrequently (incidence of 0.5–1.1%),[28] the consequences can be catastrophic. A keen understanding of skull base anatomy and close correlation with intraoperative image

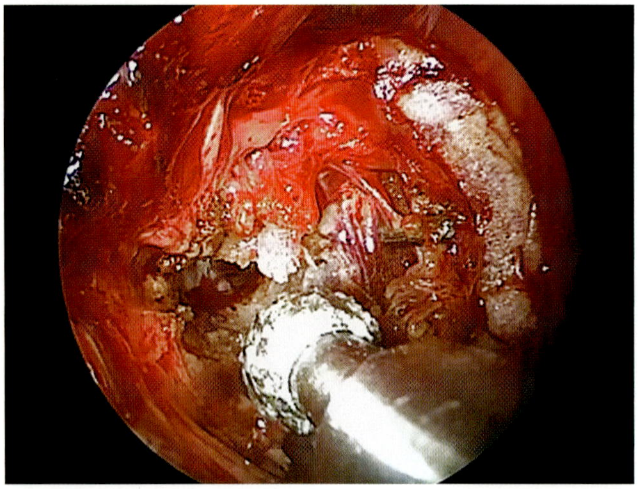

Fig. 28.7: The anterior aspect of the pterygoid plates are resected with an endoscopic diamond bur.

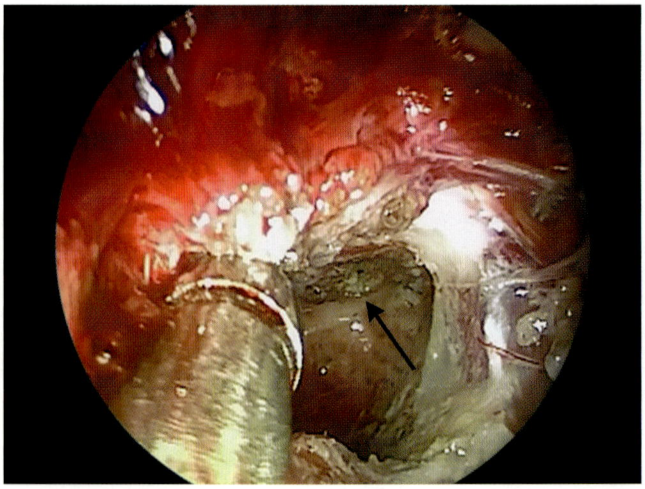

Fig. 28.8: The lateral pterygoid recess of the sphenoid sinus is exposed to gain access to the encephalocele (arrow).

guidance is paramount to anticipating and avoiding this structure. However, every skull base surgeon must familiarize themselves with the maneuvers required to gain control of such a vascular injury. Valentine and Wormald[29] used an animal simulation to delineate important steps in achieving control as quickly as possible. First, the surgical field must be controlled before the injury can be addressed. Maneuvers used to achieve this included the use of a two surgeon team, a large bore (at least 12 French) suction to keep up with the rate of bleeding, an endoscopic lens cleaning system, and placing the suction in the contralateral nare to use the posterior septum as a shield from the vascular flow. The vessel may then be clamped and sutured.

SKULL BASE DEFECT REPAIR

Whether an approach to the PPF and ITF is initiated because of an encephalocele and CSF leak or a defect is created iatrogenically from the resection of a neoplasm, the skull base surgeon must be facile with reconstruction of the skull base. This is often accomplished in a multi-layered fashion, utilizing a combination of septal bone, a tissue inlay graft such as Biodesign® (Cook Medical, Bloomington, IN) or fascia, and an overlay fascia/mucosal graft.[16] Pedicled mucosal flaps, typically obtained from the nasal septum, have been found to have a higher rate of success than free mucosal grafts in preventing recurrent CSF leak for large high flow CSF leaks from tumor resection.[30,31] Postoperatively, patients undergoing these types of extensive skull base procedures are predisposed to developing significant headache related to the low pressure of CSF. There is some evidence to suggest that replacement of some of this volume may improve the frequency of these symptoms.[32]

REFERENCES

1. El-Sayed I, Pletcher S, Russell M, et al. Endoscopic anterior maxillotomy: infratemporal fossa via transnasal approach. Laryngoscope. 2011;121:694-8.
2. Fisch U, Fagan P, Valavanis A. The infratemporal fossa approach for the lateral skull base. Otolaryngol Clin. North Am. 1984;17:513-52.
3. Fisch U, Mattox D. Microsurgery of the skull base. Stuttgart; New York: Thieme; 1988.
4. Mansour OI, Carrau RL, Snyderman CH, et al. Preauricular infratemporal fossa surgical approach: modifications of the technique and surgical indications. Skull Base. 2004; 14:143-51; discussion 151.
5. Hwang SW, Rahal JP, Wein RO, et al. Temporal craniotomy for surgical access to the infratemporal fossa. Skull Base. 2010; 20:93-9.
6. Kassam AB, Gardner P, Snyderman C, et al. Expanded endonasal approach: fully endoscopic, completely transnasal approach to the middle third of the clivus, petrous bone, middle cranial fossa, and infratemporal fossa. Neurosurg Focus. 2005;19:E6.
7. Prosser JD, Figueroa R, Carrau RI, et al. Quantitative analysis of endoscopic endonasal approaches to the infratemporal fossa. Laryngoscope. 2011;121:1601-5.
8. Harvey RJ, Sheehan PO, Debnath NI, et al. Transseptal approach for extended endoscopic resections of the maxilla and infratemporal fossa. Am J Rhinol Allergy. 2009;23:426-32.
9. Falcon RT, Rivera-Serrano CM, Miranda JF, et al. Endoscopic endonasal dissection of the infratemporal fossa: Anatomic relationships and importance of eustachian tube in the endoscopic skull base surgery. Laryngoscope. 2011;121: 31-41.

10. Fortes FS, Sennes LU, Carrau RL, et al. Endoscopic anatomy of the pterygopalatine fossa and the transpterygoid approach: development of a surgical instruction model. Laryngoscope. 2008;118:44-9.
11. Chaaban MR, Illing E, Riley KO, et al. Spontaneous cerebrospinal fluid leak repair: A five-year prospective evaluation. Laryngoscope. 2013;124:70-5.
12. Fisch U. Infratemporal fossa approach to tumours of the temporal bone and base of the skull. J Laryngol Otol. 1978; 92:949-67.
13. Borghei P, Baradaranfar MH, Borghei SH, et al. Transnasal endoscopic resection of juvenile nasopharyngeal angiofibroma without preoperative embolization. Ear Nose Throat J. 2006;85:740-3, 746.
14. Wassef SN, Batra PS, Barnett S. Skull base inverted papilloma: a comprehensive review. ISRN Surg. 2012;2012: 175903.
15. Blount A, Riley KO, Woodworth BA. Juvenile nasopharyngeal angiofibroma. Otolaryngol Clin North Am. 2011;44:989-1004, ix.
16. Alexander NS, Chaaban MR, Riley KO, et al. Treatment strategies for lateral sphenoid sinus recess cerebrospinal fluid leaks. Arch Otolaryngol Head Neck Surg. 2012;138: 471-8.
17. Selmani Z, Aitasalo K, Ashammakhi N. Fibrous dysplasia of the sphenoid sinus and skull base presents in an adult with localized temporal headache. J Craniofac Surg. 2004; 15:261-3.
18. Rossiello R, Ferrara G, Varricchio A, et al. Chondroid chordoma of the lateral skull base. ORL J Otorhinolaryngol Relat Spec. 2001;63:114-8.
19. Wang X, Yu Y, Zhang X, et al. Unusual imaging appearance of a huge intracranial dermoid cyst located across the anterior and middle skull base. J Neurolog Surg Part A Cent Eur Neurosurg. 2013;74:e185-7.
20. Smith N, Riley KO, Woodworth BA. Endoscopic Coblator-assisted management of encephaloceles. Laryngoscope. 2010;120:2535-9.
21. Woodworth BA, Palmer JN. Spontaneous cerebrospinal fluid leaks. Curr Opin Otolaryngol Head Neck Surg. 2009; 17:59-65.
22. Hendryk S, Czecior E, Misiolek M, et al. Surgical strategies in the removal of malignant tumors and benign lesions of the anterior skull base. Neurosurg . 2004;27:205-13.
23. Abdel Razek A, Mossad A, Ghonim M. Role of diffusion-weighted MR imaging in assessing malignant versus benign skull-base lesions. La Radiologia Medica 2011;116:125-32.
24. Chaaban MR, Illing E, Riley KO, et al. Acetazolamide for high intracranial pressure cerebrospinal fluid leaks. Int Forum Allergy Rhinol. 2013.
25. Hosseini SM, Razfar A, Carrau RL, et al. Endonasal transpterygoid approach to the infratemporal fossa: correlation of endoscopic and multiplanar CT anatomy. Head Neck. 2012;34:313-20.
26. Wasserzug O, Margalit N, Weizman N, et al. Utility of a three-dimensional endoscopic system in skull base surgery. Skull Base. 2010;20:223-8.
27. Farhadi M, Jalessi M, Sharifi G, et al. Use of image guidance in endoscopic endonasal surgeries: a 5-year experience. B-ENT. 2011;7:277-82.
28. Berker M, Aghayev K, Saatci I, et al. Overview of vascular complications of pituitary surgery with special emphasis on unexpected abnormality. Pituitary. 2010;13:160-7.
29. Valentine R, Wormald PJ. Controlling the surgical field during a large endoscopic vascular injury. Laryngoscope. 2011;121:562-6.
30. Chaaban MR, Chaudhry A, Riley KO, et al. Simultaneous pericranial and nasoseptal flap reconstruction of anterior skull base defects following endoscopic-assisted craniofacial resection. Laryngoscope. 2013;123:2383-6.
31. Harvey RJ, Parmar P, Sacks R, et al. Endoscopic skull base reconstruction of large dural defects: a systematic review of published evidence. Laryngoscope. 2012;122:452-9.
32. Blount A, Riley K, Cure J, et al. Cerebrospinal fluid volume replacement following large endoscopic anterior cranial base resection. Int Forum Allergy Rhinol. 2012;2:217-21

CHAPTER

29

Endoscopic Nasopharyngectomy

Ning-Wei Li, Nilesh A Vyas, Ameet Singh

INTRODUCTION

Benign and malignant lesions of the nasopharynx are uncommon tumors of the head and neck. Benign lesions, which occur most frequently in children and adolescents, include hemangiomas, angiofibromas, and minor salivary gland tumors. The most common malignant tumor of the nasopharynx is squamous cell carcinoma (SCC), which has an incidence of one in 100,000 in the general population. This epithelial malignancy has a distinct racial and geographic predilection, with its highest prevalence (over 20 times higher) in Inuit Indians, and Cantonese Chinese in Southern China and Southeast Asia.[1,2] Other rarer nasopharyngeal malignancies include lymphomas, sarcomas, melanomas, and salivary gland malignancies. Given the predominance of nasopharyngeal carcinoma (NPC) among tumors of the nasopharynx, this chapter will focus on the endoscopic management of NPC of the nasopharynx.

BRIEF ANATOMY OF THE NASOPHARYNX

The nasopharynx is an anatomical space located posterior to the nasal cavity, which lies superior to the pharyngeal isthmus/soft palate and inferior to the basisphenoid/upper clivus. The superior pharyngeal constrictor muscles and pharyngobasilar fascia define the nasopharyngeal space borders laterally and posteriorly. The pharyngobasilar fascia (a thick neck fascia) originates from the pharyngeal tubercle of the occipital bone and attaches to the medial pterygoid plates anteriorly. This fascia holds the superior pharyngeal constrictors to the skull base. The medial pterygoid plates also serve as the anatomic anterolateral border of the nasopharynx.

The auditory tube orifices lie posterior and lateral to the posterior nasal choanae. The eustachian tube orifices are surrounded by cartilage that produces a curvilinear elevation known as the torus tubarius. From the posterior aspect of the torus tubarius arises the salpingopharyngeal fold that contains the salpingopharyngeus muscle. This muscle originates from the cartilaginous torus tubarius and blends with the palatopharyngeus muscle. Posterior to the salpingopharyngeal fold is a longitudinal depression called the pharyngeal recess, or fossa of Rosenmüller. This fossa usually marks the origin of NPC. Inferior to the torus tubarius is another fold named the torus levatorius, formed by the levator veli palatini muscle. The adenoid pad, a conglomeration of lymphoid tissue, also occupies the posterior and superior portion of the nasopharynx.

STAGING OF NPC

Nasopharyngeal carcinoma was classified by the World Health Organization in 1978 into keratinizing SCC (Type I), nonkeratinizing SCC (Type II), and nonkeratinizing undifferentiated carcinoma (Type III). The classification was revised in 1991 when Types I, II, and III were changed to Type 1, 2a, and 2b. In addition, basaloid SCC was added as a subtype. Type 2b NPC is associated with Epstein-Barr virus, whereas Types 1 and 2a have been associated with alcohol and tobacco use. NPC is known for having a high rate of bilateral regional (lymph node) and distant metastasis.[2]

In a paper by Chen et al., patients with NPC were categorized as follows: recurrent rT1 tumors had tumor involvement of the nasopharyngeal cavity; rT2a patients had tumors extending to the nasal septum; rT2b patients had tumors involving the superficial parapharyngeal space; and rT3 patients had tumors involving the base of the sphenoid sinus.[1,3]

TREATMENT OF NPC

Primary Treatment

Nasopharyngeal carcinoma is a highly radiosensitive tumor and therefore radiation therapy is the primary treatment modality for newly diagnosed tumors. Current radiotherapy techniques can achieve a 5-year 72% local control rate.[2,4] Concurrent chemotherapy has shown an overall survival advantage for locoregionally advanced NPC. Combined modality treatment (radiation and chemotherapy) has resulted in 5-year local control rates of 76–91%.[1] Early disease (Stages I and II) is usually treated with radiation therapy, whereas advanced disease (Stages III and IV) is treated with concomitant chemoradiation. Surgery for primary NPC tumors has been limited to residual or persistent local disease or recurrent regional tumor after primary radiation ± chemotherapy.[5-8] However, surgery may serve a primary role for tumors with glandular or mesenchymal differentiation such as adenocarcinomas, adenoid cystic carcinomas, or sarcomas.[9,10]

Treatment for Recurrence or Residual Tumor

Recurrence rates after radiotherapy (or chemoradiation) vary from 9% to 56% based on initial tumor stage.[4,11] Treatment for recurrent or residual NPC after primary treatment includes reirradiation with external beam or brachytherapy, and/or surgery. Locoregional recurrences without distant metastasis may be salvaged and should be treated aggressively. Although reirradiation can result in a 5-year survival rate of 8–36%, it carries the risk of significant morbidity, which includes cranial nerve dysfunction, osteoradionecrosis, skull base fibrosis, and brain necrosis.[4,12,13] Late complications from reirradiation have been documented in 26–57% of patients.[1] Open nasopharyngectomy has been able to achieve similar 5-year local control rates of 40–50%.[2,7] However, surgery has also been associated with technical difficulties, morbidity and suboptimal oncologic outcomes. For example, King et al.[7] reported a 29% positive margin rate using multiple open approaches.

Traditionally, nasopharyngectomy was performed via techniques such as transpalatal, transmaxillary, midline mandibulectomy, transpterygoid, mid-facial degloving, craniofacial disassembly, facial translocation, and infratemporal approaches. Complications include palatal defects, trismus, facial scarring, dental malocclusions, facial/glossal numbness, chronic otitis media, velopharyngeal insufficiency, dysphagia, and osteomyelitis.[4]

ENDOSCOPIC NASOPHARYNGECTOMY

Traditionally, minimally invasive approaches to the nasopharynx have been limited due to poor accessibility. Advances in endoscopic instrumentation, techniques, and experience with endoscopic tumor surgery have led to the development of specific techniques for endoscopic nasopharyngectomy. Endoscopic surgery offers panoramic views, and excellent magnification thereby eliminating the morbidity of open approaches. Advantages of endoscopic approaches include improved visualization of tumor margins, elimination of facial deformity, and preservation of neurovascular function.

The oncologic principles of endoscopic nasopharyngectomy remain the same, namely complete tumor resection with negative surgical margins. Attaining these negative surgical margins is a key independent predictor of success for all sinonasal malignancies, including nasopharyngeal tumors (Figs. 29.1A and B). The challenge

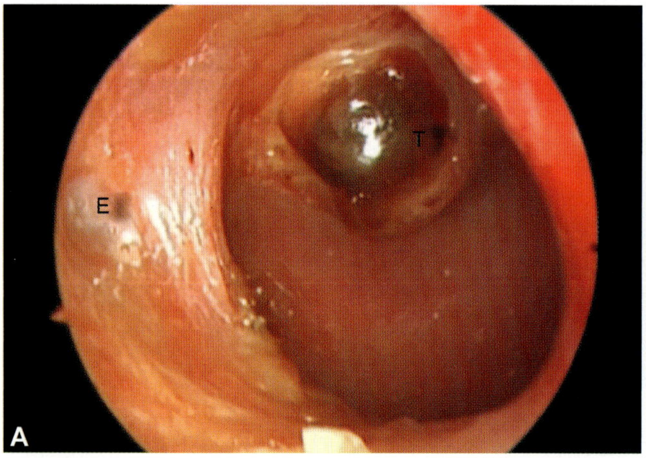

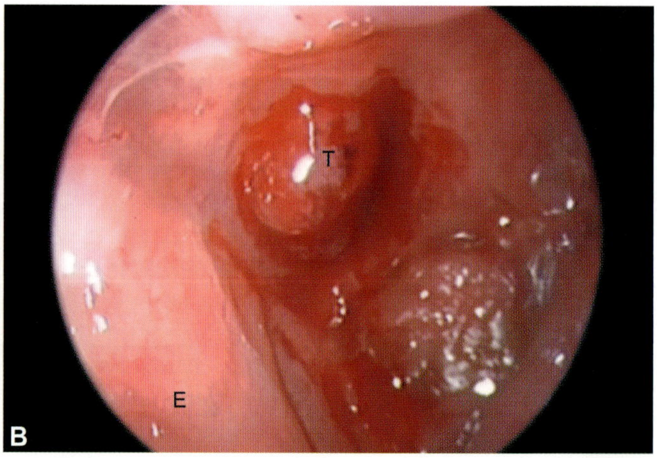

Figs. 29.1A and B: (A) Midline recurrent nasopharyngeal (rT1) tumor. For this tumor, surgical margins of 0.5–1.0 cm can be obtained with a Type I approach. (B) Tumor in right lateral wall of nasopharynx. For this tumor, attaining surgical margins of 0.5–1.0 cm may require a Type II or III approach. (T: Tumor; E: Eustachian tube).

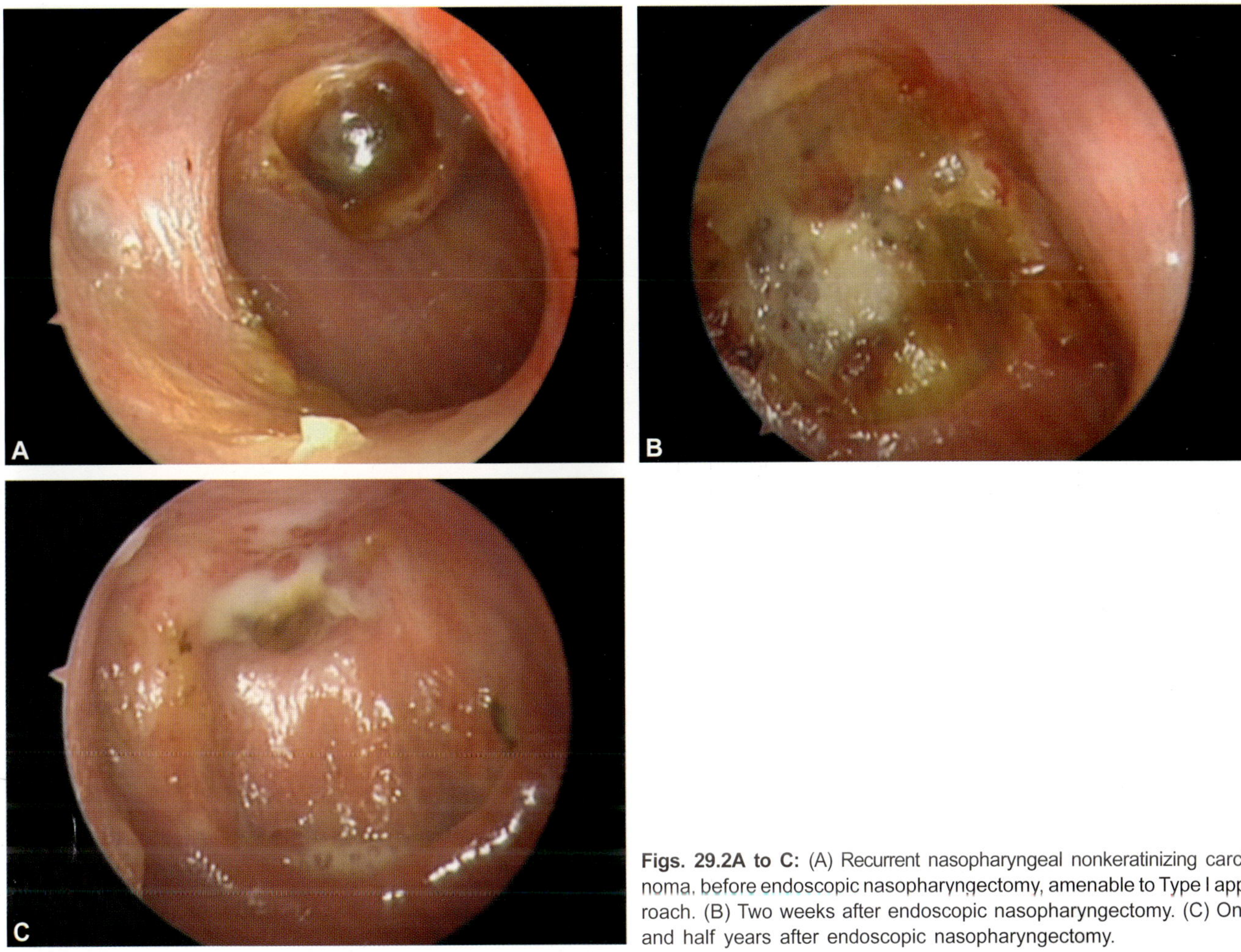

Figs. 29.2A to C: (A) Recurrent nasopharyngeal nonkeratinizing carcinoma, before endoscopic nasopharyngectomy, amenable to Type I approach. (B) Two weeks after endoscopic nasopharyngectomy. (C) One and half years after endoscopic nasopharyngectomy.

with endoscopic approaches, akin to open approaches, is that the surgeon's ability to obtain negative margins is often limited by the proximity of critical vital structures. Endoscopic approaches do, however, offer a minimally invasive exposure with excellent visualization of nasopharyngeal anatomy. This allows for the ability to attain negative margins while preserving function of uninvolved structures.

Approaches

Three modulated endoscopic approaches (Types I, II, and III) to the nasopharynx have been described by Castelnuovo et al.[14] Type I resection involves horizontal incisions along the posterior border of the torus tubarius (preserving the eustachian tube), a superior incision at the level of the atlas, and deep dissection to the ventral clivus. This approach is suitable for small tumors located centrally in the nasopharynx (Figs. 29.2A to C). The type II extirpation also entails exposure of the sphenoid sinuses and resection of the floor of the sphenoid to the clivus. Tumors extending to the roof of the nasopharynx are most suitable for a type II approach. Type III represents the most extensive removal of the nasopharynx which includes resection of the lateral nasopharyngeal wall to the parapharyngeal space, cartilaginous portion of the ET (Figs. 29.3A to C). A type III approach also requires a medial maxillectomy, pterygopalatine fossa dissection, and removal of the medial pterygoid plate. Given that the pharyngeal ICA is just posterior to the bony portion of the ET, a type III approach represents the highest risk of all three modulated approaches for catastrophic vascular injury.[14]

A more extensive endoscopic endonasal transpterygoid approach has also been described by Al-Sheibani et al.[9] where a medial maxillectomy aided by a Denker approach (removal of the anterior maxillary buttress, accessed just posterior to the nasal vestibule) is followed

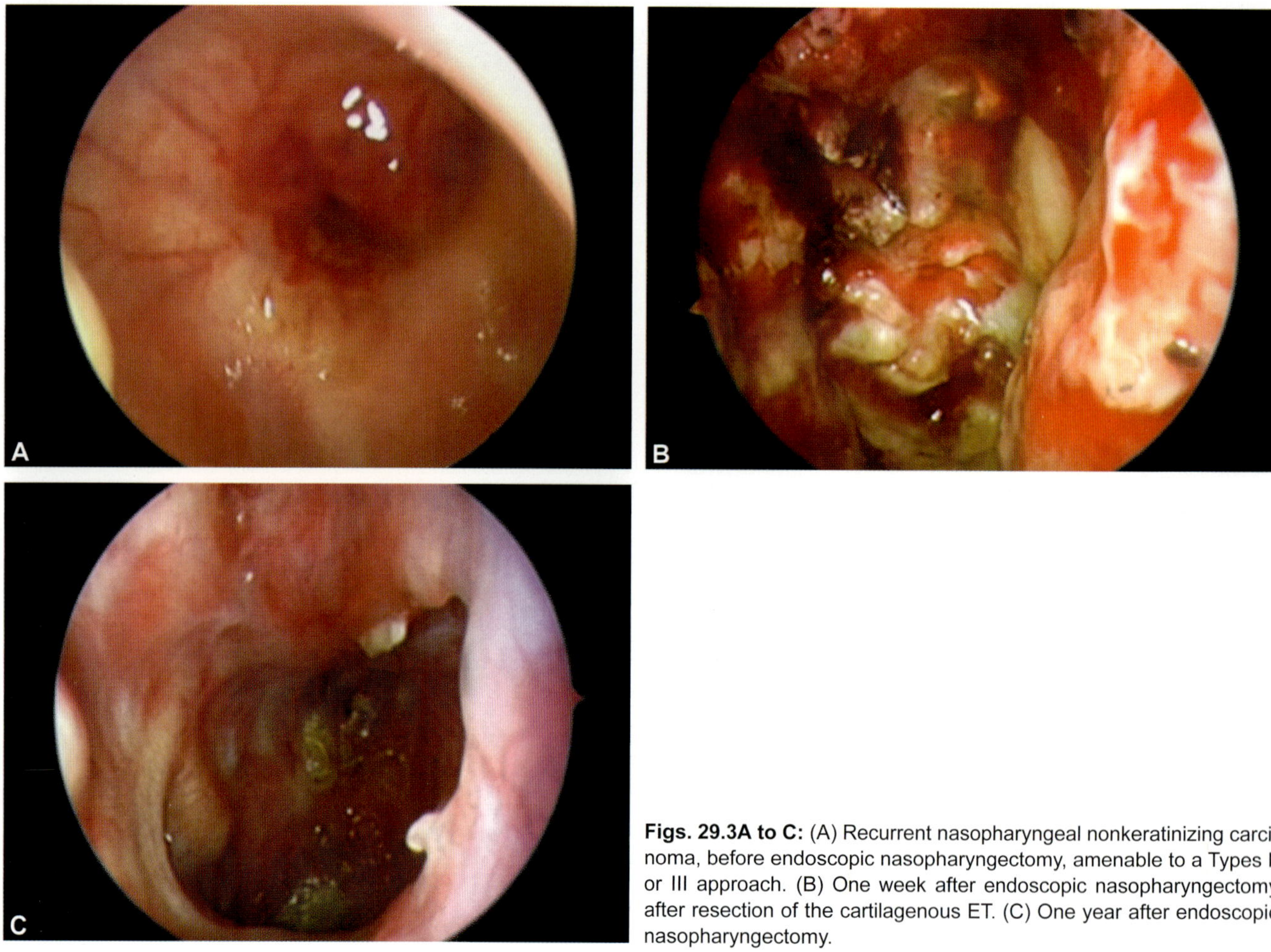

Figs. 29.3A to C: (A) Recurrent nasopharyngeal nonkeratinizing carcinoma, before endoscopic nasopharyngectomy, amenable to a Types II or III approach. (B) One week after endoscopic nasopharyngectomy after resection of the cartilagenous ET. (C) One year after endoscopic nasopharyngectomy.

by lateral mobilization of the pterygopalatine fossa. This allows the surgeon to resect the pterygoid process, and cartilagenous ET as well as to remove any tumor extending into the parapharyngeal or infratemporal fossa. This approach also allows for exposure and control of the parapharyngeal and petrous portions of the internal carotid artery. If involved with tumor, the ICA may be resected endoscopically if the artery is sacrificed preoperatively. Alternatively, an open approach may be used for this portion of the procedure.[9]

Ideal candidates for endoscopic nasopharyngectomy include benign tumors (e.g., JNA, IP), primary radioresistant tumors (Figs. 29.4A to C), or small recurrent (rT1 or rT2) NPCs without any extension to the ICA, ET, or cranial cavity.[3,13,15-17] Given the availability of more aggressive approaches to the nasopharynx, higher stage tumors with extensive ICA or lateral involvement (parapharyngeal, infratemporal fossa) now carry relative contraindications for an endoscopic nasopharyngectomy. In our experience, if the distance between the tumor and carotid artery is less than 0.5 cm, negative margins are difficult to obtain. In addition, invasion of the clival, petrous, or lateral sphenoid bone portend a poor prognosis for surgical approaches (Fig. 29.5). There is limited consensus for the ideal treatment (surgery vs. reirradiation) for higher stage (rT3) malignant tumors.[18-24]

PREOPERATIVE EVALUATION OF NPC

Physical Examination

A thorough preoperative evaluation of patients being considered for surgical treatment of residual or recurrent NPC tumor must be performed. A neurologic exam with attention to all the cranial nerves is necessary prior to operative intervention. Endoscopic examination of the sinonasal cavity is performed to document anatomic variations as well as any extension of nasopharyngeal pathology into the sinonasal cavity. Preoperative biopsy

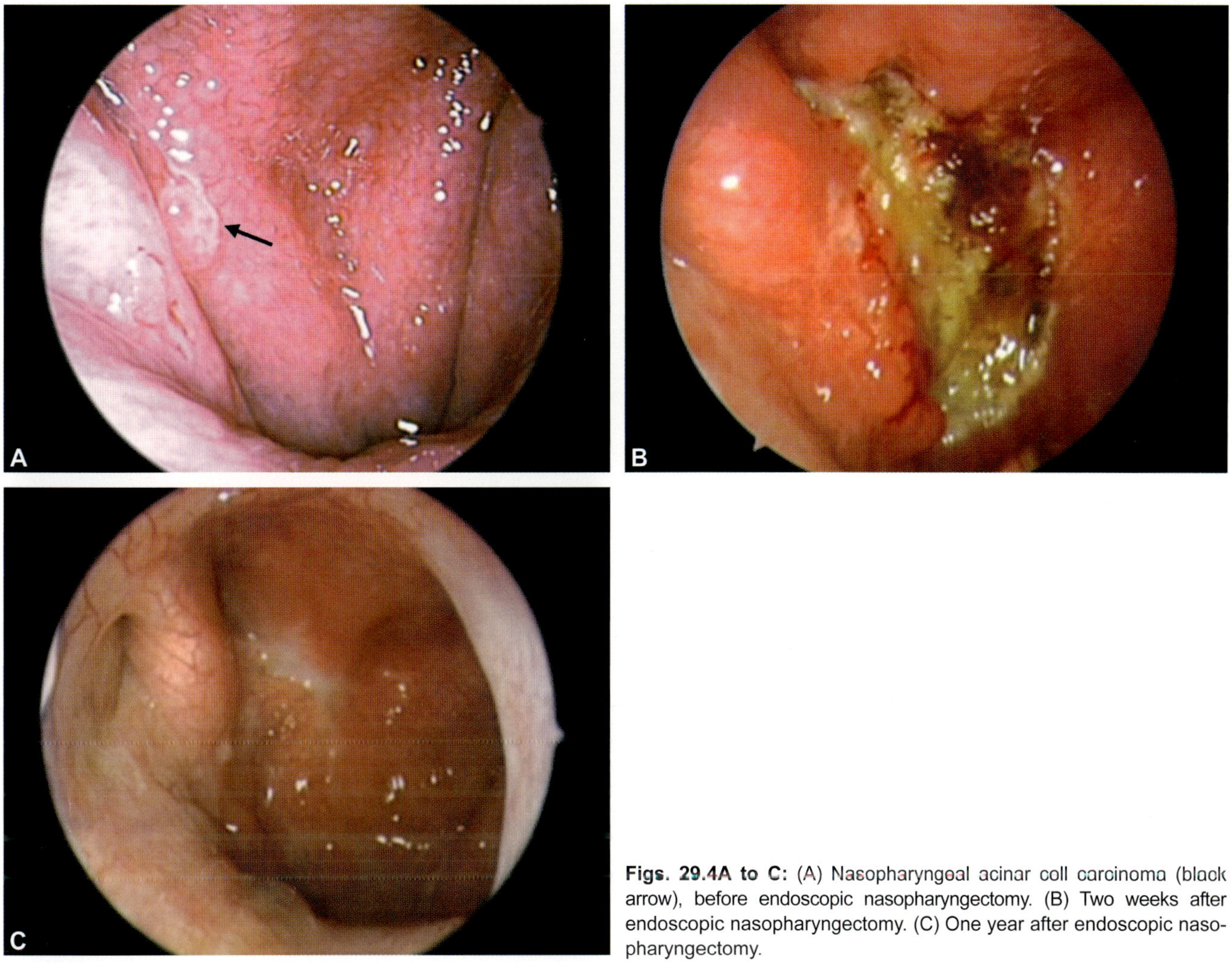

Figs. 29.4A to C: (A) Nasopharyngeal acinar cell carcinoma (black arrow), before endoscopic nasopharyngectomy. (B) Two weeks after endoscopic nasopharyngectomy. (C) One year after endoscopic nasopharyngectomy.

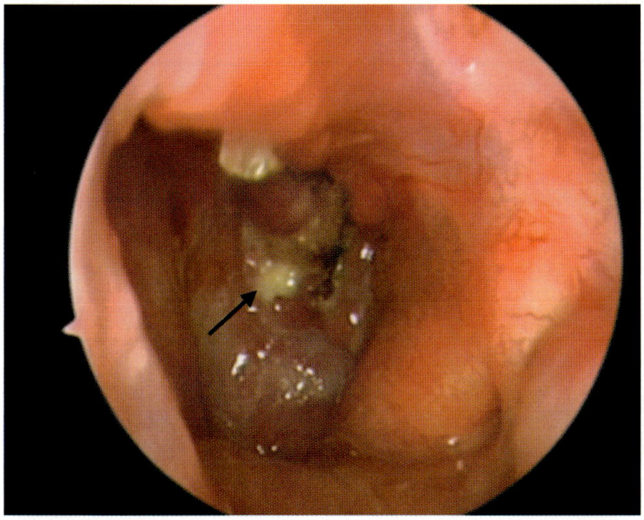

Fig. 29.5: Clival bone involvement (black arrow) with recurrent nasopharyngeal tumor.

of recurrent NPC tumor is not always necessary but should be performed if the diagnosis of residual or recurrent cases is in question.

Imaging

Edema and fibrosis of the nasopharynx after primary radiotherapy may make it difficult for the surgeon to assess the extent of local tumor. PET/CT has been shown to be more sensitive than MRI and CT in detecting recurrent or residual tumor.[1,9] Staging, however, is more accurately performed with CT and MRI. CT allows for the assessment of bony architecture including presence of skull base erosion, and location of the internal carotid arteries (ICA). MRI is important for delineating soft tissue architecture, in particular, differentiating between tumor and inflammation. Imaging (CT and MRI) also aids in performing a complete assessment of regional (cervical lymph node status) and distant metastasis. Detection of metastatic tumor can significantly alter the management strategy for recurrent carcinoma from curative to palliative.

Vascular Assessment

Preoperative assessment of the parapharyngeal and petrous segments of the ICA is critical. We find CT angiography useful for simultaneous visualization of bony and vascular structures, especially for intraoperative navigation.[25] CT angiography is helpful when tumor is involved or abuts the carotid or vertebrobasilar system. Circumferential involvement of the ICA generally precludes an endoscopic approach for NPC. However, if the ICA is sacrificed preoperatively, an endoscopic approach may still be considered. Furthermore, the ICA may be sacrificed only if a patient passes a preoperative balloon occlusion test with neuromonitoring to reduce the risk of a cerebrovascular complication (Figs. 29.6A and B). In contrast, surgical therapy may be modified or abandoned for alternate therapy if the tumor involves the ICA and the patient fails the balloon occlusion test.[26,27] Finally, although dural or minor intracranial involvement does not preclude an endoscopic endonasal approach, patients with extensive intracranial involvement are not candidates for endoscopic resection.

RESULTS OF ENDOSCOPIC NASOPHARYNGECTOMY

Multiple studies have reported favorable results with the use of endoscopic nasopharyngectomy in the treatment of recurrent or residual NPC. An early small series by Chen et al. reported a local control rate of 83.3% in 6 patients (3 rT1, 3 rT2) with a mean follow-up time of 29 months. The extent of resection included the cartilaginous ET.[16] In a larger early series, Ko et al. resected locally recurrent tumor is 28 patients (12 rT1N0, 14 rT2aN0, 2 rT2aN1) with a mean follow-up of 3–48 months. Depending on tumor involvement, the resection involved removal of the cartilaginous ET, fossa of Rosenmüller, and prevertebral muscles as necessary. The 2-year disease free survival rate was 57.6% (100% for rT1, 41.7% for rT2a tumors).[13] In a subsequent large series, Chen et al. reported a local relapse-free survival of 86.3% with a median follow-up of 24 months. Tumors were staged as T1 (n = 17), rT2a (n = 4), rT2b (n = 14), and rT3 (n = 2). None of the patients with rT1 tumors recurred, whereas one of 4 rT2a patients and four of 14 rT2b patients developed local recurrences.[3]

Endoscopic surgical resections with high rates disease-free survival have been reported for all rT1, some rT2a and a few rT2B patients with NPC.[3,13,16] In contrast, disease-free survival rates for endoscopic nasopharyngectomy for most rT2b and nearly all rT3 patients have been suboptimal.[3,13] Most early authors described limitations for endoscopic nasopharyngectomy which included difficulty in resecting larger tumors, especially if there was involvement of the fossa of Rosenmüller, cartilage of the ET, central skull base, or oropharyngeal invasion.[3,12] Other authors excluded patients where carotid artery exposure was expected,[12] or where the tumor involved cranial nerves, brain, or the carotid sheath.[3,17]

Recent authors have reported comparable results to open techniques for advanced stage tumors. Al-Sheibani

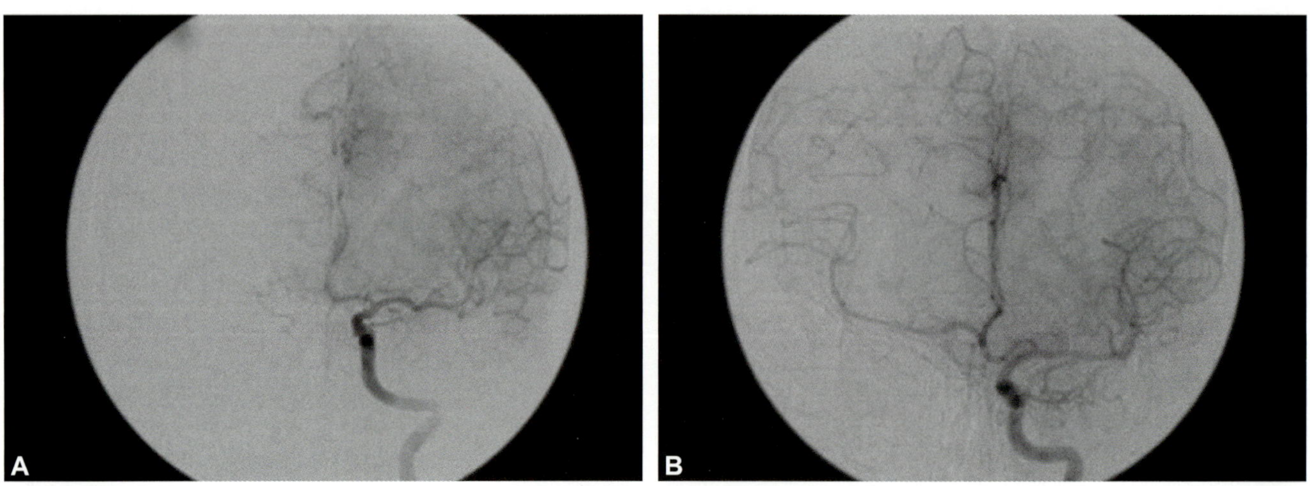

Figs. 29.6A and B: Balloon occlusion test. (A) After occluding the right common carotid artery, the circle of Willis has no communication from the left to right cerebrum. (B) After occluding the right common carotid artery, the circle of Willis has good communication from the left to right cerebrum.

reported an actuarial rate of local control of 65% for advanced stage malignant tumors at a mean follow-up of 33 months.[9]

ENDOSCOPIC TECHNIQUES

Operative Preparation

The patient is orotracheally intubated and preoperative antibiotics, usually a third generation cephalosporin with good CSF penetration (e.g., ceftriaxone) is given. The endotracheal tube is usually taped to the left (for the right-handed surgeon) and 4% cocaine (or 1:20,000 epinephrine) soaked cottonoids are placed in the nasal cavity for decongestion and vasoconstriction. The patient is positioned in a "beach-chair" position, with the bed reflexed, and the legs dropped to decrease tension on the back. The head may be placed in pins (for optical tracking navigation), or on a Mayfield holder (for electromagnetic tracking navigation). Preoperative imaging is reviewed and image guidance registration and verification is performed. The face is prepped in standard fashion. If a large surgical defect or CSF leak is anticipated, the abdomen or thigh is prepped to harvest a fat and/or rectus sheath fascia graft for a multilayered reconstruction.

Nasal Exposure

Nasal endoscopy is initiated and sites of tumor attachment to the septum, middle turbinates, inferior turbinates, nasal floor, sphenoethmoidal recesses, and septal mucosa are examined. The vertical lamella of the middle turbinates, the superior turbinates, superior septum, nasal floor, and columella are injected with a local anesthetic (e.g., 1% lidocaine with 1:100,000 epinephrine) to provide vasoconstriction. If a dural defect with a high-flow cerebrospinal fluid is anticipated, a vascularized nasoseptal flap for secondary skull base closure is harvested (*see* Chapter 30) contralateral to the bulky side of the tumor. The flap is placed in an ipsilateral enlarged maxillary antrostomy window. With large malignant nasopharyngeal tumors, the pedicle of the nasoseptal flap may not be available and an alternate vascularized flap may be necessary.

The inferior and middle turbinates are lateralized to increase the working space. If necessary, the inferior turbinates may be reduced or partially resected to provide improved access to the nasopharynx. Although middle turbinate preservation is preferred, partial or complete resection may be performed to improve access to the nasopharynx. A posterior septectomy as well as drilling the vomer flush with the hard palate is recommended to allow for unfettered access to the nasopharynx (Figs. 29.7A and B). This also allows for a binostril, four-handed approach as necessary.

Tumor Resection

Small rT1 and rT2a tumors require dissection primarily in the nasopharynx. Superior and inferior incisions are made along the basisphenoid and at the level of soft palate, respectively. Lateral incisions are made along the mucosa of the salpingopharyngeal folds incorporating

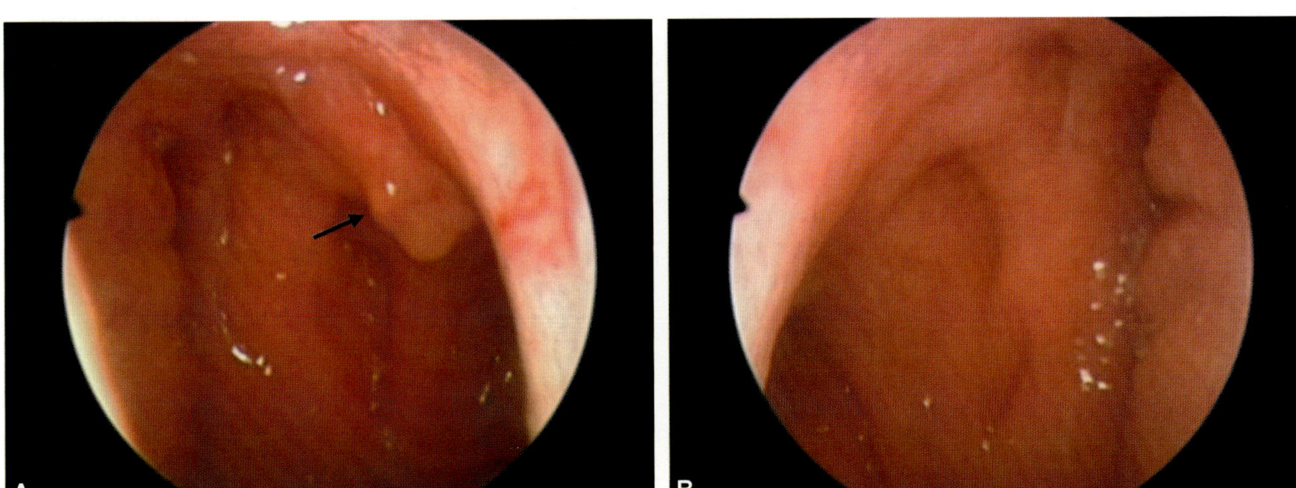

Figs. 29.7A and B: (A) Recurrent nasopharyngeal tumor (black arrow) can be seen clearly though right nasal cavity. (B) Tumor cannot be seen though left nasal cavity. This patient benefited from removal of the posterior nasal septum to obtain good visualization and access to the tumor.

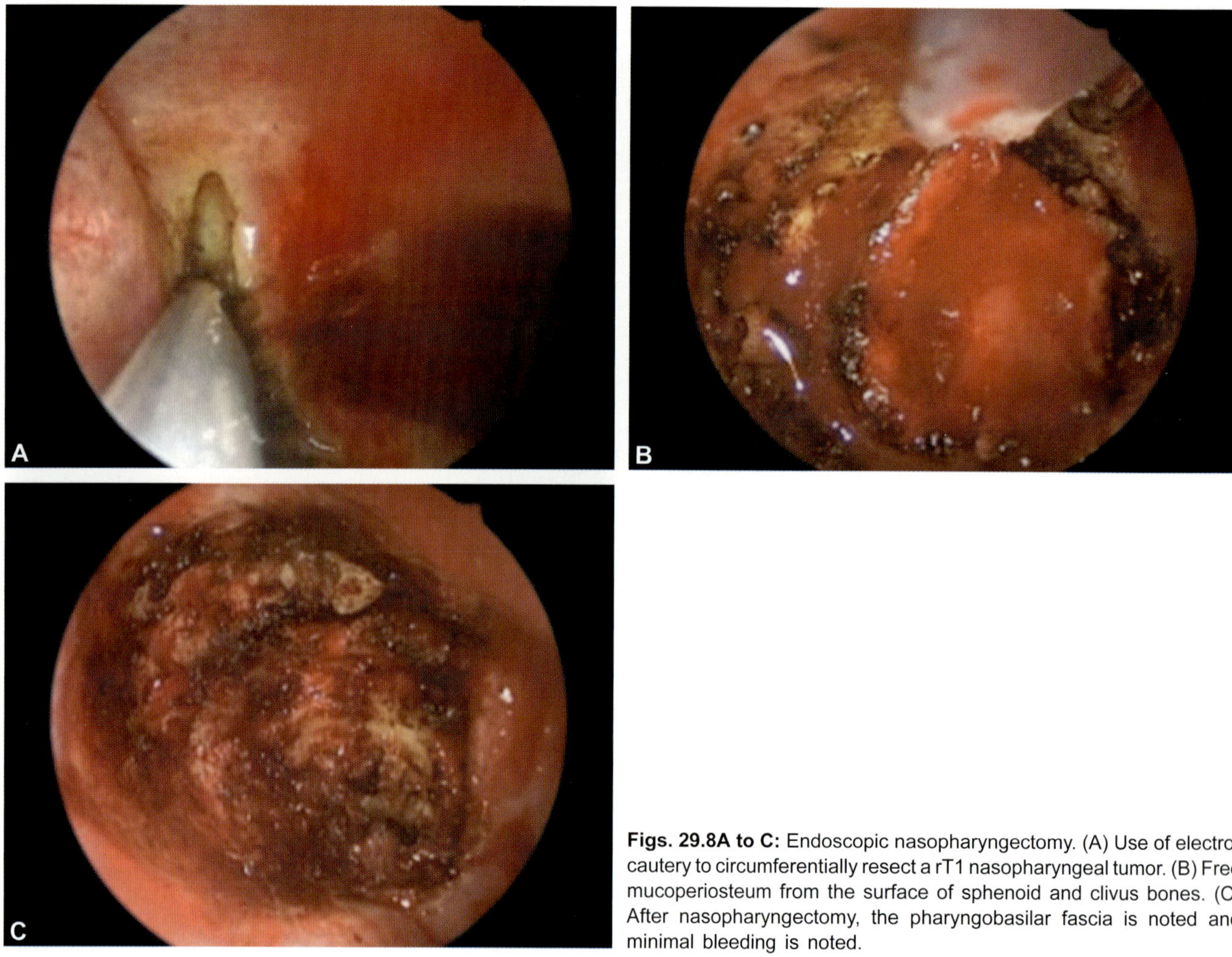

Figs. 29.8A to C: Endoscopic nasopharyngectomy. (A) Use of electrocautery to circumferentially resect a rT1 nasopharyngeal tumor. (B) Free mucoperiosteum from the surface of sphenoid and clivus bones. (C) After nasopharyngectomy, the pharyngobasilar fascia is noted and minimal bleeding is noted.

the superior aspects of the fossae of Rosenmuller (Figs. 29.8A to C). Deep dissection is performed to the level of the pharyngobasilar fascia, longus colli, and capitis muscles.[11] The anatomy of the region is often obscured secondary to previous radiation. For most rT1 and rT2a tumors, the above dissection is all that is required to obtain negative margins. These techniques require instrumentation and equipment similar to that required for endoscopic sinus surgery. Laser, mono- or bipolar cautery, high frequency diathermy, and curved blade harmonic scalpel may be used to resect the tumor. Multiple tissue samples from the superior, inferior, lateral, and central deep margins are obtained for histologic section during the procedure to establish negative margins. Hemostasis may be achieved with mono- or bipolar cautery, and a plethora of hemostatic agents.

Larger rT2 and rT3 tumors require far more exposure and dissection for complete removal. This includes complete ethmoidectomies, wide sphenoidotomies, and complete removal of the sphenoid sinus floor for adequate exposure. In addition, a modified medial maxillectomy, mobilization of ipsilateral or bilateral PPF's, and removal of the medial pterygoid plates may be necessary to accomplish adequate exposure for larger tumors. Exposure of the medial infratemporal fossa as well as infraorbital and pterygomaxillary fissures is also important for more extensive tumors. Additional equipment required for extended dissection include a high-speed drill with a variety of hybrid or coarse diamond burrs, extended length instruments (dissectors, curettes, tru-cutting instruments, Kerrison rongeurs), and micro-Doppler for internal carotid artery mapping. Although not necessary, an ultrasonic aspirator (Sonopet, Stryker) is useful for bony and soft tissue removal, especially for more fibrotic and adherent masses.

Although nasopharyngeal tumors that involve the dura or extend intracranially may be resected endoscopically, great consideration must be given to resect these tumors with open approaches or consider alternate therapy altogether. Intradural tumor extension often requires central debulking after the edges of the tumor are defined. Depending on the texture of lesion, this may be simple suction and curettage, or require more aggressive instrumentation such as a microdebrider or ultrasonic aspirator. Fibrotic and adherent tumors require retraction and sharp dissection with microscissors. Depending on the extent of the tumor, critical attention must be paid to vascular structures, specifically the carotid arteries as well as vasculature of the posterior circulation. Frequent confirmation of anatomic structures with intraoperative navigation and micro-Doppler is necessary to deliver the tumor safely. Additional techniques are described in Chapters 22, 25, and 26.

Reconstruction

Several options exist for addressing nasopharyngeal defects after surgery. If no dura is exposed after completion of the resection, bony edges, and spurs are smoothed out using diamond or rough-diamond burrs on a high speed drill. Extracranial defects may be left alone to close by secondary intention. Disadvantages of secondary intention include longstanding crusting, with poor mucociliary clearance, bacterial stasis, and chronic sinusitis. Reconstruction of a nasopharyngeal defect may also be accomplished with a free mucosa graft, or vascularized pedicled flap. Free mucosal grafts may be harvested from the nasal cavity (e.g., septum, floor) or oral cavity (e.g., buccal). Free mucosal grafts may speed up wound healing. Our preferred option for vascularized flaps is the nasoseptal flap. This may be used for reconstruction of extracranial defects as well as secondary reconstruction of skull base defects with CSF leaks. Other flaps such as inferior turbinate flap, middle turbinate flap,[28] lateral nasal wall flap, palatal flap, temporoparietal flap or endoscopic pericranial flap may also be utilized.[29,30] Vascularized flaps should be especially considered when the ICA is in close proximity or left 'bare' during extended nasopharyngectomy approaches. Reconstruction after intradural tumor resection also requires multilayered prior to a vascularized pedicled flap. A variety of techniques have been used and reported in the literature which include the gasket seal, bilayer button, and acellular dermal collagen matrix reconstruction.

Postoperative Care

Endoscopic nasopharyngectomy allows patients to resume oral intake soon after surgery with no impairment of their swallow function. Patients after extracranial endoscopic nasopharyngectomy with minimal blood loss may be discharged on the first postoperative day, with resumption of oral intake, and full swallowing function. Patients after dural resection with skull base reconstruction are monitored in the intensive care setting for complications such postoperative bleeding or CSF leak.

Complications

The most significant complication after endoscopic nasopharyngectomy is a vascular injury to the carotid artery. In the event of a carotid artery injury, bleeding is controlled with extensive packing. A Foley balloon is routinely kept on the back table in preparation for a catastrophic vascular injury. After control of hemorrhage, angiography is recommended to identify the location of bleeding. The artery may be sacrificed as long as the patient has passed the balloon occlusion test (TBO). Delayed psuedoaneurysms may be treated with endovascular stent grafts (Figs. 29.9A and B).[31-34] Minor complications after endoscopic nasopharyngectomy include otitis media with effusion, followed by headache and nasopharyngeal purulence (Fig. 29.10). Less common complications include sinusitis, aural, neck pain, dysphagia, and epistaxis.[17]

ROBOTIC NASOPHARYNGECTOMY

Recently, feasibility studies for robotic nasopharyngectomy via transoral and transnasal routes have been conducted with encouraging results.[35,36] Case reports detailing transoral or combined transnasal/transoral resection of recurrent NPC have been reported with good results. The authors discussed advantages of robotic nasopharyngectomy which included increased maneuverability and resection of the lateral extent of disease.[37]

CONCLUSION

Endoscopic nasopharyngectomy shows great promise for the treatment of nasopharyngeal tumors. Nearly all authors have noted improved cosmesis, reduced thermal damage, decreased wound infections, fistulae, trismus, and dysphagia compared with open nasopharyngectomy techniques. The maximal benefit appears to be for patients with benign tumors, radioresistant tumor and early stage recurrences (rT1, rT2a) for NPC. Equivocal benefit for endoscopic nasopharyngectomy has been demonstrated for late stage recurrences (rT2b, rT3). Long-term follow-up is necessary to ascertain if endoscopic nasopharyngectomy is comparable or more favorable than open surgical approaches or reirradiation techniques.

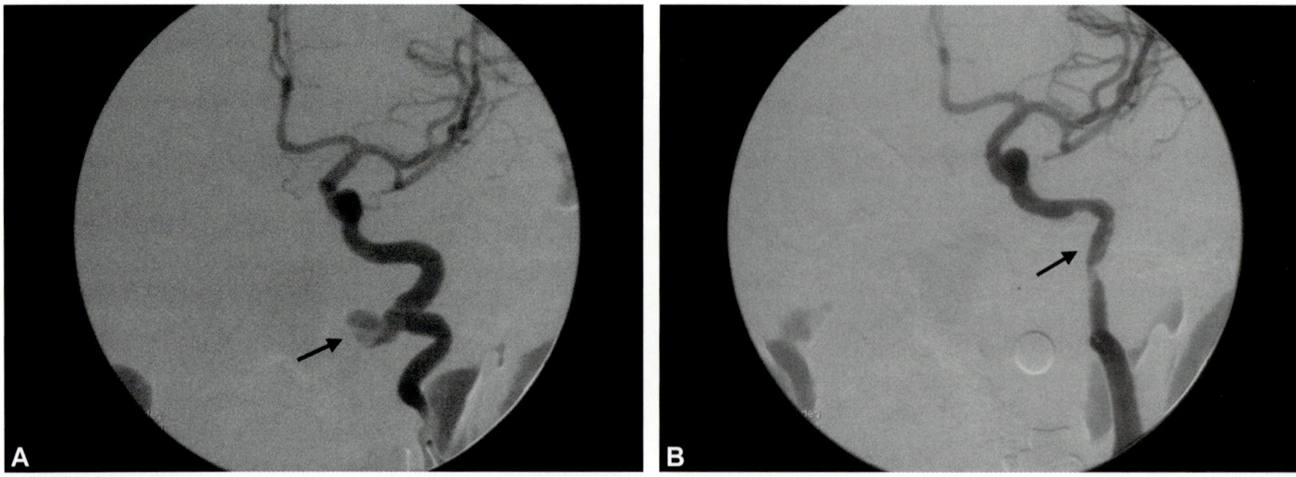

Figs. 29.9A and B: (A) Pseudoaneurysm (black arrow) at the left internal carotid artery caused after an extended endoscopic nasopharygectomy. (B) After treatement with an endovascular stent into left carotid artery, the pseudoaneurysm resolved (black arrow).[31-34]

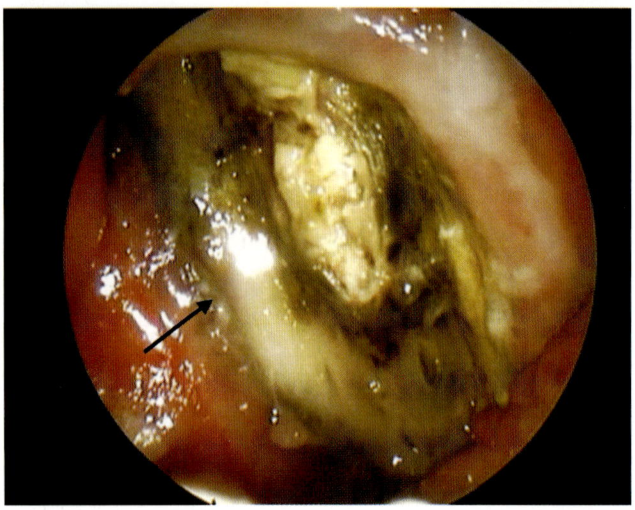

Fig. 29.10: Nasopharyngeal necrosis and purulence (black arrow) after endoscopic nasopharyngectomy requiring treatment with topical and oral antibiotics.

REFERENCES

1. Ong YK, Solares CA, Lee S, et al. Endoscopic nasopharyngectomy and its role in managing locally recurrent nasopharyngeal carcinoma. Otolaryngol Clin North Am, 2011;44(5):1141-54.
2. Spratt DE, Lee N. Current and emerging treatment options for nasopharyngeal carcinoma. Onco Targets Ther. 2012;5: 297-308.
3. Chen MY, Wen WP, Guo X, et al. Endoscopic nasopharyngectomy for locally recurrent nasopharyngeal carcinoma. Laryngoscope. 2009;119(3):516-22.
4. Tan CT, Hsiao SH, Hwang JH, et al. Potassium-titanyl-phosphate laser nasopharyngectomy with nasopharyngoscopic guidance for recurrent nasopharyngeal carcinoma. J Formos Med Assoc. 2005;104(12):960-3.
5. Fee WE Jr., Moir MS, Choi EC, et al. Nasopharyngectomy for recurrent nasopharyngeal cancer: a 2- to 17-year follow-up. Arch Otolaryngol Head Neck Surg. 2002;128(3):280-4.
6. Fee WE Jr., Roberson JB Jr., Goffinet DR. Long-term survival after surgical resection for recurrent nasopharyngeal cancer after radiotherapy failure. Arch Otolaryngol Head Neck Surg. 1991;117(11):1233-6.
7. King WW, Ku PK, Mok CO, et al. Nasopharyngectomy in the treatment of recurrent nasopharyngeal carcinoma: a twelve-year experience. Head Neck. 2000;22(3):215-22.
8. Wei WI, Kwong DL. Recurrent nasopharyngeal carcinoma: surgical salvage vs. additional chemoradiation. Curr Opin Otolaryngol Head Neck Surg. 2011;19(2):82-6.
9. Al-Sheibani S, Zanation AM, Carrau RL, et al. Endoscopic endonasal transpterygoid nasopharyngectomy. Laryngoscope. 2011;121:2081-0.
10. Yu-Shih Lai, Mu-Kuan Chen. Exclusively endoscopic resection of nasopharyngeal adenocarcinoma. Clin Exp Otorhinolaryngol. 2013;6(4):263-5.
11. Becker AM, Hwang PH. Endoscopic endonasal anatomy of the nasopharynx in a cadaver model. Int Forum Allergy Rhinol. 2013;3:319-24.
12. Yoshizaki T, Wakisaka N, Murono S, et al. Endoscopic nasopharyngectomy for patients with recurrent nasopharyngeal carcinoma at the primary site. Laryngoscope. 2005;115(8): 1517-9.
13. Ko JY, Wang CP, Ting LL, et al. Endoscopic nasopharyngectomy with potassium-titanyl-phosphate (KTP) laser for early locally recurrent nasopharyngeal carcinoma. Head Neck. 2009;31(10):1309-15.
14. Castelnuovo P, Nicolai P, Turri-Zanoni M, et al. Endoscopic endonasal nasopharyngectomy in selected cancers. Otolaryngol Head Neck Surg. 2013;149(3):424-30.
15. Singh A, Anand VK, Schwartz TH. Endoscopic approaches to the pterygopalatine fossa and infratemporal fossa. Rhinology: Diseases of the nose, sinuses, and skull base. New York: Thieme Publishers; 2012.

16. Chen MK, Lai JC, Chang CC, et al. Minimally invasive endoscopic nasopharyngectomy in the treatment of recurrent T1-2a nasopharyngeal carcinoma. Laryngoscope. 2007; 117(5):894-6.
17. Ho AS, Kaplan MJ, Fee WE Jr., et al. Targeted endoscopic salvage nasopharyngectomy for recurrent nasopharyngeal carcinoma. Int Forum Allergy Rhinol. 2012;2(2):166-73.
18. Yang TS, Ng KT, Wang HM, et al. Prognostic factors of locoregionally recurrent nasopharyngeal carcinoma—a retrospective review of 182 cases. Am J Clin Oncol. 1996; 19(4):337-43.
19. To EW, Lai EC, Cheng JH, et al. Nasopharyngectomy for recurrent nasopharyngeal carcinoma: a review of 31 patients and prognostic factors. Laryngoscope. 2002;112(10):1877-82.
20. Chen C, Fee W, Chen J, et al. Salvage treatment for locally recurrent Nasopharyngeal Carcinoma (NPC). Am J Clin Oncol. 2014;37:327-31.
21. Qiu S, Lin S, Tham IW, et al. Intensity-modulated radiation therapy in the salvage of locally recurrent nasopharyngeal carcinoma. Int J Radiat Oncol Biol Phys. 2012;83(2):676-83.
22. Chan JY, Wei WI. Recurrent nasopharyngeal carcinoma after salvage nasopharyngectomy. Arch Otolaryngol Head Neck Surg. 2012;138(6):572-6.
23. Han F, Zhao C, Huang SM, et al. Long-term outcomes and prognostic factors of re-irradiation for locally recurrent nasopharyngeal carcinoma using intensity-modulated radiotherapy. Clin Oncol (R Coll Radiol). 2012;24(8):569-76.
24. Hua YJ, Han F, Lu LX, et al. Long-term treatment outcome of recurrent nasopharyngeal carcinoma treated with salvage intensity modulated radiotherapy. Eur J Cancer. 2012; 48(18):3422-8.
25. To EW, Yuen EH, Tsang WM, et al. The use of stereotactic navigation guidance in minimally invasive transnasal nasopharyngectomy: a comparison with the conventional open transfacial approach. Br J Radiol. 2002;75(892):345-50.
26. de Vries EJ, Sekhar LN, Janecka IP, et al. Elective resection of the internal carotid artery without reconstruction. Laryngoscope. 1988;98(9):960-6.
27. Johnson MH, Chiang VL, Ross DA. Interventional neuroradiology adjuncts and alternatives in patients with head and neck vascular lesions. Neurosurg Clin N Am. 2005; 16(3):547-60, vii.
28. Chen MY, Hua YJ, Wan XB, et al. A posteriorly pedicled middle turbinate mucoperiosteal flap resurfacing nasopharynx after endoscopic nasopharyngectomy for recurrent nasopharyngeal carcinoma. Otolaryngol Head Neck Surg. 2012;146(3):409-11.
29. Hadad G, Bassagasteguy L, Carrau RL, et al. A novel reconstructive technique after endoscopic expanded endonasal approaches: vascular pedicle nasoseptal flap. Laryngoscope. 2006;116:1882-6.
30. Zanation AM, Thorp BD, Parmar P, et a;. Reconstructive options for endoscopic skull base surgery. Otolaryngol Clin North Am. 2011;44(5):1201-22.
31. Li Z, Chang G, Yao C, et al. Endovascular stenting of extracranial carotid artery aneurysm: a systematic review. Eur J Vasc Endovasc Surg. 2011;42(4):419-26.
32. Kim HO, Ji YB, Lee SH, et al. Cases of common carotid artery pseudoaneurysm treated by stent graft. Case Rep Otolaryngol. 2012;2012:674827.
33. Marine L, Sarac TP. Hybrid stent-graft repair of an iatrogenic complex proximal right common carotid artery injury. Ann Vasc Surg. 2012;26(4):574 e1-7.
34. Xiao L, Shen J, Tong JJ. Emergency stent-graft implantation for iatrogenic peripheral arterial rupture. Radiol Med. 2013;118(1):152-7.
35. Dallan I, Castelnuovo P, Montevecchi F, et al. Combined transoral transnasal robotic-assisted nasopharyngectomy: a cadaveric feasibility study. Eur Arch Otorhinolaryngol. 2012;269(1):235-9.
36. Ozer E, Waltonen J. Transoral robotic nasopharyngectomy: a novel approach for nasopharyngeal lesions. Laryngoscope. 2008;118(9):1613-6.
37. Wei WI, Ho WK. Transoral robotic resection of recurrent nasopharyngeal carcinoma. Laryngoscope. 2010;120(10): 2011-4.

CHAPTER

30

Skull Base Reconstruction

Spencer C Payne

BACKGROUND

The considerations for any surgery are not just restricted to the methods of approach to the pathology but must also include the careful thought on any necessary closure or reconstruction that may be required. This is no more true than in endoscopic skull base surgery in which the approach and removal of tumors result in a high probability of cerebrospinal fluid (CSF) leak along with its anticipated sequellae. In much the same way that the pectoralis flap and, to a certain extent, the radial forearm free flap serve as the workhorses for head and neck reconstruction, so too has the local pedicled nasoseptal flap become this for the endonasal approach. Even so, not every situation warrants the use of a pedicled flap. Nor, in many circumstances, such as with prior nasal surgery or concurrent tumor involvement, may these flaps even be available. As such the endoscopic skull base surgeon must be aware of a number of different techniques for dealing with closure and reconstruction of the sellar, parasellar, and more rostral anterior skull base. In 2001, Kaptain et al.[1] published a small series of sellar repairs utilizing intradurally placed abdominal fat along with bone or absorbable plate reconstruction of the sellar floor. Dusick et al.,[2] in 2005, described their technique with a fat and collagen sponge inlay, titanium mesh buttress, and intrasphenoidally placed fat onlay for non-adenomatous suprasellar lesions. Shortly thereafter, Couldwell et al.[3] noted their technique of fat and fascia lata inlay, absorbable plate buttress, and placement of sphenoid fat. The quoted leak rates were 0%, 21%, and 6%, respectively. It is not certain which factors, or which reconstruction, were truly predictive of success. What is certain though is that given the number of techniques and subsequent leak rates that have been described it is likely that no one technique is best for all situations.

Common to most of the described techniques is the concept of creating a multilayered reconstruction, with the choice of product for each layer left to physician discretion and familiarity. With the advent of pedicled intranasal flaps, the reconstructive techniques can roughly be divided into vascularized or free/nonvascular. For all intents and purposes, the former, as discussed in this chapter, is limited to the nasoseptal and inferior turbinate flaps. Other flaps have been described (palatal,[4] endoscopically harvested pericranial,[5] and temporalis[6]) but they are beyond the scope of this chapter and the reader is directed to the original descriptions.

NONVASCULARIZED RECONSTRUCTION

Simple Inlay–Onlay Grafting

The simplest, if not also most widely published, technique involves a combination of inlay and onlay grafting. In this sense a reconstructive layer is placed in both intracranial and extracranial planes (Figs. 30.1A to C). A variety

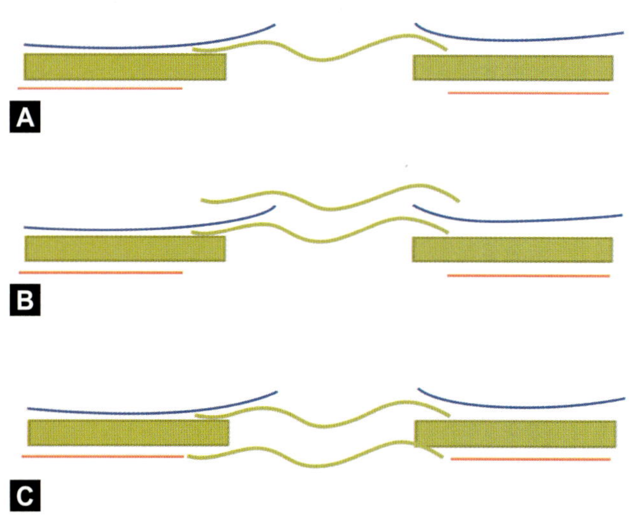

Figs. 30.1A to C: Placement of inlay/onlay grafts—(A) Extradural inlay graft; (B) intra and extradural inlay grafts, and (C) extradural inlay graft and onlay graft abutting sinus mucosa.

Table 30.1: Options for inlay/onlay grafting

Dural substitutes	
	Lyophilized acellular dermis (Alloderm®)
	Acellular collagen matrix (Duragen®, Durepair®, DuraMatrix®)
	Acellular porcine intestinal submucosa (Biodesign®)
Autologous	
	Fascia lata
	Abdominal fat
	Intranasal mucosa (only as extracranial onlay)
	Split thickness skin graft (only as extracranial onlay)
Sealants	
	Polyethylene glycol hydrogel (Duraseal®)
	Fibrin sealant (Tisseel®, Evicel®)

Table 30.2: Options for rigid buttressing

Autologous	
	Septal cartilage
	Septal bone
Manufactured	
	Titanium reconstruction mesh plates
	Absorbable reconstruction plates
	Porous polyethylene (Medpor)

Table 30.3: Reconstructive ladder

Leak characteristic or Degree	*Reconstructive options*
No leak	No reconstruction
	Simple packing of sella with dural onlay
Small weeping leak (diaphragmatic)	Dural reinforcement with inlay graft and light packing
Small weeping leak (anterior dural reflection at tuberculum)	Gland elevation with sellar packing using inlay grafts
Medium volume leak	Inlay, fat packing, onlay and rigid buttress
	Inlay basket with inlay packing, onlay and rigid buttress
Large volume/high pressure leak	Vascularized repair

of substances can be used for either of these purposes (Table 30.1). When a large volume defect is noted, especially following macroadenoma resection, the inlay graft can be paired with abdominally harvested fat as well. The use of a rigid buttress for this repair, with numerous options (Table 30.2), has also been described. In our experience, the use of various products often depends on the size and flow rate of the underlying CSF leak (Table 30.3). If no leak is noted (sellar lesions), a reconstruction can likely be deferred,[7] however the authors usually place a layer of oxidized cellulose or collagen based material, which serves a secondary purpose of aiding in coagulation. For the smaller, weeping leaks an inlay graft of collagen-based products is typically selected. For larger, higher flow leaks in the sellar and parasellar regions, we typically use a dural substitute as an inlay graft against the diaphragm with abdominal fat in a basket like configuration (Fig. 30.2). An onlay graft and usually a rigid buttress follow this.

Fig. 30.2: Sellar reconstruction for higher flow leaks—Dural substitute is placed within the sella and against diaphragm like a pouch which is filled with a fat graft. An extradural inlay graft followed by rigid buttress is then placed.

Technique

Step 1

The reconstruction starts after the surgical bed has been cleaned and hemostasis confirmed. Warm saline irrigations often provide both functions. If not, bipoloar cautery or the application of a hemostatic substance is performed.

Step 2

Next the defect size is measured. The authors find that a small plastic ruler, often supplied with a surgical marker, cut down to 2 cm works well for this.

Step 3

The dura is then circumferentially elevated off the skull base at least 1–2 mm peripherally. This is essential in order to provide an area for the edges of an extradural inlay graft to rest.

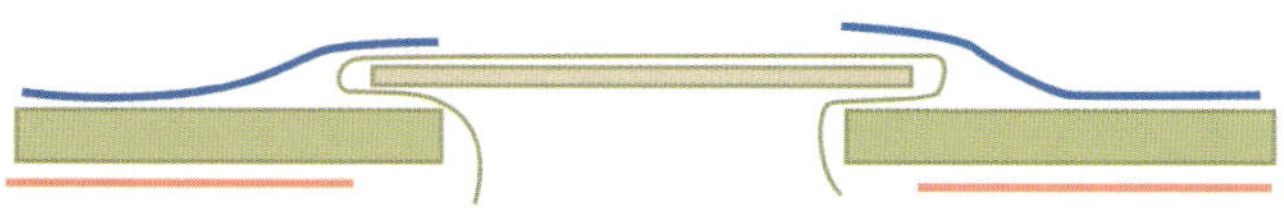

Fig. 30.3: "Jam Cap" grafting—An extradural inlay graft is placed such that its edges completely surround a rigid buttress and then extend out through the bone defect.

Step 4

If a sellar lesion has been removed the decision to provide a space occupying construction must be made. The utilization of such may help reduce hematoma formation within the cavity. Furthermore, an inlay graft will likely not adhere to the undersurface of the dura unless some tissue mass, if not cerebral cortex, is abutting its surface. Either fat or a roll/tuft of inlay material is inserted.

Step 5

The graft material is cut to shape and size and brought into the field using either small cup or bayonet forceps. After placing within the cavity the edges are tucked between the brain/rolled inlay and the dura.

Step 6

An extradural inlay graft is then cut to size and then placed between the dura and the bone of the skull base with the edges resting in the previously elevated pocket.

Step 7

A rigid buttress is placed if desired, also tucking the edges of the buttress into the epidural space that was elevated.

Step 8

An optional free mucosal graft can be placed at this time over the defect in the bone.

Step 9

The reconstruction is secured with an application of glue/sealant.

Step 10

Either absorbable or nonabsorbable packs may be placed to bolster the reconstruction if desired. This may be any variety of sponge meant for this purpose. If choosing a nonabsorbable pack, such as a polyvinyl alcohol sponge (Merocel), it should be placed within the finger of a surgical glove to facilitate later removal.

"Jam Cap" Alternate Technique

Described by Leng et al. in 2008,[8] the authors have found this to be a very helpful option. The technique may be used with or without the use of an inlay graft and may often precede vascularized reconstruction as noted below. A benefit of the technique is the ability to create an "immobile" construct which can be secured against the dural edges and bone of the skull base without the need for additional inlay packing which may otherwise be required if a large defect results.

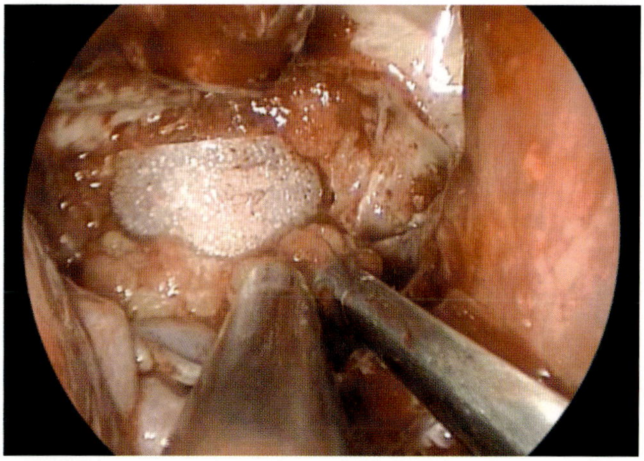

Fig. 30.4: "Jam Cap" graft with fat as inlay/onlay material—Fat can be seen around the edges of the rigid Medpor® buttress.

Steps 1–5

Proceed as above, utilizing packing and inlay grafting if desired.

Step 6

An onlay graft is cut several (2–3) mm larger than the defect and laid over the exposed bone of the defect.

Step 7

A rigid buttress, cut nearly identical in shape but slightly larger, is then placed over the onlay graft. Using small elevators, the edges of the buttress are then tucked deep to the bone circumferentially while maintaining a cuff of the onlay graft "extruding" circumferentially. The buttress is thus placed into the epidural pocket with a rim of graft material both deep and superficial to it; this creates a virtual inlay/onlay hybrid (Fig. 30.3).

Steps 8–10. As above.

As a result of this modification the graft makes significant contact with dura and skull base bone circumferentially and is quite secure. The effect is such that the skull base bone "cinches" down over the inlay graft much like a gasket seal (Fig. 30.4).

VASCULARIZED RECONSTRUCTION

Despite the myriad options for inlay and onlay grafting, significant postoperative leak rates (as noted above) were regularly reported. As endoscopic skull base tumor resection advanced, so too did the size of the dural defect and likelihood of a high-flow leak. Additionally, a high burden was placed on the nose for remucosalization to "complete" the reconstruction. Although Hirsch[9] had originally described the use of a septal rotation flap for endonasal repair of a CSF leak in 1952, it was not until 2006[10] that a truly pedicled septal flap was described. The obvious benefit of such techniques is the immediate reconstruction of the mucosal layer of the nose and anticipated acceleration of "water-tightness." Consequently, since the introduction of the nasoseptal flap by Hadad and Bassagasteguy many centers have reported a significant reduction in their postoperative leak rates after adoption of this technique in to their algorithms.

Nasoseptal Flap

Based on the posterior septal branch of the sphenopalatine artery (*see* Chapter 2), the posterior portion of the nasoseptal flap is a true axial flap. Given the rich anastomotic network of the septum the flap is able to be harvested as far superior as the nasal vestibule. Despite the more "random" nature of the caudal portion of the septum this region is adequately perfused more often than not. The flap can further encompass tissue superiorly from 1 to 2 cm inferior to the nasal vault (to preserve olfaction) and be extended to the junction of the septum and nasal floor or even out laterally under the inferior turbinate for particularly large defects. As such the flap can provide substantial coverage to ventral skull base defects extending as anterior as the posterior table of the frontal sinus and spanning from lamina to lamina.

Technique

Harvest: This is performed at the beginning of the procedure as accidental violation of the pedicle could nullify its potential use. We prefer to harvest the flap from the patient's right side unless substantial deviation or spurring of the septum may make this difficult.

1. An approach to the sphenoid ostium is first performed as described in Chapter 28. Care is taken not to injure the mucosa overlying the sphenoid face.
2. An extended insulated needle tip bovie (set at 10) is utilized. The tip is angled to 90°.
3. The inferior limb of the incision is made first. Starting laterally, on the clival bone above the choana the incision is brought medially on to the septum (Fig. 30.5).
4. The incision is take down along the posterior aspect of the septum, coursing anteriorly along the vomer to the nasal floor (Figs. 30.6A and B).
5. Depending on the desired width of the flap, the incision is carried laterally along the nasal floor.

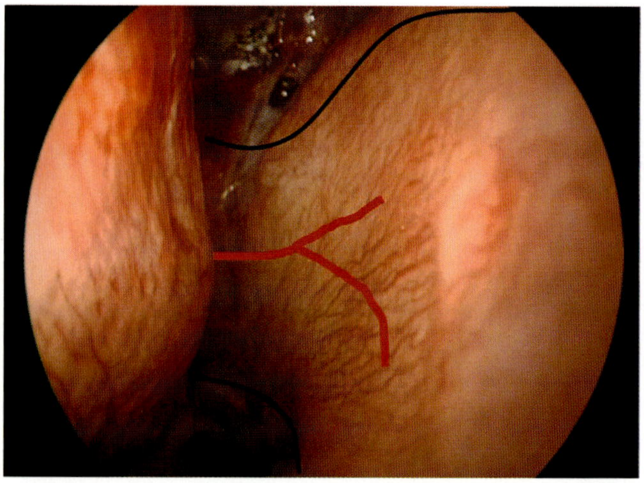

Fig. 30.5: Posterior septal incisions for the septal flap (black lines)—The inferior incision is just above the choana and the superior incision is just below the sphenoid ostium. The location of the posterior septal artery is represented by the red line.

6. The incision is then brought as anteriorly as needed, maximally to behind the squamous-mucosal junction of the vestibule.
7. The superior limb of the incision is then made. Starting at a level just below the sphenoid ostium, the incision is started laterally and brought across the sphenoid face and on to the septum (Fig. 30.5).
8. The incision is brought superiorly in an s-shaped fashion on to the posterior septum to 1–2 cm below the cribriform (Fig. 30.7).
9. It is then carried anteriorly to the level of the head of the inferior turbinate and a vertical incision dropped to connect to the inferior limb (Fig. 30.8).
10. A suction elevator is then used to elevate in a subperichondrial/periosteal plane. It is often easier to first free up the inferior incision as well as the incisions across the sphenoid face as these areas may be more difficult to address after the majority of the flap has been elevated.
11. After elevating from anterior to posterior, the flap is then tucked into and stored in the nasopharynx (Fig. 30.9). Alternatively the flap can be stored in the maxillary sinus (after wide antrostomy) should the surgery require dissection of the clivus or nasopharynx.
12. Take care to prevent spinning of the flap on its pedicle. Additionally attempt to prevent excessive folding of the flap as over the course of the surgery, minor retraction of the flap may result in "stiffening" of any folds making later placement of the flap difficult.

Flap Inset:

1. The area is cleaned of any residual mucosa and a care is taken that there is exposed bone circumferentially

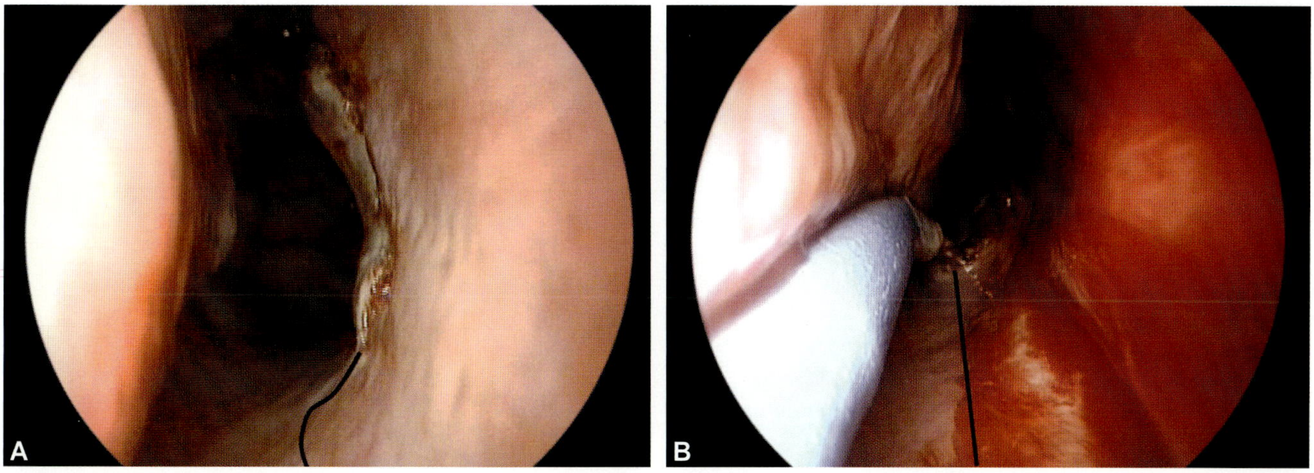

Figs. 30.6A and B: Inferior incision—(A) The incision is carried down the posterior aspect of the vomer and then (B) extended anteriorly along the septal floor (black line).

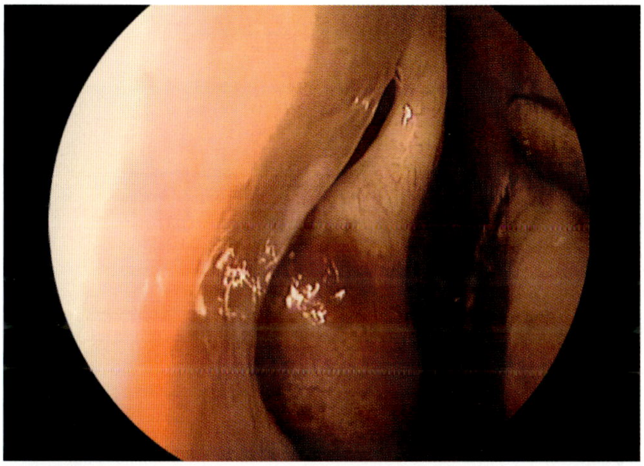

Fig. 30.7: Superior incision—The superior incision is carried anteriorly at least 1 cm inferior to the nasal vault/cribriform to preserve olfaction.

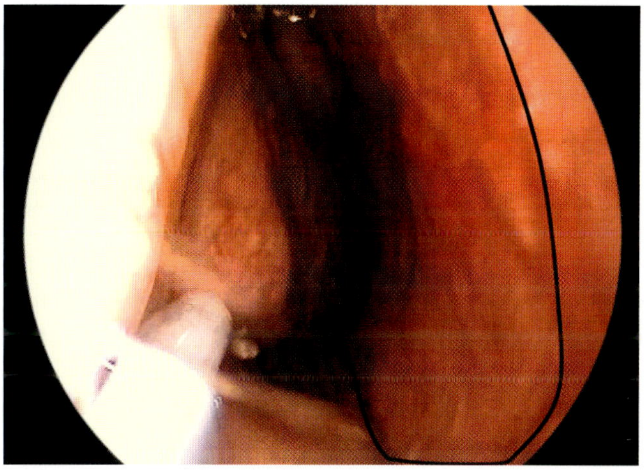

Fig. 30.8: Caudal/anterior incision (black line).

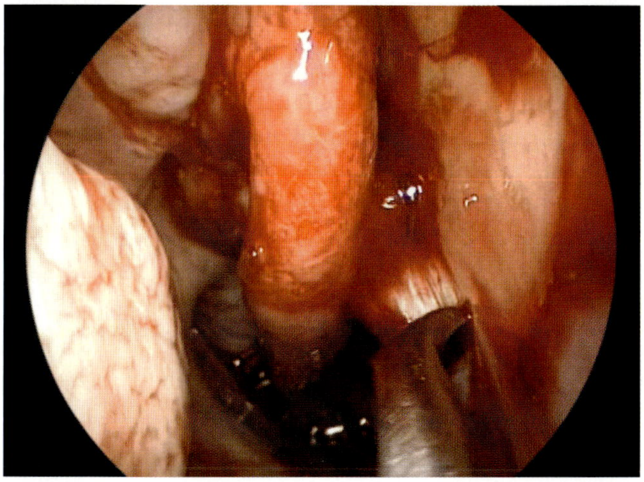

Fig. 30.9: Nasoseptal flap stored in the nasopharynx—Note the bulge of the pedicle extending inferiorly into the nasopharynx.

around the defect. (In lieu of complete stripping of the sphenoid sinus we prefer to elevate the mucosa peripherally until the edges are able to rest along the sides of the flap.)

2. Any intracranial inlay or onlay flap is performed as desired. Given the hardiness of the flap these are often not necessary but a rigid buttress can help prevent brain pulsations from causing dislodging of the flap.
3. The flap is brought out of where it was stored and placed over the defect. It is imperative that the flap lay directly on bone circumferentially around the defect (Fig. 30.10).
4. Strips of surgical are then placed along the edges of the flap. This serves the dual role of providing any hemostasis from flap edges as well as helping to secure the flap in position (Fig. 30.11).

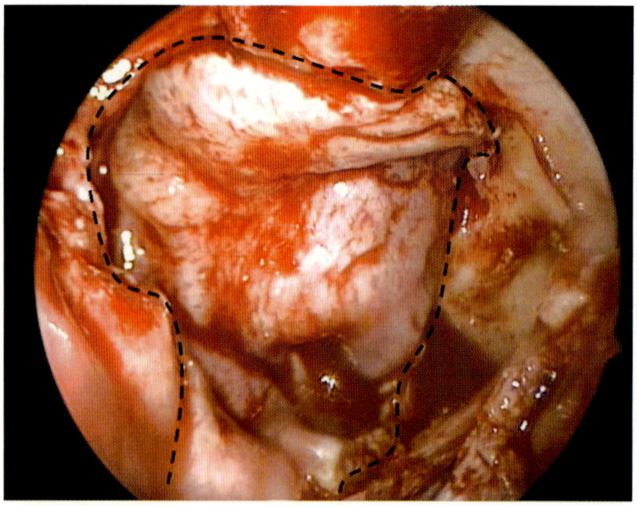

Fig. 30.10: Septal flap in place—The dashed line indicates the edges of the nasoseptal flap for easy visualization; the edges are on bone and abutting elevated sphenoid mucosa.

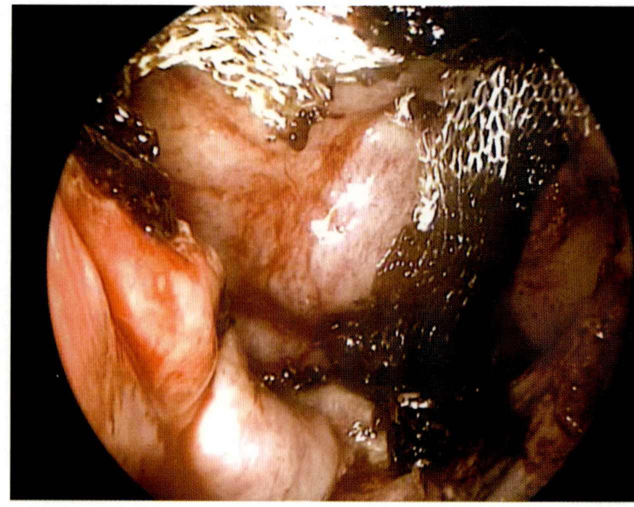

Fig. 30.11: Surgicel strips placed along edges.

5. Any area where the flap may tend to tent off the bone (e.g., corners of the sinus such as the clival recess) are then packed with gelfoam.
6. Sealant such as Duraseal or fibrin glue is then applied.
7. The septal donor site is then addressed. There are a variety of options for this (see below).
8. The reconstruction can then be reinforced with packs constructed of polyvinyl acetate (Merocel) covered in finger of a surgical glove placed bilaterally. Sutures tied to the ends of the glove are brought out of the nose and either secured with steri-strips or tied around a dental roll placed in front of the columella.

Rescue Flap Approach Alternative

In situations where the use of the septal flap is possible, but not definitive, a rescue flap approach can be used. This approach is actually a modification of the original sellar/parasellar approach and is described in Chapter 24.

Donor Site

Three options exist at present for managing the donor site. If left to granulate on its own the septal cartilage and bone will remucosalize over the course of 8–12 weeks.[11] It has been reported that this results in significant morbidity to the patient but this has not necessarily been our experience. Our preference is to use a silastic sheet (0.020″ thick) cut to shape and placed over the donor site (Fig. 30.12). It is then sutured in place to the columella with 4-0 nylon. It is removed 3 weeks later.

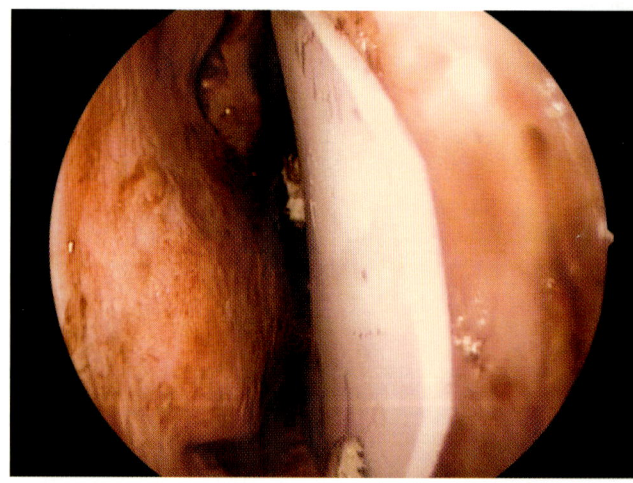

Fig. 30.12: Silastic sheet placed on septal flap donor site.

A second option that has been described is the contralateral reverse rotation flap.[12] With this method the entire posterior bony septum is removed and the contralateral septal mucosa is incised and separated from the back of the nose and nasal floor. It is then rotated anteriorly around the posterior aspect of the cartilaginous septum and sutured or stapled in place. One series indicated that this resulted in 98% mucosalization within 2 weeks of surgery and reduced the number of necessary debridements.[13] The theoretical downside, however, may be an increased effect on nasal airflow and smell as well as increased operative time. Furthermore, while it results in earlier return of functioning cilia, at least initially these cilia may be beating in an anterior direction.

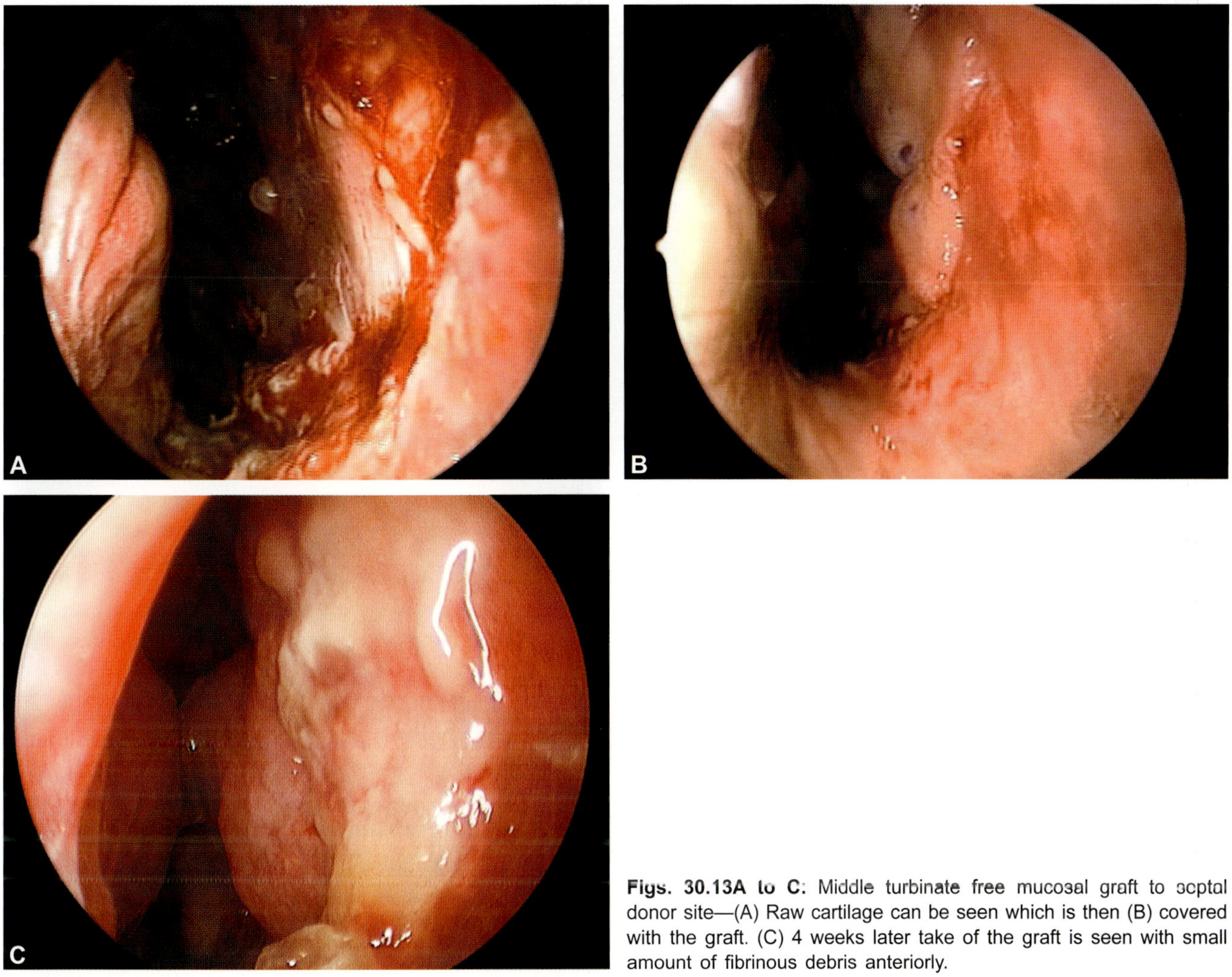

Figs. 30.13A to C: Middle turbinate free mucosal graft to septal donor site—(A) Raw cartilage can be seen which is then (B) covered with the graft. (C) 4 weeks later take of the graft is seen with small amount of fibrinous debris anteriorly.

For many, it is standard to remove the middle turbinate before proceeding with skull base approaches. While it is not our standard practice to do so (*see* Chapter 24), if the middle turbinate is to be resected, its mucosa can be secondarily utilized as a free graft to the caudal septum.[14] Upon removal of the turbinate its mucosa is marked to ensure recognition of the epithelial side after harvest. Then using a 15 blade scalpel, Cottle elevator and tissue forceps the mucosa is elevated off the medial and lateral surfaces first, followed by its attachment along the inferior aspect of the turbinate. It is then applied to the donor site and smoothed out endoscopically with either a ball tipped probe or a small 45 degree ring curette. It can then be sutured or stapled in place (Figs. 30.13A to C). Alternatively, as originally described, it can be secured in place after bilateral placement of Doyle nasal splints with through and through prolene sutures.

Inferior Turbinate Flap

A limitation of the septal flap, however, is the distinct probability of its being involved by the lesion being resected. Further, if prior surgery has occurred in this area, and/or a posterior septectomy already exists, the vascular supply and hence, viability of the flap may be at risk. A significant option in these instances, especially for more rostral defects, is the inferior turbinate flap. Having previously been used for septal and nasal reconstruction, the inferior turbinate has a long history of providing mucosal coverage to areas of need. It was not until 2007[15] and 2009[16] however when its use for skull base reconstruction was first described. While offering just as hardy a reconstruction, the harvest of the flap can be difficult compared with the NSF and it offers a reduced length and width thus limiting its use to clival and sellar defects.

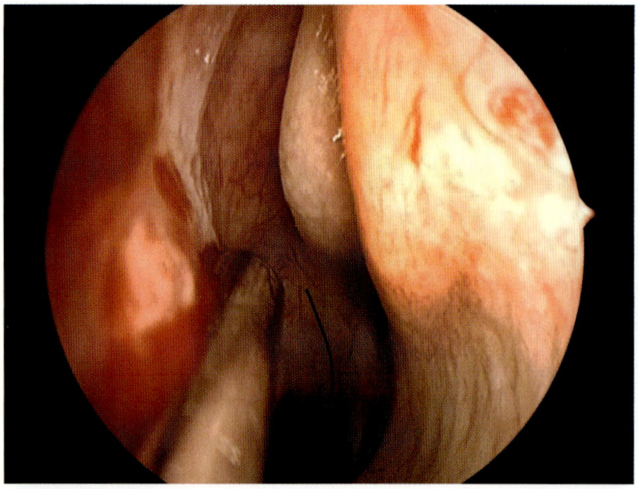

Fig. 30.14: Incision to isolate vessels for IT flap—Line indicates where to make incision on the lateral wall to dissect and isolate vessels running to inferior turbinate.

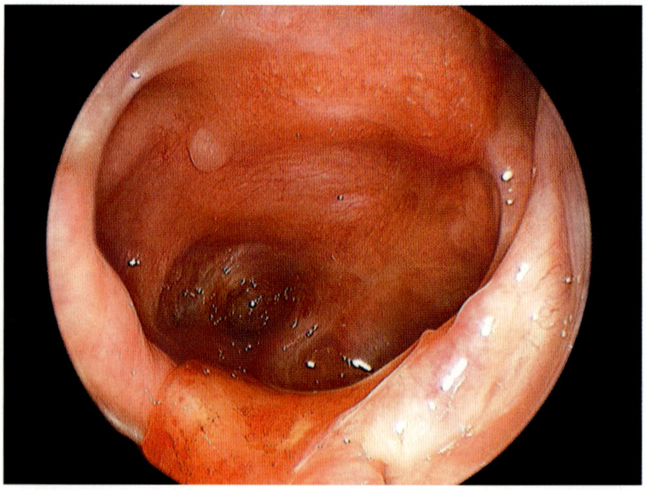

Fig. 30.15: Healed nasoseptal flap from above at 8 weeks—Some areas of granulation are noted over the area of the prior pedicle.

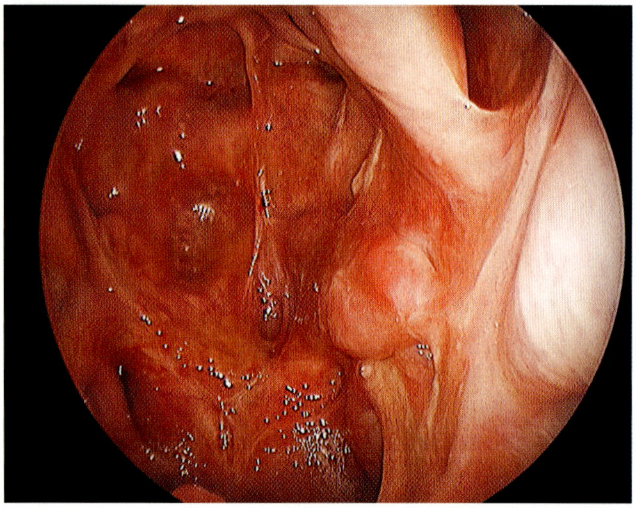

Fig. 30.16: Healed inferior turbinate flap at 12 weeks—Repair of a clival defect from chordoma resection. Note the pedicle of the inferior turbinate reversed into the inferior aspect of the sphenoid sinus where it was used to cover an exposed paraclival ICA.

Technique

Steps

1. Identify the sphenopalatine foramen and artery (SPF and SPA). A vertical incision can be made in the lateral nasal cavity wall superior to the inferior turbinate, and anterior to the tail of the middle turbinate (Fig. 30.14). Elevate the mucosa off the bone and locate the crista ethmoidalis, a triangular wedge of bone extending medially. The SPF and SPA should be immediately behind this. The bone can be removed with Kerrison rongeurs.
2. Identify the posterolateral nasal artery as it branches off the SPA and follow it inferiorly into the inferior turbinate. This prevents accidental transection of the pedicle.
3. Two parallel horizontal incisions are then made, one along the inferior margin of the turbinate and the second just above the turbinate on the lateral wall over the maxillary fontanelles. (For greater width the incisions can be modified to higher on to the lateral wall or more laterally into the inferior meatus.)
4. A vertical incision then joins the horizontals over the head of the inferior turbinate.
5. Elevate the flap using Freer, Cottle, or suction elevators as desired from anterior to posterior.
6. Place flap over defect utilizing layers as desired.

POSTOPERATIVE MANAGEMENT

Saline nasal irrigations are employed after the third postoperative day. This helps prevent confusion regarding salty taste and/or discharge immediately following surgery. Activity is restricted usually based on the underlying procedure but commonly includes only light activity without heavy lifting or straining for 4–6 weeks. As long as irrigations are performed regularly, debridements are usually only necessary at the 2–3 and 8 week marks. As noted previously, the vascularized flaps are quite hardy. They are almost usually completely healed at the 8 week mark (Figs. 30.15 and 30.16) however if no grafting is performed of the donor site, the septum can often demonstrate persistent crusting (Fig. 30.17). For this reason, we recommend 3 months of saline irrigation at a minimum.

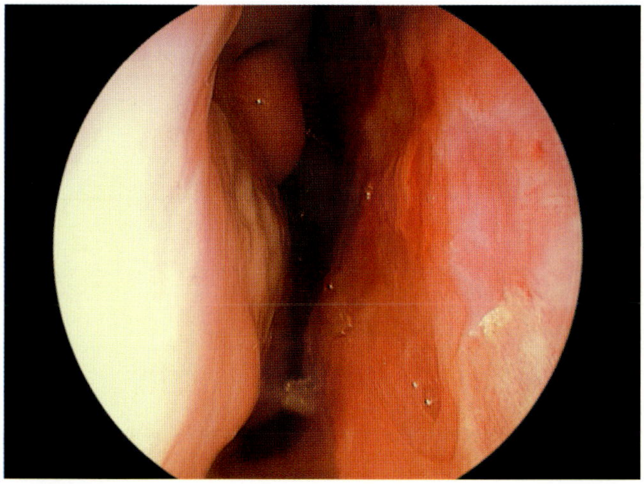

Fig. 30.17: Persistent crusting at septal donor site—This should resolve by the 12 week mark.

CONCLUSION

A variety of reconstructive options are available to the endoscopic skull base surgeon. It is important to balance complexity of reconstruction with the expected degree of defect size and CSF flow rate or pressure.

REFERENCES

1. Kaptain GJ, Kanter AS, Hamilton DK, et al. Management and implications of intraoperative cerebrospinal fluid leak in transnasoseptal transphenoidal microsurgery. Neurosurgery. 2011;68(1 Suppl Operative):144-50.
2. Dusick JR, Esposito F, Kelly DF, et al. The extended direct endonasal transsphenoidal approach for nonadenomatous suprasellar tumors. J Neurosurg. 2005;102:832-41.
3. Couldwell WT, Kan P, Weiss MH. Simple closure following transphenoidal surgery: Technical note. Neurosurg Focus. 2006;15:E11.
4. Oliver CL, Hackman TG, Carrau RL, et al. Palatal flap modifications allow pedicled reconstruction of the skull base. Laryngoscope. 2008;118:2102-6.
5. Zanation AM, Snyderman CH, Carrau RL, et al. Minimally invasive endoscopic pericranial flap: a new method for endonasal skull base reconstruction. Laryngoscope. 2009; 119:13-8.
6. Fortes FSG, Carrau RL, Snyderman CH, et al. Transpterygoid transposition of a temporoparietal fascia flap: A new method for skull base reconstruction after endoscopic expanded endonasal approaches. Laryngoscope. 2007;117:970-6.
7. Sonnenburg RE, White D, Ewend MG, et al. Sellar reconstruction: is it necessary? Am J Rhinol 2003;17:343-6.
8. Leng LZ, Brown S, Anand VK, et al. "Gasket-seal" watertight closure in minimal-access endoscopic cranial base surgery. Neurosurgery. 2008;62(2):342-3.
9. Hirsch O. Successful closure of cerebrospinal fluid rhinorrhea by endonasal surgery. AMA Arch Otolaryngol 1952;56: 1-12.
10. Hadad G, Bassagasteguy L, Carrau RL, et al. A novel reconstructive technique after endoscopic expanded endonasal approaches: Vascular pedicle nasoseptal flap. Laryngoscope. 2006;116:1882-6.
11. Kassam AB, Thomas A, Carrau RL, et al. Endoscopic reconstruction of the cranial base using a pedicled nasoseptal flap. Neurosurgery. 2008;63:ONS44–ONS52; discussion ONS52-ONS53.
12. Caicedo-Granados E, Carrau RL, Snyderman CH, et al. Reverse rotation flap for reconstruction of donor site after vascular pedicled nasoseptal flap in skull base surgery. Laryngoscope. 2010;120:1550-2.
13. Kasemsiri P, Carrau RL, Ottoa BA, et al. Reconstruction of the pedicled nasoseptal flap donor site with a contralateral reverse rotation flap: Technical modifications and outcomes. Laryngoscope. 2013;212:Epub 11 Mar 2013.
14. Kimple AJ, Leight WD, Wheless SA, et al. Reducing nasal morbidity after skull base reconstruction with the nasoseptal flap: free middle turbinate mucosal grafts. Laryngoscope. 2012;122:1920-4.
15. Fortes FSG, Carrau RL, Snyderman CH, et al. The posterior pedicle inferior turbinate flap: a new vascularized flap for skull base reconstruction. Laryngoscope. 2007;117:1329-32.
16. Harvey RJ, Sheahan PO, Schlosser RJ. Inferior turbinate pedicle flap for endoscopic skull base defect repair. Am J Rhinol Allergy. 2009;23:522-6.

Index

Note: Page numbers followed by *f* and *t* indicate figures and tables respectively.

F

G

H

I

J

K

L

M

N

O

P

R

S

T

U

V

W